BD Chaurasia's *dream*

Human Embryology

Second Edition

Arushi Khurana

MBBS

Resident Physician
Internal Medicine
University of Connecticut, School of Medicine
USA

Indu Khurana

MBBS MD

Senior Professor
Postgraduate Institute of Medical Sciences
Pt BD Sharma University of Health Sciences
Rohtak, Haryana

Edited by

Krishna Garg

MBBS MS PhD FIMSA FIAMS FAMS

Ex-Professor and Head
Department of Anatomy
Lady Hardinge Medical College, New Delhi

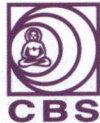

CBS

CBS Publishers & Distributors Pvt Ltd

New Delhi • Bengaluru • Chennai • Kochi • Kolkata • Mumbai
Hyderabad • Nagpur • Patna • Pune • Vijayawada

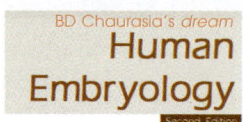

ISBN: 978-81-239-2046-7

Copyright © Arushi, Indu Khurana

Second Edition: 2012
Reprint: 2013, 2014, 2016, 2017
First Edition: 2010

Published by Satish Kumar Jain and produced by Varun Jain for
CBS Publishers & Distributors Pvt Ltd
4819/XI Prahlad Street, 24 Ansari Road, Daryaganj, New Delhi 110 002, India.
Ph: 23289259, 23266861, 23266867   Website: www.cbspd.com
Fax: 011-23243014   e-mail: delhi@cbspd.com; cbspubs@airtelmail.in.
Corporate Office: 204 FIE, Industrial Area, Patparganj, Delhi 110 092
Ph: 4934 4934   Fax: 4934 4935   e-mail: publishing@cbspd.com; publicity@cbspd.com

Branches

• **Bengaluru:** Seema House 2975, 17th Cross, K.R. Road,
  Banasankari 2nd Stage, Bengaluru 560 070, Karnataka
  Ph: +91-80-26771678/79   Fax: +91-80-26771680   e-mail: bangalore@cbspd.com
• **Chennai:** 7, Subbaraya Street, Shenoy Nagar, Chennai 600 030, Tamil Nadu
  Ph: +91-44-26680620, 26681266   Fax: +91-44-42032115   e-mail: chennai@cbspd.com
• **Kochi:** Ashana House, No. 39/1904, AM Thomas Road, Valanjambalam,
  Ernakulam 682 016, Kochi, Kerala
  Ph: +91-484-4059061-65   Fax: +91-484-4059065   e-mail: kochi@cbspd.com
• **Kolkata:** 6/B, Ground Floor, Rameswar Shaw Road, Kolkata-700 014, West Bengal
  Ph: +91-33-22891126, 22891127, 22891128   e-mail: kolkata@cbspd.com
• **Mumbai:** 83-C, Dr E Moses Road, Worli, Mumbai-400018, Maharashtra
  Ph: +91-22-24902340/41   Fax: +91-22-24902342   e-mail: mumbai@cbspd.com

Representatives

• **Hyderabad** 0-9885175004   • **Nagpur**   0-9021734563   • **Patna** 0-9334159340
• **Pune**   0-9623451994   • **Vijayawada** 0-9000660880

Printed at: Nutech Print Services - India, Faridabad

Editor's Foreword

Embryology, an interesting and essential component of the study of human anatomy, is a complex subject not so easy to understand and conceptualize. It gives me immense pleasure to edit the second edition of the book and to write the Foreword for such a comprehensive work which has made it easy to understand, retain and reproduce the basic concepts of human development. Further, I am delighted to know that like the Eklavya, Dr Arushi, ably helped by Senior Professor Indu Khurana, has taken the challenge of fulfilling the dream of a great teacher, late Dr BD Chaurasia.

The book covers the subject in a systematic manner. The concept of organizing the text in three sections: General Embryology, Systemic Embryology and Applied Embryology, is unique and provides insight of the subject. The text is complete and up-to-date with recent advances, including developments in the molecular biology and genetics in relation to human embryology.

I am very impressed by the abundant tables and flow charts provided in the text for an easy assimilation. The clear line diagrams presented in an attractive colour format provide vivid and lucid details, and are the real asset for the book. With vast experience as a teacher and author of anatomy, I have edited the text of the second edition to the best of my ability. I can vouch with confidence that the features of this wonderful book make it an indispensable text for medical and dental students. Candidates preparing for entrance examinations would also find it an authentic reference source for knowledge of human embryology. I foresee a great scope for this unique venture.

Krishna Garg

Preface

Embryology, the study of development of human before birth, is not only fascinating but an indispensable foundation step for the medical students. Advances in molecular biology and genetics in relation to embryology have further enhanced the scope of this branch of medical science in providing an insight into many otherwise baffling problems encountered by the medical doctors.

It is unequivocal that the subject of embryology is very interesting but at the same time not very easy to understand and conceptualize. To write an easy to understand yet comprehensive book on embryology was a dream of the great author, Dr BD Chaurasia which could not be fulfilled due to his sudden demise. Mr SK Jain, Managing Director, CBS Publishers and Distributors Pvt Ltd, New Delhi, approached the authors with this unfulfilled dream of late Dr BD Chaurasia. The authors took this challenge and made sincere efforts in bringing out this project *Human Embryology* and dedicated it to the great teacher and author of anatomy. In fact this book owes its existence to the dream of late Dr BD Chaurasia. This maiden venture of the authors deals with the fundamentals of the subject, therefore, for advanced and detailed study it is advisable to consult some standard reference works.

Organization of the book

The book has been organized into three sections:

❑ *Section I: General Embryology* begins with introduction to embryology and developmental biology. This section covers the general aspects of embryology from formation of gametes to the fetal stage of development.

❑ *Section II: Systemic Embryology* is devoted to the development of various systems of the human body.

❑ *Section III: Applied Embryology* includes a chapter on teratology and prenatal diagnosis.

Salient features of the book

❑ *Mind map of the chapter,* i.e. a brief list highlighting the topics covered, given in the beginning of each chapter, provides a quick overview of the chapter contents and organizational logic.

❑ *Organization of the text* is such that the students can easily understand, retain and reproduce it. Various levels of headings, subheadings, bold face and italics given in the text will be helpful in conceptualizing as well as later in the quick revision of the text.

❑ *Text content* is complete and up-to-date with recent advances, including the molecular aspects. To be true, some part of the text is in more detail than the requirement of undergraduate students. But this very feature of the book makes it a useful handbook for the postgraduate students of anatomy as well as medicine and surgery.

❑ *Occurrence of congenital anomalies* has been correlated with the normal developmental steps, wherever possible.

❑ *Illustrations* are in abundance. The clear line diagrams presented in an attractive colour format provide vivid and lucid details.

❑ *Tables and flow charts* have been included, wherever possible, for highlighting the important information.

Acknowledgements

Undoubtedly, ventures like this can never be accomplished without the generous help of an army of well-wishers and learned people. First, the authors like to bow to the great authors and publishers who have produced so many exhaustive and authentic publications on this topic by which the authors were enlightened and able to conceptualise the text and figures for the present work. We are grateful to Dr Krishna Garg, ex-Professor and Head, Department of Anatomy, Lady Hardinge Medical College, New Delhi, for editing and authenticating the text from her vast experience of more than 40 years of teaching, and research.

The present book is surely not intended to be a substitute for the standard reference works. Second, we are grateful to Mr SK Jain, Managing Director, CBS P&D, who considered us worth fulfilling this dream. Third, we are grateful to Prof AK Khurana, who virtually made it possible for us to complete this arduous work. Our thanks are also due to Sr Prof Sushma Sood, Head of the Department of Physiology; Sr Prof Sudha Chhabra, Head, Department of Anatomy; Dr SK Srivastava, Prof of Anatomy; Dr Manjit, Dr Naresh and Dr Jai for their cooperation; and Sr Prof CS Dhull, Director, PGIMS, and Sr Prof SS Sangwan, Vice-Chancellor, Pt BD Sharma University of Health Sciences, Rohtak, for providing a working atmosphere. We also want to convey our sincere thanks to Dr Usha Dhall, Professor of Anatomy, and Principal, Maharaja Agarsen Medical College, Agroha, for her guidance. The editorial team comprising Mrs Ritu Chawla, Mrs Jyoti and Mr PS Ghuman, headed by Mr YN Arjuna, Senior Director, Publishing, CBS P&D, needs to be complemented for their untiring efforts. We shall also like to acknowledge the unparalleled skills of Mr Majumdar, an artist par excellence; Mr. Mahesh Gupta, a wonderful typesetter; and Mr Vinod Jain, an efficient Production Director of CBS P&D, New Delhi.

Disclosure

The authors have made sincere efforts to verify the correctness of the text. However, in spite of the best efforts, ventures of this kind are not likely to be free from human errors, some inaccuracies, ambiguities or typographic mistakes. All the readers (students as well as teachers) are, therefore, requested to send their valuable feedback and suggestions, the importance of which cannot be overemphasized by us in mere words.

Arushi
Indu Khurana

Contents

Other Books in the Series

General Embryology

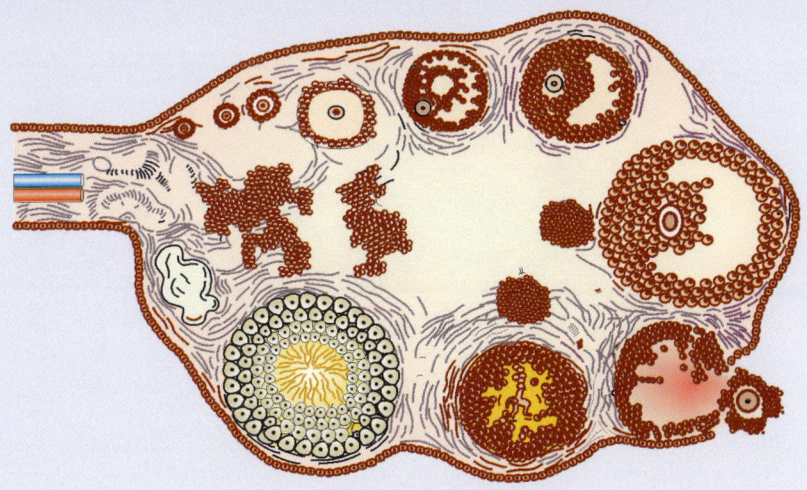

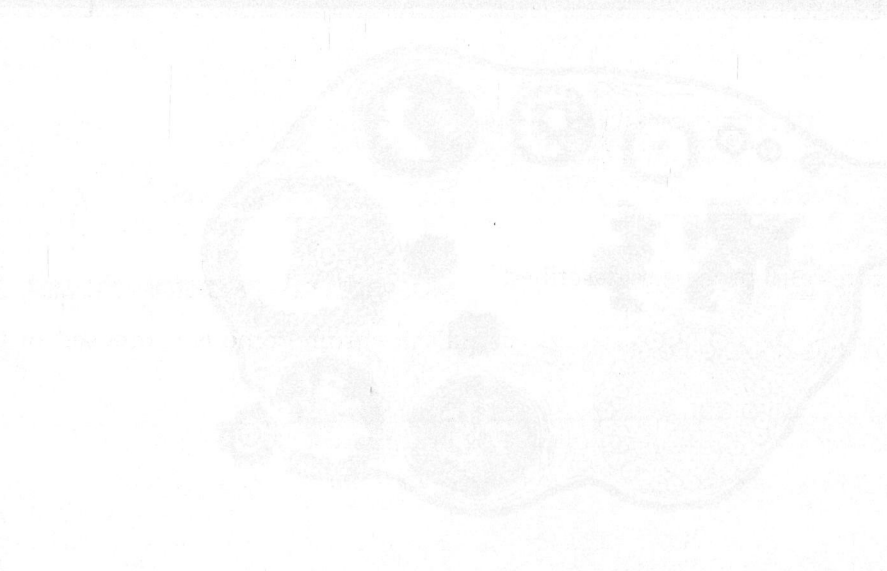

Developmental Biology and Embryology: Introduction and Control

DEVELOPMENTAL BIOLOGY

Chromosomes
- Morphology of chromosomes
- Structure and functions of DNA and RNA

Genes
- General considerations
- Gene expression
- Regulation of gene expression

Cell division and cell cycle
- Cell cycle
- Comparison of mitosis and meiosis

EMBRYOLOGY : AN INTRODUCTION

Outlines of human development

- Prenatal development
- Postnatal development

CONTROL OF DEVELOPMENT

Processes controlling development
- Cell differentiation
- Regulated cell migration
- Induction
- Apoptosis

Outlines of molecular control of development
- Molecular control of early embryonic development
- Molecular control of gastrulation
- Molecular control of development of various system organs

DEVELOPMENTAL BIOLOGY

Developmental biology refers to study of structures and processes involved in the development of a new individual. Such structures and processes, described here briefly, include:

- Chromosomes, DNA and RNA,
- Genes, and
- Cell cycle.

CHROMOSOMES

Waldeyer in 1888 coined the term chromosomes to denote the thread-like structures present in the nucleus of eukaryotic cells during division. It is now established that the chromosomes are responsible for the transmission of the hereditary information from one generation to next. There are 46 chromosomes (23 pairs in all the dividing cells of the body except the gametes (sex cells) which contain only 23 chromosomes (haploid number).

MORPHOLOGY OF CHROMOSOMES

Each chromosome is composed of two chromatids connected at the *centromere*. Each chromatid consists of two *chromonemes*. *Telomeres* are the terminal ends of chromosomes DNA molecule.

Functional types of chromosomes. There are three types of eukaryotic chromosomes:

- *Autosomes* are the chromosomes present in somatic cells. The number of autosomes in a cell is fixed and is expressed as 2n or *diploid number*.
- *Sex chromosomes* are present in the sex cells and are responsible for determining the sex of individual.

- *Supernumerary or redundant chromosomes* are also found in eukaryotic cells but their occurrence is quite uncommon.

Chemical structure of chromosome

The chromosomes are mainly composed of DNA. The chromosome also contains RNA, basic proteins called histones, complex proteins including enzymes, some organic phosphorus compounds and inorganic salts. The amount of DNA in a haploid cell is half the amount present in a diploid cell of the same species. Further, the concentration of DNA in any cell remains constant in every circumstances. An important feature of DNA is that it is metabolically stable.

STRUCTURE AND FUNCTIONS OF DNA AND RNA

DNA

DNA, i.e. deoxyribonucleic acid is a molecule of inheritance and thus may be regarded as the reserve bank of genetic information. DNA is exclusively responsible for maintaining the identity of different species of organisms for millions of years.

Structure of DNA

DNA is a polymer of four monomeric deoxyribonucleotides namely deoxyadenylate (dAMP), deoxyguanylate (dGMP), deoxycytidylate (dCMP) and deoxythymidylate (dTMP). Each deoxyribonucleotide in turn is composed of a nitrogenous base purines or pyrimidines (A, G, C or T), a pentose sugar, i.e. deoxyribose and a phosphate. Each molecule of DNA has equal number of adenine and thymine residues (A=T) and equal number of guanine and cytosine residues (G=C). This is known as *Chargaff's rule*.

Watson-Crick model of DNA structure. The salient features of Watson-Crick model of DNA (now known as B-DNA) are (Fig. 1.1):

- *Double helix structure.* Each DNA molecule is right handed double helix composed of two polydeoxyribonucleotides chains (strands) twisted around each other on a common axis.
- *Antiparallel chains.* The two chains of each DNA molecule are antiparallel, i.e. one chain runs in the 5' to 3' direction while the other in 3' to 5' direction.
- *Dimensions.* The width of a double helix is 20Å (2 nm). Each turn (pitch) of the helix contains 10 pairs of nucleotides, each placed at distance of about 3.4Å (0.34 nm), thus each turn is 34Å (3.4 nm) in dimension.
- *Arrangement of base, sugar and phosphate molecule.* Each chain has a sugar phosphate backbone with

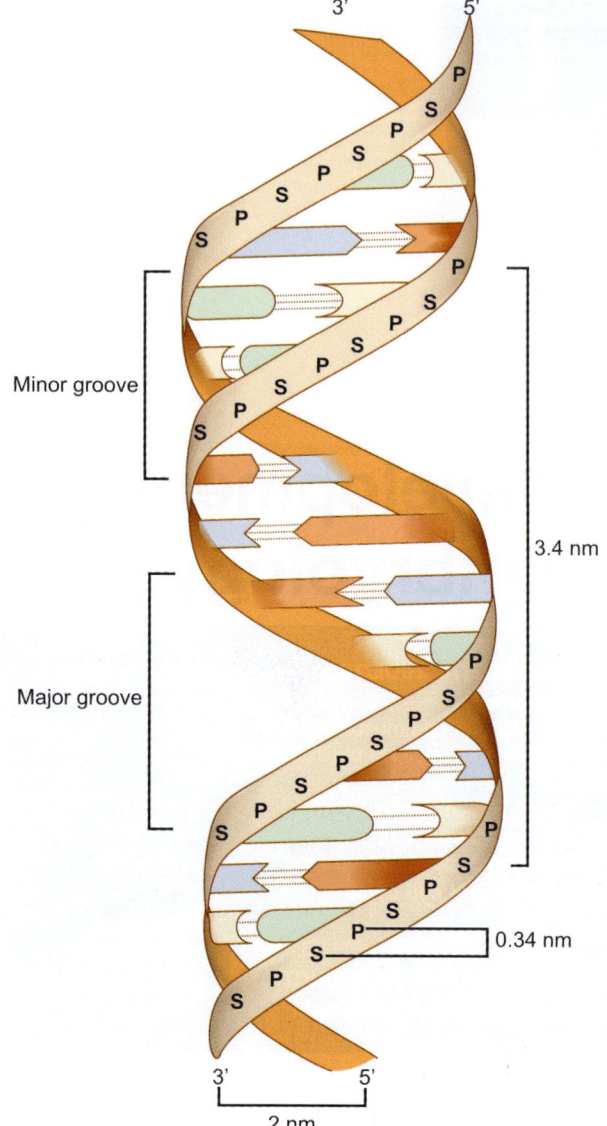

Fig. 1.1: Watson-Crick model of DNA structure.

bases which project at right angles and hydrogen bond with the bases of the opposite chain across the double helix (Fig. 1.2).

- *Complementary chains.* The two polynucleotide chains are not identical but complementary due to base pairing.
- *Genetic information.* The genetic information resides in one of two strands known as template strand or sense strand. The opposite strand is antisense strand.

Organization of DNA in the cell

In human cells the DNA is found in association with positively charged protein molecules called *histones*. Each DNA helix combines with group of 8 histone molecules to form structures known as *nucleosomes* which have a appearance of 'beads and string'. These nucleosomes, and the DNA strands linking them, are packed closely together to produce a 30 nm diameter

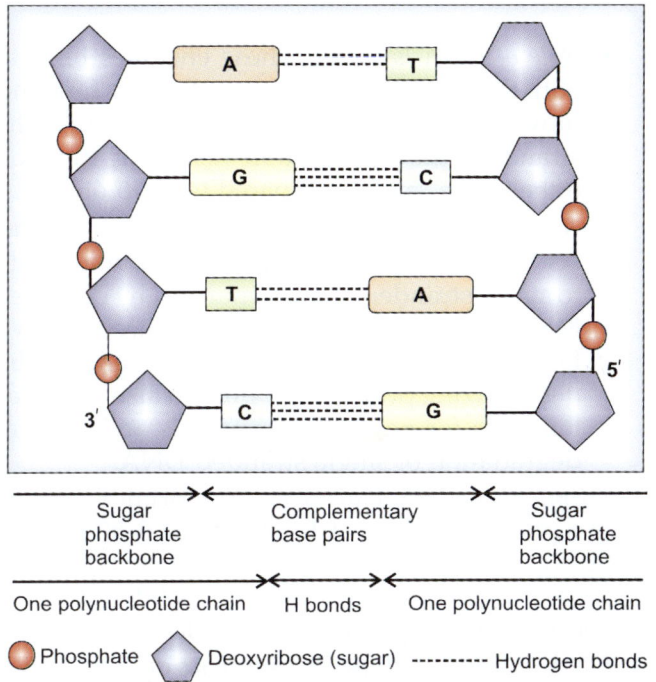

Fig. 1.2: Diagrammatic structure of straightened chains of DNA.

helix with about six nucleosome per turn. This is known as 30 nm fibre or the *solenoid fibre*. The solenoid fibres in turn coil to form *chromatin fibres* which are further coiled and packed in the form of *chromatin* in which form DNA is present in the chromosome (Fig. 1.3).

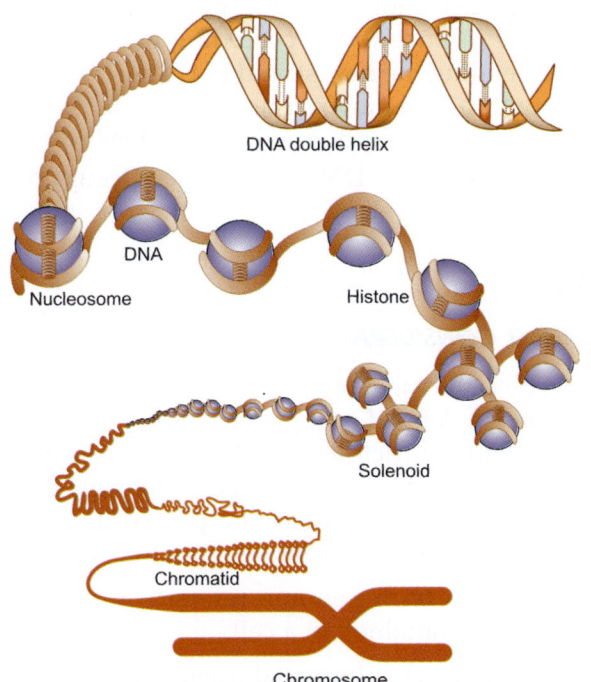

Fig. 1.3: Diagrammatic organization of DNA in chromosome of the human cell.

RNA

Structure of RNA

RNA is a polymer of ribonucleotides held together by 3′, 5′-phosphodiester bridges. Though RNA molecule like that of DNA is composed of nucleotides consisting of a base sugar and phosphate but has following structural differences:

- *Single strand.* RNA is commonly single stranded structure unlike DNA. However in certain forms of RNA this strand may fold at certain places to give a double stranded structure if complementary base pairs are in close proximity.
- *Ribose sugar.* The sugar molecule in RNA molecule is ribose in contrast to deoxyribose.
- *Base.* The pyrimidine base in a RNA molecule is uracil in place of thymine of a DNA molecule.
- *Chargaff's rule.* Due to the single stranded structure Chargaff's rule is not obeyed, i.e. there is no specific relation between purine and pyrimidine contents.

Types of RNA

Following types of RNAs have been recognised:

Nuclear RNA (nRNA) also known as premessenger RNA is the initial transcript of a gene nRNA is longer than mRNA because it contains introns that are removed (*spliced out*) as the mRNA *moves from the nucleus to the cytoplasm.*

Messenger RNA (mRNA). In the human cell it is synthesized in the nucleus and enters the cytoplasm to participate in protein synthesis.

Transfer RNA (tRNA). There are about 20 species of tRNA corresponding to 20 amino acids present in protein structure. The structure of tRNA resembles that of cloves leaf with four arms. tRNA delivers amino acids for protein synthesis.

Ribosomal RNA (rRNA). rRNAs are present in ribosomes (factories of protein synthesis). It is believed that rRNAs play a significant role in binding of mRNA to ribosomes in protein synthesis.

DNA Replication

DNA replication is a process by which each original DNA molecule gives rise to two copies with identical structure. The method by which the DNA replicates is called *semiconservation replication* since each new double helix retains (conserves) one of the two strands of the original DNA double helices. Steps involved in the DNA replication are (Fig. 1.4):

1. *Initiation of replication.* The site from where the replication of DNA is initiated is called *origin of*

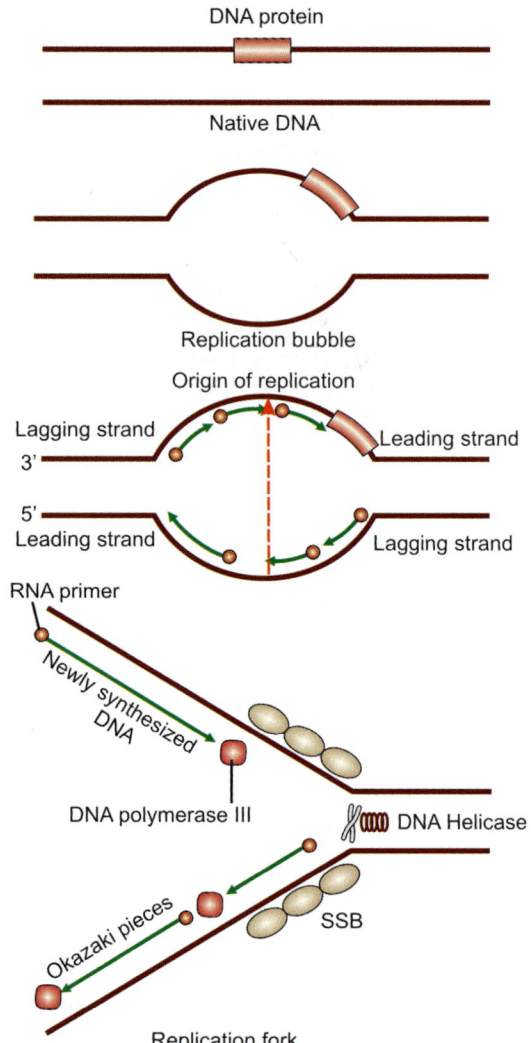

Fig. 1.4: Simplified diagram showing main steps of DNA replication.

replication. In prokaryotes, DNA replication initiates from only one site hence called mono-repliconic replication and in eukaryotes it starts from multiple sites *(multirepliconic replication)*. The origin of replication mostly consists of A-T base pairs. When a specific binding protein (DNA protein) binds to the site of replication then there occurs separation of double stranded DNA, and separated strands of DNA form a bubble at the site of origin.

2. *Formation of replication fork and replication eye.* The next step in the DNA replication is unwinding of double helix leading to formation of either Y-shaped *replication fork*, (when DNA replication initiates from the terminal end of the double helix), or q-shaped replication eye, (when DNA replication starts from the intercalary position). This step is controlled by an enzyme called *helicase* and a protein called *single strand binding* (SSB) protein.

- *Role of DNA helicases.* These enzymes bind to both the strands of DNA at replication fork and move along the DNA helix and separate the strands of the DNA double helix. The function of helicases can be compared to a zip opener.

- *Role of single strand DNA binding (SSB) proteins.* As the name indicates SSB protein binds only to single stranded DNA (separated by helicase). Main function of this protein is to keep the two DNA strands separate hence also called helix destabilizing protein. SSB protein also provides template for new DNA synthesis and prevent degradation of single stranded DNA.

3. *Formation of RNA primer.* RNA primer consists of a short fragment of RNA (about 5–50 nucleotides). It is required for synthesis of new DNA. The RNA primer is synthesised on DNA template by specific *RNA polymerase* (primase).

4. *DNA synthesis along the replication fork.* DNA replication occurs simultaneously in both the leading as well as lagging strands of Y-shaped replication fork and is of two types:

- *Continuous DNA replication.* In the leading strand DNA polymerase III binds to the single stranded DNA and starts to move along the strand. Each time it meets the next base on DNA, free nucleotides approach the DNA strand, and one with the correct complementary base hydrogen bonds to the base in the DNA. The free nucleotide is then in place by the enzyme until it binds to the preceding nucleotide thus extending the new strand of DNA. The enzyme continues to move along one base at time with new DNA strand growing as it does so.

- *Discontinuous DNA replication.* Occurs in the lagging strand.

GENES

GENERAL CONSIDERATIONS

The gene is the functional unit of DNA. A gene could therefore be defined as a piece of DNA which codes for a protein. In strictest sense the gene can be defined as the DNA code for a polypeptide. Since some proteins are made up of more than one polypeptide chains and are therefore coded for by more than one genes.

Genome. The term genome refers to total genetic information contained in a cell.

Human genome. For human the genome is essentially equivalent to all of the genetic information which is present in a single set of 23 chromosomes.

Human genome project (1990-2003). The human genome project (HGP) which completed on April 14, 2003 has accomplished the following goals:

- Identified all the *approximate 35,000 genes in human DNA.*

- Determined the sequences of 3 billion chemical base pairs that make the human DNA.

- Disproved the one gene–one protein hypothesis. In other words, concluded that through a variety of mechanisms a single gene may give rise to many proteins.

Functional genomics. Understanding the functions of genes and other parts of genome is known as functional genomics.

Comparative genomics. Comparative genomics is the analysis and comparison of genome from different species.

Constitutive and inducible genes. The genes are generally considered under two categories:

- *Constitutive.* The products (proteins) of these genes are required all the time in a cell. Therefore, the constitutive genes (or housekeeping genes) are expressed more or less at constant rate in almost all the cell and, further, they may not be subjected to regulation, e.g. enzymes of citric acid cycle.

- *Inducible genes.* The concentration of the proteins synthesized by inducible genes is regulated by various molecular signals. An inducer increases the expression of these genes while a repressor decreases, e.g. tryptophan pyrrolase of liver is induced by tryptophan.

GENE EXPRESSION: CENTRAL DOGMA

As mentioned above each cell of human body contains entire genome, yet the genetic expression is very selective and different patterns of protein synthesis occur in different tissues. Not only this, even in the same tissue there is wide variation in the proteins produced during the course of development.

The expression of genetic material occurs through the production of proteins. This involves two consecutive steps—transcription and translation. In transcription the genetic information, stored in DNA, is transferred to an RNA intermediate, which in turn uses this information to direct the synthesis of proteins during translation. This unidirectional flow of information was described by FHC Crick in 1958 as the *central dogma of molecular biology* (Fig. 1.5). However, an important modification of this information flow was given by David Baltimore and H Temin, who described reversible sequence through reverse

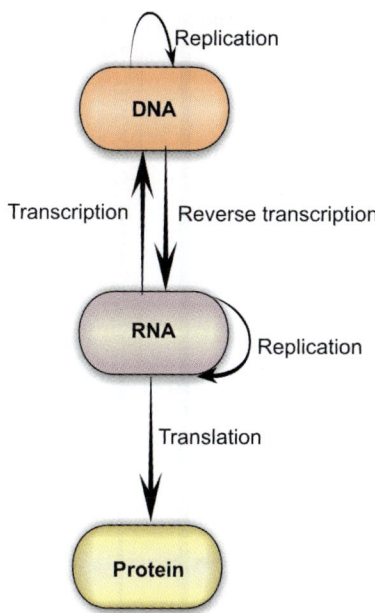

Fig. 1.5: Central dogma: The flow of genetic information.

transcription or teminism in the presence of transcripts (*revised central dogma*).

Transcription

Transcription is a process in which RNA is synthesized from DNA. All types of RNAs (nRNA, mRNA, tRNA and rRNA) are produced through transcription. The transcription process is selective, i.e. the entire molecule of DNA is not expressed in transcription, but the RNAs are synthesised only for selected regions of DNA. The strand of DNA that directs the synthesis of mRNA via complementary base pairing is called the *template strand* or coding strand or sense strand, and the other strand is known as noncoding strand or antisense strand. Transcription is accomplished by an enzyme *RNA polymerase* that gets physically associated with DNA. Only one type of such an enzyme is found in prokaryotes in contrast to eukaryotes (where three different forms of RNA polymerase are found). RNA I, II and III catalyse the synthesis of rRNA, mRNA and tRNA respectively.

Promotor sites. RNA polymerase binds to a region of DNA called promotor site. In eukaryotes, a sequence of DNA bases has been identified. This sequence, known as *Hogness box* or TATA box (Fig. 1.6) is located on left about 25 nucleotides away (upstream) from the starting site of mRNA synthesis. There also exists another site of recognition between 70 and 80 nucleotides upstream from the start of transcription. This second site is referred to as *CAAT box.* One of these two sites (or sometimes both) helps RNA polymerase II to recognize requisite sequence of DNA for transcription.

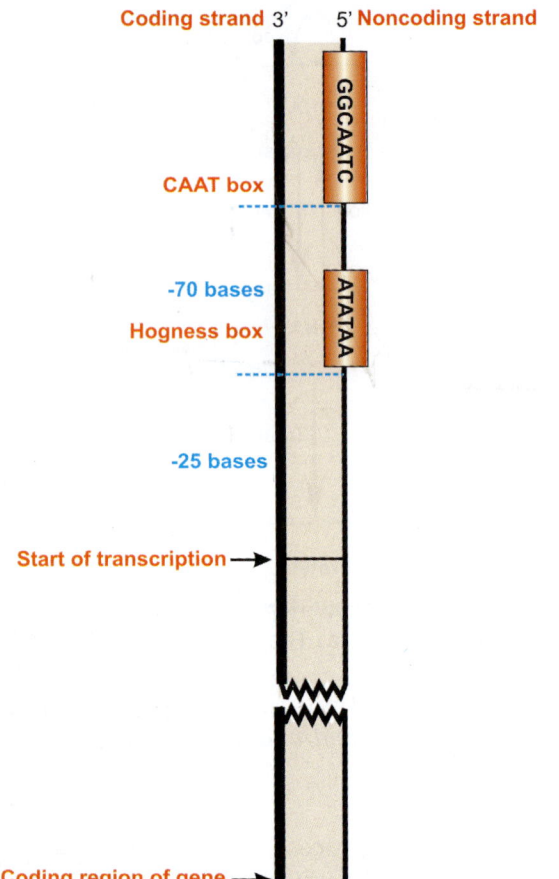

Coding strand 3'   5' Noncoding strand

GGCAATC

CAAT box

-70 bases

ATATAA

Hogness box

-25 bases

Start of transcription →

Coding region of gene →

Fig. 1.6: Promotor sites of DNA in eukaryotes.

Salient features of transcription in eukaryotes vis-a-vis prokaryotes are:

- Transcription in eukaryotes unlike prokaryotes occurs within the nucleus and mRNA moves out of the nucleus into the cytoplasm for translation.
- The initiation and regulation of transcription in eukaryotes is more extensive than prokaryotes.

Post-transcriptional modifications

- The mRNA in eukaryotes is processed from the primary RNA transcript; a process called maturation which includes:
  - Releases of the introns and joining with two adjacent ex ons to produce mature mRNA.
  - *RNA editing.* Besides, these two post-transcriptional modifications, RNA editing may also take place before translation begins.

Reverse transcription refers to formation of DNA from RNA. The enzyme reverse transcriptase is responsible for this process. The DNA so formed is complementary (cDNA) to viral RNA can be transmitted to host DNA. Reverse transcription is known to occur in retroviruses which include human immunodeficiency virus that cause AIDS.

Translation: Biosynthesis of proteins

Translation is the process by which genetic message carried by mRNA from the DNA is converted in the form of a polypeptide chain having specific sequence of amino acids. Before discussing the process of translation, it will be worthwhile to know something about genetic code.

Genetic code

Process by which the information coded in the mRNA is decoded into polypeptide is referred to as *deciphering the genetic code.* Dr Hargobind Khorana shared 'Nobel Prize' in 1968 with Nirenberg and Holly for the discovery of genetic code. The genetic code (codons) is formed by three nucleotides (triplet) base sequences in mRNA. The codons are formed of four nucleotide base (A, G, C and U). These four bases produce 64 different combinations of three base codons. Of the 64 codons, the 61 codons code for 20 amino acids found in proteins and the three codons (UAA, UAG and UGA) are *termination codons* which act as stop signals in protein synthesis. The codons AUG and sometimes GUG act as *initiating codons.*

Characteristics of genetic code are:

- *Universality,* i.e. same codons are used to code for the same amino acids in all the living organisms with a few exceptions.
- *Specificity,* i.e. a particular codon always codes for the same amino acid, e.g. AUG is the codon for methionine.
- *Non-overlapping,* i.e. the genetic code is read from a fixed point as a continuous base sequence.
- *Degenerate,* i.e. one amino acid is coded by more than one codons. The codons that designate the same amino acid are called synonyms.

Process of protein biosynthesis

The process of protein synthesis, i.e. translation, in addition to mRNA requires amino acids tRNA, energy sources (ATP and GTP) and protein factors. Protein synthesis occurs over ribosomes which are also called *protein factories.* The protein biosynthesis involves three processes:

I. *Activation of amino acids.* Amino acids are activated and attached to tRNA in a two-step reaction. A group of enzymes, namely aminoacyl tRNA synthetases are required for this process. In the first step an amino acid reacts with ATP in the presence of specific amino acid tRNA to form *enzyme-AMP-amino acid complex.* This complex then reacts with a specific tRNA and the amino acid is transferred to 3' end of the tRNA to form aminoacyl tRNA.

II. *Translation proper* involves three steps—initiation, elongation and termination.

1. *Initiation.* The translation of mRNA begins with the formation of initiation complex.

2. *Elongation.* Ribosomes elongate the polypeptide chain by a sequential addition of amino acids to the growing carboxyl end.

The elongation process is repeated again and again with addition of one amino acid each time till signal for termination is reached.

3. *Termination* of polypeptide synthesis is evoked by a nonsense or termination codon (UAA, UAG or UGA).

III. *Post-translational modifications.* The proteins synthesized in translation are, as such not functional. Many changes take place in the polypeptides after the initiation of their synthesis or, most frequently after the protein synthesis is completed. Post-translational modification include:

- Proteolytic degradation, and
- Covalent modifications (phosphorylation, hydroxylation and glycosylation).

Alternate splicing

Alternate splicing refers to the process by which different proteins can be produced from a single gene.

- *Spliceosomes,* complexes of nRNAs carry out the process of alternate splicing.
- *Splicing isoforms* or splice variants, or alternative splice forms is the term used to denote the proteins derived from the same gene.
- The process affords the opportunity for different cells to use the same gene to make proteins specific for that cell type. For example, isoforms of the WT1 gene have different functions in gonadal versus kidney development.

REGULATION OF GENE EXPRESSION

As discussed earlier, each nucleated somatic cell in the body contains full genetic message, yet there is great differentiation and specialization in the functions of various types of adult cells. It is because of the fact that there exists a full proof system for regulation of gene expression that maintains orderly growth in cells and prevents uncontrolled growth. The genes are controlled both spatially and temporally. The regulation of gene expression is thus absolutely essential for growth, development and differentiation of an organism. A positive regulator increases the gene expression whereas a negative regulator decreases.

Regulation of gene expression in eukaryotes

The regulation of gene expression in eukaryotes is very complex and involves various mechanisms. Some of the mechanisms are:

1. *Gene amplification.* In this mechanism the expression of gene is increased several folds. An example of gene amplification in humans includes development of drug resistance by the malignant cells to long-term administration of methotrexate. This occurs by amplifying the gene coding for dihydrofolate reductase.

2. *Gene rearrangement.* The process of gene rearrangement is responsible for the generation of 10 billion antigen specific immunoglobulins.

3. *Regulation of gene expression through transcription factors.* Transcription factors are products of other genes and hence mediate transregulation by binding to specific DNA segments. This specific interaction of protein to DNA in over 80% of the non-transcription factors is brought about by one of the four DNA-binding motiffs: zinc finger motiff, Lucine zipper-motiff, helix-turn-helix motiff, and helix-loop-helix motiff.

4. *Regulation of gene through mRNA.* Gene expression is also regulated by regulation of synthesis, transport, processing and stability of mRNA.
   - mRNAs may be selectively translated, and
   - Proteins made from the mRNA may be differently modified.

CELL DIVISION AND CELL CYCLE

The division of pre-existing cells leads to increase in the number of cells. The cell multiplication is an essential feature of development and growth. Two kinds of cell division known are:

- Mitosis, and
- Meiosis.

CELL CYCLE

The cells proliferate in response to extracellular growth factors, passing through a repeated sequence of events known as the *cell cycle.* It has three main stages (Fig. 1.7):

- Interphase
- Mitosis or M-phase, and
- Cell division.

A. INTERPHASE

Interphase refers to the period between two successive divisions. This is a period of synthesis and growth. Interphase includes three sub-phases (Fig. 1.7A):

- G_1-phase,
- S-phase, and
- G_2-phase

G_1-phase. The gap period between M-phase and S-phase is called *G_1-phase.* During this phase cytoplasm increases in volume. It includes the *G_1 check points,* when damage to the DNA is repaired and the cell checks that its environment is favourable before committing itself to S-phase.

G_0-phase. Most body cells are not actively dividing and are arrested at G_0-phase within G_1-phase. Cells can remain in G_0-phase for years before recommencing division. The G_0 block is imposed by *mitosis-suppressor proteins.*

S-phase. S-phase refers to phase of *DNA synthesis.* The replication of DNA during S-phase has already been described (see page 5). After replication of DNA each chromosome exists as a pair of *chromatids* joined together by a *centromere* (Fig. 1.7A). At this stage the cell is 4n (4 copies of each DNA molecule 2 in each chromosomes of a homologous pair). During this phase chromosome material is in the form of very loosely coiled threads called *chromatin.* Centrioles have replicated (Fig. 1.7A).

G_2-phase. This is the gap between S-phase and M-phase. The G_2 *check point* during this phase allows the cell to check that DNA replication is complete before proceeding to mitosis (M-phase).

B. MITOSIS (M-PHASE)

Mitosis is the process by which a cell nucleus divides to produce two daughter nuclei containing identical sets of chromosomes to the parent cell. It is usually followed immediately by division of the whole cell to form two daughter cells. Mitosis with cell division results in an increase in cell numbers and is the method by which growth, replacement and repair of cell occur in eukaryotes. It is important to note that mammalian cells will proliferate only if stimulated by *extracellular growth factors* secreted by other cells.

Mitosis or M-phase is divided into following phases (Fig. 1.7B):

1. *Prophase.* This is usually the longest phase. During this phase:
   - Chromosomes, each consisting of two identical chromatids, begin to contract and become visible within the nucleus.
   - Centrioles move to opposite poles of the cells.
   - Short microtubules may be seen radiating from the centrioles. These are called *asters.*
   - The nucleoli disappear as their DNA passes to certain chromosomes.
   - At the end of prophase the nuclear envelop is no longer visible as it breaks up into small vesicles which disperse.
   - A spindle is formed.

2. *Metaphase* is characterized by:
   - Linning up of chromosomes around the equator of spindle attached by their centromeres to the spindle fibres (microtubules).
   - A metaphase plate is created due to above alignment of chromosomes.

3. *Anaphase* is a very rapid stage and in this phase:
   - The centromeres split into two and the spindle fibres pull the daughter centromeres to opposite poles.
   - The separated chromatids are pulled along behind the centromeres, and the separated chromatids now become independent chromosomes. Thus, at this stage the cell can be said to possesses forty-six pairs of chromosomes.

4. *Telophase.* In this phase:
   - The separated chromatids (now considered to be chromosomes) which have reached the poles of the cell, uncoil and lengthen to form chromatin again, losing the ability to be seen clearly.
   - The spindle fibres (microtubules) degenerate and the centrioles replicate.
   - A nuclear envelop reforms around the chromosomes at each pole and nucleoli reappear.

C. CYTOKINESIS (CELL DIVISION PHASE)

The cell membrane contracts around the mid-region between the poles, creating a *cleavage furrow* which leads to division of cytoplasm into two and eventually separates the two daughter cells.

Role of mitosis

Cell division by mitosis plays following roles:

1. *Genetic stability.* Mitosis produces two nuclei which have the same number of chromosomes as the parent cell. Since these chromosomes were derived from parental chromosomes by the exact replication of their DNA, they will carry the same hereditary information in their genes. Daughter cells are genetically identical to the parent cell and no variation in genetic information can therefore

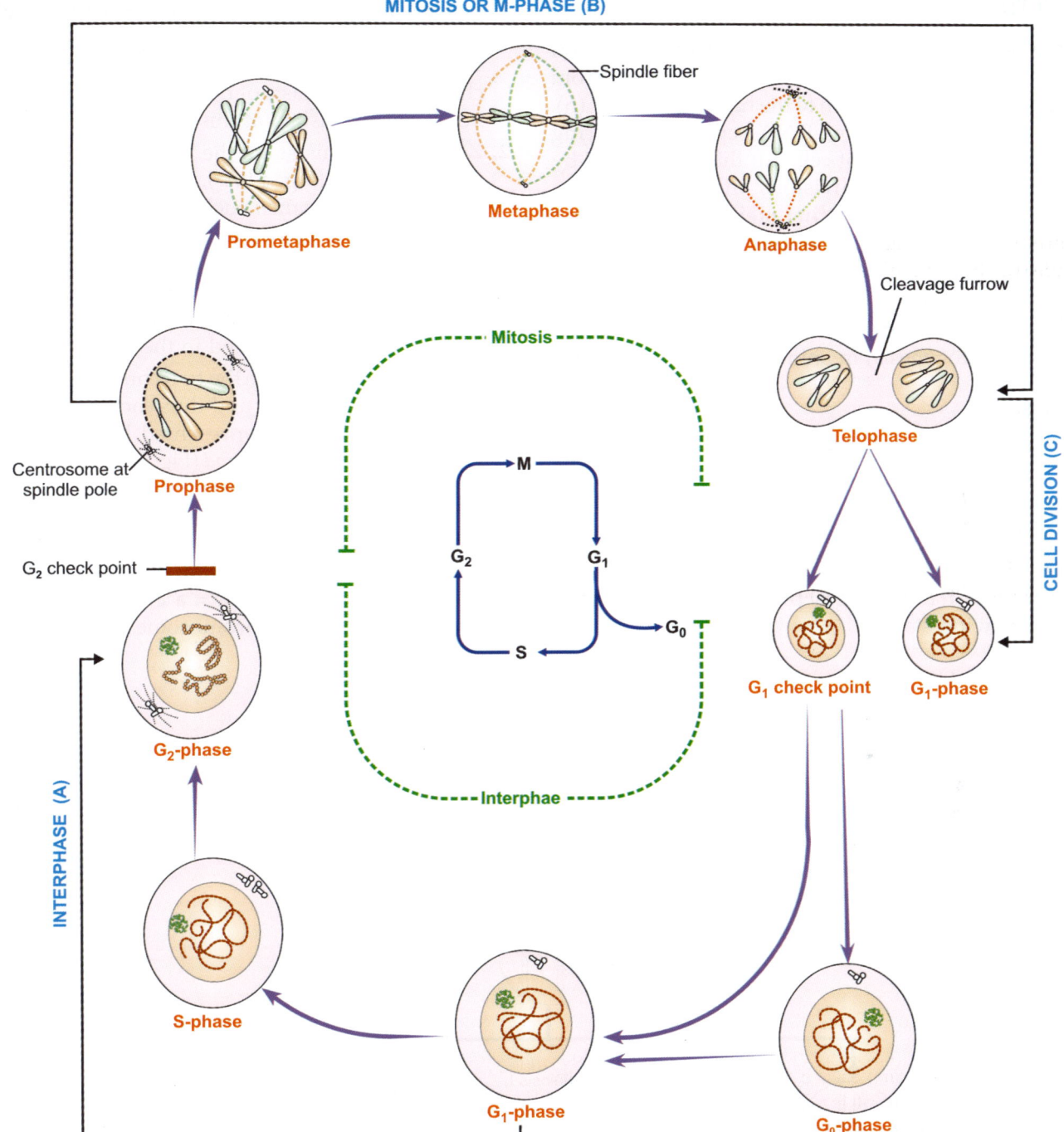

Fig. 1.7: The cell cycle consisting of: interphase A, mitosis phase B and phase of cell division C.

be introduced during mitosis. This results in genetic stability within populations of cells derived from the same parental cells.

2. *Growth.* The number of cells within an organism increases by mitosis and this is the basis of growth in multicellular organisms.

3. *Cell replacement.* Replacement of cells and tissues also involves mitosis. Cells are constantly dying and being replaced, an obvious example being in the skin.

4. *Regeneration.* Some animals are able to regenerate whole parts of the body, such as legs in crustacea and arms in starfish. Production of the new cells involves mitosis.

5. *Asexual reproduction.* Mitosis is the basis of asexual reproduction, the production of new individuals of a species by one parent organism. Many species undergo asexual reproduction.

MEIOSIS

Meiosis (*meio, to reduce*) is a form of nuclear division in which the chromosome number is halved from being diploid number (2n) to the haploid number (n). Like mitosis, it involves DNA replication during interphase in the parent cell, but this is followed by *two cycles* of nuclear divisions and cell divisions, known as **meiosis I (the first meiotic division)** and **meiosis II (the second meiotic division).** Thus a single diploid cell gives rise to four haploid cells (Fig. 1.8).

Meiosis occurs during the formation of sperms and eggs (gametogenesis) in animals.

MEIOSIS I

Phases of meiosis I are (Fig. 1.9):

Prophase I

Prophase I involves reciprocal exchange between maternal and paternal chromatids by the process of *crossing over*. It is the longest phase and can be divided into following stages:

1. *Leptotene.* In this stage chromosomes become visible as long threads attached at each end to the nuclear envelop (like mitosis). Although each chromosome consists of two chromatids, these can not be distinguished at this stage (Fig. 1.9A$_1$).

2. *Zygotene.* In this stage the homologous chromosomes pair up (Fig. 1.9A$_2$). This process is called *synapsis* or *conjugation* each pair is called *bivalent*. One of the pair comes from the male parent and one from the female parent. Each member of the pair is in the same length, their centromeres are in the same positions and they usually have the same number of genes arranged in the same order.

3. *Pachytene.* In this stage the two chromatids of each chromosome separate and thus each *bivalent* (pair of chromosomes) is represented by four double helices and is called a *tetrad* (Fig. 1.9A$_3$). Then there occurs *crossing over, i.e.* one or both chromatids of each paternal chromosome crosses over with those from the mother is what is known as a *synaptonemal complex* (Fig. 1.9A$_4$). The point of crossing over are called *chiasmata* (chiasma = a cross). As a result, genes from parental chromosome may swap with

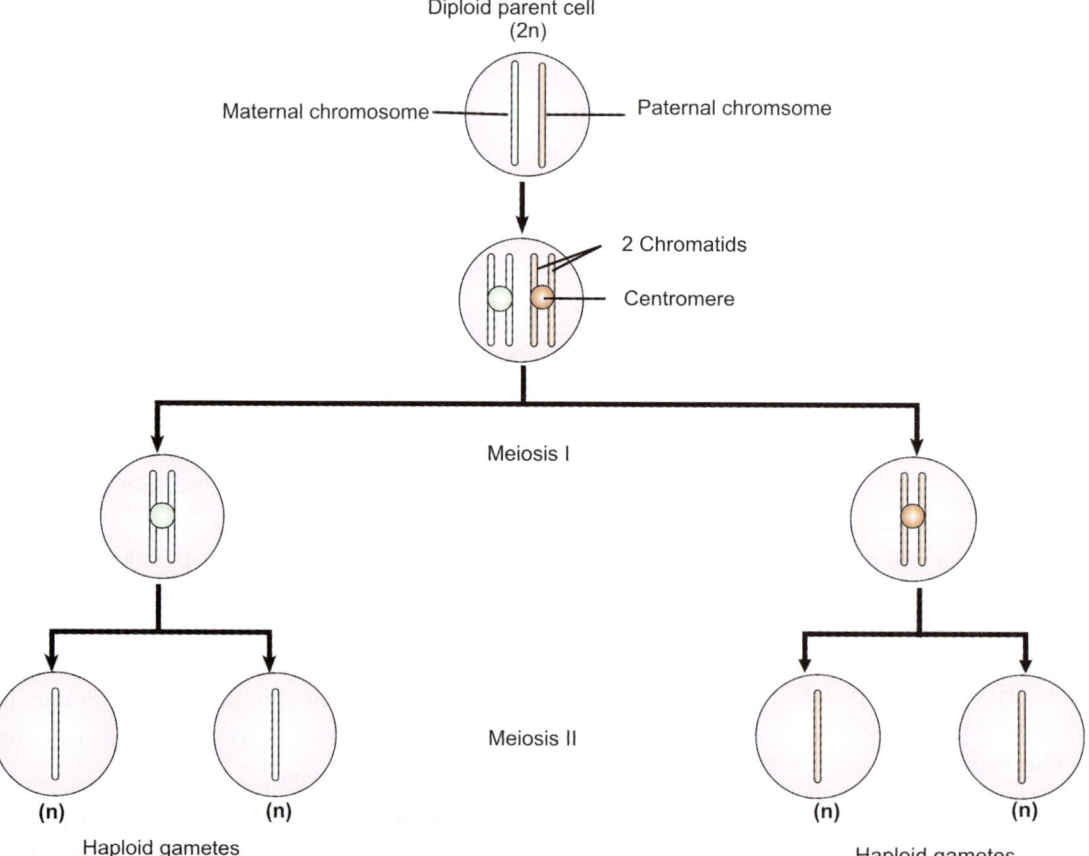

Fig. 1.8: The basic characteristics of meiosis showing one chromosome duplication followed by two nuclear and cell divisions. Note that, as for mitosis, chromosomes may be single or double structures. When double the two parts are called chromatids.

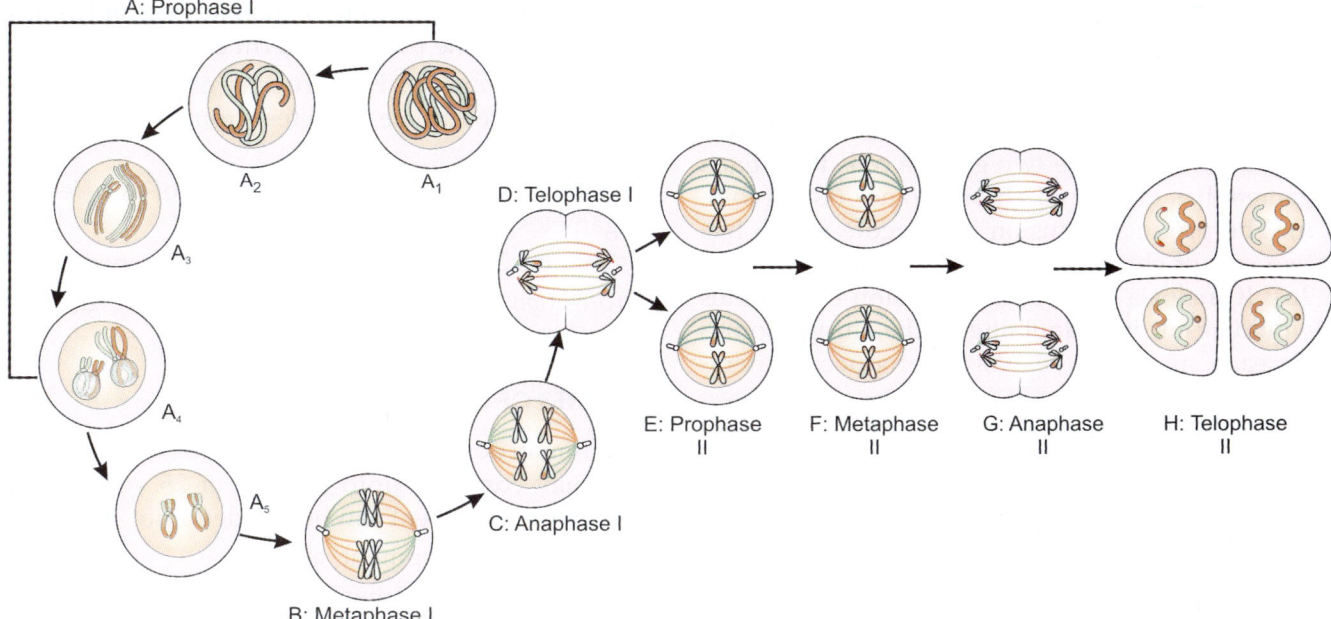

Fig. 1.9: Phases of meiosis: A, prophase I, leptotene, (A₁), zygotene (A₂), pachytene (A₃), diplotene (A₄), diakinesis (A₅); B, metaphase I; C, anaphase I; D, telophase I; and phases of meiosis II: E, prophase II; F, metaphase II; G, anaphase II, and H, telophase II.

genes from the maternal chromosome leading to new gene combinations in the resulting chromatids. Every chromosome pair undergoes at least one cross-over.

4. *Diplotene.* In this stage the chromatids separate except in the regions of crossing over or chiasmata (Fig. 1.9A₄).

5. *Diakinesis.* In this stage the reorganized chromosomes begin to move apart. Each bivalent can now be seen to contain four chromatids linked by a common centromere, while non-sister chromatids are linked by chiasmata (Fig. 1.9A₅).

Metaphase I

The bivalents become arranged around the equator of the spindle, attached by their centromeres (Fig. 1.9B).

Anaphase I

Spindle fibres pull homologous chromosomes, centromeres first, towards opposite poles of the spindle (unlike mitosis there is no splitting of the centromeres). This separates the chromosome into two haploid sets, one set at each end of the spindle (Fig. 1.9C).

Telophase I

The telophase is similar to mitosis, i.e. (Fig. 1.9D):

• The homologous chromosomes which have reached at opposite poles of the cells uncoil and lengthen to form chromatin again, losing the ability to be seen clearly.

• The spindle fibres usually disappear.

• A nuclear envelop reforms around the chromosomes at each pole.

• *Cytokinesis* and *cleavage* then occurs and two daughter cells are formed.

Thus, at the end of meiosis I each daughter cell contains 23 chromosomes (1-n), each consisting of two chromatids (i.e. 2C).

MEIOSIS II

Phases of meiosis II (Fig. 1.9E to H) are:

Interphase II. There is a transient interphase I after meiosis I. This differs from the usual interphase in that no chromosome replication occurs in this phase (since the daughter cells after meiosis I already posses two chromatids each).

Prophase II, metaphase II, anaphase II, telophase II and cytokinesis are similar to the phases of mitosis in that pair of chromatids (bivalents) linked at their centromeres become aligned at the metaphase plate and are then drawn into separate daughter cells following replication of the centromeric DNA.

Unlike mitosis, because of the crossing over that has occurred during the meiosis I, the daughter cells are not identical in genetic content. Further, the daughter cells at the end of meiosis II contain 23 chromosomes (1-n), each consisting of a single chromatid (IC) (Fig. 1.9H).

Role of meiosis

The meiotic division plays following roles:

1. *Sexual reproduction.* Meiosis occurs in all organisms carrying out sexual reproduction. During fertilization the nuclei of the two gamete cells fuse. Each gamete has one set of chromosomes (is haploid, n). The product of fusion is a zygote which has two sets of chromosomes (the diploid condition, 2n). If meiosis did not occur fusion of gametes would result in a doubling of the chromosomes for each successive sexually reproduced generation.

2. *Genetic variation.* Meiosis also provides opportunities for new combinations of genes to occur in the gametes. This leads to genetic variation in the offspring produced by fusion of the gametes. Meiosis does this is two ways, namely independent assortment of chromosomes and crossing over in meiosis I.

COMPARISON OF MITOSIS AND MEIOSIS

The biologically significant differences between mitosis and meiosis are really between mitosis and meiosis I. Meiosis II is almost identical to mitosis. Therefore, Table 1.1 summarizes the comparison of mitosis and meiosis I.

EMBRYOLOGY: AN INTRODUCTION

Human embryology refers to the study of development of a new human embryo and fetus from fertilization of ovum up to the time of delivery.

Gametogenesis refers to formation of male and female gametes from the primitive germ cells. It includes:

- *Spermatogenesis,* i.e. process of formation of spermatozoa (male gametes) from the spermatogonia, and
- *Oogenesis,* i.e. process of formation of ova (female gametes) from the oogonia.

  Chapter 2 includes details of gametogenesis.

Fertilization, i.e. fusion of male and female gametes initiates embryogenesis.

OUTLINES OF HUMAN DEVELOPMENT

The human development which begins with fertilization may continue upto the age of 25 years. Thus human development can be divided into:

- Prenatal development, and
- Postnatal development.

Prenatal development

Prenatal period extends from fertilization of the ovum up to the delivery and is also called *gestation period* (average duration 280 days or 10 lunar months and range is 250 to 310 days). Embryology refers to developmental changes during this phase.

Phases of prenatal development

Period of prenatal (before birth) development can be divided into three main phases:

- *Pre-embryo or germinal phase* (day 0–weeks 3). During this phase zygote develops and forms the trilaminar germ disc.

	Mitosis	Meiosis
Prophase	• Homologous chromosomes remain separate. • No formation of chiasmata • No crossing over	• Homologous chromosomes pair up. • Chiasmata form • Crossing over may occur.
Metaphase	• Pairs of chromatids line up on the equator of the spindle.	• Pairs of chromosomes line up on the equator.
Anaphase	• Centromeres divide • Chromatids separate • Separating chromatids identical.	• Centromeres do not divide. • Whole chromosomes separate • Separating chromosomes and their chromatids may not be identical due to crossing over.
Telophase	• Same number of chromosomes present in daughter cells as parent cells. • Both homologous chromosomes present in daughter cells if diploid.	• Half the number of chromosomes present in daughter cells. • Only one of each pair of homologous chromosomes present in daughter cells.
Occurrence	• May occur in haploid, diploid or polyploid cells. • Occurs during the formation of somatic (body) cells and some spores. • Also occurs during the formation of gametes in plants.	• Only occurs in diploid or polyploid cells. • Occurs during formation of gametes or spores.

Table 1.1: Comparison of mitosis and meiosis

- *Embryo phase* (weeks 4–8). During this phase there occurs differentiation and formation of most of the tissues and organs of the body.
- *Fetal phase* (weeks 9–40).

Stages of pre-embryo (germinal) phase and embryo phase of human development. The embryonic development (pre-embryo phase and embryo phase, i.e. day 0 to weeks 8) has been described in 23 stages by Carnegie because of the variable period it takes for embryos to develop certain morphological characteristics. Salient features of the 23 stages of human development are summarized in Table 4.1 (page 58).

Fetal phase of development. The fetal period (weeks 9–40) of development begins after the embryonic period and ends when the fetus is completely outside the mother (i.e. after birth). During fetal phase of development there occurs complete development of placenta and rapid growth of the tissues and organs formed during the embryo phase of development without much tissue differentiation.

Postnatal development

Development does not stop at birth, i.e. it is a continuous process. Most developmental changes are completed by the age of 25 years. Postnatal period of development can be divided into following phases:

Neonate or newborn refers to an infant from birth to one month of age.

Infancy refers to the period of one year after birth.

Childhood is the period after one year of age until puberty (sexual maturity).

Puberty is the period when secondary sex characteristics develop and capability of sexual reproduction is attained. In girls, puberty occurs between 12 to 15 years of age and in boys between 13 to 16 years.

Adolescence refers to the period of rapid physical and sexual maturation. It is the period from about 12 to 19 years of age.

Adulthood is attained between 18 to 21 years, when an individual is physically, sexually and mentally matured. During adulthood, i.e. between 21 to 25 years of age, ossification of the most of the bones and body growth is completed.

CONTROL OF DEVELOPMENT

PROCESSES CONTROLLING DEVELOPMENT

Several processes which control differentiation and ensure synchronised development include:

- Cell differentiation,

- Regulated cell migration,
- Induction, and
- Apoptosis.

CELL DIFFERENTIATION

Totipotent cells are present in the zygote during first few days before the embryo develops. Each such cell is capable of forming a normal embryo or developing into any of the more than 200 cell types in the body.

Pluripotent cells are present in the blastocyst, including the early embryo. They are capable of forming a variety of cell types, but not a whole individual. They are genetically programmed to follow more specific development paths.

Multipotent cells are present as some undifferentiated stem cells in adult organs and act as source of new cells. These can be cultured to form entirely different tissues than in their organ of origin but are thought to have less flexibility in differentiation than embryonic stem cells.

REGULATED MIGRATION OF CELLS

Most events in the embryogenesis involve the association, dissociation, and migration of cells. The interrelated processes involve dynamic changes in the molecules expressed in cell membranes. Cell adhesion molecules (CAMS) cause cells to aggregate. Their inactivation is a requirement of the initiation of cell migration, but control of migration pathway is very complex. Following factors play role in cell migration:

- *Connective tissue fibres* often help to guide the cells for migration a process termed *contact guidance.*
- *Chemical signals* may attract cells and induce migration,
- *Hyaluronic acid,* is a connective tissue protein that binds water and creates a favourable environment for cell migration.

INDUCTION

Induction is the interaction between two separate histological tissues or primordia in the embryo that result in morphological differentiation. One tissue usually induces the other, but one or both can participate in subsequent organogenesis. The signals for induction process travel from one cell to another by any of the following methods:

- Diffusion of signaling molecules from one cell to other.
- Extracellular matrix mediated signaling, and
- Direct cellular contact between the two embryonic tissues.

Growth factors: The signaling molecules

Growth factors are a group of more than 50 naturally occurring proteins that bind to specific cell receptors to stimulate cell division, differentiation and other functions, related to control of tissue proliferation. Thus, the growth factors act as cell signaling molecules for induction of cellular differentiation. Some growth factors can stimulate only one cell type (e.g. nerve growth factor), whereas other have broad specificity. Some common growth factors can be grouped as below:

1. **Fibroblast growth factors (FGFs).** These are particularly important for:
   - Angiogenesis,
   - Axon growth,
   - Mesoderm differentiation (limb development (FDFs- 2, 4 and 8).

2. **WNT proteins.** There are about 15 WNT proteins. These are particularly important for:
   - Regulating limb patterning,
   - Regulating mid-brain development, and
   - Regulating some aspects of somites and urogenital differentiation.

3. **Hedgehog proteins.** There are three hedgehog proteins genes, desert, Indian and sonic hedgehog.

   Sonic hedgehog is particularly important for:
   - Limb patterning,
   - Neural tube induction and patterning,
   - Somite differentiation and
   - Gut regionalization.

4. **Transforming growth factor β (TGF-β) super family**

   The TGF-β super family has over 30 members.
   - *TGF-β members* are particularly important for extracellular matrix formation and epithelial branching that occurs in the development of lungs, kidneys and salivary glands.
   - *Bone morphogenic proteins (MBPs)* belonging to this family induce bone formation and is involved in regulating cell division, cell death (apoptosis), and cell migration among other functions.

5. **Epidermal growth factor (EGF)** is concerned with growth and proliferation of cells of ectodermal and mesodermal origin.

6. **Nerve growth factors** (NGFs) stimulate the growth of sensory and sympathetic neurons.

7. **Insulin like growth factors (IGFs)**
   - *IGF-1* act as a factor for bone growth, and
   - *IGF-2* is a fetal growth factor.

Morphogens, e.g. retinoic acid, neurotransmitters and products of Wnt genes are reported to trigger a cascade of events in the reacting cells, and in many cases, the initial process is activation of homeobox genes. These genes code for transcription factors that then regulate expression of other genes.

Growth factor receptors

Growth factor receptors are present in the cell membrane. They recognize and respond to specific growth factors which act as cell signaling molecules for induction of cellular differentiation. Two types of growth factor receptors known are:

1. **Transmembrane receptors** are present within the cell membrane and protein in nature. They bind to the signaling molecules on the outer side of the membrane and initiate *tyrosine kinase* activity on the inner side of membrane. This is followed by the activation of cytoplasmic protein kinases.

2. **Notch receptors.** These play important role in the induction process during embryonic development. These are involved in *juxtacrine signaling* in which a protein on one cell surface interacts with a receptor on adjacent cell surface. Juxtacrine signaling is involved in:
   - Neuronal differentiation,
   - Blood vessel specification, and
   - Somite segmentation.

APOPTOSIS

Apoptosis, an extremely important process of normal development, refers to programmed cell death. It is initiated in mitochondria in response to a variety of stimuli. Cytochrome C and other molecules are released into the cytoplasm, triggering a cascade of reactions involving a number of cystein proteases called caspases. The result is the condensation of chromatin in the nucleus and the degradation of DNA. There may also be caspase-independent mechanisms for apoptosis that act in very early development.

Some roles played by apoptosis in development are highlighted below:

- Disappearance of a large number of tissues and structures during development is an obvious function of apoptosis. Fingers and toes are formed by the elimination of tissue between them.

- The lumen of vessels, ducts, hollow organs, other spaces in the body are formed via apoptosis.

- In nervous system large number of neurons are lost by apoptosis to allow for the proper connections and functions of the remaining cells.

MOLECULAR CONTROL OF DEVELOPMENT

Today, the genome of fertilized ovum is held to contain all the information necessary for the development of a new individual. In other words the development proceeds as per the plans in the chromosomes of sperm as well as ovum. The products of genes controlling embryogenesis are mostly transcriptional factors that regulate the expression of other genes. Most of the information about genetic control of development has come from studies in other organisms, especially *Drosophila* fruit flies. From fruit flies to humans, it appears that similar genetic controls predetermine the shape of living things.

Genes controlling development

Three hierarchial groups of genes controlling development have been identified in *Drosophila*. These include:

- Maternal effect genes,
- Segmentation genes, and
- Homeotic genes.

1. *Maternal effect genes.* These genes begin producing their proteins within the oocyte before fertilization. The gene products have an asymmetrical accumulation in the early rounds of cell division that is responsible for the establishment of the morphological axes in the embryos. With fertilization, mRNA from a specific gene is translated into its corresponding protein. This diffuses from the cranial pole, and with colinear proteins of other mRNAs, bring about steeply falling morphogenic gradients, defining the *craniocaudal and dorsoventral axes*. A similar system operates from the caudal end of the egg.

2. *Segmentation genes* of the Hox gene family are responsible for defining the segments, i.e. the establishment of the repeating morphological patterns in the embryo. Segmentation is expressed throughout the embryo in the formation of:

- Cranial and spinal nerves,
- Vertebral column and ribs,
- Early muscle development, and
- Pattern of blood vessel formation.

Segmentation of the embryonic head is more obvious than anywhere else in the embryo, with neuromeres in the hindbrain, somites and somitomeres, and the pharyngeal arches of mesoderm.

3. *Homeotic genes.* These genes are activated by the segmentation genes to determine the fate of segments. Thus the differentiation of the embryonic segments is controlled by homeotic genes.

Homeobox gene clusters

Homeobox (Hox) genes are a group of genes present in all vertebrates and represent the genes controlling development in *Drosophila* which have been well conserved during evolution. Over hundreds millions of years of evolution, these genes have been duplicated twice, and thus in human they exist as four copies: Hox-A, Hox-B, Hox-C and Hox-D. Genes in each cluster are numbered 1 to 13 and lie on a separate chromosome as shown below:

Gene cluster	Total number of genes	Chromosome location
Hox-A	11	7 p
Hox-B	9	17 q
Hox-C	9	12 q
Hox-D	9	2 q

Paralogus group is formed by genes with the same number, but belonging to different clusters, for example Hox-A4, Hox-B4, Hox-C4 and Hox-D4 form a paralogus group of genes.

Cranial-to-caudal patterning of the derivatives of all three germ layers is determined by the Hox genes. Thus, the Hox genes play role in the development of all systems.

Paired-box (pax) genes, eight in number have been identified in humans through their homology with *Drosophila* paired box sequences. They encode DNA-binding proteins, which act as transcription control factor, and play an important role in the development across the animal kingdom.

OUTLINES OF MOLECULAR CONTROL OF DEVELOPMENT

A brief account of molecular control of development can be organized as below:

A. *Molecular control of early embryonic development*

- Molecular control of establishment of the axes of the embryo.
- Molecular control of segmentation process.
- Molecular control of determination of fate of segments.

For details see page 17 and 45.

B. *Molecular control of gastrulation*

For details see page 44.

C. *Molecular control of systemic development*

- Molecular regulation of neural induction (see page 245).
- Molecular regulation of somite differentiation. (see page 45).
- Molecular regulation of nerve differentiation in the spinal cord (see page 245).
- Molecular regulation of limb development (see page 125).
- Molecular regulation of bone development (see page 95).
- Molecular regulation of muscle development (see page 96).
- Molecular regulation of cardiac development (see page 221).
- Molecular regulation of lung development (see page 202).
- Molecular regulation of gut tube development (see page 153).
- Molecular regulation of liver induction (see page 159).
- Molecular regulation of pancreas development (see page 161).
- Molecular regulation of renal development (see page 179).
- Molecular regulation of facial development (see page 143).
- Molecular regulation of eye development (see page 272).

Gametogenesis and Female Sexual Cycle

GAMETOGENESIS

As mentioned earlier embryology refers to study of the development of an individual before birth. Fusion of male and female gametes initiates embryogenesis. This chapter is devoted to *gametogenesis,* i.e. formation of male and female gametes from the primitive germ cells. The gametogenesis, thus, includes:

- Spermatogenesis, and
- Oogenesis.

SPERMATOGENESIS

Spermatogenesis refers to the process of formation of spermatozoa from the primitive germ cells (spermatogonia).

CHARACTERISTIC FEATURES OF SPERMATOGENESIS

- Spermatogenesis begins at puberty and continues throughout adult life to decline in old age.
- The majority of the spermatogonia undergo continuous mitotic division to provide additional stem cells.
- Only a minority of the spermatogonia undergo further differentiation by meiosis, a process unique to germinal epithelium.
- Each differentiating spermatogonium develops into 512 spermatids.
- Spermatogenesis does not occur simultaneously in all the parts of testes. At any one moment, some areas of the seminiferous tubules are active while others are in resting state.

- In humans, it takes an average of 74 days to form a mature sperm from a primitive germ cell.
- The spermatozoa formed in the seminiferous tubules are non-motile structures.
- The spermatozoa undergo process of maturation while passing through the male genital tract, and acquire the ability of fertilization of an ovum (capacitation) in the female genital tract.

PHASES OF SPERMATOGENESIS

The phases of spermatogenesis are as follows (Fig. 2.1):

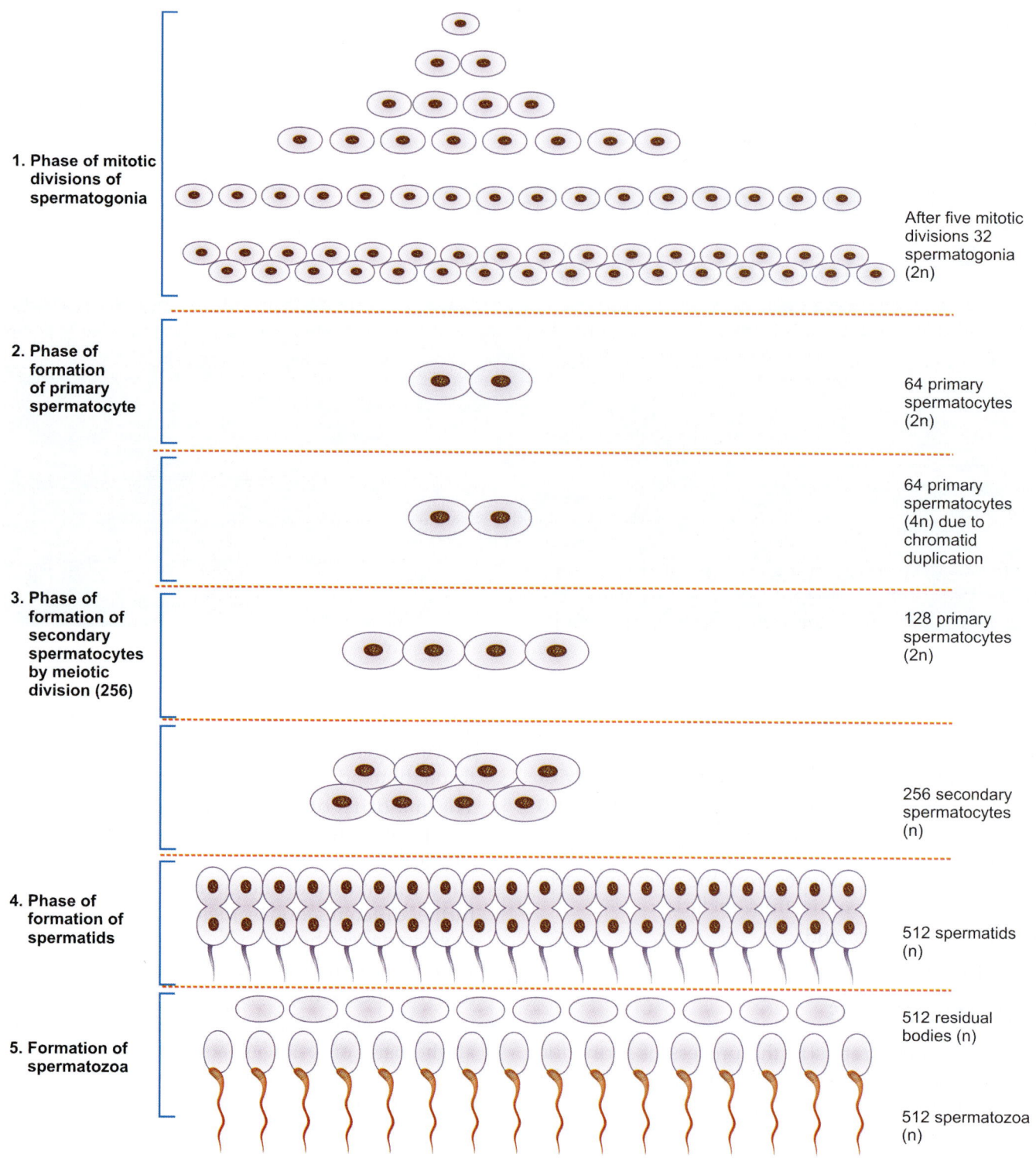

1. Phase of mitotic divisions of spermatogonia

After five mitotic divisions 32 spermatogonia (2n)

2. Phase of formation of primary spermatocyte

64 primary spermatocytes (2n)

64 primary spermatocytes (4n) due to chromatid duplication

3. Phase of formation of secondary spermatocytes by meiotic division (256)

128 primary spermatocytes (2n)

256 secondary spermatocytes (n)

4. Phase of formation of spermatids

512 spermatids (n)

5. Formation of spermatozoa

512 residual bodies (n)

512 spermatozoa (n)

Fig. 2.1: Phases of spermatogenesis.

1. *Phase of mitotic division of spermatogonia.* Spermatogonia or the primitive germ cells (44+XY) serve as a pool of undifferentiated stem cells from which develop the spermatozoa. These cells lie near the basal lamina of seminiferous tubules. Three main types of spermatogonia are described:

   - *Dark type-A (AD) spermatogonia* (also called type A1) represent a reserve of resting stem cells. They have dark staining oval nuclei. They divide to form more dark type-A cells and also some light type-A cells (or A2 cells).
   - *Light or pale type-A (AP) spermatogonia* have light staining oval nucleus. They divide to form more light type-A spermatogonia and also some spermatogonia of type-B.
   - *Type-B spermatogonia* have spherical nucleus. Each type of spermatogonium divides mitotically 5 times to form 32 type-B spermatogonia. The division occurs in the basal compartment of the seminiferous tubule. Due to incomplete cytokinesis, all cells derived from a single spermatogonium remain connected through cytoplasmic bridges and are synchronized in subsequent cell divisions. The connections remain throughout till the formation of individual spermatozoa.

2. *Phase of formation of primary spermatocytes by mitotic division.* The 32 type-B spermatogonia (44+X+Y) undergo mitosis to form 64 primary spermatocytes (44+X+Y). Primary spermatocytes are large cells with large nucleus having diploid number of chromosomes (2n).

3. *Phase of formation of secondary spermatocyte by meiotic division.* Each primary spermatocyte undergoes meiotic division:

   - In the prophase of meiotic division (when chromatids duplicate), each primary spermatocyte is represented as tetraploid number of chromosomes (4n). In this phase they remain for about 22 days.
   - After first reduction division (meiosis), the 64 tetraploid primary spermatocytes (4n) are converted into 128 primary spermatocytes with diploid number of chromosomes (2n).
   - The 128 primary spermatocytes (meiosis) to form 256 secondary spermatocytes having haploid number of chromosomes (n), i.e. either 22+X or 22+Y. Therefore, 50% of sperms will have X chromosome and other 50% will have Y-chromosome.
   - Size of secondary spermatocyte is quite small as compared to primary spermatocyte.

4. *Phase of formation of spermatid.* Each secondary spermatocyte divides mitotically to give rise to two spermatids. Thus, a total of 512 spermatids are formed from a single spermatogonium.

   - *Early spermatid* is a small round cell with spherical nucleus containing haploid number of chromosomes.
   - *Late spermatids* are formed when the early spermatids undergo changes in the shape and orientation of organelles.

5. *Phase of formation of spermatozoon (spermiogenesis)*

   - The spermatids do not divide further but undergo morphological changes to form sperms or spermatozoa. The spermatid undergoes changes in the shape and orientation of its organelles. The spermatids mature into spermatozoa in the deep folds of the cytoplasm of the Sertoli cells. During this process the components of spermatid which take part in forming spermatozoon are (Fig. 2.2):

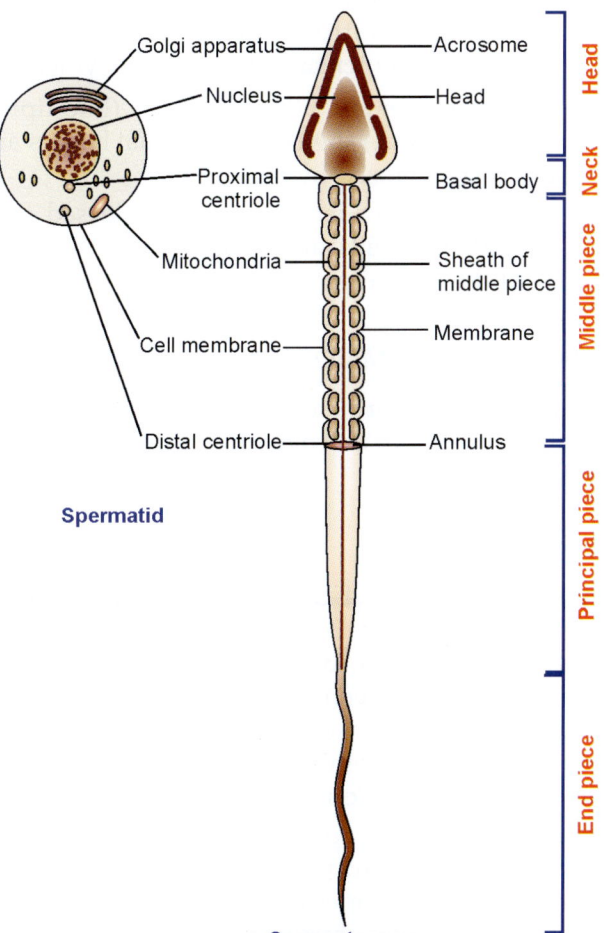

Fig. 2.2: Derivatives of different parts of spermatozoon from that of spermatid.

- Nucleus undergoes condensation and changes its shape to form head of the spermatozoon.
  - The nuclear proteins are replaced by protamine which surround the chromatins and thus protect them from mutagenic factors.
  - The centriole divides into two parts, the distal part forms the axial filament and the proximal part forms the basal body. In the beginning both the parts lie close to each other but later they migrate away. The region earlier occupied by the centriole later on forms the neck of a spermatozoon.
- *The Golgi apparatus* forms the cap-like structure covering anterior 2/3 of the head (acrosome). It contains proteolytic enzyme (hyaluronidase) and other proteases, which help the sperm in penetration of an ovum during fertilization.
- *Mitochondria* surround the tail part of the sperm lying wrapped in a sheath and provide energy for movements of the spermatozoon.
- *Cell membrane* of the spermatid persists as covering of the spermatozoon. The membranes of late spermatids and of sperms contain germinal angiotensin converting enzyme.
- *The cytoplasm and other organelles* (like lipids, ribosomes, etc.) shed off as residual bodies and are phagocytosed by Sertoli cells.
  - The mature spermatozoa are released from the Sertoli cells and become free in the lumen of the seminiferous tubules.

STRUCTURE OF SPERMATOZOON

A fully formed spermatozoon is an intricate motile cell about 55–65 µm in length. It comprises following parts (Fig. 2.3A).

Head

The head is about 4–5 µm long, flattened from anterior to posterior. It is oval when seen from the front, but appears to be pointed (somewhat like a spear-head) when seen from one side. It is mainly composed of condensed nucleus with a very thin cytoplasmic cell membrane layer around it. It is surrounded by acrosome.

Acrosome is a thick cap-like structure which covers the anterior two-third part of the head. It is formed mainly from lysosome-like organelle containing a number of enzymes (hyaluronidase, proteolytic enzymes and acid phosphatase) which help the sperm in penetrating ovum during fertilization.

Neck

It is a narrow constricted part. It contains a funnel-shaped basal body and a spherical centriole.

Basal body, it is also called *connecting piece*, because it helps to establish an intimate union between the head and remainder of the spermatozoon through its convex articular surface which fits into a depression called the *implantation* fossa present in the head.

The basal body is made up of nine segmented rod-like structures which become continuous with the axial filaments present in the tail.

Tail

Tail of the sperm is the motile portion and is also called the flagellum. It can be divided into three parts:
- Middle piece,
- Principal piece, and
- End piece.

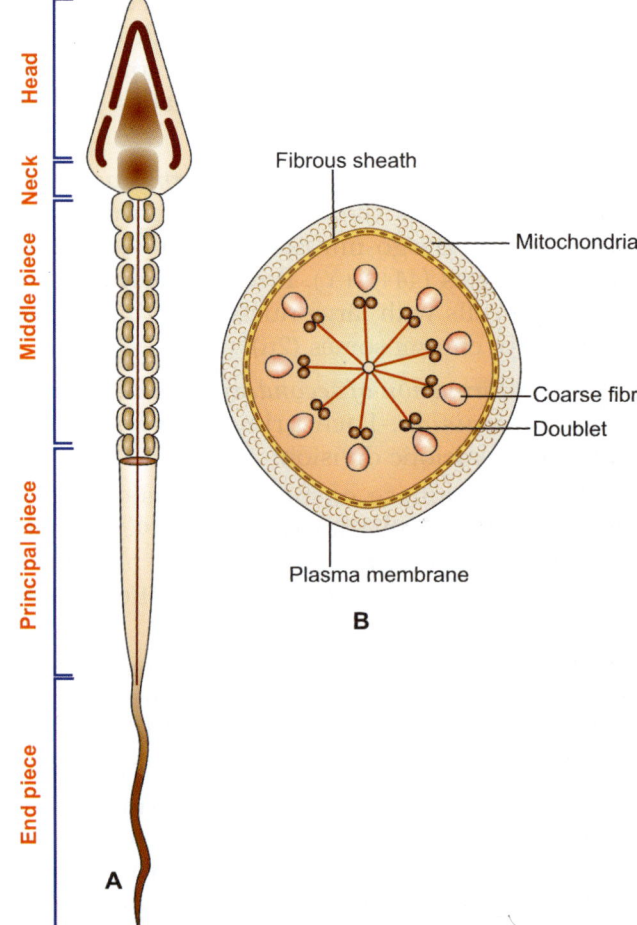

Fig. 2.3: Structure of mature human spermatozoon (A) and transverse section of the middle piece of tail part showing its detailed structure (B).

Structure

The tail of the sperm consists of following components:

Axoneme or *axial filament.* It forms the central skeleton of the tail. The axoneme begins just behind in the neck and extends through the entire length of tail. It is made up of nine pairs (doublets) of microtubules arranged in a circle, surrounding central pair (Fig. 2.3B). This structure is similar to that of a cilia. To and fro movements of the tail result due to rhythmic longitudinal sliding motion between the anterior and posterior tubules that make up axoneme.

Coarse fibrils. The nine petal-shaped coarse fibrils are present, one each just outside each doublet of microtubules (Fig. 2.3B). These coarse fibrils are present in the *middle piece* and principal piece, but do not extend into the end piece of tail.

Fibrous sheath is present outside the coarse fibrils.

Mitochondria. In the region of middle piece, i.e. proximal part of tail, the fibrous sheath is surrounded by spirally arranged mitochondria in abundance. The mitochondria synthesize ATP which supplies energy for the motility of tail.

Plasma membrane encloses the entire sperm.

STORAGE OF SPERMATOZOA

About 120 million sperms are formed each day. A small quantity of them is stored in the epididymis but most of them are stored in vas deferens and ampulla of vas deferens. They can remain stored maintaining their fertility for about a month.

MATURATION AND CAPACITATION OF SPERMATOZOA

Role of epididymis. The fully formed spermatozoa are released into the lumen of seminiferous tubules, from where they reach the epididymis after traversing the rete testis and efferent ducts of testes. Epididymis is the site of extra testicular maturation of spermatozoa. When the sperms arrive in the epididymis they are non-motile. They acquire some motility only after passing through the epididymis. The epididymal secretions required for this maturation are androgen dependent.

Role of seminal vesicles and prostate gland. The secretions of seminal vesicles and the prostate have a stimulating effect on sperm motility, but the spermatozoa become fully motile only after ejaculation.

Role of female genital tract. When introduced into the vagina, spermatozoa reach the uterine tubes much sooner than their own motility would allow,

suggesting that contraction of uterine and tubal musculature exert a sucking effect.

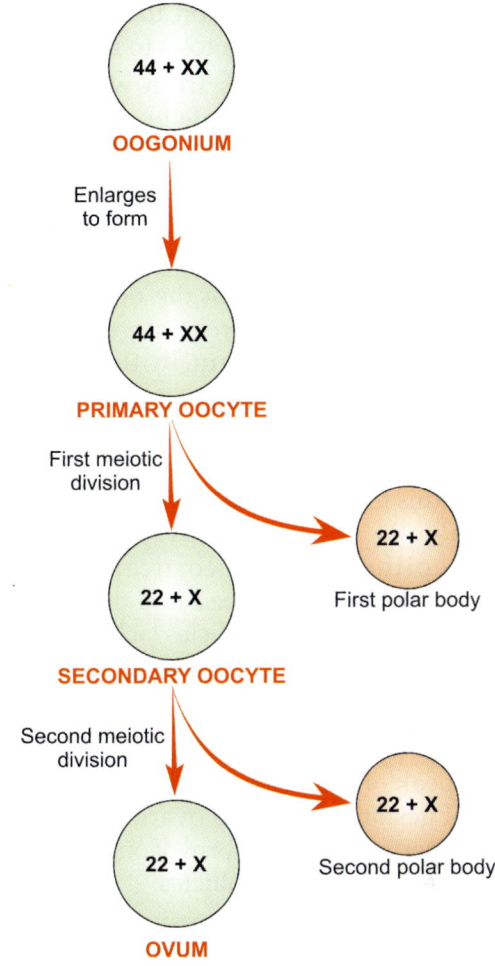

Fig. 2.4: Steps of oogenesis.

Spermatozoa acquire ability to fertilize the ovum only after they have been in the female genital tract for sometime (1 to 10 hours). This final step in their maturation is called capacitation.

OOGENESIS

Oogenesis refers to the process of formation of ova from the primitive germ cells (Fig. 2.4).

Phases of oogenesis include:
- Fetal oogenesis,
- Postnatal oogenesis,
- Prepubertal oogenesis, and
- Pubertal oogenesis.

1. Fetal oogenesis

Unlike the fetal testis (in which spermatogenesis begins at puberty), the fetal ovary begins oogenesis by 10 weeks of gestation.

Primitive germ cells. When the bipotential gonads differentiate into ovaries in genetic female (44 + XX) embryo (in the absence of testis determining factor, i.e. TDF) by 10th week of gestation, the primitive germ cells increase in number by mitosis to form oogonia.

Oogonia are the stem cells from which ova are derived. The oogonia proliferate by mitosis to form primary oocytes. The process begins at 15 weeks and reaches a peak between 20 and 28 weeks gestation.

The oogonium is unique in that it is the only female cell in which both X chromosomes are active.

Primary oocytes formed from the oogonia, enter a prolonged prophase (*diplotene stage*) of the first meiotic division and remain in this state until ovulation occurs after puberty.

Primordial follicles. The *diploid primary oocytes* become enveloped by single layer of flat granulosa cells and in this form are called *primordial follicles* (the granulosa cells are formed by proliferation of coelomic epithelium, i.e. cortical cells). Each primordial follicle is enveloped in a thin membrane called the *basal lamina.* The follicles lack a direct blood supply.

- The primordial follicle is fundamental in reproductive unit of the ovary.
- During peak of development (between 20 and 28. weeks of gestation) the two ovaries contain about 7 million germ cells in the form of oogonia, primary oocytes and primordial follicles.
- Many germ cells undergo atresia (involution) and at term only 2 million germ cells are present, most

of which have developed into primordial follicles, some are as oogonia and primary oocytes.

2. Postnatal and prepubertal oogenesis

- The number of primordial follicles present in the ovaries at birth, rapidly diminishes thereafter.
- By 6 months postpartum all of the oogonia have been converted into primary oocytes and primordial follicles.
- No new ova are formed after birth.
- By the onset of puberty (at about 12–13 years of age) the two ovaries contain about 3,00,000 primordial follicles.

3. Pubertal oogenesis

- After puberty the oogenesis or formation of ovum occurs in a highly cyclic fashion, once every 28 days till menopause.
- Every month, in each ovary, more than one primordial follicles start undergoing maturation process but only one reaches maturity and the rest undergo atresia at different stages of development (Fig. 2.5). Thus throughout the whole normal reproductive life of about 30 years (from 13 to 42 years) about 450 ova are expelled and the remainder degenerate.
- The different stages of maturation of primordial follicle into graafian follicle (*folliculogenesis*) are described in the ovarian cycle (see page 26).
- The primary oocytes which is in the prophase of first meiotic division since fetal life completes

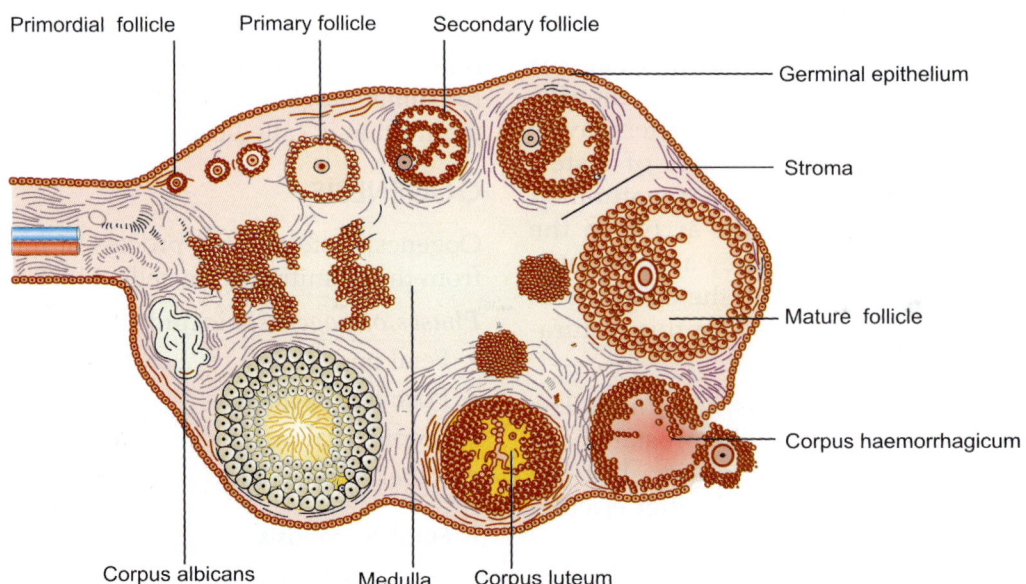

Fig. 2.5: Schematic histological section of adult ovary depicting various stages of development of follicles, ovulation, corpus haemorrhagicum and corpus luteum.

the first meiotic division just before ovulation. As a result *secondary oocyte* containing most of the cytoplasm and *first polar body* are formed. The first polar body soon fragments and disappears.

- The *secondary oocyte* (haploid cell) immediately begins the *second meiotic division* but this division stops at metaphase and is completed only if the mature ovum (ootid) is fertilized by a sperm. At that time the *second polar body (polocyte)* is extruded and the fertilized ovum proceeds to form a new individual. Fertilization normally occurs in the ampulla of fallopian tube.

Pubertal oogenesis versus spermatogenesis

From the above description of pubertal oogenesis and spermatogenesis (page 19), the following can be concluded:

- In contrast to the male who produces spermatogonia and primary spermatocytes continuously throughout life, the female cannot form oogonia beyond 28 weeks gestation and must function with a declining pool of oocytes.
- Meiosis in the female results in the formation of one viable oocyte. In contrast, each primary spermatogonium in the male ultimately gives rise to 64 spermatozoa.
- Oogenesis in the female begins in *utero* in response to *meiosis-stimulating factor,* whereas in the male, spermatogenesis is arrested at the spermatogonial stage in response to *meiosis-inhibiting factor.*

ABNORMALITIES IN FORMATION OF GAMETES

ABNORMALITIES OF FORM

Abnormalities of spermatozoa include:
- *Giant spermatozoa,* i.e. too large spermatozoa
- *Dwarf spermatozoa,* i.e. too small spermatozoa.
- *Spermatozoa with duplicated parts,* i.e. the head, body or tail of spermatozoa may be duplicated.

Abnormalities of ovum include:
- Ovum may have an unusually large nucleus or two nuclei.
- Two oocytes may be seen in one follicle.

FEMALE SEXUAL CYCLE

The study of female sexual cycle is essential to understand the *development during first week, i.e. ovulation to implantation.* The sexual life span of a female can be divided into three periods:

1. *Birth to puberty.* During this period primary and accessory female sex organs remain quiescent. Puberty occurs between 12 and 14 years of age.
2. *Puberty to menopause.* With the onset of puberty the female sexual cycle starts which repeats every 28 days. The occurrence of first menstrual cycle is called *menarche.* The permanent stoppage of menstrual cycle is called *menopause,* which occurs at the age of about 45 to 50 years. The period between menarche and menopause is called *reproductive period.* During this period females have rhythmical sexual cycles.
3. *Postmenopausal period* extends after menopause (45 to 50 years) to rest of the life. During this period the female sexual cycle ceases.

Female sexual cycle refers to monthly rhythmic sexual cycle occurring in females during the normal reproductive period.

Components of human female sexual cycle. During each female sexual cycle, rhythmical changes occur in ovaries and accessary sex organs—uterus, cervix and vagina. The components of female sexual cycle are:

- Ovarian cycle,
- Endometrial cycle,
- Changes in cervix uteri,
- Changes in vagina,
- Other changes during sexual cycle, and
- Changes in gonadotropin secretion, i.e. hormonal control of female sexual cycle.

Duration of female sexual cycle is usually 28 days. But under physiological conditions it may vary between 20 and 40 days. Traditionally first day of the menstrual bleeding is taken as the 1st day to each component of female sexual cycle.

OVARIAN CYCLE

Ovarian cycle refers to rhythmic changes occurring in ovaries during each female sexual cycle of about 28 days (range 20–40 days). During each cycle a single mature ovum is released from the ovary. Ovarian changes occurring during the female sexual life completely depend on the gonadotropic hormones (FSH and LH) which are secreted by the anterior pituitary. Both FSH and LH stimulate ovarian target cells by combining with highly specific FSH and LH receptors present on their membranes. FSH and LH activate cyclic adenosine monophosphate (cAMP)—second messenger system in the cell cytoplasm. However some effects of hormones cannot be attributed entirely to cAMP system. The ovarian cycle can be divided into three phases:

- Preovulatory phase or follicular phase,
- Ovulation, and
- Postovulatory phase or luteal phase.

A. PREOVULATORY PHASE

Preovulatory or follicular phase of the ovarian cycle extends from the 5th day of the cycle till the time of ovulation (which takes place at about 14th day of the cycle). Thus, this phase generally lasts for 8–9 days (but may vary from 10 to 25 days).

- Changes in the ovary during preovulatory phase or follicular phase are mostly under the influence of follicule stimulating hormone (FSH) from the anterior pituitary. Luteinizing hormone (LH) also helps in maturation of the follicle in the latter part of follicular phase (for details see hormonal control of female sexual cycle).
- During this phase of each cycle (of about 28 days), some 10–15 primordial follicles start maturing, but only one follicle matures fully and the rest undergo atresia (atrophy) at different stages of development. The process of maturation of follicle is called folliculogenesis.

Phases of folliculogenesis

The follicles at different stages of maturation are (Figs 2.5 and 2.6):

1. *Primordial follicles* are the fundamental reproductive units of ovary. At the time of puberty both ovaries contain about 3,00,000 primordial follicles.
   - Primordial follicles are formed in fetal life. Each primordial follicle consists of the primary oocyte in prophase of the first meiotic division surrounded by a single layer of spindle-shaped (flat) cells called the granulosa cells.
   - Both the granulosa cells and the primary oocyte are enveloped in a thin membrane called basal lamina (Fig. 2.6A).
   - The primordial follicles lack a direct blood supply.
   - The granulosa cells of the primordial follicle are believed to provide nutrition to the ovum (primary oocyte) throughout the childhood (from birth to puberty). These cells also secrete *oocyte maturation inhibiting factor* (OMIF) which keeps the ovum in immature stage till puberty. At the onset of puberty, under the influence of FSH and LH, the primordial follicles start growing and convert into primary follicles.

2. *Primary follicle.* The primary follicle is formed when the primordial follicle undergoes following developmental changes (Fig. 2.6B):
   - *Granulosa cells*, which are flat (spindle-shaped) in primordial follicle become columnar and undergo mitotic division to form a multilayered stratum granulosum.
   - *Oocyte enlarges* and becomes about 20 µm in size.
   - *Zona pellucida*, a homogeneous membrane appears consisting of glycoprotein between the granulosa (follicular) cells and the oocyte. With the appearance of zona pellucida the follicle is now referred to as a multilaminar primary follicle.

3. *Secondary follicle* is formed from the primary follicle when following changes occur (Fig. 2.6C):
   - *Granulosa cells* undergo further proliferation.
   - *Oocyte* further increases in size upto 100 µm. Its nucleus becomes larger and vesicular, forming germinal spots.

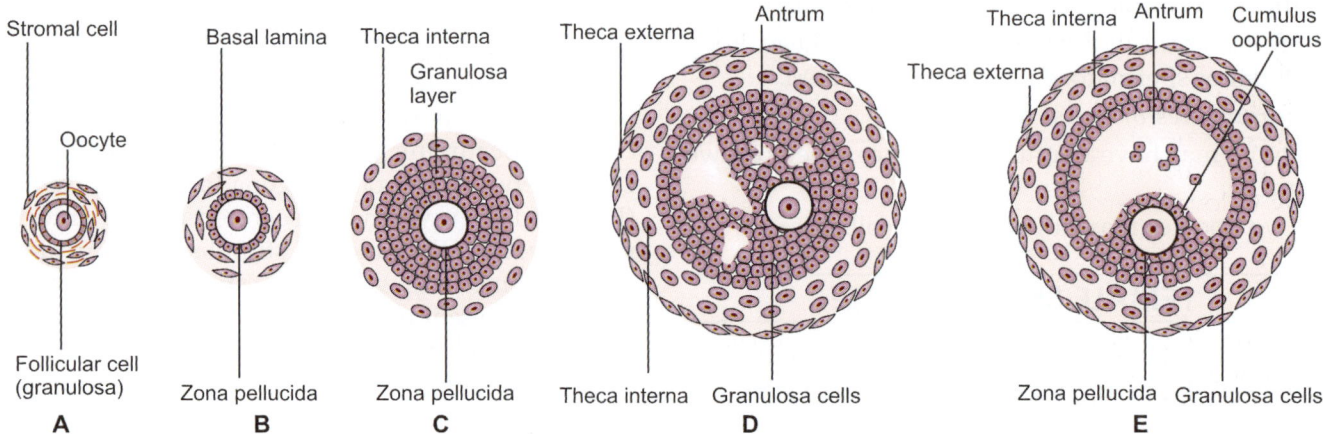

Fig. 2.6: Phases of folliculogenesis.

- *Theca folliculi* or follicular sheath is formed outside the basal lamina from the spindle-shaped cells from the stroma of cortex in ovary. The theca folliculi consist of an inner rim of secretory cells called *theca interna* and an outer rim of thickly packed fibres and spindle-shaped cells called *theca externa* (that merges with the surrounding stroma).
- *Independent blood supply* consisting of arterioles that do not penetrate the basal lamina is acquired by the secondary follicles.

4. *Tertiary follicle* is characterized by following features:

- *Formation of antrum.* After proliferation, the granulosa cells start secreting follicular fluid, this causes cavity to be formed in the stratum granulosum (cavitation), which is called antrum or follicular cavity. The fluid filled in the antrum is called liquor folliculi which also contains oestrogen. The granulosa cells continue to proliferate and the size of follicle is increased (Fig. 2.6D).
- *Changes in theca folliculi.* The theca cells proliferate more rapidly. The theca interna is transformed into theca interstitial cells which will become steroidogenic cells which synthesize and secrete androgens (androstenedione) in response to gonadotropins (FSH and LH).
- *Blood vessels* of the follicle do not penetrate the zona pellucida and thus the oocyte and the granulosa remain avascular.
- Upto this stage follicular growth is mainly stimulated by FSH alone.

5. *Graafian (antral) follicle.* After about 7th day of sexual cycle one of the tertiary follicle increases in size in response to gonadotropins (both FSH and LH) and forms the mature follicle called graafian or antral or vesicular follicle (Fig. 2.6E). It is uncertain how one follicle is selected to become the mature graafian follicle in this follicular phase of the cycle, but it seems to be related to the ability of the follicle to secrete the oestrogen inside it that is needed for final maturation. Rest of the follicles degenerate and become atrophied by apoptosis. A fully matured graafian follicle is characterized by following features:

- *Size* of the follicle increases markedly to about 2 to 5 mm. The growth of the graafian follicle is accomplished by granulosa and theca proliferation. It extends through the whole thickness of cortex of ovary. At one place, it encroaches upon the tunica albuginea and bulges out of the surface of the ovary into the peritoneal cavity.

- *Antrum becomes larger* and distended with fluid. With the enlargement of follicles, the follicular fluid collects in such a large amount that it surrounds the ovum all around except at one point. As a result the ovum covered by a layer of cells called *corona radiata* remains in contact with granulosa cells only at a hill like area called *cumulus oophorus*.
- *Theca interna becomes more prominent.* The thickness of theca interna becomes double with rich network of capillaries. The oestrogen secreting cells of theca interna increase and are called the cells of theca glands.
- *Formation of secondary oocyte.* Just prior to ovulation, the primary oocyte of the fully matured graafian follicle completes the first meiotic division (which began in fetal life at about 20th, 28th week of gestation, i.e. before birth), and forms the secondary oocyte with a haploid nucleus and the first polar body.

B. OVULATION

Ovulation refers to release of secondary oocyte from the ovary (following rupture of graafian follicle) into the peritoneal cavity. It usually occurs *14 days after the onset* of menstruation, i.e. *early on day 15* in a normal 28 days cycle (Fig. 2.7).

Process of ovulation involves following sequence of events (Fig. 2.7A):

- *LH surge and ovulatory peak of FSH.* The ovulation is caused by a LH surge at midcycle in response to an elevation in plasma oestradiol concentration (150 picograms per ml).
- *Onset of LH surge* (a relatively precise indicator of ovulation) occurs 34 to 36 hours before ovulation.
- *Peak of the LH surge* occurs 12 to 24 hours before ovulation (secretion of LH increases 6–10 fold).
- *Immediately before the LH peak*, oestradiol levels in the plasma fall.
- *Ovulatory peak of FSH* (2–3 fold increase in secretion) occurring 2 days prior to ovulation is thought to be stimulated by progesterone. FSH increases the granulosa cell LH receptors.

Changes in graafian follicle. The LH and FSH produce following changes in graafian follicle before ovulation (Fig. 2.7B):

- *Rapid swelling of the follicle* is caused by FSH and LH a few days before ovulation. There occurs a rapid growth of new blood vessels into the follicle wall and prostaglandins are secreted into the follicular tissue. Both these cause diffusion of

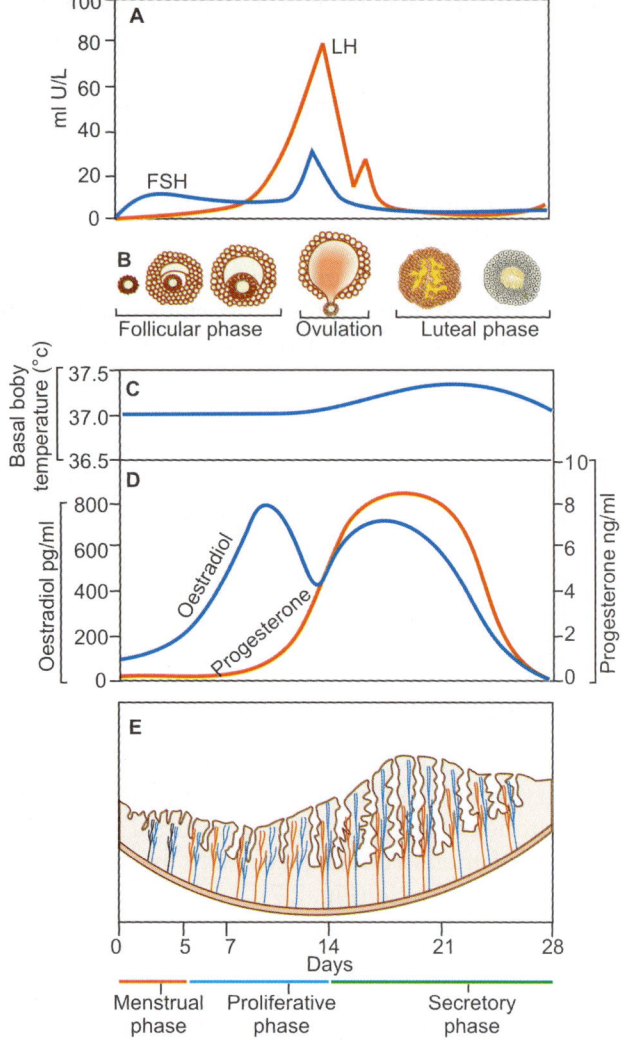

Fig. 2.7: Correlation of plasma concentration of gonadotropins (FSH and LH) (A), ovarian cycle changes (B), basal body temperature (C), ovarian hormones (D), and endometrial changes (E), during female sexual cycle.

plasma into the follicular fluid and further swelling of the follicle.

- *Formation of stigma.* Due to rapid swelling of the follicle, its outer wall is stretched forming a very thin avascular area (stigma) over the most convex point of the follicle which protrudes like a nipple in the peritoneal cavity.

- *Release of proteolytic* enzymes from the lysosomes in the theca externa cells is activated by the progesterone.

- *Dissolution of capsular* wall and its further weakening is caused by the proteolytic enzymes.

- *Rupture of graafian follicle.* The simultaneous stretching and enzymatic dissolution of the follicular wall leads to degeneration of *the stigma.* Within 30 minutes of protrusion, fluid begins to ooze from the stigma followed soon by rupture of

follicle with release of ovum (secondary oocyte) surrounded by corona radiata into the peritoneal cavity near the fimbriated end of fallopian tube. Thus, usually only one ovum is released from any one of two ovaries during each sexual cycle. The released ovum enters the fallopian tube through its fimbriated end.

Determination of ovulation time

Ovulation usually occurs 14 days after the onset of menstruation, i.e. early on day 15 in a normal 28-day cycle. The ovulation time can be determined by following indirect methods:

1. *From basal body temperature.* The basal body temperature falls slightly (0.3 to 0.5°C) just prior to ovulation and increases slightly after ovulation. Therefore, the time of ovulation can be determined by measuring the morning temperature from rectum or vagina for few days during mid period of menstrual cycle (Fig. 2.7C).

2. *From hormonal excretion in urine.* The urinary excretion of end products of oestrogen like oestrone, oestradiol and 17 β-oestradiol increases to the peak at the time of ovulation and that of end products of progesterone-like pregnanediol increases after ovulation. Therefore, time of ovulation can be determined by estimating their urinary levels for few days during mid period of menstrual cycle.

3. *From hormonal levels in plasma.* The plasma content of FSH, LH, oestrogen and progesterone is measured during mid period of menstrual cycle and time of ovulation is determined from following observations (Fig. 2.7D):
   - LH and oestrogen levels are increased and FSH level is decreased at the time of ovulation.
   - Progesterone level is increased after ovulation.

4. *By ultrasound scanning* the process of ovulation can be recorded.

Anovulatory Cycles

The ovarian cycles during which ovulation does not occur are called unovulatory cycles. If LH surge occurring prior to ovulation is not of sufficient magnitude, ovulation does not occur. First few cycles after puberty may be unovulatory.

C. POSTOVULATORY PHASE

Postovulatory phase also called luteal phase of ovarian cycle is of remarkably constant period of about 14 days. Therefore, retrospectively the time of ovulation can be estimated by subtracting 14 days from the total duration of the menstrual cycle. This phase is characterized by following events (Fig. 2.5):

Formation of corpus haemorrhagicum. Following ovulation, the outer wall of the graafian follicle collapses and promptly fills with blood forming the so-called corpus haemorrhagicum. Minor bleeding from the follicle into the abdominal cavity may cause peritoneal irritation and fleeting lower abdominal pain (mittelschmerz).

Formation of corpus luteum. Soon, the granulosa cells and theca cells of the follicle lining begin to proliferate, and the clotted blood is rapidly replaced with yellowish lipid-rich *luteal cells*. This process is called *luteinization* and the total mass of the cells is now called *corpus luteum*. LH is responsible for luteinization. The lutein cells secrete large amount of progesterone and also oestrogen to a lesser extent. Seven days after ovulation, i.e. by 22nd day of menstrual cycle the corpus luteum attains a diameter of about 1.5 cm. The progesterone secreted by these have a strong negative feedback effect on the anterior pituitary gland to decrease secretion of both LH and FSH. The fate of corpus luteum depends on whether or not pregnancy occurs.

Formation of corpus albicans. If there is no fertilization and pregnancy does not occur, the corpus luteum begins to involute (regress) after 24th day of the sexual cycle and is eventually replaced by a whitish scar tissue, called the corpus albicans. This involution occurs due to falling levels of FSH and LH and also the hormone *inhibin* secreted by the lutein cells. With the involution of corpus luteum, on 26th day of the normal female sexual cycle, levels of oestrogen, progesterone and inhibin fall. This removes feedback inhibition of the anterior pituitary consequently the FSH and within a few days LH secretion begins and the next ovarian cycle is initiated.

Corpus luteum of pregnancy. However, if the ovum released is fertilized and pregnancy occurs, then the corpus luteum formed during postovulatory phase persists and serves as the major source of oestrogen and progesterone till the 3rd month of pregnancy when the placenta takes over its endocrine function.

ENDOMETRIAL CYCLE

Endometrial cycle refers to the cyclic changes occurring in the endometrium during active reproductive period (menarche to menopause) in females leading to recurrent monthly bleeding per vaginum (menstruation). These cyclic changes in the endometrium are brought about by the cyclic production of oestrogens and progesterone by the ovaries. Strictly speaking the menstrual cycle is synonymous with female sexual cycle and includes cyclic changes in all the female reproductive organs. However, in day-to-day practice the term menstrual cycle is used for cyclic changes in the endometrium. Menstrual is a Latin word meaning mensis, i.e. lunar month of 28 days. Though the menstrual cycle for description purposes is considered to be of 28 days, but the cycle is by no means as regular as the name suggests. The menstrual cycles of 25 to 35 days are also regarded as normal cycles.

PHASES OF ENDOMETRIAL CYCLE

Conventionally, 1st day of the bleeding is considered to be the first day of endometrial cycle. The endometrial cycle of 28 days can be divided into three phases (Fig. 2.7E):

- Menstrual phase (1st to 5th day),
- Proliferative phase (6th to 14th day), and
- Secretory phase (15th to 28th day)

For the purpose of better understanding the menstrual phase is described last of all.

Proliferative phase

Extent of proliferative phase, also known as pre-ovulatory phase of endometrial cycle is from day 6th to 14th day. It follows the phase of menstruation, after which only a thin basal layer of original endometrium is left.

Hormone responsible for changes in the endometrium during this phase is oestrogen secreted by the developing graafian follicle in the ovary. Thus, proliferative phase of endometrial cycle coincides with the follicular phase of ovarian cycle (Fig. 2.7D).

Changes in endometrium, which occur under the influence of oestrogens during proliferative phase are (Fig. 2.7E):

1. Epithelial cells are stimulated to grow and re-epithelialise the endometrial surface.

2. Thickness of endometrium, which is less than 1 mm at the end of menstrual phase increases to 3–4 mm at the end of the proliferative phase.

3. Mitosis of the stratum basale regenerates the stroma of stratum functionale.

4. Angiogenesis in the stratum functionale leads to proliferation of blood vessels which become the spiral arterioles that profuse the stratum func-tionale.

5. Endometrial glands are stimulated to grow. The glands contain glycogen but they are nonsecretory.

6. Ovulation occurs at the end of this phase.

Secretory phase

Extent of secretory phase (also known as post-ovulatory phase of endometrial cycle) is from day 15th to 28th day.

Hormones responsible for changes in the endometrium during this phase are both oestrogens and progesterone secreted by the *corpus luteum* formed after ovulation. Thus, the secretory phase of endometrial cycle coincides with the luteal phase of ovarian cycle (Fig. 2.7D).

Changes in the endometrium, which occur under the influence of oestrogen and progesterone during this phase are:

- *Additional proliferation of cellular stroma* is caused by oestrogens.
- *Differentiation of the endometrium* is promoted by progesterone causing elongation and coiling of endometrial mucous glands. These glands become secretory and secrete thick viscous fluid containing glycogen.
- *Blood supply* of endometrium further increases as progesterone promotes spiralling of blood vessels.
- *Two characteristic features of endometrium* in secretory phase thus are prominent corkscrew-shaped glands and increased vascularity.
- *Thickness* of endometrium increases to 5–6 mm at the end of secretory phase. Thus the thickened endometrium with large amounts of nutrients is ready to provide appropriate conditions for implantation of ovum during this phase.
- *If fertilization does not occur* and there is no pregnancy, the corpus luteum in the ovary involutes to form corpus albicans and on day 26th of the menstrual cycle the levels of oestrogen and progesterone fall suddenly and mark the end of secretory phase of endometrial cycle.

Menstrual phase

The menstrual phase of endometrial cycle is also called bleeding phase. The average duration of this phase is 3–5 days, but it may be as short as 1 day and as long as 8 days in a normal woman.

Cause of bleeding and sequence of events. About 24 hours before the end of menstrual cycle, there is sharp decline in the plasma levels of oestrogen and progesterone, which is responsible for menstrual bleeding. The sequence of events is:

- *Intense spasm of spiral arteries* occurs leading to hypoxia and ischaemia. This effect is mediated via local production of *leukotrienes* and *prostaglandins*.
- *Necrosis of stratum functionale of the endometrium* and of the walls of the spiral arteries occurs as a result of ischaemia.
- *Blood vessels get open up* due to necrosis of their wall resulting in seepage of blood into the surrounding endometrial necrotic tissue.
- *Separation of necrotic tissue* starts gradually from the underlying basal viable tissue and ultimately it is sloughed off. The necrosis and sloughing does not occur simultaneously in whole of the uterus rather it occurs in patches and is completed in 3–5 days.
- *Endometrial debris* contains necrosed sloughed off tissue, blood, serous fluid and large amount of prostaglandins and fibrolysins.
- *Average amount of blood loss during each* menstrual cycle is 30 ml. Normally, it may vary from slight spotting to about 80 ml, and is affected by factors like endometrial thickness and the conditions which affect clotting mechanism.
- *Menstrual blood immediately gets clotted inside the uterine cavity but soon gets liquefied* by fibrolysins present in endometrial debris. This is the reason that menstrual blood does not normally contain blood clots unless the flow is excessive.
- *The prostaglandins* of the endometrial debris cause further spasm of spiral arteries and also produces contractions of myometrium.
- During menstrual phase about 2/3rd of the superficial endometrium is sloughed off and only a thin basal layer (2 mm thick) is left behind.

Pre-embryo Phase of Development (First to Third Week)

INTRODUCTION

As mentioned earlier, the development of a new individual involves three phases:

- Pre-embryo phase or germinal phase (day 0–week 3),
- Embryo phase (Weeks 4–8), and
- Fetal phase (weeks 8–38).

Pre-embryo phase of development (days 0–21) forms the content of this chapter. This phase of development can be further divided into following stages:

- Ovulation (all ready described on page 27).
- Fertilization and implantation (days 0–7).

- Stage of bilaminar germ disc (second week of development), and
- Stage of trilaminar germ disc (third week of development).

Note. While describing embryology, a day-to-day, week-to-week and month-to-month account is given of the major events. However, it must be realized that embryos of the same fertilization age do not necessarily develop at the same rate. Indeed, considerable differences in the rate of growth have been reported at every stage of development. Therefore, the time frame in chronology of embryological events is just for conceptualization only.

FERTILIZATION AND IMPLANTATION

FERTILIZATION

Fertilization refers to fusion of male and female gametes (i.e. spermatozoon and ovum). It takes place in the middle segment (ampulla) of the fallopian tube. It involves following events:

Transport of gametes

Before fertilization, the ovum and sperms reach the ampulla for fertilization.

Transport of ovum. At the time of ovulation the ovum is directly expelled into the peritoneal cavity and then enters into the fallopian tube.

Mechanism: The fimbriae of the fallopian tube are internally lined by ciliated epithelium. When ovulation occurs, the fimbriae of infundibulum encircle the surface of ovary, rub it, and pick up the ovum and then direct it towards the ostium by continuous beating of cilia. The contractions of smooth muscle fibres present in the wall of fallopian tube also help in transport of the ovum. These contractions are increased at the time of ovulation under the influence of oestrogen.

Structure of ovum. The released mature ovum (Fig. 3.1) consists of oocyte (containing 23 unpaired chromosomes) surrounded by the inner membranous layer called zona pellucida consisting of glyco-proteins and on its outer side surrounded by corona radiata consisting of granulosa cells arranged in multilayers. These cells are held together by matrix composed of hyaluronic acid.

Fate of ovum. The ovum is held up at ampulla isthmic junction for 2–3 days. It remains viable for 6–24 hours after ovulation. During this period if viable sperm

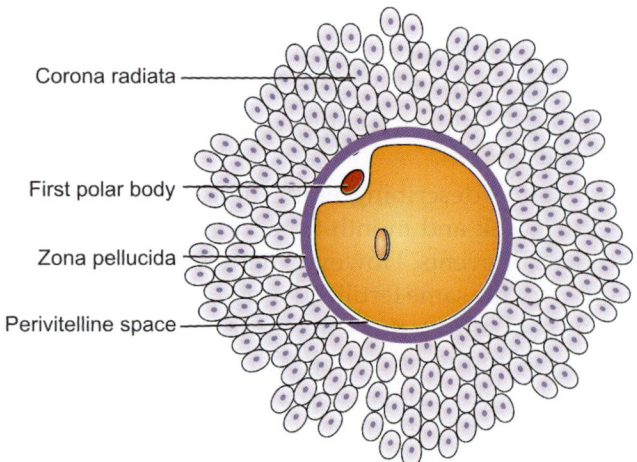

Fig. 3.1: Structure of a mature ovum at the time of ovulation.

Corona radiata

First polar body

Zona pellucida

Perivitelline space

penetrates it then fertilization takes place and leading on to pregnancy. On the other hand, if fertilization does not occur, the ovum dies out and degenerates.

Transport of sperms in the female genital tract. After ejaculation, several million sperms (average—200 million sperms per ejaculation) get deposited in the vagina. Out of these about 50–100 sperms manage to reach on to ovum and only one is able to penetrate it. This is because of several factors that affect the transportation and accessibility of the sperm to ovum.

Motility of sperms. After ejaculation normal sperm shows flagellar movements in the fluid medium at a rate of 1–4 mm/min. Therefore, in 30–60 minutes, they are able to reach the fallopian tube. The motility of sperms in turn depends on:

- pH of the fluid medium,
- Cervical mucus secretions,
- Fluid currents,
- Temperature, and
- Hormones.

i. *pH of medium.* Neutral and alkaline pH enhances the activity of sperms, but it is greatly depressed in even mild acidic medium. The vaginal fluid is acidic, hence immediately sperm activity is inhibited and sperms become non-motile. The alkaline semen (pH 7.5) neutralizes the vaginal acidic fluid. Therefore, in less than 60 min after ejaculation sperms again become active and their activity increases in cervix and in the body of uterus for next 25–40 hours.

ii. *Cervical secretion.* The cervical secretion acts as a mechanical barrier for sperms. The nature of cervical secretion depends upon the hormonal concentrations in the plasma. During proliferative phase of menstrual cycle and at the time of ovulation (under the influence of high level of oestrogen) cervical secretion becomes thin and watery, which favours the passage of the sperms. The morphologically abnormal sperms cannot pass through cervical mucus barrier and get entrapped within the fluid.

iii. *Fluid currents.* The vaginal and uterine cavity represent a vast sea in which currents are set up by ciliary movements towards exterior (antagonistic direction), which further resists sperm motility.

iv. *Temperature.* With rising temperature the activity of sperms increases but their life span is shortened. In ejaculated semen the maximum life span of sperm is 24–48 hours at body temperature. At lower temperature, however, semen can be stored for several weeks and at –100°C sperms can be preserved for many years.

v. *Hormones.* Local release of hormones as well as high concentration of certain hormones in the blood affect sperm transport. These include:

- *Oxytocin.* During coitus, stimulation of female genitalia leads to reflex release of oxytocin from the neurohypophysis; oxytocin causes propulsive movements of uterus, which help to aspirate seminal fluid from vagina into the fallopian tube.
- *Oestrogen.* It makes the cervical secretion thin and watery thus favours transport of sperms.
- *Prostaglandins.* Prostaglandins present in the semen (contributed by seminal vesicle fluid) also increase female genital tract movements.
- *Progesterone.* After ovulation, progesterone present in the follicular fluid is released which further stimulates sperm motility.

Sperm capacitation

Sperm capacitation refers to the process that makes a sperm to fertilize an ovum. Immediately after ejaculation in female genital tract the sperm undergoes certain changes, which enable it to fertilize an ovum. It takes about 1–10 hours (capacitation period). Sperm capacitation occurs due to removal of certain factors, which normally remain quiescent in male genital tract. These are:

- *Cholesterol contents of acrosomal membrane.* In the male genital tract the acrosomal membrane remains very tough because of high cholesterol contents. Whereas in the female genital tract the cholesterol contents of acrosomal membrane decrease and it becomes weak leading to easy release of enzymes from the head.
- *Calcium ions.* The membrane of sperm becomes permeable to calcium ions. The influx of Ca^{2+} acts by two ways: it makes the flagellar movements of the sperms more strong and whipish (hyper-activation of sperms) and secondly it triggers the release of enzymes from the acrosome.

Fusion of gametes

The fusion of ovum and sperm involves the following steps:

i. Chemoattraction. Chemoattraction of the sperms to ovum occurs by substances produced by the ovum.

ii. Penetration of sperm through ovum coverings. The sperm passes through two layers (corona radiata and zona pellucida) before it reaches the oocyte.

Penetration of corona radiata (Fig. 3.2A). It is made possible by release of enzyme hyaluronidase and other proteolytic enzymes present on the acrosome of the sperm and hyperactivation of the sperm.

- The hyaluronidase polymerizes the hyaluronic acid present in the intercellular matrix holding granulosa cells, and
- The proteolytic enzymes digest away the proteins of the structural tissues.

Hyperactivation of sperms (increased flagellar movements) produces penetrating thrust on the ovum due to vigorous lashing of sperm's tail.

Binding of sperm to zona pellucida. After passing through multilayered granulosa cells (corona radiata) many sperms make contact with zona pellucida by binding to receptor protein called *zona pellucida glycoprotein* (ZP_3) (Fig. 3.2B). The binding of sperm to ZP_3 triggers acrosomal reaction.

Acrosomal reaction (Fig. 3.2C). It involves release of acrosin (protease enzyme) from anterior membrane of acrosome of the sperm. Acrosin opens the penetrating pathway for passage of sperm head into the perivitelline space (space between zona pellucida and oocyte membrane). For effective penetration by the sperm the acrosomal reaction should take place at the zona pellucida because the life span of acrosomal reacted sperm is very short. If it takes place outside zona pellucida, the sperm cannot pass through this membrane.

The acrosomal reaction is also important for actual fusion of sperm cell with oocyte membrane.

iii. Fusion of sperm with oocyte (Fig. 3.2D). The equatorial region of acrosome is considered to be the site of initial contact between sperm and oocyte membrane (vitelline membrane). *Fertilin* is a protein present on acrosomal reacted sperm which interacts with the protein present on vitelline membrane and within 30 minutes the membranes of sperm and oocyte fuse, and genetic material of sperm enters into the oocyte and cause fertilization and embryo begins to develop.

Only one sperm can enter into the oocyte, and further entry of sperms is prevented by the activation of ovum.

iv. Ovum activation. Fusion of membranes of the gametes leads to ovum activation, which involves following events:

- *The membrane potential of the ovum decreases* (depolarization), which is followed by some structural changes in the zona pellucida.
- *Release of calcium* from intracellular egg reserve leads to exocytosis of the cortical granules (situated near the oocyte membrane) into the perivitelline space (Fig. 3.2E).
- *Vitelline block to polyspermy.* The spread of cortical granules along the perivitelline membrane

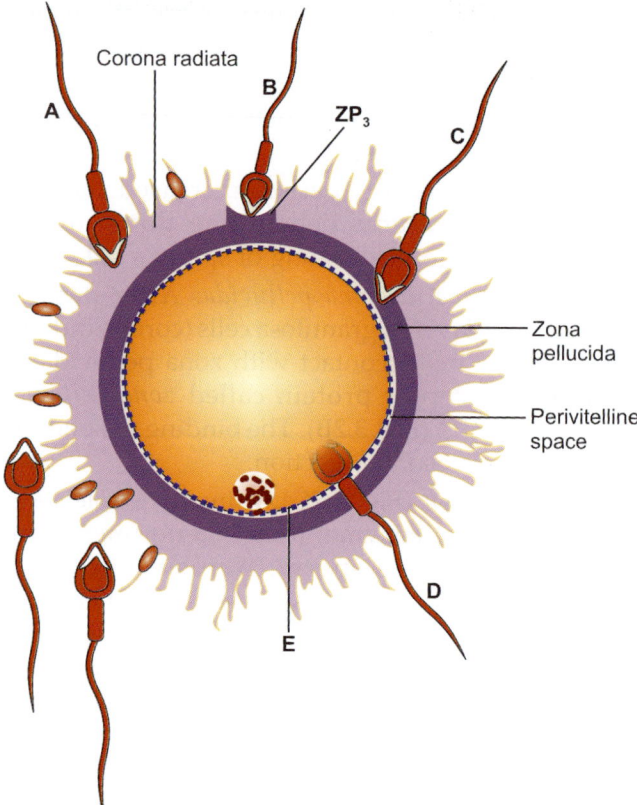

Corona radiata

A B ZP₃ C

Zona pellucida

Perivitelline space

D

E

Fig. 3.2: Sequential events of fertilization of an ovum by the sperm: A, penetration of corona radiata; B, binding of sperm to zona pellucida; C, acrosomal reaction; D fusion of sperm with oocyte; and E, discharge of cortical granules into perivitelline space producing vitelline block to polyspermy.

prevents further entry of sperm into the ovum. This is called vitelline block to polyspermy.

• *Zona blockade to polyspermy.* The cortical granules contain certain substances like glycosidases and proteases. Glycosidases cause alterations in the ZP_3 receptor protein of the zona pellucida and proteases degrade the ZP_3. Both of these mechanisms cause loss of affinity of sperm for zona pellucida and thus prevent polyspermy. This is called zona block to polyspermy.

FIRST WEEK OF DEVELOPMENT

First week of development begins immediately after fertilization. Changes seen during this week include:

• Cleavage of zygote
• Formation of morula, transportation to uterine cavity and conversion into blastocyst, and
• Implantation of blastocyst.

Cleavage of zygote (0 to 3 days)

The fertilized and activated ovum (zygote) is much larger (140 μm) than an average cell and starts dividing immediately. The process of repeated mitotic division of the zygote within the zona pellucida, resulting in rapid increase in the number of cells, is called *cleavage*. The cells formed are called *blastomeres.* In humans and other mammals, due to scanty deutoplasm there occurs *holoblastic or total cleavage* in which whole ovum is involved in cleavage.

Site and duration of cleavage. The cleavage occurs in the *uterine tube* (Fig. 3.3) upto 3 days after fertilization.

Stages of cleavage are as follows (Figs 3.3 and 3.4):

• *Two cells-stage.* The first cleavage division gives rise to two cells of unequal size after about 30 hours of fertilization (Fig. 3.4A).
• *Three cells-stage.* The larger cell divides to form the three cells-stage.
• *Four cells-stage.* Then the smaller cell also divides into two. In this way 2 large and 2 small cells are formed after about 40–50 hours of fertilization (Fig. 3.4B).
• *Eight cells-stage* is reached after further cleavage.
• *Twelve cells-stage* is reached after about 72 hour of fertilization.

Formation of morula, transportation in uterine cavity, and its conversion into blastocyst

Morula. At about sixteen cells-stage, the blastomeres tightly align themselves against each other to form a compact ball of cells called morula (mulberry) (Fig. 3.4C). The process of compaction leads to segregation of inner cells (which form inner cell mass) from the surrounding cells (which form the *external cell mass*).

Transportation of morula into the uterine cavity then occurs (Fig. 3.3). The transportation is assisted by the fluid currents and ciliary movements of epithelial cells of the fallopian tube and uterus.

Formation of blastocyst. In the cavity of uterus, the fluid from the lumen of uterus (uterine milk) seaps through the zona pellucida and outer-cell-mass of the morula. With continued accumulation of fluid the morula is converted into a cyst structure called blastocyst. The blastocyst, thus consists of (Fig. 3.4D):

• *Zona pellucida* is the outer covering,
• *Embryoblast,* is a group of clustered blastomeres, formed from inner-cell mass of the morula (Fig. 3.4E). It is attached to one pole of the blastocyst and later give rise to tissues of the embryo proper and some extraembryonic tissues, and
• *Trophoblast* is a thin outer layer of cells formed from the outer-cell-mass of the morula. The trophoblast covering the embryonic pole of the blastocyst is

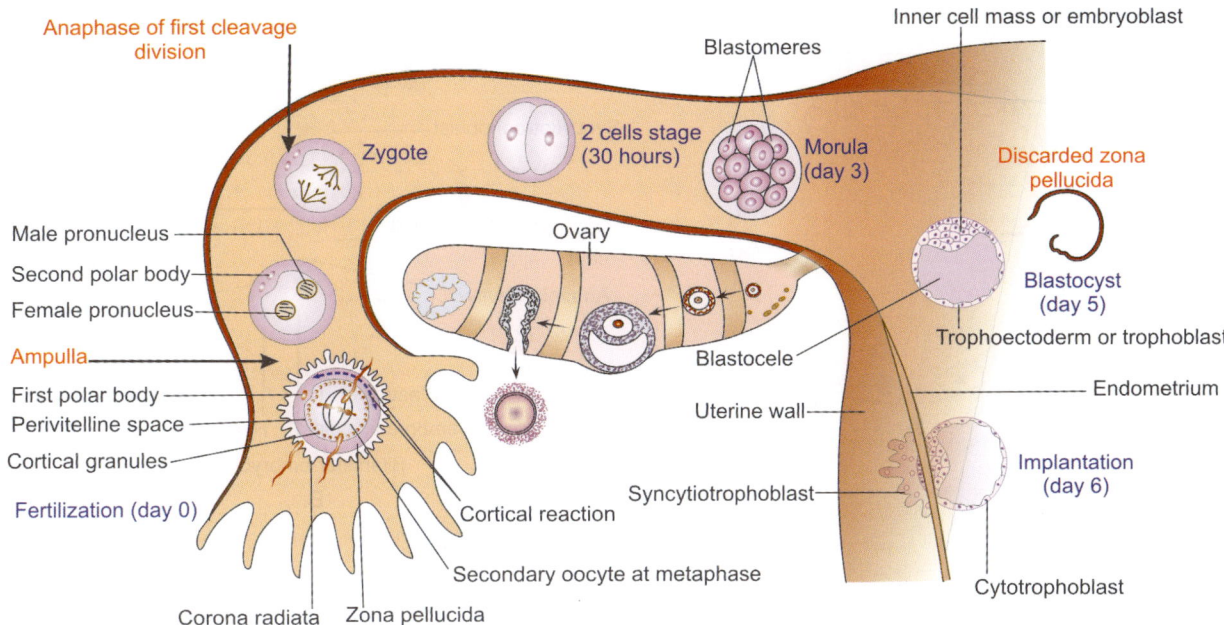

Fig. 3.3: Events during first week of development: Ovulation, fertilization, formation and implantation of the blastocyst.

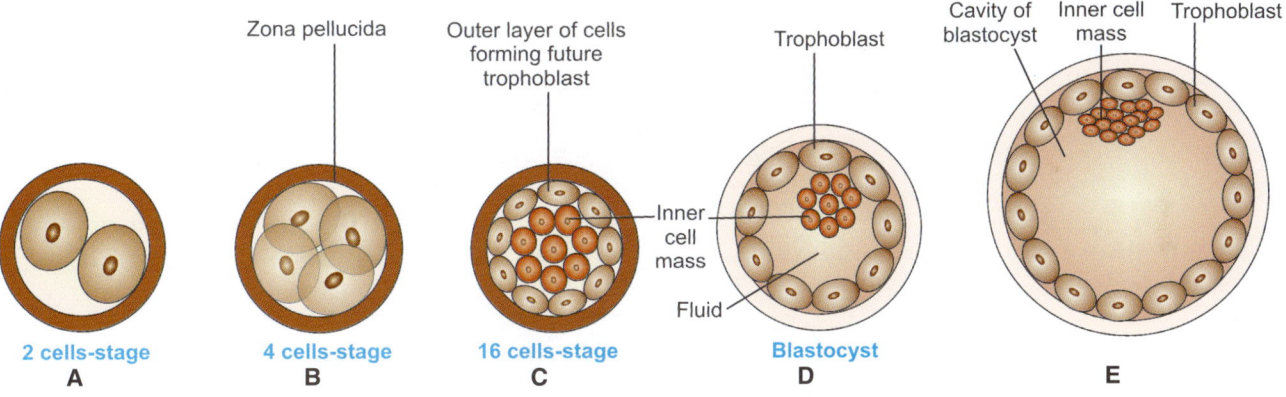

Fig. 3.4: Stages of formation of blastocyst.

called *polar trophoblast* and that occupying the rest of wall including embryonic pole is called mural trophoblast. It later contributes to extraembryonic structures and embryonic part of placenta.

- *Blastocele* is the fluid filled space inside the blastocyst. A fully developed blastocyst consists of about 107 cells arranged as below:
- *Embryoblast* is formed by only 8 cells,
- *Polar trophoblast* is formed by about 30 cells, and
- *Mural trophoblast* consists of 69 cells.

Implantation of the blastocyst in the endometrium

- *Blastocyst floates* in the cavity of uterus for some time (Fig. 3.3) and in the mean time.
- *Zona pellucida disappears* exposing the trophoblast layer.

- *Endometrium of uterus* is in the meanwhile converted into decidua by enlargement of stromal cells which become vacuolated and filled with glycogen and lipids.
- *Sticky polar trophoblast then adheres* with the hormonally prepared endometrium (now called decidua). This adhesion process is assisted by the interaction of a chemical substance, pentasaccharide lacto-N-fucopentose-1 on the epithelium and its receptors on the trophoblasts (Figs 3.3 and 3.5). The blastocyst then erodes and burrows into the decidua with the help of proteolytic enzymes secreted by the trophoblast.
- *Blastocyst grows deeper* in the decidua progressively till it is completely burried under the mucosa (Fig. 3.5). The *implantation* or *embedding* of the blastocyst takes place on 6th or 7th day after fertilization.

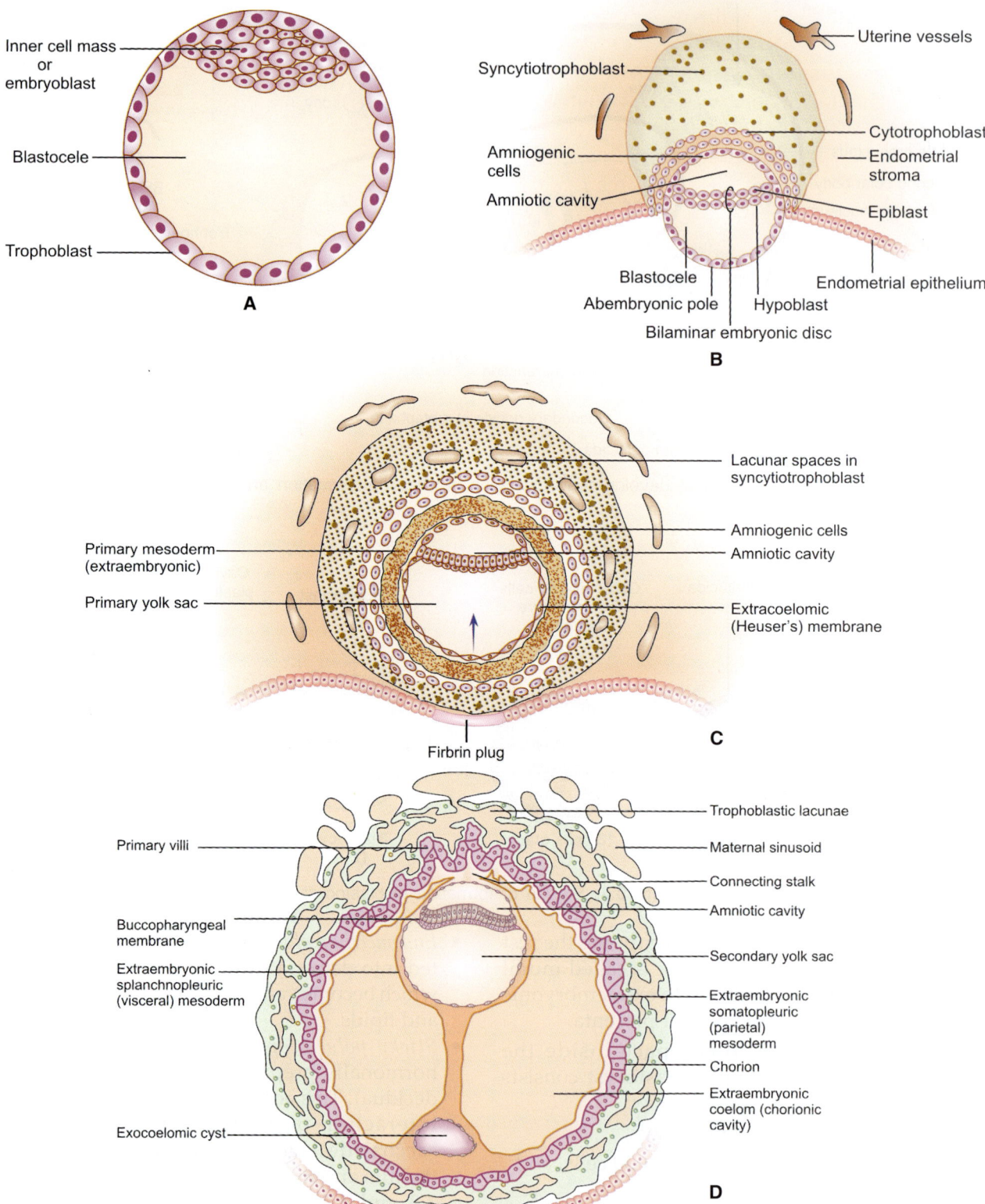

Fig. 3.5: Implantation of blastocyst in endometrium and formation of bilaminar disc, amniotic cavity and yolk sac : A, blastocyst at the time of implantation consisting of embryoblast, trophoblast and blastocele; B, differentiation of embryoblast into a bilaminar disc consisting of two layers (epiblast and hypoblasts); C, differentiation of amniogenic cells and amniotic cavity. Note formation of exocoelomic membrane and primary yolk sac. Also note differentiation of trophoblast into cytotrophoblast and syncytiotrophoblast, and development of lacunae in syncytiotrophoblast; D, establishment of uteroplacental circulation, formation of chorionic cavity and chorion and of primary and secondary villi.

- *Site of implantation* normally is dorsal wall near the junction of fundus with the body of the uterus. But implantation anywhere in the upper part of uterine cavity is considered normal.
- *Source of nutrition* for the embedded embryo till placenta takes up the function are glycogen and lipid filled decidual cells.

CLINICALLY APPLIED ASPECTS

ABNORMAL IMPLANTATION

Abnormal implantation of blastocyst may be extrauterine or intrauterine.

1. *Extrauterine implantation* (ectopic pregnancy) is usually followed by death of embryo. Extrauterine sites are:
   - *Ovary,* is rare site of ectopic implantation.
   - *Abdominal cavity.* Rarely implantation may occur in the peritoneal lining of the pouch of Douglas.
   - *Uterine tubes* are not an infrequent site of abnormal implantation. Tubal ectopic pregnancy is usually followed by rupture of the uterine tube, which is an emergency and may even cause death of the mother due to alarming haemorrhage.
2. *Intrauterine abnormal implantation* occurs in the lower part of the uterine cavity overlaping the internal Os. Such abnormal implantation results in *placenta praevia,* which produces severe haemorrhage in the later part of gestation and during parturition.

IN VITRO-FERTILIZATION (IVF)

In vitro-fertilization (IVF) and transfer of cleaving zygote into the uterus, popularly known as test tube boby technique, is presently being increasingly used in women, who fail to conceive normally.

Steps of IVF are:
- *Maturation of ovarian follicles* by administration of gonadotropins.
- *Collection of oocytes* by aspiration from follicles is done by laparoscopic technique.
- *Fertilization* of aspirated oocytes by the sperms collected is allowed to occur in a petridish containing culture medium. Fertilization and cleavage of zygote are monitored microscopically.
- *Transfer of cleaving zygote* during the four-to-eight cell stage is done into the uterine cavity with the help of catheter. The patient should remain in supine position for several hours.

SURROGATE MOTHER

In this technique after invitro fertilization (IVF) as described above, the cleaving zygote is implanted in the uterine cavity of some other woman. The other woman (surrogate mother) bears the embryo and fetus and delivers it to the natural mother at birth. This is done when the natural mother is unable to continue pregnancy due to uterine disorders.

CONTRACEPTION

Aims of contraception. Contraception refers to prevention of pregnancy. The aims of contraception are:

- The main aim of contraception is family planning to check the enormous increase in population growth, which is the root cause of socioeconomic problems of poor and developing countries, like India.
- Certain contraceptive measures are important to prevent the sexually transmitted diseases like AIDS.
- Contraceptives are also recommended on medical grounds to control the stress of pregnancy, labour and lactation in women suffering from heart diseases, etc.

Methods of contraception can be broadly grouped as:
- Spacing methods, and
- Terminal methods.

A. Spacing methods

The spacing methods increase the gap between two pregnancies. These include:
- Natural methods,
- Barrier methods,
- Contraceptive pills, and
- Intrauterine contraceptive devices.

I. Natural methods

1. *Rhythm method* is also known as *calender method* or *safe period method* or natural method. This method of contraception depends on the time of ovulation. In a woman having regular menstrual cycle, ovulation occurs on 14th day of the cycle. After ovulation, ovum remains viable for 48–72 hours. Similarly, after ejaculation sperms remain alive for 24–48 hours. Thus pregnancy occurs only if coitus is performed during this period. This is the period of high fertility and is called as *dangerous period.*

Therefore, to avoid pregnancy intercourse should be avoided in the dangerous period. Rest of the cycle, i.e. 5–6 days after bleeding phase of menstrual cycle and 5–6 days before the next cycle is the *safe period* (period of least fertility). This method of contraception is successful only if menstrual cycles are regular and woman knows the exact time of ovulation by keeping a record of basal body temperature.

2. **Coitus interruptus:** It is the oldest method of voluntary fertility control. In this method male withdraws the penis before ejaculation into the vagina and tries to prevent deposition of semen into the vagina. This method needs practice and discipline. The failure rate is high.

II. Barrier methods

Barrier methods of contraception prevent the meeting of ovum and sperms after coitus. These include:

1. Mechanical barriers
1. **Male condom** made of latex is the most commonly used barrier technique worldwide. Modern condoms also contain chemical spermicides. The condom is worn on erect penis before intercourse.
2. **Female condom,** made of polyurethane which lines the vagina is also available.
3. **Diaphragm and cervical cap** are other barrier devices applied on the cervix in females.

2. Chemical barriers

Chemical barriers refer to spermicidal agents which can destroy the sperms when applied in the female genital tract before coitus. The common spermicidal agents used are: Ricinoleic acid (oldest), Nanoxynol-9, and Octoxynol-3. These spermicidal agents are available in various forms such as: foam tablets, pastes, creams, jellies, and vaginal sponges.

3. Combined methods

As mentioned above, mechanical barriers (condoms, diaphragm and cervical caps) along with spermicidal agents give good protection.

III. Contraceptive pills

1. **Female oral contraceptives.** Oral contraceptives are most widely used contraceptive measure by the women all over the globe. These are recommended in women of younger age group (upto 35 years).

Mechanism of action. In general oral contraceptives contain synthetic preparation of oestrogen and progesterone and when taken orally, the plasma concentration of these hormones rises. The raised levels of these hormones by their negative feedback effect, act on anterior pituitary to inhibit the release of gonadotropins (FSH and LH) and thus inhibit ovulation.

2. **Male pills** are also available which inhibit spermatogenesis. These are not much popular.

IV. Intrauterine contraceptive devices

Intrauterine contraceptive devices (IUCDs) are inserted into the uterine cavity for long-term contraception. The devices are usually made up of inert materials like plastic, polythene and metal.

Copper-T

Copper-T is the most commonly used IUCD in India. As the name indicates it is made up of copper and its shape resembles the letter T. Like Lippe's loop it is also attached with a nylon thread (tail) (Fig. 3.6).

B. Terminal methods

Terminal method of contraception provide permanent sterilization. These include:

1. **Tubectomy.** Tubectomy is the permanent method of sterilization in female and is recommended only when the family is completed. In it fallopian tubes are cut and then cut ends are ligated and buried as shown in Fig. 3.7.
2. **Laparoscopic tubal occlusion.** In this procedure the fallopian tubes are occluded using silicon rubber bands, Fallope rings or Hulka-Clemens clips. This method is much quicker and simple and hospitalization is not required.
3. **Vasectomy.** Vasectomy is a simple operation employed for permanent sterilization in males. In

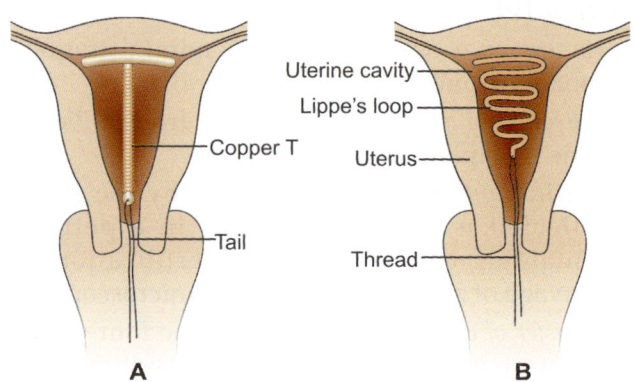

Fig. 3.6: Intrauterine contraceptive devices; A, copper T; and B, Lippe's loop.

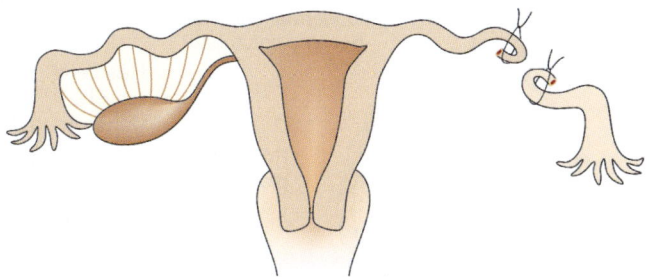

Fig. 3.7: Steps of female sterilization (tubectomy).

it about one cm piece of vas deferens is removed after clamping. Then both the ends are ligated and sutured so that they face away from each other (Fig. 3.8). This procedure reduces the risk of recanalization later on. After vasectomy sperm production and hormones are not affected but entry of the sperms into the semen is prevented.

4. *No scalpel vas occlusion* is a newer technique, which is quite safe, convenient and is acceptable to males. In it elastomer is injected into the vas deferens, which gets hardened in situ within 20 minutes and plugs the vas (occludes it).

STAGE OF BILAMINAR GERM DISC (SECOND WEEK OF DEVELOPMENT)

The stage of bilaminar germ disc formation approximately occurs during second week of development. The events of this stage of development, for the purpose of convenience can be described under following headings:

• Changes in the embryoblast.
• Development of extraembryonic membranes and cavities, and
• Endometrial changes

A. CHANGES IN THE EMBRYOBLAST

As described above, during implantation the blastocyst is formed of inner cell mass called as *embryoblast* (located at one pole) and the outer cell

mass called as *trophoblast* (Fig. 3.5A). Following changes occur in the embryoblast during 2nd week of development:

Formation of bilaminar disc

On 8th day after ovulation the embryoblast is converted into a *bilaminar disc* consisting of following two layers (Fig. 3.5B):

• *Epiblast*, the upper layer, is thick and composed of regularly arranged columnar cells. It is continuous at the periphery with amnion (see below).
• *Hypoblast*, the lower layer, is thin and made of irregularly arranged polyhedral cells. It is continuous at its periphery with the yolk sac.

Formation of prochordal plate

At the end of second week some of the cubical cells of hypoblast near the margin of the disc become columnar and form the so called prochordal plate. The appearance of the prochordal plate determines the central axis of the embryo (i.e. enables us to divide the embryo into right and left halves), and also enables us to distinguish its future head and tail (Fig. 3.9).

Formation of primitive streak

By the end of the second week, soon after the formation of prochordal plate, the *primitive streak* is formed by the proliferation of some of the epiblast cells near the caudal end of the embryonic disc. It appears as a clump of cells in the midline between the epiblast and hypoblast (Fig. 3.10).

B. DEVELOPMENT OF EXTRAEMBRYONIC MEMBRANES AND CAVITIES

Changes in the trophoblast

After embedding of blastocyst in the endometrial stroma the trophoblast differentiates into two layers (Fig. 3.5C):

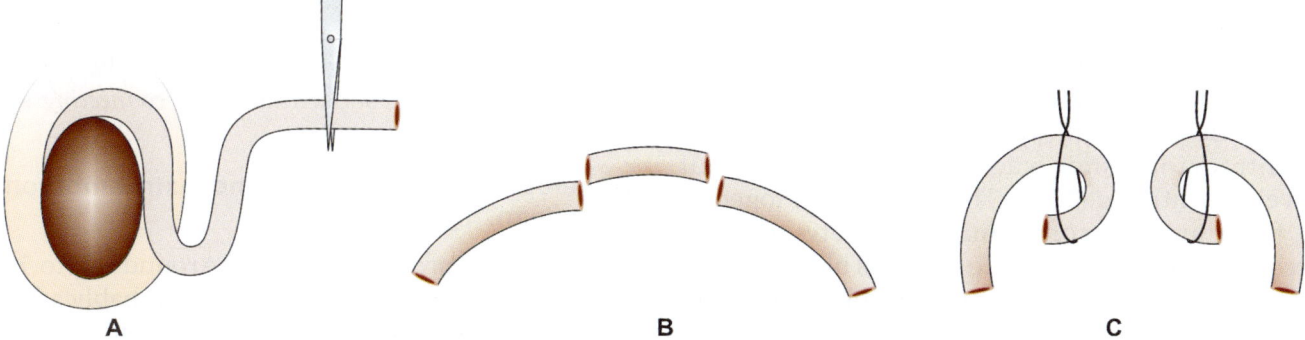

A   B   C

Fig. 3.8: Steps of male sterilization (vasectomy).

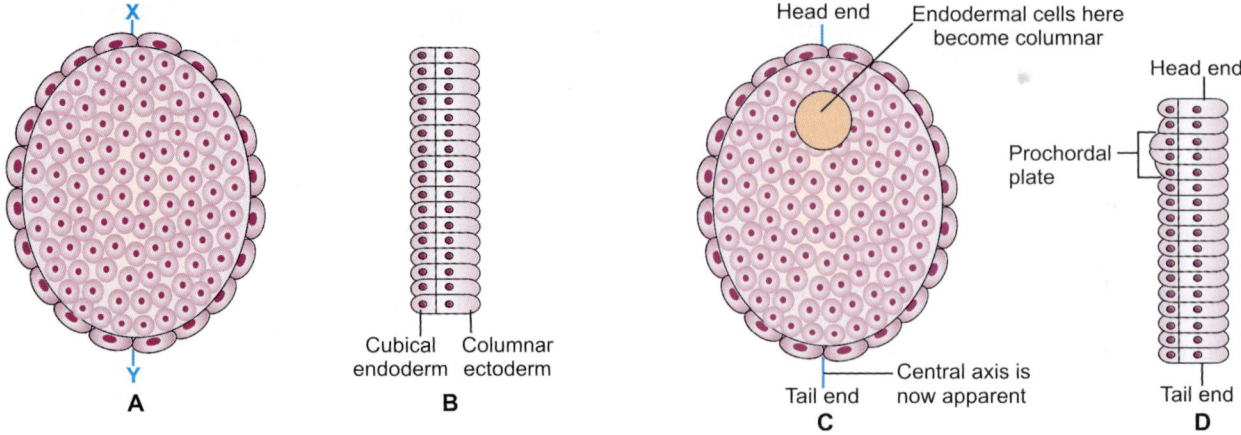

Fig. 3.9: Dorsal view and transverse section of bilaminar disc, respectively, before (A and B) and after (C and D) formation of prochordal plate by conversion of cubical cells of hypoblast near the margin of disc into columnar cells. XY represents central axis.

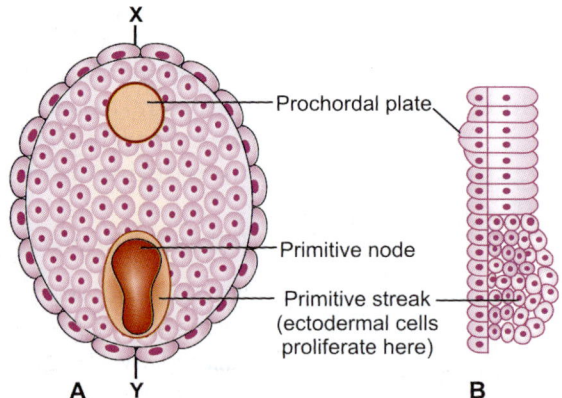

Fig. 3.10: Dorsal view (A) and transverse section (B) showing formation of primitive streak by proliferation of epiblast cells near the caudal end of embryonic disc.

Cytotrophoblast, the actively proliferating layer lies on the inner or embryonic side. Cells called *extra-embryonic mesoblasts* are formed along the inner surface of the cytotrophoblast. Their origin is controversial.

Syncytiotrophoblast, the outer layer of trophoblast, erodes maternal tissues. The maternal capillaries in the vicinity become congested with blood cells and dilate to form *sinusoids.* The syncytiotrophoblast erodes the walls of the sinusoids and becomes continuous with their endothelial lining. By day 2 lacunae develop in the syncytiotrophoblast by fusion of intracytoplasmic vacuoles (*lacunar stage* of development) (Fig. 3.5C). The lacunae join together to form an intercommunicating network that becomes continuous with the maternal blood vessels. By the end of 2nd week the maternal blood begins to flow through the lacunar network, establishing the primitive *uteroplacental circulation* (Fig. 3.5D).

Formation of amnion and amniotic cavity

Early in the second week a membrane called amnion begins to form by delamination from the cyto-trophoblast. The cells forming amnion (amniogenic cells) are a layer of thin squamous cells. This layer is continuous with the epiblast layer of bilaminar disc and encloses a space above the disc called amniotic cavity (Fig. 3.5C). The amniotic cavity is filled by amniotic fluid or liquor amnii. Later, the amniogenic cellular layer of amnion is covered by the parietal extra-embryonic mesoderm and the *connecting stalk* is attached to it.

Development of yolk sac and extraembryonic mesoderm

Formation of primary yolk sac. Around 9th to 10th day of development, flattened cells, probably arising from the hypoblast (or according to some workers from trophoblast), form a thin membrane, known as *exocoelomic (Heuser's) membrane,* that lines the inner surface of cytotrophoblast (of blastocystic cavity). This membrane, together with the hypoblast, encloses the cavity known as *primary yolk sac* (Fig. 3.5C).

Development of extraembryonic mesoderm: By 11th to 12th day of development the cells of the trophoblast give origin to a mass of cells called the *extraembryonic mesoderm* (or primary mesoderm). These cells form a fine loose connective tissue, which comes to occupy the space between the trophoblast externally and the amnion and exocoelomic (Heuser's) membrane internally. This mesoderm is called extraembryonic mesoderm as it lies outside the embryonic disc and does not give rise to any tissues of the embryo proper (Fig. 3.5C).

Further changes in extraembryonic mesoderm. Soon many cavities appear in the extraembryonic mesoderm which coaleace to form a large cavity known as *extraembryonic coelom (chorionic cavity).* This cavity surrounds the primary yolk sac and amniotic cavity except where the germ disc is connected to the trophoblast by the connecting stalk (Fig. 3.5D). This cavity divides the extraembryonic mesoderm into two layers:

- *Extraembryonic somatopleuric or parietal mesoderm,* which lines the inside of cytotrophoblast and the outside of amnion, and
- *Extraembryonic splanchnopleuric or visceral mesoderm,* which lines the outside of the yolk sac.

Formation of secondary or definitive yolk sac. By the end of second week the lower part of the primary yolk sac pinches off, resulting in a smaller sac next to the embryonic disc called the *secondary (definitive) yolk sac.* The detached remnant in the extraembryonic coelom is called the *exocoelomic cyst.*

Formation of chorion

By the end of the second week the extraembryonic somatopleural mesoderm fuses with the overlying cytotrophoblast to form a membrane called the *chorion.* The chorion encloses the embryo proper and all of the other extraembryonic membranes (Fig. 3.5D). Meanwhile, the extraembryonic coelom expands and forms a large cavity known as *chorionic cavity.* The only place where extraembryonic mesoderm traverses the chorionic cavity is the connecting stalk with development of blood vessels, this stalk will become the *umbilical cord.*

It is important to note that only a portion of chorion together with the adjacent endometrium will form the placenta in subsequent weeks.

Further changes in chorion. By thirteenth day of development finger like projections called *villi* appear in the chorion. These villi are formed by the cells of cytotrophoblast which proliferate locally and penetrate into the syncytiotrophoblast. Such cellular masses surrounded by syncytial covering are called *primary villi* (see Fig. 6.2). By the end of second week some of the cell masses change into columns of cells that have a core of extraembryonic mesoderm. For a short period the core is avascular and is called a *secondary villus.*

C. ENDOMETRIAL CHANGES

Decidual reaction. After implantation the endometrium is called decidua. The stroma cells of endometrium get enlarged, become vacuolated and filled with glycogen and lipids. These cells are called decidual cells. Therefore this change in stroma cell is called decidual reaction. The stored glycogen and lipids are the source of nutrition for the embryo till placenta takes up this function.

STAGE OF TRILAMINAR GERM DISC (THIRD WEEK OF DEVELOPMENT)

The stage of trilaminar disc formation is marked by changes during third week of development. The events during this stage of development for the purpose of convenience can be described under following groups:

A. Changes in embryo proper.

B. Changes in the extraembryonic membranes and cavities.

C. Changes in the mother.

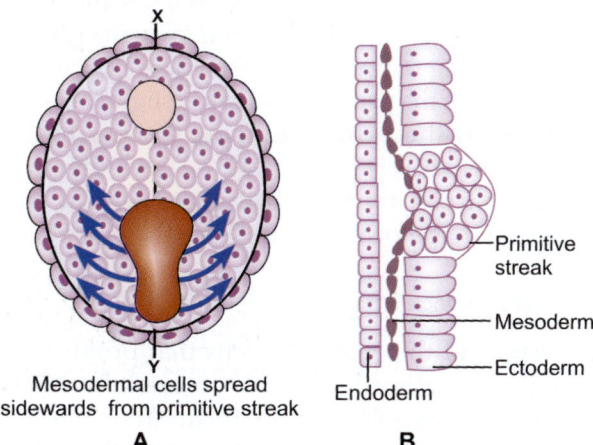

Fig. 3.11: Formation of embryonic mesoderm from the cells of primitive streak; A, is the dorsal (amniotic) view; and B; is the section along axis XY in A.

A. CHANGES IN THE EMBRYO PROPER

Changes in the embryo proper during third week of development includes:

- Establishment of embryonic axes
- Gastrulation
- Neurulation
- Development of somites
- Development of intraembryonic coelom
- Early development of cardiovascular system.

In the embryo establishment of the body-axes, anteroposterior, dorso-ventral and right to left takes place before and during the period of gastrulation. As described on page 44 the establishment of a bilaterally symmetrical segmented body plan with cranio-caudal, right-left and dorso-ventral axes has been well studied in *Drosophila* and is presumed in humans to be controlled by three sets of genes:

- Maternal effect genes,
- Segmentation genes, and
- Homeotic genes (for details see page 17).

I. Gastrulation: Formation of germ layers

As described above, the embryonic disc at the end of second week is a bilaminar disc consisting of epiblast and hypoblasts. At the beginning of third week there occurs, the most characteristic event, the gastrulation, which establishes all the three germ cells, changing the embryonic disc from a bilaminar to a trilaminar structure. During this period, the embryo may be referred to as a gastrula. Events during gastrulation are:

1. Formation of primitive groove

Primitive streak formed by the end of 2nd week, becomes clearly, visible as a narrow groove with slightly bulging regions on either side (Fig. 3.10). The cephalic end of the primitive streak is slightly elevated and is called the primitive node. Concurrently, a narrow groove *primitive groove* — develops in the primitive streak that is continuous with a small depression in the primitive node — the *primitive pit*.

2. Formation of germ cells

Invagination of the epiblastic cells that proliferate in the region of primitive streak occurs between the epiblast and hypoblast and forms the *embryonic mesoderm* (Fig. 3.11). According to a view, the epiblast, through the process of gastrulation, is the source of all three germ layers in the embryo (i.e. ectoderm, mesoderm and endoderm). According to this view:

- Some cells of the epiblast after invagination displace the hypoblast and form the embryonic *endoderm*.
- Some epiblast cells which after invagination come to lie between the epiblast and newly created endoderm form the *mesoderm,* and
- The cells remaining in the epiblast then form *ectoderm*.

3. Formation of notochord

Notochord a bud like structure formed early in the third week, in the region extending from the cranial end of the primitive streak to the caudal end of prochordal plate (Fig. 3.12). It develops from the mesenchymal cells from the primitive node.

Steps involved in the formation of notochord are (Fig. 3.12):

- *Formation of notochordal process.* Mesenchymal cells in the primitive node (*prenotochordal cells*) multiply and pass cranially in the midline, between the ectoderm and endoderm upto the caudal margin of prochordal plate and form a median cellular cord the notochordal process (Fig. 3.12A to C).
- *Formation of notochordal canal.* The primitive pit extends into the notochordal process converting it into notochordal canal (Fig. 3.12D to F). Soon the floor of notochordal canal begins to develop an opening through which it communicates with the yolk sac. Through the primitive pit the notochordal canal communicates with the amniotic cavity.
- *Formation of notochordal plate.* Gradually the opening in the floor of the notochordal canal coaleace and thus the floor disappears completely. In this way the notochoral canal is converted into the flat notochordal plate (Fig. 3.12G, H, I).
- *Formation of definitive notochord.* Soon the notochordal plate again assumes the shape of a tube and is eventually converted into a solid rod by proliferation of the notochordal cells (Fig. 3.12J, K, L). This definitive notochord becomes detached from the endoderm of the yolk sac, which again become a continuous layer.

Fate and Significance of Notochord

- The notochord is an intricate structure around which the vertebral column is formed. However, the notochord does not give rise to vertebral column.
- The developing notochord induces the overlying embryonic ectoderm to thicken and form the *neural plate* (the primordium of central nervous system).
- The notochord degenerates and disappears as the bodies of vertebrae form, but parts of it persist in the region of each intervertebral disc as the *nucleus pulposus*.

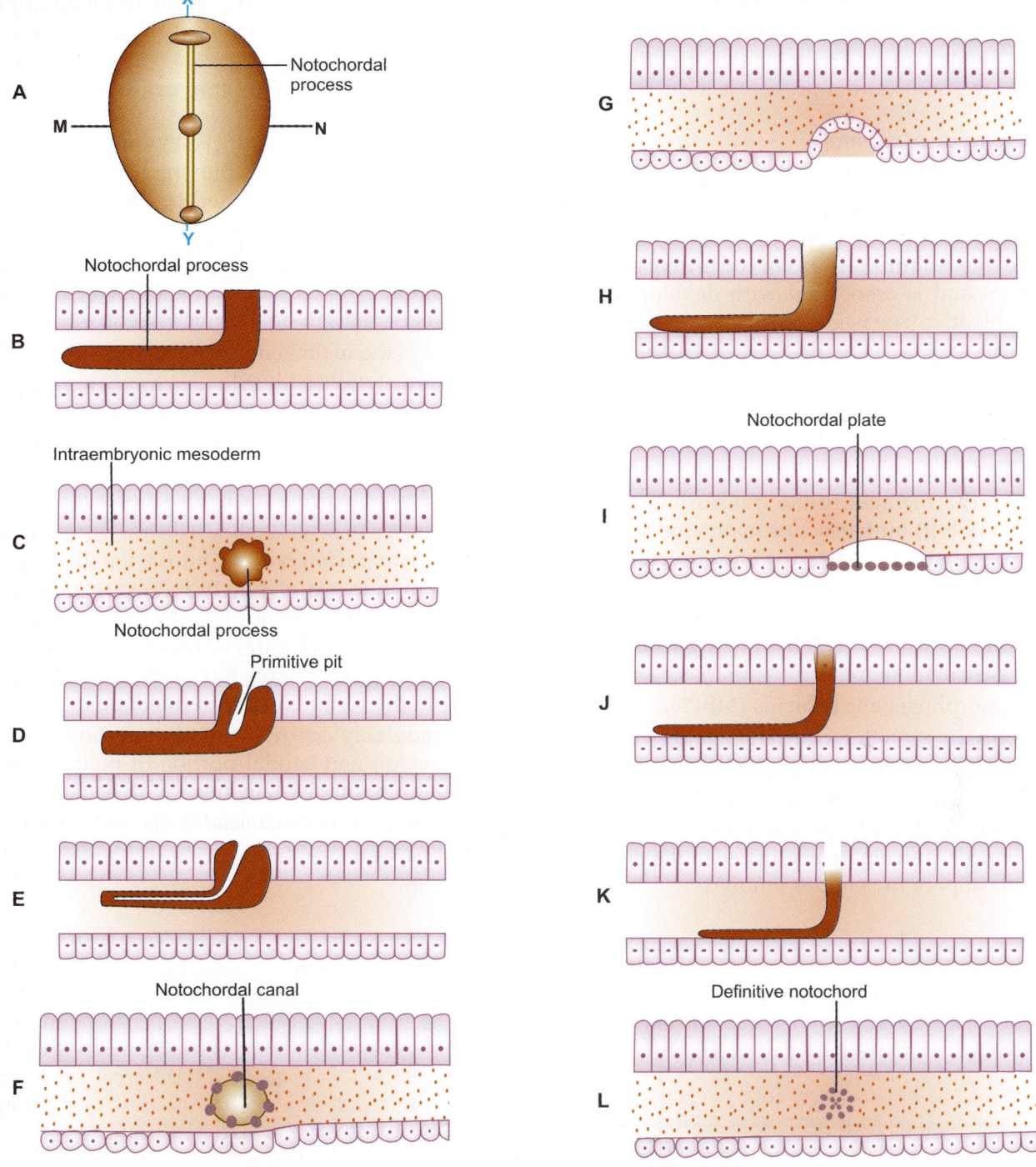

Fig. 3.12: Steps in the formation of notochord: A, B, C, notochordal process is formed by mesenchymal cells from primitive node passing cranially in the midline between ectoderm and endoderm; D, E, F, notochordal canal is formed by extension of primitive pit into the notochordal process; G, H, I, notochordal plate is formed by coalesence of the walls of canal; J, K, L, definitive notochord (A, D, G, J = dorsal view of embryonic disc; B, E, H, K = sections along axis XY in A; C, F, I and L = Sections along axis MN in A).

4. Spread of mesoderm and formation of buccopharyngeal and cloacal membranes

During gastrulation, the embryonic mesoderm spreads throughout the embryonic disc between the ectoderm and endoderm except at following places

where the ectoderm and endoderm are fused and the embryonic disc remains a bilaminar structure here (Fig. 3.13):

- The area of prochordal plate, which later forms the *buccopharyngeal membrane* (future site of the oral cavity).

- A small circular area caudal to the primitive streak which forms the *cloacal membrane* (future site of anus).
- In the median plane cranial to the primitive node, where the notochordal process is located.

5. Appearance of allantois

A tiny diverticulum called the allantois appears in the caudal wall of secondary yolk sac on about day 16. It extends into the connecting stalk. In human embryo the allantois is involved in early blood formation and is associated with development of urinary bladder (see page 183).

Molecular control of gastrulation

Gastrulation starts after the formation of primitive streak. Cephalic and caudal ends of the embryo are established before the primitive streak is formed.

Nodal gene, a member of the transforming growth factor β (TGF β), initiates and maintains formation of primitive streak. After formation of primitive streak a number of genes regulate process of gastrulation.

Signaling molecules which play significant role during gastrulation are:

- Bone morphogenetic proteins (MBPs),
- Fibroblastic growth factor (FGF), and
- Transcription factor, PIT X 2.

Primary organizer, i.e. the structure which controls the systematic development in human refers to the *primitive node,* a structure analogues to the dorsal lip of the blastopore in xenopus embryo.

Signaling molecules involved in the induction of this organizer include:

- Wnt family (Wnt-3),
- Paired type homeobox transcription factor mix, and
- Fibroblast growth factor (FGF) family.

Fate map of epiblast cells moving through the node and streak is predetermined by their position to become specific types of mesoderm and endoderm.

Head organizing centre. Controls the formation of head region by expression of the following genes by the cephalic margin of anterior visceral endoderm:

- *LIM 1* is the main gene; its knocking out produces an animal without head.
- *OTX 1, OTX 2, and HESX 1* and the *secreted factor cerebrus* are the other genes involved in organization of head region.
- *Nodal gene* expression is also necessary for the development of cranial structures.

Trunk organization centre controls the formation of trunk region by expression of following genes:

- *T-box genes* (Tbx 6 and brachury), which control formation of trunk paraxial lateral plate mesoderm.
- *Fibroblast growth factor 9 (FGF-9)* appears to play role in the formation of intermediate mesoderm.

Tail organizing centre forms the mesoderm of the sacral region and caudal portion of neural tube by expression of following genes:

- Brachury (its mutation leads to caudal dysgenesis),
- Wnt 5a, and
- Wnt 5b.

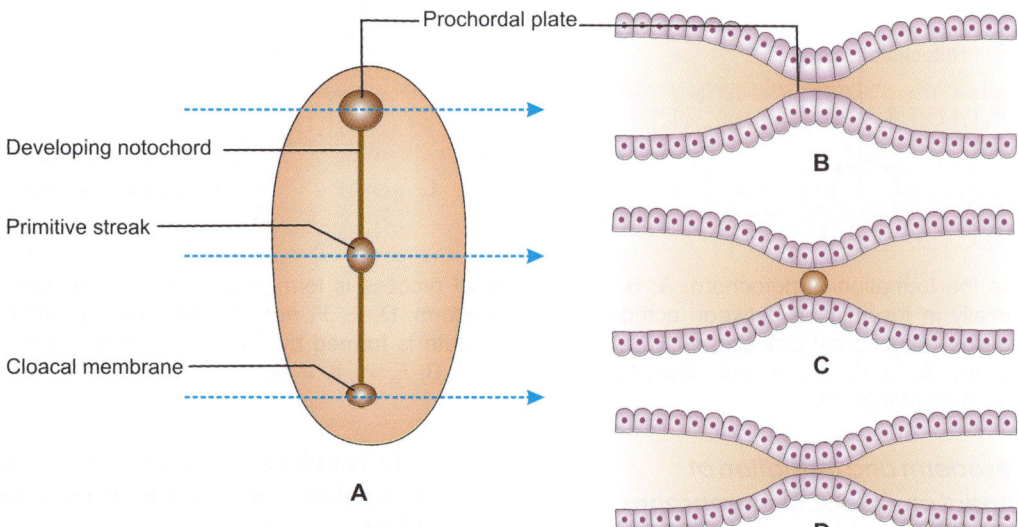

Fig. 3.13: A, Spread of mesoderm and formation of buccopharyngeal and cloacal membranes; B, note that the mesoderm comes to lie between the ectoderm and endoderm in all parts of the embryonic disc, except at prochordal plate; C, region of notochord; and D, at cloacal membrane.

II. Neurulation

Formation of neural tube

Neurulation refers to process of neural plate formation and its infolding to form neural tube. Steps involved in formation of neural tube are (Fig. 3.14):

- *Neural plate* is formed by the thickening of ectoderm overlying the notochord, and therefore extends from the prochordal plate to the primitive node (Fig. 3.14A and B). It is the first appearance of nervous system.

- *Neural groove,* a longitudinal furrow appears in the neural plate, which is bound on each side by *neural folds* (Fig. 3.14C and D).

- *Neural tube,* the primordium of the central nervous system, is formed by fusion of the neural folds in the midline dorsally (Fig. 3.14 E and F). Neural tube is soon divisible into a cranial enlarged part that forms the brain, and a caudal tubular part which forms the spinal cord (For details see page 248).

Neural crest formation

When the neural folds fuse to form the neural tube, the neuroectodermal cells migrate dorsolaterally and proliferate to form the neural crest between the surface ectoderm and neural tube (Fig. 3.14). The neural crest gives rise to ganglia of cranial and spinal nerves and some other structures (see page 243).

Molecular Regulation of Neurulation

Induction of neural plate is regulated by inactivation of bone morphogenic protein 4 (BMP4).

Inactivation of BMP4 is caused by:

- *Noggin, chordin, and fallistatin* secreted by the node, notochord and prechordal mesoderm in the cranial region.

- *WNT 3a and FGF* in the hind brain and spinal cord region.

III. Development of somites

- The intraembryonic mesoderm located on each side of the notochord (Fig. 3.15A) proliferates and is arranged in three columns — paraxial mesoderm, intermediate mesoderm and lateral plate mesoderm — which are continuous with each other (Fig. 3.15B).

- Towards the end of the third week, the paraxial mesoderm differentiates and begins to divide into pairs of somites (Fig. 3.15C).

- Somites are segmentally arranged with first pair forming near the cranial end of the embryo in the future occipital region by the end of third

week. Then about 3 pairs of somites are formed per day and by the end of 5th week about 42 to 44 somite pairs are formed (4-occipital, 8 cervical, 12 thoracic, 5 lumbar, 5 sacral and 8 to 10 coccygeal) (Fig. 3.15D).

- The somite number is used to determine the relative age of embryos in the somite period.

- Eventually the somites will give rise to major components of the skeletal, muscular and integumentary systems.

Molecular regulation of somite differentiation

Signals for somite differentiation are derived from surrounding structures, including the notochord, neural tube, epidermis and lateral plate mesoderm.

Regulation of somite differentiation is as below:

- *Sclerotome formation* from the ventromedial portion of the somites is induced by the secreted protein products of the *noggin* genes and *sonic hedgehog* (SHH) produced by the notochord and floor plate of neural tube.

- *Vertebrae formation* is regulated by a cascade of cartilage and bone-forming genes initiated by the transcription factor PAX-1 which is expressed by the sclerotome cells.

- *Dermomyotome differentiation* from the somite is caused by expression of PAX3, regulated by WNT proteins from the dorsal neural tube.

- *Myogenic differentiation* is induced by MYOD, a member of the family of myogenic regulatory factors (MRFs). The MYOD activates transcription of muscle specific genes.

IV. Formation of intraembryonic coelom

As described above the paraxial mesoderm undergoes segmentation to form the somites. At the same time small isolated spaces appear in the lateral plate mesoderm (Fig. 3.15B). These spaces coalesce to form one large horse-shoe shaped cavity, the *intraembryonic coelom* (Fig. 3.15C). There are two halves of this cavity (one on either side of midline) which are joined together cranial to the prochordal plate forming U-shaped coelomic cavity. Initially the intraembryonic coelom is a closed cavity (Figs 3.16A and B), but soon it communicate with the extraembryonic coelom (Figs 3.16C and D).

Divisions of lateral plate mesoderm. With the formation of intraembryonic coelom, the lateral plate mesoderm is divided into two layers:

- *Somatopleuric or parietal layer* which is in contact with ectoderm and is continuous with the extra embryonic mesoderm covering the amnion.

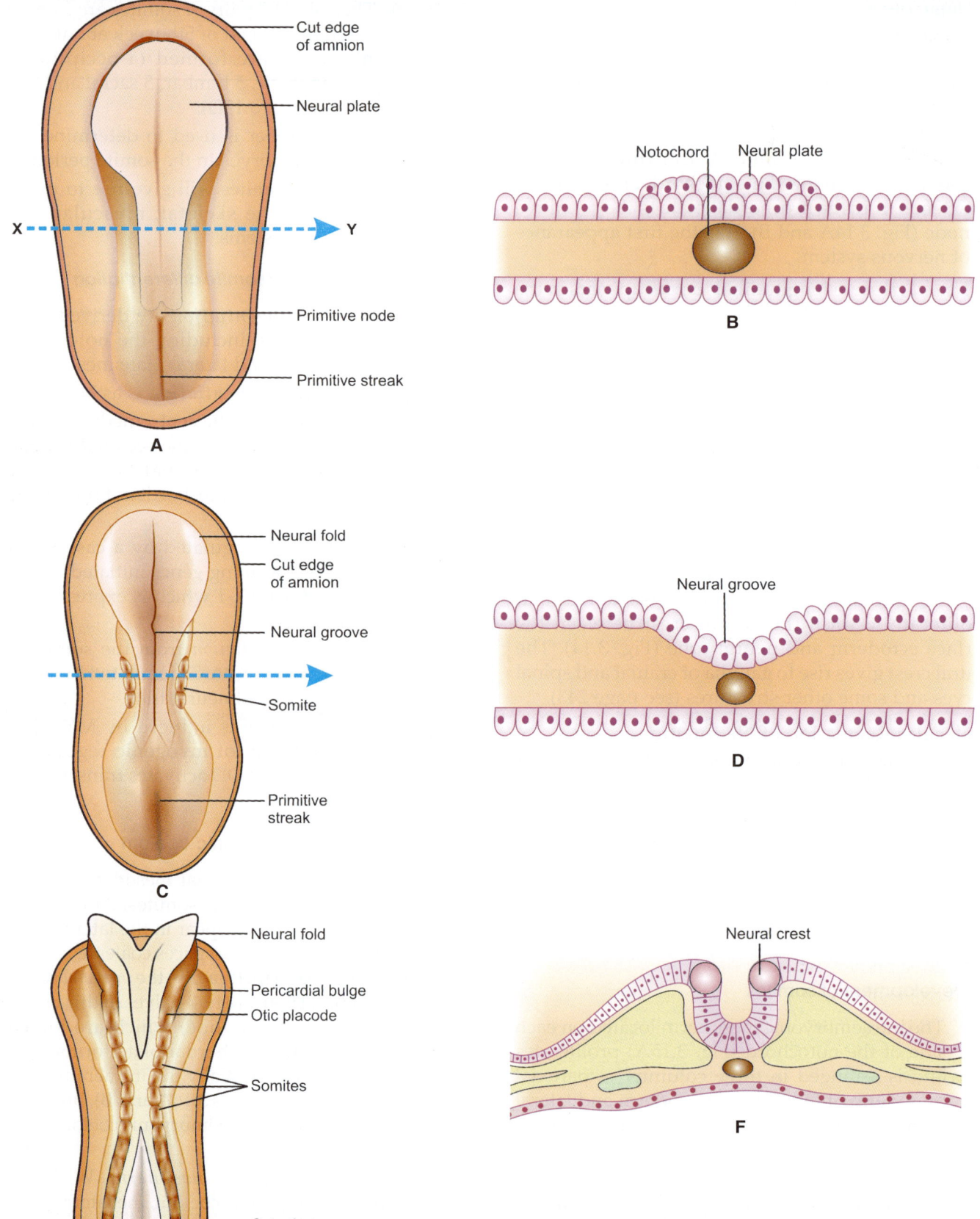

Fig. 3.14: Stages in the formation of neural tube: A and B, formation of neural plate; C and D, formation of neural groove and folds; E and F, formation of neural tube. A, C and E are dorsal views of embryo and B, D and F are sections across the axis XY.

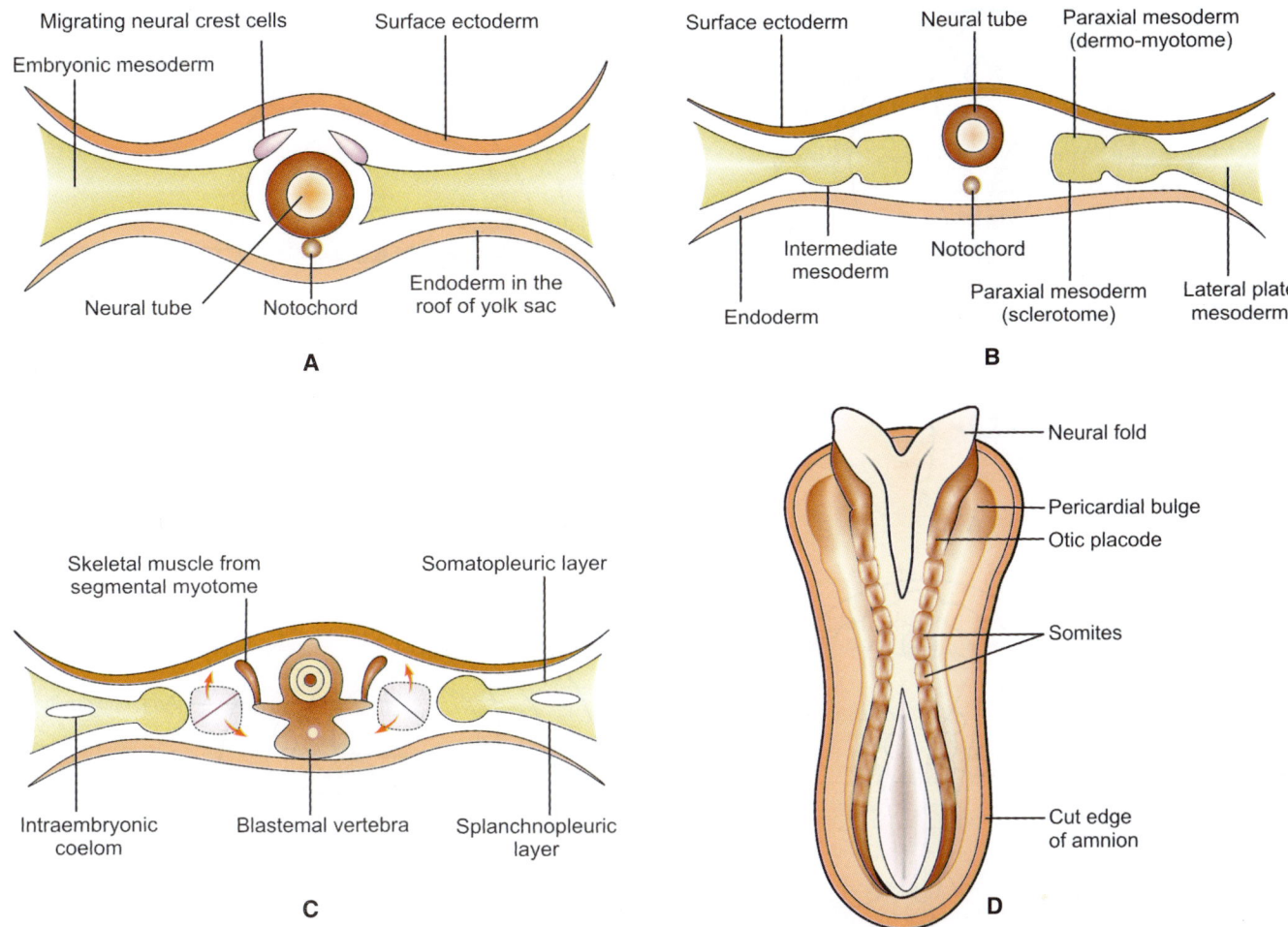

Fig. 3.15: Schematic transverse sections to show formation of somites and intraembryonic coelom: A, embryonic mesoderm arranged on each side of notochord; B, differentiation of embryonic mesoderm into three columns of: paraxial, intermediate, and lateral plate mesoderm; C, formation of somites from paraxial mesoderm; D, dorsal view of the embryo depicting arrangement of somites.

- *Splanchnopleuric or visceral layer,* which is in contact with the endoderm and is continuous with the extraembryonic mesoderm covering the yolk sac.

Divisions of intraembryonic coelom. During the second month the intraembryonic coelom is divided into three body cavities :

- Pericardial cavity,
- Pleural cavity, and
- Peritoneal cavity

  For further details see page 96.

V. Early development of cardiovascular system

The development of cardiovascular system starts at the beginning of third week. Early development of cardiovascular system during this period includes:

- Formation of blood vessels.
- Formation of primordial blood cells.
- Formation of primordial cardiovascular system.

Formation of blood vessels

Extraembryonic blood vessels begin to form at the beginning of third week in the extraembryonic mesoderm of the yolk sac, connecting stalk, and chorion (Fig. 3.17).

Embryonic blood vessels start developing after 2 days of extraembryonic blood vessels.

Process of blood vessel formation includes vasculogenesis and angiogenesis.

- *Vasculogenesis.* Mesenchymal cells differentiate into angioblasts which proliferate to form isolated clusters of cells (blood islands). Spaces appear within these blood islands and get lined with endothelium derived from the mesenchymal cells and thus form a network of endothelial channels (vasculogenesis).
- *Angiogenesis.* Further proliferation of vessels occurs by budding from the above formed endothelial channels (angiogenesis).

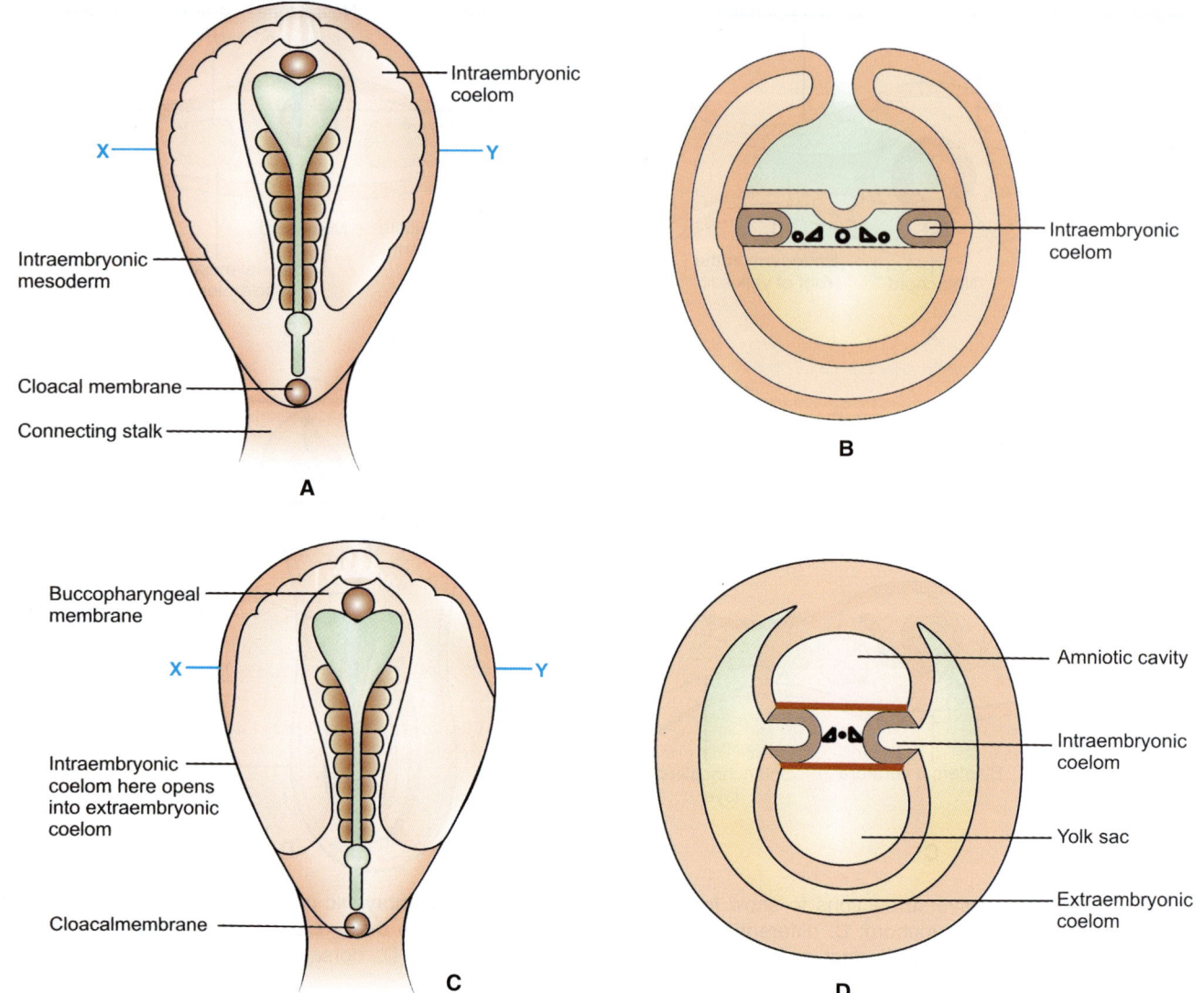

Fig. 3.16: U-shaped intraembryonic coelom formed in lateral plate mesoderm is initially a closed cavity (A and B) but soon communicates with extraembryonic coelom (C and D).

Formation of primordial blood cells

Primordial blood cells (haemangioblasts) are derived from the endothelial cells of the vessels in the walls of yolk sac, and allantois at the end of third week. Blood formation in the embryo starts in fifth week.

Note: Fetal and adult blood cells are derived from different hematopoietic progenitor cells (hemangio-blasts).

Formation of primordial cardiovascular system

Primordial cardiovascular system is formed by the end of third week and consists of :

Tubular heart. It is formed by fusion of two heart tubes which develop from that part of visceral intraembryonic mesoderm (cardiogenic area or cardiogenic plate) which forms the floor of that part of intraembryonic coelom which forms pericardial cavity (Fig. 3.17)

Vessels which connect to embryo (dorsal aorta and its branches), yolk sac (vitelline artery and vein), umbilical cord (umbilical artery and vein),

Note: For details and related figures see page 208.

B. CHANGES IN THE EXTRAEMBRYONIC MEMBRANES AND CAVITIES

Further development of chorionic villi

Secondary villi are formed in the early third week. This occurs by penetration and growth of mesenchymal cells into the core of primary villi formed in 2nd week of development (Fig. 6.2G).

Tertiary villi are formed by the end of third week. This occurs by differentiation of mesenchymal cells

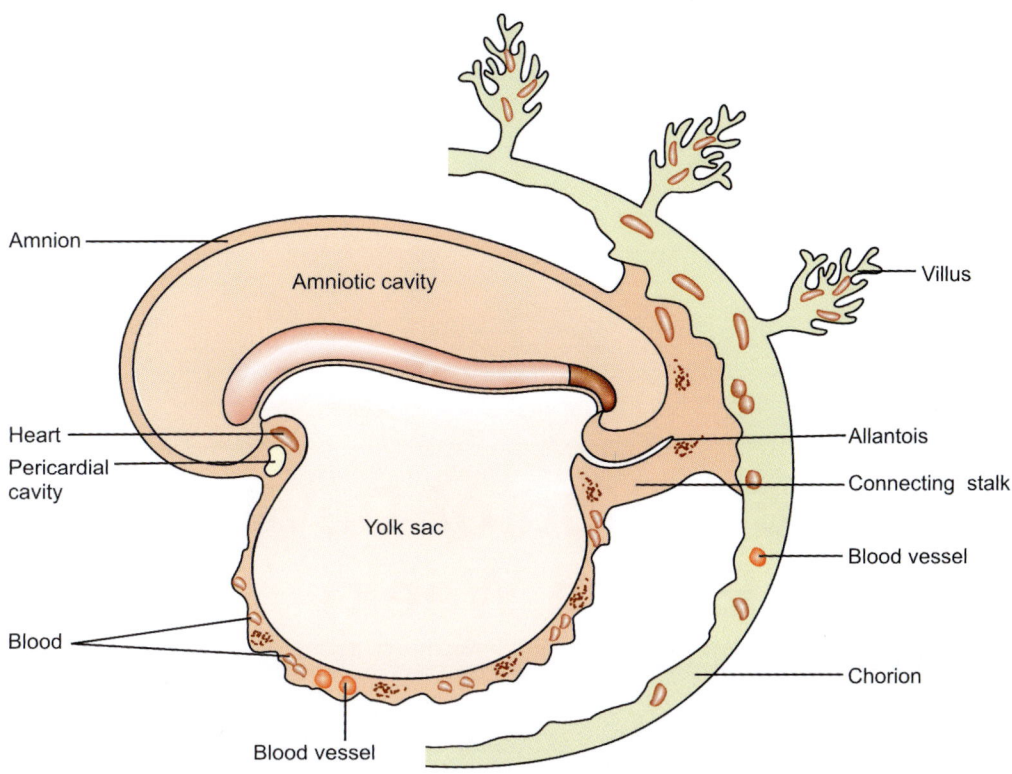

Fig. 3.17: Extraembryonic blood vessels formation in the villi, chorion, connecting stalk and wall of yolk sac in a presomite embryo of appoximately 19 days. Note the formation of primitive heart and pericardial cavity.

of core of secondary villi into capillaries and blood cells. These capillaries then fuse to form arterio-capillary networks and make contact with capillaries developing in the mesoderm of chorionic plate and in the connecting stalk (Fig. 6.2H). These vessels in turn soon become connected with intraembryonic circulatory system. In this way the placenta is connected with the embryo and is ready to supply the embryo proper with essential nutrients and oxygen derived from the maternal blood.

Anchoring versus free villi. Concurrently, with the development of tertiary villi, the cytotrophoblast cells of these villi, proliferate and penetrate through the syncytiotrophoblast to form a *cytotrophoblastic shell,* which gradually surrounds the chorionic sac and attaches it firmly to the maternal endometrial tissue. Such villi which are attached on one side to the chorionic plate and on the other side to the maternal tissue (decidua basalis) are called *anchoring or stem villi* (Fig. 6.2I). Certain villi which branch from the sides of anchoring villi and protrude into the inter villi space are called free or *branch or terminal villi.* Thus the main exchange of nutrients and waste products between the maternal and embryo blood occurs through the walls of the branch villi.

Note: For details and related Figures see page 71 and 72.

Changes in Chorionic Cavity and Connecting Stalk

- *Chorionic cavity* show no significant changes except enlargement.
- *Connecting stalk* becomes bit narrow and allantois extends further into the connecting stalk.
- *Allantois* becomes a distinct, endodermally lined duct caudal to the *cloacal* membrane.

C. CHANGES IN MOTHER

1. *Amenorrhea,* the first symptom of pregnancy, is known to the mother in the beginning of third week of development.

2. *Normal bleeding of pregnancy,* i.e. Hartman's sign is seen in 20 to 25% of all pregnancies. This occurs due to erosion of the endometrial vessels during normal implantation and placentation.

3. *Breast changes* in the form of tenderness and /or tingling sensations are commonly noted by the end of third week.

4. *Frequency of urination* is often increased.

5. *Constipation* may occur in some of the pregnant women.

6. *Human chorionic gonadotropin* (HCG) levels are increased in serum and urine. These form the basis of positive pregnancy tests by the end of third week.

Embryonic Period of Development (Fourth to Eighth Week)

INTRODUCTION
FOLDING OF EMBRYO
Position of structures in embryonic disc
Effects of folding of embryo
- Formation of folds
- Formation of primitive gut
- Expansion of amniotic cavity
- Effect or relative position of structures of embryo

CHANGES IN GERMINAL LAYERS AND THEIR DERIVATIVES
Phases of organogenesis
Induction
Derivatives of germinal layers

- Derivatives of ectoderm
- Derivatives of mesoderm
- Derivatives of endoderm

DEVELOPMENTAL STAGES OF HUMAN PRE-EMBRYO AND EMBRYO AND ESTIMATION OF EMBRYONIC AGE
- Human developmental stages
- Estimation of embryonic age

KEY EVENTS DURING FOURTH TO EIGHTH WEEKS OF DEVELOPMENT
- Fourth week : Somite and neural tube period
- Fifth week : Early pharyngeal arch and limb bud period.
- Sixth week : Late pharyngeal arch and limb bud period.
- Seventh week and eighth week : Late embryonic period

INTRODUCTION

The embryonic period of development extends from fourth to eighth week of gestation and is also called *period of organogenesis*. During this period the main organ systems are developed from the three germinal layers. Concurrently with the development of organ systems of the body and establishment of major internal structures, there occur major changes in the external features, i.e. shape and size of the embryo as well. Thus by the end of period of organogenesis (i.e. by the end of eighth week of development) internally most of the organ systems are developed; however, the function of most of them is negligible except for the cardiovascular system; and externally the major features of human appearance are recognizable. During the fetal period (third month to birth) there occurs rapid growth of the body and maturation of the tissue organs established during period of organogenesis (fourth to eighth week).

The period of organogenesis can be divided into various stages of development with different phases. However, before discussing the phases and stages of organogenesis, it will be worthwhile to know the different derivatives of the three germinal layers. Hence, the topic of organogenesis can be discussed as:

- Folding of embryo and its effects on positions of other structures.

- Changes in germinal layers and their derivatives.

- Developmental stages of human pre-embryo and embryo and estimation of embryonic age.

- Key events during fourth to eighth week of development.

FOLDING OF EMBRYO

Folding of trilaminar embryonic disc which starts in the beginning of 4th week is the key event in the formation of body form and development of gastrointestinal tract. Folding of embryo occurs simultaneously in two planes:

- Folding in median plane or cephalocaudal folding, and
- Folding in horizontal plane or lateral folding.

RELATIVE POSITION OF VARIOUS STRUCTURES IN EMBRYONIC DISC

Before discussing the effects of folding of embryo on various structures, it will be worthwhile to revise their relative position in the flat embryonic disc. Just before folding the relative position of various structures from cranial to caudal end of embryonic disc is as follow (Fig. 4.1A to C):

- *Septum transversum,* formed by mesoderm lying cranial to the intraembryonic coelom.
- *Pericardial cavity* developing from the cranial part of intraembryonic coelom and
- *Cardiogenic plate,* i.e. developing heart from the underlying visceral mesoderm.
- *Prochordal plate,* formed by enlarged columnar endodermal cells. Prochordal plate along with overlying ectoderm forms buccopharyngeal membrane.
- *Neural plate,* formed by thickening of ectoderm in the median plane.
- *Primitive streak,* formed by thickening of ectoderm.
- *Cloacal membrane,* formed by fusion of ectoderm and endoderm in the caudal end of embryonic disc.

EFFECTS OF FOLDING OF EMBRYO

Formation of head fold, tail fold and lateral folds

Cephalocaudal folding, i.e. folding of embryo in the median plane is caused mainly by the rapid longitudinal growth of the central nervous system. Folding at the cranial end producing *head fold,* and folding at the caudal end producing *tail fold* occurs simultaneously. As a result the cranial and caudal ends of the embryonic disc move ventrally (Fig. 4.1D and F).

Lateral folding or transverse folding or folding in horizontal plane of the embryonic disc is produced by rapidly growing spinal cord and somites. Folding of the sides of embryonic disc occurs simultaneous with cephalocaudal folding and produces right and left lateral folds. These lateral folds convert the embryonic disc into cylindrical embryo and are primordia of ventrolateral wall of the body (Fig. 4.1E and G).

Formation of primitive gut

With the formation of head and tail folds, a continuously larger portion of the yolk sac lined by endoderm is incorporated into the body of the embryo proper and forms the *primitive gut* from which most of the gastrointestinal tract is developed. Primitive gut can be divided into three parts by the wide communicating stalk which connect the primitive gut with the yolk sac (Fig. 4.1E).

Foregut refers to the part of primitive gut cranial to the communicating stalk. It is the primordium of pharynx, esophagus, etc. Buccopharyngeal membrane temporarily bounds the cranial end of foregut. Soon this membrane ruptures and the foregut communicates with the amniotic cavity.

Hindgut refers to the part of primitive gut which is caudal to the communicating stalk and lies in the tail fold. It is the primordium of descending colon. The cloacal membrane temporarily bounds the caudal end of the hindgut. With folding of embryo some part of the allantois is also incorporated in the body of embryo. This part of allantois along with caudal most part of hindgut forms the *cloaca* (Fig. 4.1F), which is primodium of urinary bladder and rectum.

Midgut. The part of the gut between foregut and hindgut is called midgut (primodium of small intestine). As mentioned above, initially this part of the gut communicates with the yolk sac by way of broad stalk. However, progressively this communication becomes narrower and is called *omphalomesenteric* or *vitelline duct.* At the same time the yolk sac also becomes small and inconspicuous and is called *definitive yolk sac.* With the formation of lateral folds the embryo comes to be enclosed all around by the ectoderm except in the region through which the vitelline duct is passing. This opening on the ventral wall is called *umbilical opening.*

Expansion of amniotic cavity

As the embryonic disc folds on itself, the amniotic cavity enlarges greatly, it obliterates most of the extraembryonic coelom, and comes to surround the embryo on all sides and the amnion also forms the epithelial covering of the umbilical cord. In this way the embryo now floats in the amniotic fluid which fills the cavity (Fig. 4.1F and G).

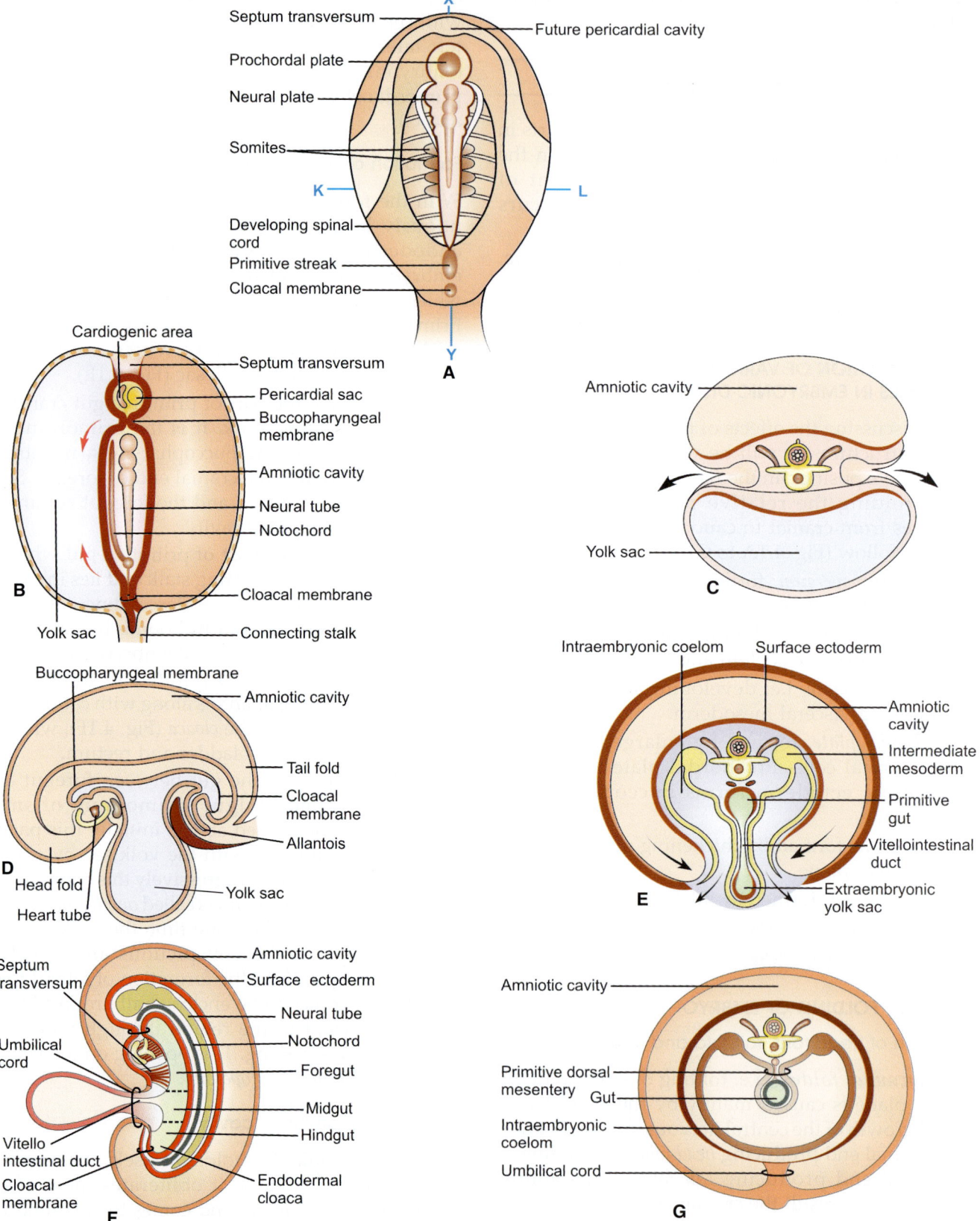

Fig. 4.1: Folding of embryo: Note positions of embryonic disc structures before folding (A), dorsal (amniotic) view, (B) section along XY axis in A; and (C) section along KL axis in A. Also note the effect of formation of head and tail folds (D) and lateral fold (E, F and G).

Effects of folding on relative position of various structures of embryo

Formation of the head and tail folds and lateral folds produce following changes (Fig. 4.1):

Enlarged cranial end of neural tube, which will form the brain, becomes the most cranial structure after folding. It enlarges very rapidly and forms cranially a bulging on the ventral aspect of the embryo.

Buccopharyngeal membrane (region of prochordal plate) comes to close the cranial end of the foregut. It forms the floor of a depression called *stomodaeum* which lies between the bulges produced by developing brain cranially and developing pericardial cavity caudally.

Pericardial cavity shifts ventrally with the formation of headfold and comes to lie ventral to the foregut. It enlarges rapidly and form a conspicuous bulging on the ventral side of the embryo.

Developing heart (from the visceral mesoderm in the floor of developing pericardial cavity), after formation of head fold, comes to lie in the roof of pericardial cavity.

Septum transversum, the most cranial structure in the embryonic disc, comes to lie caudal to the developing heart folding. The diaphragm and liver develop in relation to it in later course of development.

Primitive streak becomes an inconspicuous structure present near the tail end of embryo.

Cloacal membrane closes the distal end of hind gut and faces ventrally after folding.

CHANGES IN GERMINAL LAYERS AND THEIR DERIVATIVES

As studied earlier, during gastrulation, three germinal layers, i.e. ectoderm, mesoderm and endoderm are formed. During week 4th to 8th the three germinal layers differentiate into various tissues and organs, so that by the embryonic period the beginning of all the main organ systems have been established.

PHASES OF ORGANOGENESIS

During organogenesis, the cells of each contributing germinal layer pass through three phases:

First phase: Growth. During this phase cells of each germinal layer divide and divide with elaboration of cell products.

Second phase: Morphogenesis. During this phase the proliferated cells migrate and aggregate and give shape, size and other morphological features of the organs. Morphogenesis is an elaborate process during which many complex interactions occur in an orderly sequence between the cells of all the three germinal layers.

Third phase: Differentiation. During this phase there occurs differentiation, i.e. maturation of various physiological functions and processes specific to different tissue organs enabling them to perform their precise functions.

INDUCTION

Induction refers to the process of interaction between the developing tissues which results in stimulation of one of the interacting tissue to show the further developmental changes. In fact, the induction is the main underlying process which occurs repeatedly during organogenesis. Before studying the changes in the germinal layers and their derivatives it will be worthwhile to know about the process of induction.

Examples of induction include:

- *Notochord* induces the overlying ectodermal cells to form neural plate following process of neurulation.
- *Optic vesicles* induce the overlying surface ectoderm to get converted into lens placode and thus formation of crystalline lens.
- *Ureteric buds* induce the overlying metanephric tissue to form kidney.

Normal versus abnormal induction. It has been observed that normal induction results in normal development and failure of induction or abnormal induction results in absence of development or abnormal development, respectively.

Molecular mechanism of induction

The induction is thought to occur through transfer of signal from one tissue to the other through signaling molecules (substances).

Methods of transfer of signaling molecules from the inducing tissue to the stimulated tissue are (Fig. 4.2):

1. Diffusion of signaling molecules

Diffusion of signaling molecules occurs from the inductor cell to the reacting cell. The cell to cell signaling through the diffusable molecules is also called paracrine induction (Fig. 4.2A). Diffusible signaling molecules, also known as *paracrine factors* include: growth and differentiation factors (GDFs).

Growth factors: The signaling molecules

For details see page 16.

2. Matrix-mediated interaction

The signal is mediated through a non-diffusable extracellular matrix secreted by the inductor tissue with which the reacting tissue comes in contact (Fig. 4.2B).

Matrix mediated interaction is also called *juxtacrine interaction or signaling.*

Methods of juxtacrine signaling are:

- *Protein receptor signaling:* In this the protein on one cell surface interacts with a receptor on an adjacent cell.
- *Legend-receptor signaling.* In this the legend in the extracellular matrix secreted by one cell interacts with their receptors on the adjacent cells.
- *Direct signaling through gap junctions* in the interacting cells. Such signaling is particularly important in tightly connected cells like epithelia of gut and neural tube.

3. Cell contact mediated signal transfer

Cell contact mediated signal transfer occurs by physical contact between the inductor and reactor tissue (Fig. 4.2C).

DERIVATIVES OF GERMINAL LAYERS

This chapter includes changes occurring in three germinal layers during embryonic period. Details of development of various tissue organs from these germinal layers are described in the section on special embryology. However, all the derivatives of each layer (even if they develop in later period) are listed here for the purpose of concept making summarized in Fig. 4.3.

Changes in Ectoderm and Its Derivatives

Ectoderm, the outer of the three germ layers, gives rise to those organs and structures that maintain contact with the outside world. As studied, during neurulation some of the ectodermal cells form *neuroectoderm* and the rest form surface ectoderm:

Surface ectoderm

Changes in surface ectoderm are:

- *Formation of otic placode:* Otic placodes appear as two thickening in cephalic region which are soon converted into disc vesicles which in turn form inner ear (for details see page 274).
- *Formation of lens placodes:* Lens placodes also appear as bilateral thickening in the cephalic region. These invaginate to form *lens vesicles* which will form crystalline lens of the eye. This coincides with the appearance of *otic vesicles* from the prosencephalon (For details see page 268).
- *Appearance of folds and invaginations* in the surface ectoderm results in formation of mucous membranes lining the various cavities and structures such as oral cavity, nasal cavity, etc.

Derivatives of surface ectoderm include:

Skin and appendages: Epidermis, hair, nails, sweat glands, sebaceous glands.

Mucous membrane of:

- Oral cavity
- Nasal cavity and paranasal sinuses
- Lower part of anal canal
- Terminal part of male urethra
- Outer surface of labia minora and whole of labia majora.

Eye

- Epithelium of cornea, conjunctiva, iris and ciliary body.
- Crystalline lens.

Ear

- Outer layer of tympanic membrane
- Epithelial lining of membranous labyrinth including the special end organs.

Glands

- *Exocrine glands:* Sweat glands, sebaceous glands, parotid (and other salivary) glands, mammary gland and lacrimal gland.

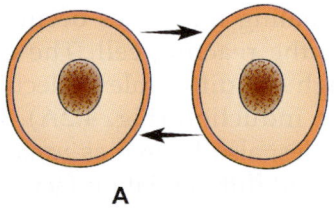 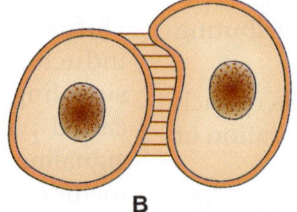 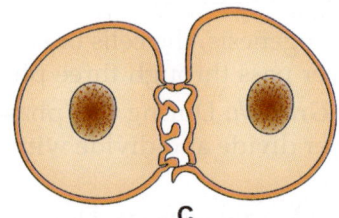

A   B   C

Fig. 4.2: Methods of transmission of cell-to-cell signals for induction: A, diffusion of signaling molecules; B, matrix mediated signaling; C, cell contact mediated interaction.

- *Endocrine glands:* Anterior part of pituitary gland.
Teeth: Enamel.

Neuroectoderm

Neuroectoderm is converted into *neural tube* and neural crest (see page 241).
Neural tube gives rise to:
- Central nervous system
- Retina
- Pineal body
- Posterior part of pituitary gland.

Neural crest gives rise to:
- Cranial and sensory nerves and ganglia
- Adrenal medulla
- Pigment cells
- Pharyngeal arch cartilages
- Head mesenchyme and connective tissue
- Bulbar and conal ridges in heart.

Changes in Mesoderm and Its Derivatives

As described in Chapter 3, formation and division of mesoderm occurs during third week of development. Derivation of various divisions of mesoderm are summarized here.

Paraxial mesoderm

The paraxial mesoderm is organized into segments, called as *somitomeres* that give rise to *mesenchymes of head* and are further organised into *somites*. Somites give rise to:
1. *Myotomes,* which give rise to striated skeletal muscles of trunk and limbs
2. *Dermatomes,* which give rise to dermis of skin, and
3. *Sclerotomes,* which give rise to skeleton except cranium.

Intermediate mesoderm

The intermediate mesoderm is organized into: nephrotomes and nephrogenic cord.
Nephrotomes. These are segmentally arranged clusters of cells in the cervical and thoracic region.
Nephrogenic cord. This is an unsegmental mass of intermediate mesoderm cells.
Derivatives. Nephrotomes and nephrogenic cord give rise to:
- *Urinary organs:* Kidneys, ureters, trigone of bladder, posterior wall of part of female urethra, posterior wall of the upper half of prostatic part of male urethra, and the inner glandular zone of prostate.

- *Reproductive organs:* In males — testes, epididymis, ductus deferens, seminal vesicles, ejaculatory duct and in female — ovaries, uterus, uterine tubes and upper part of vagina.

Lateral plate mesoderm

Lateral plate mesoderm is divided into following two layers with the formation of intraembryonic coelom (page 45, Fig. 3.15C):
- Somatopleuric or parietal layer, and
- Splanchnopleuric or visceral layer

Somatopleuric or parietal layer along with overlying ectoderm forms lateral and ventral walls of the body.
Tissues contributed by parietal layer mesoderm include:
- All connective tissues including loose areolar tissue filling the interstices between other tissues.
- Superficial and deep fascia.
- Ligaments, tendons and aponeurosis.
- Dermis of skin.
- Specialized connective tissues like adipose tissue, reticular tissue, cartilage and bone.
- All muscles.

Splanchnopleuric or visceral mesoderm gives rise to:
- Lining mesothelium of pleural, peritoneal and pericardial cavities, and of tunica vaginalis.
- Blood and lymph cells.
- Wall of heart, blood vessels and lymph vessels.

CHANGES IN ENDODERM AND ITS DERIVATIVES

Changes in endoderm. As discussed above with folding of the embryonic disc the endoderm forms the epithelial lining of primitive gut and the intraembryonic portions of the allantois and vitelline duct.

Derivatives of endoderm. Eventually the endoderm gives rise to:

Lining epithelia of following structures:
- *Gastrointestinal tract* including gallbladder, extrahepatic duct system and pancreatic duct.
- *Pharyngotympanic tube,* middle ear, inner layer of tympanic membrane, mastoid antrum and air cells.
- *Respiratory tract,*
- *Genitourinary tract:* Urinary bladder except trigone (mesodermal), female urethra except part of its posterior wall (mesodermal) male urethra except part of the posterior wall of prostatic urethra (mesodermal) and except the part of the penile urethra lying the glans (ectodermal). Part of vagina, vestibule and inner surface of labia minora.

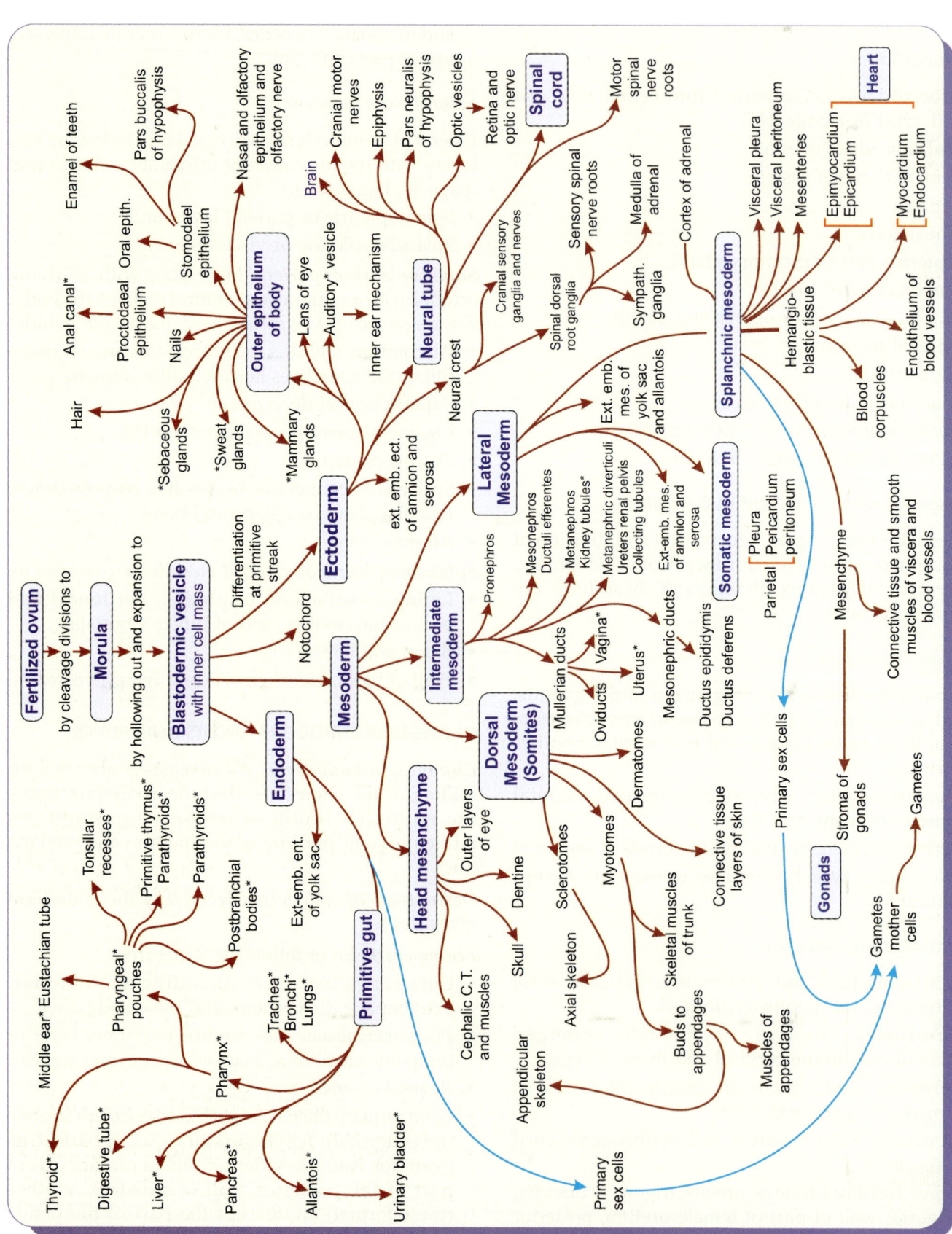

Fig. 4.3: Summary of derivation of various parts of the body by progressive differentiation from three primary germinal layers.

Glandular tissue
- *Endocrinal glands* such as thyroid, parathyroids, and islets of langerhans.
- *Exocrinal glands* such as liver, pancreas, glands in walls of gastrointestinal tract, greater part of prostate (except inner glandular zone) and its female homologues.

Reticular tissue of thymus and tonsils.

DEVELOPMENTAL STAGES OF HUMAN PRE-EMBRYO AND EMBRYO AND ESTIMATION OF EMBRYONIC AGE

HUMAN DEVELOPMENTAL STAGES

Carnegie has described 23 stages of development of human pre-embryonic and embryonic period (Day 0 to week 8). Criteria for labelling developmental stages are summarized in Table 4.1. The Carnegie embryonic staging system is used internationally.

ESTIMATION OF EMBRYONIC AGE

A. Direct method

The embryonic age can be determined accurately from the precise data of coitus and menstrual history, which helps in knowing the date of fertilization. The oocyte is usually fertilized within 12 hours after ovulation, and coitus must have occurred within 24 hours preceding fertilization. However, usually precise data is not available. A pregnant woman usually will see her obstetrician when two successive menstrual bleeds have failed to occur and by that time the recollection of coitus is usually vague.

The obstetricians calculate the date of birth 280 days or 40 weeks from the first day of last normal menstrual period (DLMP).

B. Indirect methods

Indirectly the age of human embryo can be estimated from the size and external features. The size and external features of the embryo, however, are variable and only give approximatives to the real age. The indirect methods include:

1. *Number of somites.* Between 20 to 30 days of development the age of the embryo is usually expressed in somites as below:

Number of somites	Approximate age (days)
1–4	20
4–7	21
7–10	22

Number of somites	Approximate age (days)
10–13	23
13–17	24
17–20	25
20–23	26
23–26	27
26–29	28
34–36	30

2. *Size of the embryo* is usually considered a method for approximately estimating the age of the embryo between 5th to 8th week of development. It may also be considered for smaller embryos of pre-somite period.

Methods of measuring size of embryos include:
- *Greatest length (GL)* refers to the measures of straight embryos during third and early fourth week of development (Fig. 4.4A).
- *Crown-rump length (CRL)* or the sitting height is commonly used to measure older embryos. It is the measurement from the vertex of the skull to the breech (i.e. mid point between apices of buttocks (Fig. 4.4B). The approximate age from CRL can be estimated as below :

CRL (mm)	Approximate age (weeks)
5–8	5
10–14	6
17–22	7
28–30	8

- *Neck-rump length (NRL)* is used in embryos which are markedly flexed (Fig. 4.4C).
- *Crown-heel length (CHL)* or standing height or total length is sometimes measured for 8 weeks embryo (Fig. 4.4D).

Note: The CRL and CHL are also used in estimating the approximate age of foetus as well.

3. *Carnegie embryonic staging system.* Size of embryo alone may be an unreliable criterion because some embryos may grow faster or slower. This is especially true for embryos recovered after a spontaneous abortion, which may undergo a progressive slower rate of growth prior to death. The carnegie embryonic staging system, used internationally employs the characteristic external features along with the size (Table 4.1).

KEY EVENTS DURING FOURTH TO EIGHTH WEEKS OF DEVELOPMENT

Depending upon the major events various periods of development are named as below:
- *Fourth week:* Somite and neural tube period.

Table 4.1 : Human developmental stages*

Carnegie Stage	Length (mm)	Age (Days)**	Somites	Characteristics
1	0.1	0–1	—	Fertilized uncleaved zygote
2	0.1–0.2	2–3	—	segmentation=two cells to morula
3	0.1–0.2	4–5	—	Unimplanted, free-floating blastocyst
4	0.2–0.3	6–7	—	Implantation
5	0.3–0.5	8–11	—	Progression into endometrium
6	0.2–0.5***	12–14	—	Embryonic disc, villi, and yolk sac appear
7	0.3–0.7	15–16	—	Primitive streak appears
8	0.5–2.0	17–18	—	Neural folds elevate
9	1.5–3.0	19–20	1–3	Head fold appears
10	2.0–3.0	21–23	4–12	Neural fold fusion begins, heart begins to beat
11	2.5–3.0	23–25	13–20	Two branchial arches, foregut, hindgut, optic evagination
12	3.0–4.0	21–29	21–29	Arm buds appear, neural tube closed, optic cup
13	4–5	28–30	40 (complete no.)	Leg buds appear, heart chambers, lung buds, metanephric bud
14	6–7	30–32	—	Lens invagination, septum primum, gonadal ridge
15	7–8	32–34	—	Lens vesicle closed, external ears becoming recognizable
16	9–10	35–36	—	Eye pigment appears, hand plate, hypophysis, liver
17	11–14	37–40	—	Finger rays, foot plate, ear defined, somites less apparent superficially
18	14–16	40–42	—	Eyelid, finger rays notched, toe rays, nerve plexuses
19	17–20	42–44	—	Head more erect, limbs extend forward, muscles developing, duodenum closed
20	21–23	45–46	—	Fingers, scalp plexus present, optic nerve, septum secundum
21	22–24	46–48	—	Hands meet over heart region, corpus striatum, thalamus, heart valves
22	25–27	48–50	—	Fingers overlap those of opposite hand, duodenum reopened
23	28–30	50–52	—	Head erect and rounded, scalp plexus reaching head vertex, ossification begins

*   From Streeter GL (1959) : *Developmental Horizons in Human Embryos.* Carnegie Institution of Washington, Washington, D.C.; Rahilly R. (1973) : *Developmental Stages in Human Embryos. Part A : Embroys of the First Three Weeks (Stages 1 to 9).* Carnegie Institution of Washington, Pub. 631, Washington, D.C.

**   Gestational age in days established from Iffy L, Shepard TH, Jakobovits A, Lemire RJ, and Kerner P (1967): The rate of growth in young human embryos of Streeter's horizon XII to XXIII, *Acta Anat. 66 : 178–186.*

***   Stage six refers to embryonic disc only, stage 5 refers to overall size. Stages thereafter refer to crown-rump length.

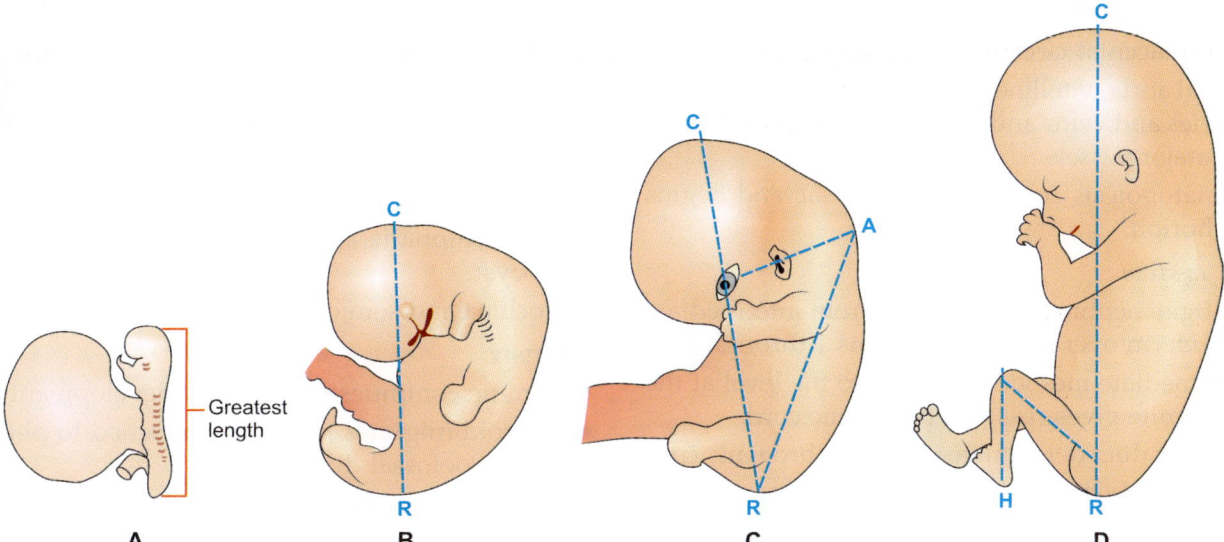

Fig. 4.4: Methods of measuring embryos : A, greatest length; B, crown-rump length; C, neck-rump length, and D, crown heal length.

- *Fifth week:* Early pharyngeal arch and limb bud period.
- *Sixth week:* Late pharyngeal arch and limb bud period.
- *Seventh week and eighth week:* Late embryonic period.

Key events during fourth to eighth week of development are mentioned below briefly.

FOURTH WEEK: SOMITE AND NEURAL TUBE PERIOD

Embryo (Fig. 4.5A)

External body form

- Embryo changes from disc-shaped to tubular by folding.
- Head and neck regions appear disproportionately large.
- Prominent pericardial elevation early in week.
- Hepatic elevation later in week.
- Limb buds appear late in week.
- Umbilical cord begins to take form.

Nervous system

- Neural folds fuse to form neural tube by 22nd or 23rd day.
- Anterior neuropore closes by 26th day.
- Histogenesis of neural tube begins.
- Neural crest is differentiated.
- Mesencephalic flexure becomes evident.

Special senses

- Otic placode appears early in week.
- Placode is transformed to otocyst by end of week.

- Optic vesicles appear as lateral grooves in the prosencephalon.
- Ectoderm overlying optic vesicle forms lens placode.

Pharynx

- Pharyngeal arches, grooves and clefts appear.
- Thyroid diverticulum appears.
- Anlagen of tongue present.
- Buccopharyngeal membrane breaks down.

Pulmonary system

- Laryngotracheal groove appears at midweek.
- Groove delaminates from foregut.
- Caudal extension of groove bifurcates to form lung buds.

Digestive system

- Esophagus and stomach delineated.
- Hepatic diverticulum appears and grows into septum transversus.
- Gallbladder diverticulum appears.
- Dorsal pancreatic bud appears.
- Urorectal septum arises late in the week to begin division of the cloaca.

Mesenteries and intraembryonic coelom

- Primitive dorsal and ventral mesenteries formed.
- Most of primitive ventral mesentery soon disappears to form single peritoneal cavity.
- Pericardial cavity formed but remains joined to peritoneal cavity by the pericardioperitoneal canals.

Cardiovascular system

- Primitive heart forms and begins beating early in the week.

- Aortic arches formed.
- Fetal-placental circulation begun.
- Dorsal aorta, vitelline arteries and veins, umbilical arteries and veins and the cardinal system of veins are major vessels.
- Hematopoiesis continues in yolk sac and begins in chorion.

Renal system
- Vestigial nephrotomes develop from intermediate mesoderm over somatic segments 1 through 7.
- Intermediate mesoderm caudal to the level at the 8th somite gives rise to nephrogenic cord.
- Nephric duct delaminates from nephrogenic cord over somatic segments 9 through 14.
- Nephric duct is at first solid but later canalized.
- Nephric duct grows caudally to joins the cloaca.
- Nephrogenic cord gives rise to primitive nephric vesicles which become functional nephrons.

Placenta
- Placenta is functional with both fetal and maternal circulation through placenta being established.
- Cytotrophoblastic shell defined.
- Maturation changes begin.

FIFTH WEEK: EARLY PHARYNGEAL ARCH AND LIMB BUD PERIOD
Embryo (Fig. 4.5B)

External body form
- Head becomes prominent.
- Limb buds exhibit basic plan of limb, forelimb and hand or foot.
- Face develops.

Nervous system
- Pontine flexure appears.
- Telencephalic vesicles appear.
- Ventricular system essentially established.
- Cerebellar thickenings appear.
- Most brain centers and fiber tracts begin differentiation.
- Spinal nerves formed.
- Cranial nerves developing.

Special senses
- Olfactory placodes appear and develop into olfactory pits.
- Olfactory pits abut on walls of cerebral hemispheres and roof of stomodaeum.
- Bucconasal membrane breaks down forming primitive internal nares.

- Primitive nasal septum formed.
- Optic cup formed with ventral optic fissure.
- Two layers of optic cup meet to form primitive retina.
- Lens placode becomes lens vesicle.
- Primary vitreous body formed.
- Endolymphatic appendage formed from wall of otocyst.
- Cochlea and semicircular canals begin forming.

Pharynx
- Tongue continues growth and development.
- Thyroid migrates remaining attached to pharynx by thyroglossal duct.
- Parathyroids and thymus develop.
- Tubotympanic recess formed from first pouch.
- Cervical sinus formed externally.

Pulmonary system
- Laryngotracheal tube separated from esophagus.
- Primary, secondary and tertiary bronchi formed by bifurcation of lung buds.

Digestive system
- Esophagus elongates.
- Stomach forms greater and lesser curvatures and rotates.
- Ventral pancreas appears and migrates to meet with dorsal pancreas.
- Midgut loop formed and begins rotation.
- Spleen develops in dorsal mesogastrium.

Mesenteries and intraembryonic coelom
- Greater and lesser omenta formed.
- Mesentery expanded with midgut loop forming fan-shaped structure.
- Mesenteric attachments of liver apparent.

Cardiovascular system
- Shift of sino-atrial orifice to right.
- Septum primum forms in roof of primitive atrium.
- Ostium primum formed by advancing septum primum.
- Ostium primum obliterated, ostium secundum appears.
- Septum secundum forms to right of septum primum.
- Foramen ovale formed.
- Muscular portion of interventricular septum appears.
- Aorticopulmonary septum forms.
- Septation of heart completed by formation of membranous portion of interventricular septum.

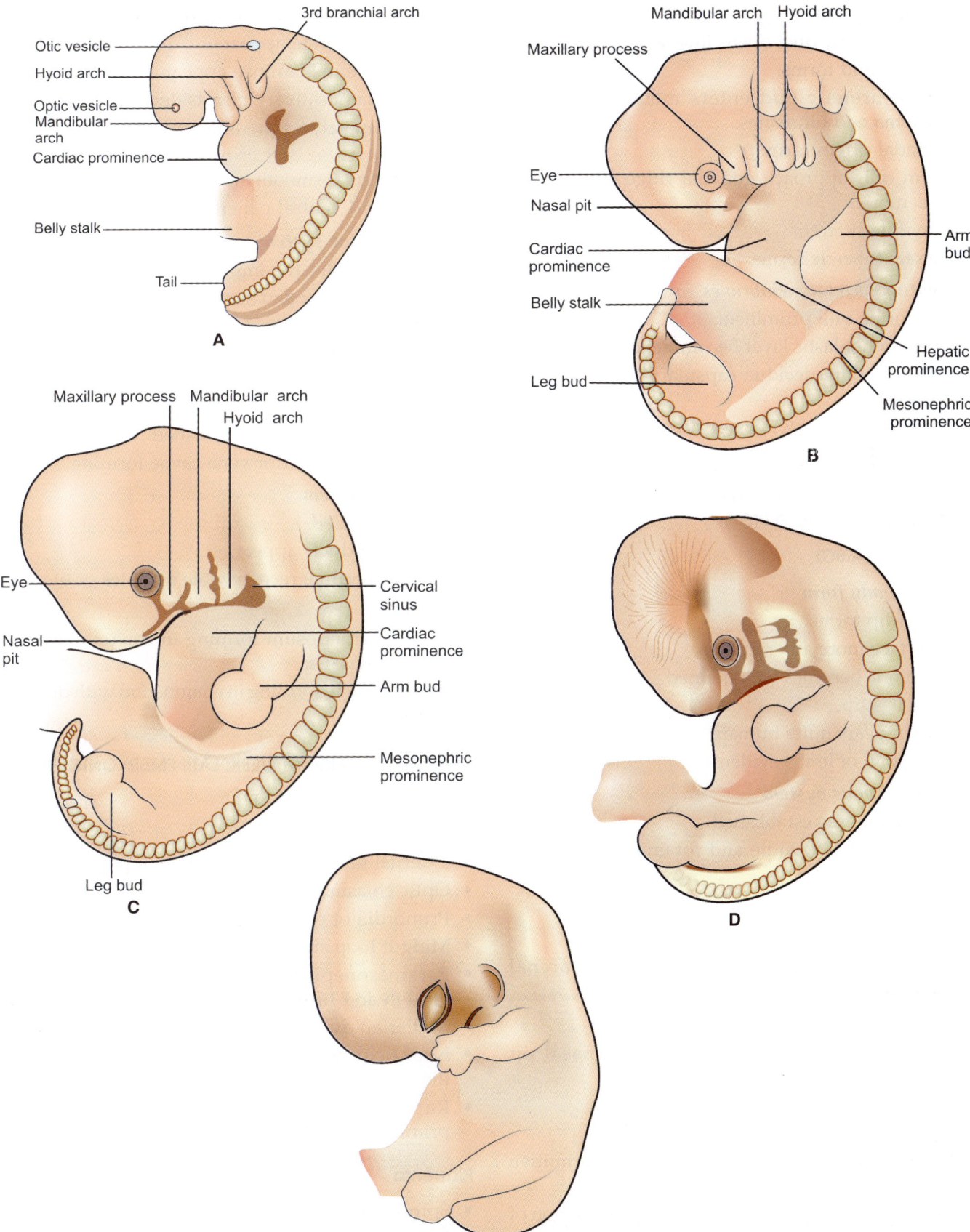

Fig. 4.5: Cardinal features during embryonic phase of development: A, 4-week old embryo; B, 5-week old embryo; C, 6-week old embryo; D, 7-week old embryo; and E, 8-week old embryo.

Urogenital system
- Patent nephric duct opens into urogenital sinus.
- Ureteric bud forms.
- Tip of ureteric bud enters metanephrogenic blastema and bifurcates.
- Gonadal ridges form.
- Germ cells approach gonadal ridge from dorsal mesenteries.
- Gonad indifferent.
- Genital tubercle forms.

Placenta and fetal membranes
- Anchoring villi prominent.
- Cytotrophoblastic layer becoming less prominent.
- Villi adjoining decidua capsularis becoming less prominent.
- Intervillous space not yet directly supplied by endometrial arterioles.

SIXTH WEEK: LATE PHARYNGEAL ARCH AND LIMB BUD PERIOD

Embryo (Fig. 4.5C)

External body form
- Upper lip forms.
- Eyes face more anteriorly.
- Ear pinna becomes well defined.
- Nose has tip.
- Face appears quite human.
- Basic plan of limbs evident.

Central nervous system
- Simple reflexes established.
- Foramen of Magendie and foramina of Luschka formed.

Autonomic nervous system
- Basic plan of system established.
- Migrating neural crest cells form suprarenal medulla.

Special senses
- Olfactory neuroblasts develop from nasal pit epithelium.
- Initial differentiation of retina.
- Optic nerve fibers reach chiasma.
- Cornea, iris and ciliary body appear in primitive form.
- Condensation of mesoderm indicates formation of sclera and extrinsic eye muscles.
- Otic capsule beginning chondrification.
- Precartilaginous condensation in ossicles.

Alimentary and respiratory systems
- Secondary palate appears.
- Primary dental laminae appear.
- Primordia of salivary glands develop.
- Approximately 8 generations of lung bud division present.
- Inner, circular smooth muscle layer develops in gut.
- Dorsal and ventral pancreatic segments fuse.

Cardiovascular system
- Septation of heart complete.
- Atrioventricular and semilunar valves develop.
- Sinus venosus absorbed into the wall of right atrium.
- Pulmonary vein absorbed into the wall of left atrium.
- Venosus system markedly modified.
- Basic arterial pattern established.
- Superior and inferior vena cavae forming.

Urogenital system
- Cloaca divided.
- Müllerian ducts appear.
- Gonads become recognizable as testes or ovaries.

Placenta
- Chorion frondosum forming in conjunction with decidua basalis.
- Chorion laeve forming in conjunction with decidua capsularis.

SEVENTH AND EIGHTH WEEK: LATE EMBRYONIC PERIOD

Embryo (Fig. 4.5D and E)

- Eyelids grossly evident.
- External nares closed by epithelial plugs.
- Optic chiasma well established.
- Primordia of palatine tonsils appear.
- Midgut loop still herniated.
- Paramesonephric or müllerian ducts complete growth and fuse.
- Müllerian duct begins to degenerate in the male.
- Nephric or wölffian duct begins to degenerate in the female.
- Rathke's pouch completely separated from primitive mouth.

Placenta

- Spiral arterioles are topped.
- Blood enters intervillous space under pressure.
- Cotyledons begin formation.
- Invasiveness of trophoblast cease.

Fetal Period of Development (Ninth Week to Birth)

GENERAL CONSIDERATIONS
- Main characteristics of growth during fetal period

HIGHLIGHTS OF DEVELOPMENT DURING FETAL PERIOD
- Key events during third month
- Key events during fourth month

- Key events during fifth month
- Key events during sixth month
- Key events during third trimester months
- Full term fetus and expected date of delivery

APPLIED ASPECTS
- Low birth weight baby
- Prenatal screening techniques

GENERAL CONSIDERATIONS

It is customary to use the term fetus for the growing embryo from the commencement of the third month (9th week) to the end of gestation (normal birth, usually 38 weeks after fertilization). Though the distinction is arbitrary but usually by the beginning of 9th week the developing embryo acquires all the characteristics which can be recognized later in development and the embryo gives an unmistakably human appearance.

Main characteristics of growth during fetal period

Main characteristics of fetal period of development are:

Body growth is very rapid.

Differentiation of tissues occurs rapidly leading to maturation of the organ system.

Growth in length is particularly striking during 3rd, 4th and 5th months (approximately 5 cm/month), and at the end of first half of intrauterine life the crown-rump length (CRL) is approximately 15 cm, i.e. about half of the total length of the new born (Table 5.1 and Fig. 5.1).

Weight of the fetus increases rather slow during first half of intrauterine life and by the end of 5th month is usually less than 500 gm. The weight increases considerably during second half of intrauterine life particularly during last 2½ months (@ approximately 700 gm/month), when about 50% of the full term weight (average 3200 gm) is added (Table 5.1).

Head growth is peculiarly slow compared to the growth of rest of the body during whole of the fetal period. This accounts for the following changing ratio between the head size and fetal length (Fig. 5.2):

- *At the beginning of 3rd month,* the head constitutes about one half CRL (i.e. head : CRL :: 1:1).

- *At the beginning of 5th month,* the size of the head is about one third of CHL (i.e. head : CHL :: 1:3).

- *At birth,* the size of head is about one-fourth of CHL (i.e. head : CHL :: 1:4).

Table 5.1. Growth in length and weight during the fetal period

Period of growth	Crown-rump length (CRL) in cm (approximate)	Weight (gm) (approximate)
3rd month (week 9–12)	8	45
4th month (week 13–16)	14	200
5th month (week 17–20)	19	450
6th month (week 21–24)	23	800
7th month (week 25–28)	27	1500
8th month (week 29–32)	30	2200
9th month (week 33–36)	34	2900
9½ month (week 37–38)	36	3300

HIGHLIGHTS OF DEVELOPMENT DURING FETAL PERIOD

There is no formal staging system for the fetal period; however it is customary to consider the development changes during fetal period as below:

- Key events during third month of gestation.
- Key events during fourth month of gestation.
- Key events during fifth month of gestation.
- Key events during sixth month of gestation.
- Key events during third trimester of gestation.

KEY EVENTS DURING THIRD MONTH

Fetal growth and changes in external form

Length of fetus increases rapidly. The crown-rump length (CRL) nearly doubles, i.e. increases from 50 to 80 mm and the crown-heal length (CHL) becomes about 95 mm (Fig. 5.1).

Weight of the fetus increases from about 10 gm in the beginning of third month to about 45 gm by the end of this month.

Head grows slowly as compared to the body and is still about 1/2 of fetal body length (Fig. 5.2).

Face becomes more human-looking with following changes occurring by the end of third month.

- *Forehead* is high and prominent and the face is wide.
- *Eyes* which are widely separated and located laterally at 9 weeks, come to lie on the ventral aspect of face by the end of 12 weeks. The eyelids meet and remain fused throughout the period.
- *Ears* which are initially low set come to lie close to their definitive position at the side of head.

Trunk region becomes relatively more slim, the liver region is less protuberant and the hernia of the midgut into the extraembryonic coelom in the region of umbilical cord is reduced.

Limbs show following changes:

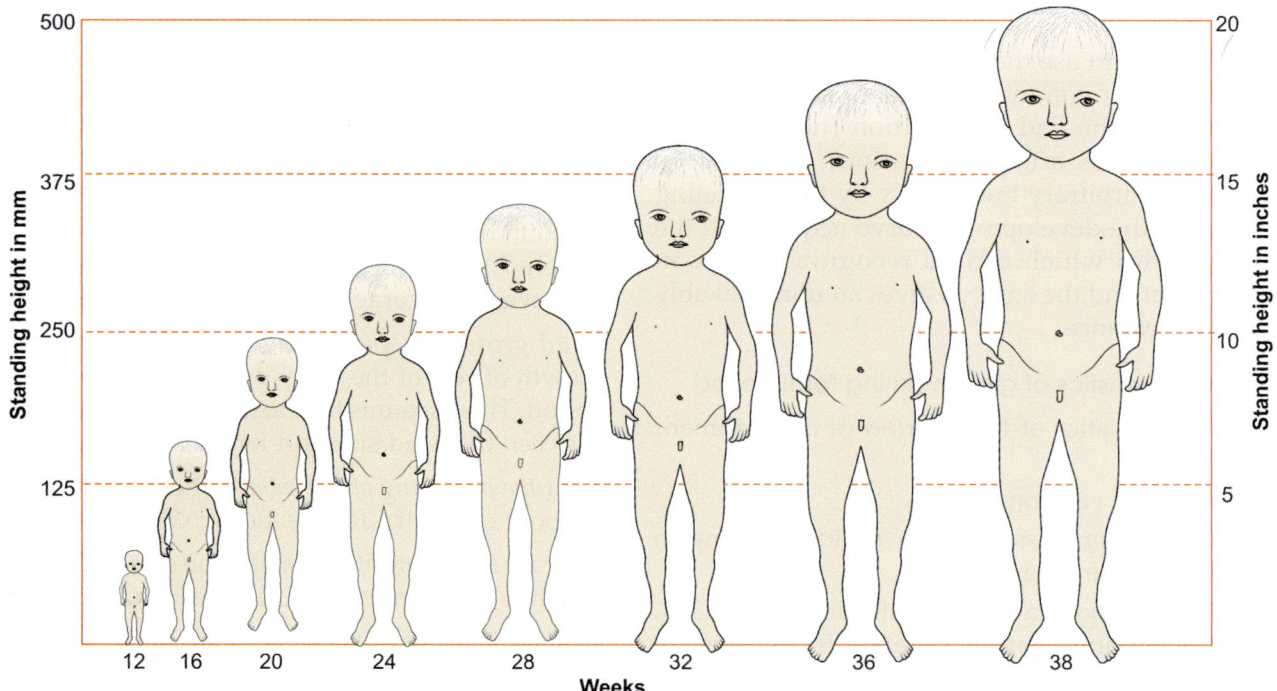

Fig. 5.1: Growth in length of human fetus.

- *Upper limbs* attain their final relative length. Nails are well indicated by furrows on the dorsal aspects of tips of fingers.
- *Lower limbs* are less well developed, and the toes are still spread out fanwise and their nails are only represented by slight furrows.

Growth and development of organ systems

Skeletal system shows following changes:

- *Primary ossification centers* appear in the long bones and skull bones.
- *Bone marrow* begins to continue in the humerus and begins to form in some other bones.

Urogenital system shows marked changes:

- *Degeneration of mesonephric tubules* and early generation of metanephric tubules continue. Degeneration of wölffian ducts in females and Müllerian ducts continue in males.
- *External genitalia* of male and female, which appear similar in the 9th week, develop to such a degree by the end of 12 weeks, that the sex of the fetus can be determined by external examination (ultrasound).
- *Urine formation* begins between 9th and 12th weeks and urine is discharged into the amniotic fluid. The fetus reabsorbs some of the amniotic fluid by swallowing.

Haemopoiesis, at nine weeks, occurs mainly in the liver. By the end of 12 weeks, this activity is decreased in the liver and begins in the spleen and bone marrow of humerus and some other bones.

Integumentary system shows following changes:

- *Epidermis* is established early in the third month and the complete fetal surface is covered with a layer of periderm.
- *Dermis* differentiation begins in the later months and melanocytes appear.
- *Hair*–Towards the end of third month a much more extensive crop of very fine fetal hair (lanugo), appears in the region of forehead and eyebrow.
- *Nails*–Primordia of digital nails appear by about the middle of the month.

Nervous system. Essential events are:

- *Histogenesis* of the cerebral cortex continues as does organization of brain and brainstem nuclei.
- *Cervical and pontine flexures* become progressively less pronounced with the pontine flexure disappearing by the end of month.

Digestive system: The key events are:

- *Return of the herniated midgut* loop to the abdominal cavity is the most significant event for this organ system (as also mentioned above in the trunk).
- *Glands begin to develop* in the mucosa of esophagus, stomach and small intestine.

Respiratory system. The key event is chondrification of the lobar bronchi.

Changes in placenta and fetal membranes

- *Amnion* expands rapidly and nearly fills the chorionic cavity.
- *Chorionic cavity* or extra-embryonic coelom is nearly obliterated by the end of the month due to expansion of amnion.
- *Placental changes* are:
  - Chorion frondosum become well defined fetal part of placenta.
  - Decidua basalis becomes the maternal part of placenta.
  - Cotyledons are formed and reach 1/10 definitive size.
  - Cytotrophoblast layer continues to disappear.

KEY EVENTS DURING FOURTH MONTH

Fetal growth and changes in external form

Crown-rump length (CRL) or sitting height of the fetus is about 140 mm by the end of 4th month (Fig. 5.1).

Weight of the fetus increases to about 200 gm by the end of month.

Facial and other external body features not only look human like, but the differences between fetus at his age and adult become progressively less pronounced. Salient facial changes are:

- *Head* is still disproportionately large but the head and body length ratio is further reduced to 1:3 (Fig. 5.2).
- *Eyes,* while still widespread, but the orbital axis angle is reduced. Eyelids still remain fused with periderm.
- *Chin* is formed due to development of the mandible.
- Indentation between nose and forehead is further reduced.
- *Ear pinnae* have characteristic appearance.
- *External nares* are patent by the end of month.
- *Limbs* reach a point where they are essentially proportional to each other and to the trunk. *Nails,* which appeared in the third month, continue to differentiate. *Scalp hair* patterning is determined during 14 to 16 weeks.

Fetal movements. Fetus begins active movements by the end of 4th month. Awareness to the mother of

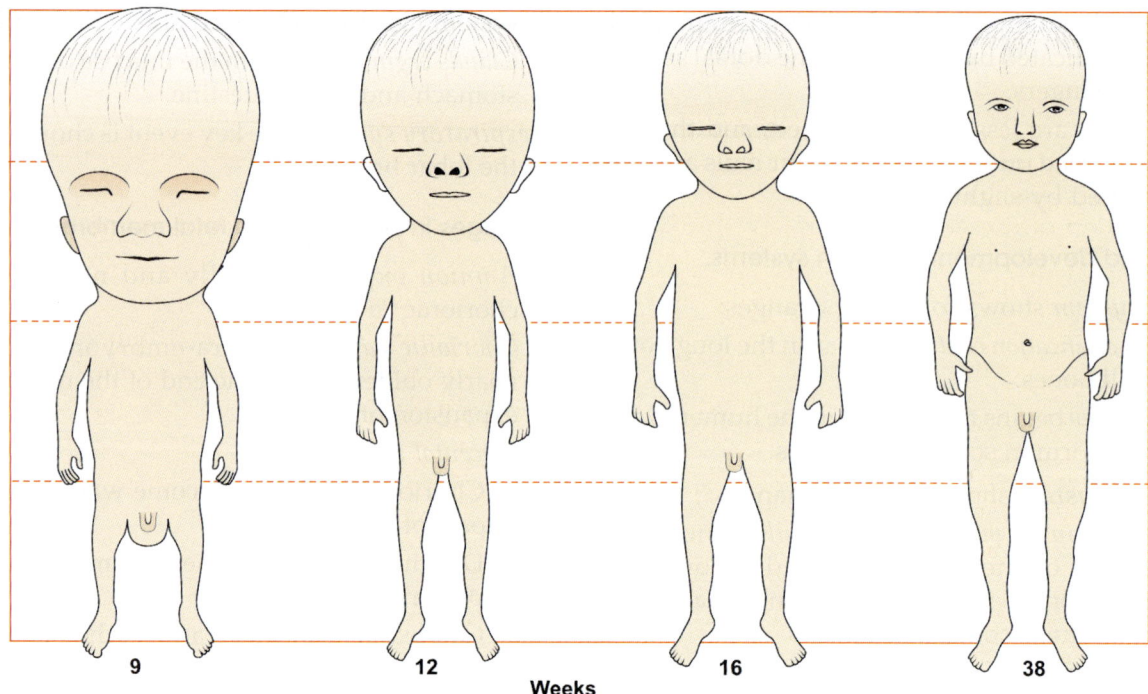

Fig. 5.2: Changing ratio of head size with fetal length during fetal period.

fetal movement is referred as *quickening*. These first movements are the cause of excitement on the part of mother.

External genitalia become unequivocally male or female and diagnosis is certain. The genitalia are still not complete at this time but subsequent changes are limited to relative minor modifications.

Skeletal system. Ossification centers appear in some other bones. Fetal skeleton becomes detectable on X-rays film by about 14th weeks.

Changes in placenta and fetal membranes

Placenta is essentially defined by the end of 4th month. Growth and hypertrophy of the cotyledons system continues through this month. Placenta and fetus are approximately equal in weight by the end of this month.

Amnion completes the obliteration of the extra-embryonic coelom by a loose fusion with the chorion.

Chorion. Formation of the chorion leave is completed. Fusion of chorion leave with the decidua parietalis leads to obliteration of the uterine cavity by 14 to 15th week.

KEY EVENTS DURING FIFTH MONTH

Fetal growth and changes in external form

Crown-rump length (CRL): Growth of the fetus is bit slowed down but the CRL increases by 50 mm by the end of month (i.e. increases from 140 mm to 190 mm) (Fig. 5.1).

Weight of the fetus increases from about 200 gm at the end of 4th month to about 450 gm by the end of 5th month.

External features. The fetus continues to appear more and more human. *Limbs, head and trunk* reach their final relative proportions.

- *Umbilical cord* is displaced cephalic due to striking expansion of the infra-umbilical region of the trunk.
- *Chin, nose and ear pinnae* become more pronounced.
- *Eyes* become frontally placed and by the end of month the epithelial fusion of eyelids begins to breakdown, although separation of eyelids does not occur until the 7th month.

Skin shows following changes:

- *Vernix caseosa,* a greasy, cheese like material covers the skin. It consists of a mixture of fatty secretions from the fetal sebaceous glands and dead epidermal cells and protects the delicate fetal skin.
- *Hair*—By the end of 5th month the fetal body is covered with fine downy hair (lanugo).
- *Brown fat* is formed during 8th month and is the site of heat production particularly in the newborn infant.

Genitourinary system shows following features:

- *In the male fetus,* the testes begin to descend by 20th week, but they are still located on the posterior abdominal wall. The external genitalia continue to advance towards a definitive state specifically, the phallus continues to elongate and the prepuce becomes well defined.

- *In the female fetus,* uterus is formed by 18th week and canalization of vagina begins. By the end of this month the female external genitalia attain the final form. The ovaries exhibit a secondary proliferation of mesenchyme and sex cords, and many primordial ovarian follicles containing oogonia are formed.

Placental changes

- *Morphogenesis* of placenta is completed by the beginning of 5th month. No major structural changes occur during this period.
- *Weight* of the placenta increases progressively.
- *Placental circulation.* The fetal component of the placental circulation begins with the paired umbilical arteries. Hydrostatic pressure in intervillous space is 5 to 10 mm of Hg and in villous capillaries is 15 to 30 mm of Hg.

KEY EVENTS DURING SIXTH MONTH

Changes in fetus

Crown-rump length (CRL) increases to about 230 mm by the end of sixth month, *weight* of the fetus increases remarkably and reaches upto about 800 gm by the end of month, which is about one-fourth of the average weight of the term fetus.

External features. By the end of sixth month the face is more infant like.

- *Eye brows and eyelids* are well formed.
- *Eye movements:* Rapid eye movements (REM) begin at 21 weeks and blink startle responses have been reported at 22 to 23 weeks.
- *Head* remains disproportionately large but relatively less so than previously as head, trunk and limbs continue to approach the characteristic adult proportions.
- *Umbilicus and pubic arch* exhibit a further spatial separation due to continued expansion of infra-umbilical region.
- *Skin* is characteristically wrinkled markedly, presumably, due to its more rapid growth than the underlying connective tissue. It has a deep pink to reddish hue, and is covered with darker lanugo.
- *Limbs:* Finger nails are present by the end of this month.

Respiratory system. Secretory epithelial cells in the interalveolar walls of the lungs start secreting *surfactant,* a surface active lipid that maintains the patency of the developing alveoli of the lung. The fetus begins to make some feeble respiratory movements and if delivered at this time may make attempts to breathe *ex utero.*

Nervous system. The layers of cerebral cortex are all defined. Myelination of the cord continues.

Haematopoiesis in the spleen is minimal early in the month but decreases rather markedly by the end of month. By about mid-month hematopoiesis begins in the sternum.

Genitourinary system. Vaginal lumen is completed and ovarian sex cords are well defined.

- *Renal pelvis* exhibits establishment of subdivisions.

Digestive system. Key events are:

- *Stomach glands* exhibit limited function
- *Pancreas* begins to produce proteolytic enzymes.

Placental changes

- No major structural change.
- Progressive growth with increase in weight.
- Becomes typically discoid in shape and covers the bulk of either the anterior or posterior uterine wall.
- Abnormal configuration of the placenta may be established in some cases, e.g. bipartite placenta, succenturiate placenta, fenestrated placenta, membranous placenta, circumvallate placenta, etc. (for details see page 77).

KEY EVENTS DURING THIRD TRIMESTER (7TH, 8TH AND 9TH MONTHS)

The key events of third trimester (7th, 8th and 9th months) can be considered combinedly because this is a period primarily of growth and maturation, and developmental events during this period are not necessarily contigent on continuation of life *in utero.*

Fetal growth and changes in external form

Crown-rump length (CRL) becomes approximately:

- 270 mm by the end of 28 weeks,
- 300 mm by the end of 32 weeks,
- 340 mm by the end of 36 weeks, and
- 360 mm by the end of 38 weeks.

Weight shows spectacular increase with an average gain of 25 gm per day. As a result the weight increases from about 800 gm by the end of 8th month to about 3000–3400 gm by end of term.

Facial and other external body features

- *Body contours and skin.* Contours of the fetus become rounded due to progressive deposition of subcutaneous fat and thickening of skin. Thus the wrinkled reddish skin noted earlier gradually disappears.

- *Eyelids* are separated during the seventh month.
- *Face* continues to appear more human and by the end of eighth month, the fetus, except perhaps the size, looks quite like any term fetus.
- *Vellus hair* on the body, particularly on the scalp, become more and more prominent while Lanugo hair is gradually shed.
- *Vernix caseosa* continues to accumulate over the last trimester and is seen to cover the term fetus.
- *Limbs.* The lower extremity grows progressively, but even at full term it is not as long as the upper. Finger-nails project beyond the finger tips and the toe-nails reach the end of toes till the end of third trimester.

Organ systems

- Muscular, digestive, cardiovascular and urinary system are essentially functional at term.
- *Respiratory system* is defined but the alveoli do not develop until after term.
- *Hematopoiesis* in the liver reaches a maximal level about the 28–30th week and then begins to decline rather sharply and becomes non-existent at term.
- *Testes* begin to descend in the scrotum in seventh month and the descent is completed before term.
- *Nervous system:* Myelination of the cord continues and that of brain begins prior to term.

FULL TERM FETUS AND EXPECTED DATE OF DELIVERY

Full term fetus

- *Weight.* Near birth a full-term fetus normally weights a little over 7 lbs (3000 gm), although any weight between 5 lbs and 10 lbs is within normal range. Heredity appears to be more significant in determining the weight of full-term fetus than does maternal diet.
- *Length.* The total body length is about 20 inches (50 cm); the sitting height (CRL) is about 12–13 inches (30–33 cm) (Fig. 5.1).
- *Head circumference* is about 12–13 inches (30–33 cm).
- *Chest circumference* is normally rather less than that of head.
- *Abdomen circumference* at the umbilical level approximates that of chest.
- *Arms and trunk* are longer than the legs.
- *Testes,* in the male fetus are normally in the scrotum at the time of birth.
- *Organ systems,* mostly are functional at full-term, they lack the latitude necessary for rapid and

adequate adaptation to environmental changes which occur during birth. In other words the newly born infant's physiological processes are capable of sustaining life given the safety of a well-controlled external environment and the nature of that external environment is dependent on prenatal manipulation.

Expected date of delivery

Expected date of delivery (EDD) can be calculated by two methods:

1. *From date of fertilization.* EDD is most accurately indicated as 266 days or 38 weeks after fertilization. However, usually it is not possible to know the exact date of fertilization. This is because, by the time the women contact her obstetrician, her recollection about the date of coitus is vague.
2. *From date of last menstrual period.* Practically, most obstetricians calculate the EDD as 280 days or 40 weeks after the first day of last menstrual period (DLMP). However, this also not fool proof method. This method is accurate in women with regular 28 days menstrual cycle, but when cycles are irregular, miscalculations about EDD are most likely.

Premature and postmature fetuses. In general most fetuses are delivered within 10–14 days of calculated EDD.

- *Premature* delivery is labelled when the fetus is born before 34 weeks of gestation.
- *Postmature* delivery is labelled when the fetus is born after 38 weeks of gestation.

APPLIED ASPECTS

LOW BIRTH WEIGHT BABY

According to world health organisation (WHO) definition.

Low birth weight baby is one whose birth weight is less than 2500 gm irrespective of the gestational age.

- *Very-low birth weight* infant weighs less than 1500 gms, and
- *Extremely low birth weight* infant weighs 1000 gm or less.

Types of low birth weight babies according to the gestational age are:

- *Preterm low birth weight baby.* The growth potential is normal and is appropriate for the gestational period.
- *Small for gestational age (SGA).* This term is used to designate the newborn with birth weight less than

10th percentile or less than two standard deviation for their gestational age. A fetus of SGA may be:

- Constitutionally small or due to pathological process (intrauterine growth restriction).

Intrauterine growth restriction

Intrauterine growth restriction (IUGR) is labelled when birth weight is below the tenth percentile of the average for the gestational age due to some pathological process. Such babies have increased prenatal mortality and morbidity.

Causes of IUGR

1. *Maternal causes* include:
   - *Malnutrition.* Deficiency of glucose, amino acids and oxygen in mother during pregnancy is a common cause of IUGR.
   - *Maternal diseases* like anaemia, hypertension, thrombophilia, heart disease, chronic renal disease collagen vascular diseases are common causes of IUGR.
   - *Toxin intake,* such as alcohol, smoking, cocaine, heroin and certain drugs, is associated with IUGR.

2. *Fetal causes,* which lead to failure of utilization of substrates from the maternal blood crossing through placenta are associated with IUGR. These include:
   - *Structural anomalies,* either cardiovascular, renal or other.
   - *Chromosomal anomalies* such as triploidy and aneuploidy. Trisomies (13, 18, 21) and Turner's syndrome are commonly observed.
   - *Infections,* e.g. by TORCH agents (toxoplasmosis, rubella, cytomegalovirus and herpes simplex) and malaria.

- *Multiple pregnancies.* Individuals of twin, triplet, and other multiple births usually weigh considerably less than infants resulting from a single pregnancy. This occurs due to mechanical hindrance to growth and excessive fetal demand.
- *Placental dysfunction or defects* (e.g. infarction, placenta praevia, placenta circumvallete, etc.) decrease the exchange of nutrients from the maternal blood and may cause IUGR.
- *Idiopathic.* In about 40% cases the cause of IUGR is unknown.

PRENATAL SCREENING TECHNIQUES

Various prenatal screening techniques are available for assessing the status of fetus and diagnosing certain diseases and developmental anomalies before birth.

Aims of prenatal diagnosis are to recommend any of the following:

- *Assurance to the parents,* when fetus is growing well.
- *Medical termination of pregnancy* may be recommended in early stage when severe anomalies incompatible with postnatal life are diagnosed (e.g. absence of most of brain).
- *Medical treatment* may be recommended in selected cases, e.g. administration of drugs to correct cardiac arrhythmia or thyroid disorders.
- *Surgical correction* of some anomalies in utero is also possible, e.g. surgical establishment of opening of the ureters into the bladder in fetuses that have ureters which do not open into the bladder.

METHODS OF PRENATAL SCREENING

For details see page 294.

Placenta, Umbilical Cord, and Fetal Membranes

PLACENTA
Formation
Placental membrane: exchange between maternal and fetal blood
- Uterine circulation
- Circulation of the placenta
- Exchange between maternal and fetal blood
- Variation anomalies of placenta

UMBILICAL CORD
- Primitive umbilical cord
- Definitive umbilical cord

FETAL MEMBRANES AND AMNIOTIC FLUID
- Fetal membranes
- Amniotic fluid
- Fetal membranes in twins

PLACENTA

Placenta is a temporary organ formed during pregnancy. It forms an important circulatory link between the mother and fetus.

Note: Since the formation of placenta is related to the implantation, so it will be worthwhile to revise this related text (page 34) before proceeding further.

FORMATION OF PLACENTA

The placenta consists of two major portions:
- Maternal part of placenta, (derived from decidua), and
- Fetal part of placenta (derived from chorion)

DECIDUA: ROLE IN FORMATION OF PLACENTA

Decidua refers to the functional layer of endometrium after implantation of the blastocyst stage of the fertilized ovum *(gravid endometrium).* The term *decidua* (meaning falling off) is used for this part of

endometrium, as it separates from the remainder of uterus and falls away during *child birth.*

Decidual reaction refers to the changes in the endometrium which convert it into decidual cells. Due to effect of increasing progesterone levels in maternal blood, the stromal cells of endometrium get converted into decidual cells by becoming enlarged, vacuolated and filled with glycogen and lipids. The stored glycogen and lipid are the source of nutrition for the embryo till placenta takes up this function.

Parts of decidua are named as below (Fig. 6.1):
- *Decidua basalis* or decidual plate refers to the part where maternal part of placenta is to develop.
- *Decidua capsularis* is that part of the decidua which overlies the embryo and separates it from the uterine cavity.
- *Decidua parietalis* refers to the part of the decidua lining the rest of uterine cavity.

Note: As the conceptus enlarges in due course of development the decidua capsularis bulges into the

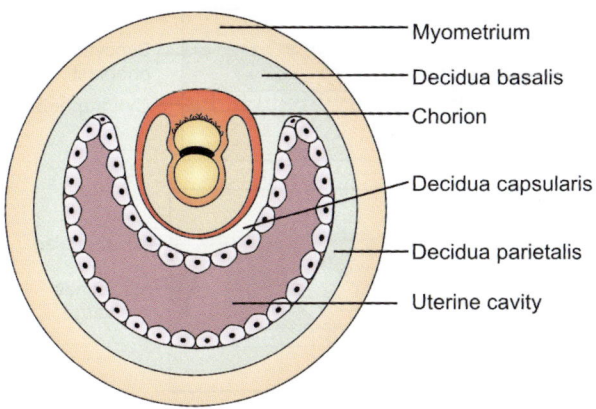

Fig. 6.1: Parts of decidua.

uterine cavity and ultimately fuses with the decidua parietalis and thus obliterates the uterine cavity.

Changes in the decidua basalis: In the region of decidua basalis the maternal blood vessels proliferate, grow, become congested with blood and dilate to form sinusoids.

CHORION: ROLE IN PLACENTA FORMATION

The fetal part of placenta is developed from the *chorion,* a membrane formed by fusion of trophoblast cells with underlying extraembryonic mesoderm (page 39 and revise the related text).

Formation of fetal part of placenta can be discussed as below:

- Formation of chorion
- Formation of villi and intervillous spaces in the chorion.
- Formation of chorion frondosum

Formation of chorion

See page 41 (revise the related text before proceeding further).

Formation of intervillous spaces and stages of villi

As described in the pre-embryo stage of development the trophoblast differentiates into two layers (Fig. 6.2B).

- *Cytotrophoblast.* It is the actively proliferating layer that lies on the inner or embryonic side.
- *Syncytiotrophoblast.* It is formed by cells that lie on the outside, i.e. in relation to the decidua basalis. These cells loose their cell boundaries, and thus one continuous sheet of cytoplasm containing many nuclei is formed (hence the name syncytium).

Steps involved in the formation of intervillous spaces and villi

1. *Lacunar stage of development.* The syncytiotrophoblast grows rapidly and intracytoplasmic

vacuoles appear, fusion of which leads to formation of lacunae (small cavities) (Fig. 6.2C). The lacunae progressively increase in size and communicate with each other. The partitions of syncytium which separate the various lacunae are called *trabeculae* (Fig. 6.2D). The syncytium concurrently grows into the surrounding decidua (endometrium) and erodes the walls of the maternal sinusoids and thus the sinusoids and lacunar spaces become continuous. Thus the trabeculae formed of syncytiotrophoblast are surrounded by maternal blood filled lacunar spaces (Fig. 6.2E).

2. *Stage of primary villi.* Subsequently the cells of cytotrophoblast proliferate locally and penetrate into the trabeculae formed by syncytiotrophoblast. Such cellular masses surrounded by layer of syncytium are called *primary villi,* and the surrounding lacunar spaces filled with maternal blood are now called *intervillous spaces* (Fig. 6.2F).

3. *Secondary villi* are formed in the early third week. This occurs by penetration and growth of mesenchymal cells into the core of primary villi formed in 2nd week of development (Fig. 6.2G).

4. *Tertiary villi* are formed by the end of third week. This occurs by differentiation of mesenchymal cells of core of secondary villi into capillaries and blood cells. These capillaries then fuse to form arterio-capillary networks and make contact with capillaries developing in the mesoderm of chorionic plate and in the connecting stalk (Fig. 6.2H). These vessels in turn soon become connected with intraembryonic circulatory system. In this way the placenta is connected with the embryo and is ready to supply the embryo proper with essential nutrients and oxygen derived from the maternal blood.

Anchoring versus free villi. Concurrently, with the development of tertiary villi, the cytotrophoblast cells of these villi, proliferate and penetrate through the syncytiotrophoblast to form a *cytotrophoblastic shell,* which gradually surrounds the chorionic sac and attaches it firmly to the maternal endometrial tissue. Such villi which are attached on one side to the chorionic plate and on the other side to the maternal tissue (decidua basalis) are called *anchoring or stem villi (Fig. 6.2I).* Certain villi which branch from the sides of anchoring villi and protrude into the intervillous space are called free or *branch or terminal villi.* Thus the main exchange of nutrients and waste products between the maternal and embryo blood occurs through the walls of the branch villi.

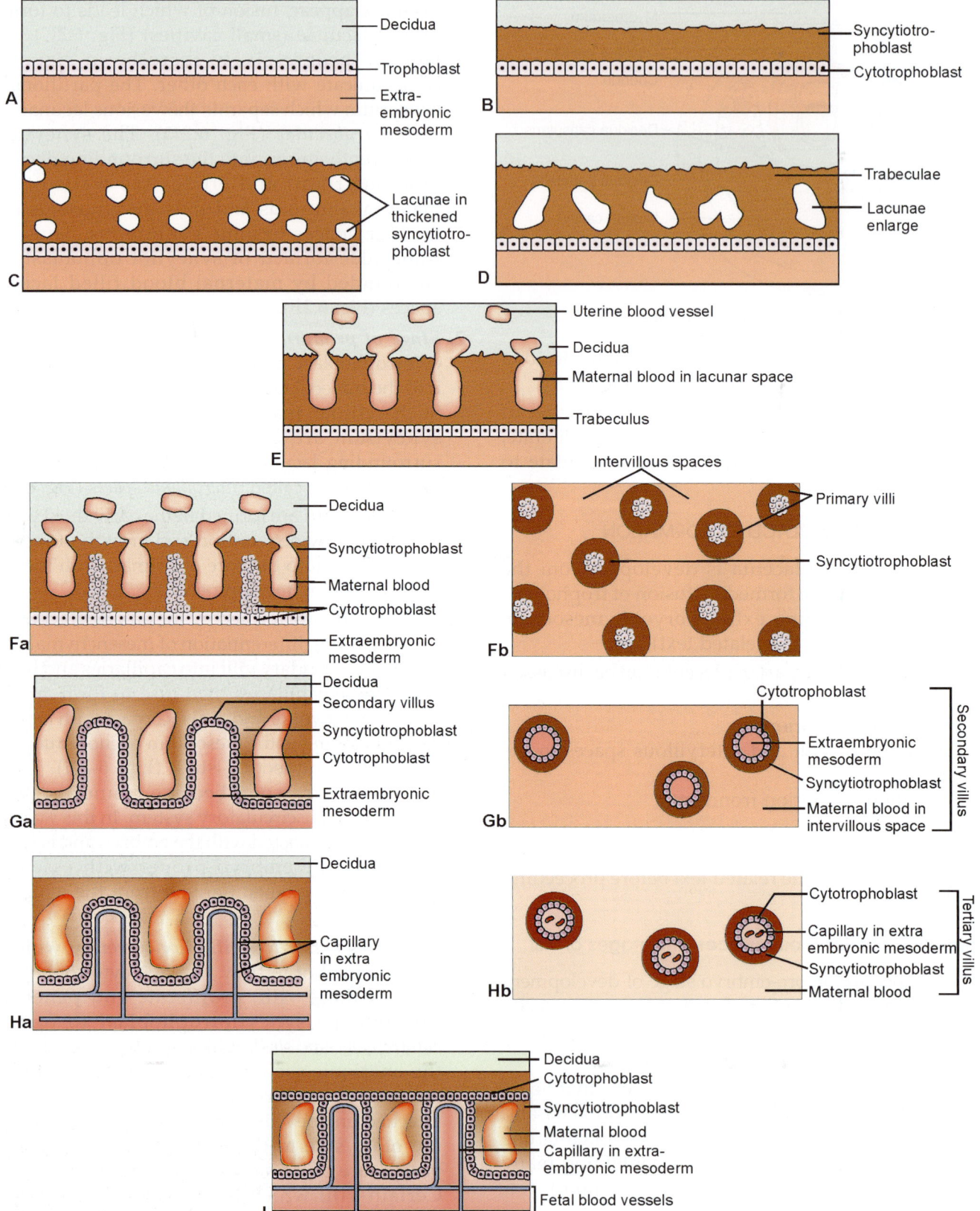

Fig. 6.2: Formation of villi and intervillous space: A, trophoblast in contact with decidua; B, trophoblast differentiates into two layers: cytotrophoblast and syncytiotrophoblast; C, appearance of lacunae in syncytiotrophoblast; D, enlargement of lacunae and formation of trabeculae; E, trabeculae surrounded by lacunae filled with mother's blood after erosion of maternal sinusoids by the syncytium; F, formation of primary villi; G, formation of secondary villi; H, formation of tertiary villi; and I, formation of anchoring versus free villi.

Formation of chorion frondosum

Initially the *chorionic villi* are formed as off shoots from the surface of trophoblast all around and grow into surrounding decidua (Fig. 6.3A). As pregnancy advances the chorionic villi growing in the decidua basalis continue to grow and form the so called *chorion frondosum* (bushy chorion), which will ultimately form the fetal part of placenta. While the chorionic villi projecting in the decidua capsularis are transitory and degenerate, by the third month of gestation, this part of chorion becomes smooth and is called *chorion* laevae (Fig. 6.3B).

FORMATION OF PLACENTAL SEPTA AND COTYLEDONS

Placental septa, the wedge shaped projections from decidua basalis, grow into the intervillous spaces.

Cotyledons. The placental septa divide the fetal part of the placenta into irregular convex areas called cotyledons. Each cotyledon consists of two or more stem villi and their many branch villi. The cotyledons form the different compartments; however, there is free communication between the compartments because the septa do not reach the chorionic plate (Fig. 6.4). The fully formed placenta has about 60 to 100 such cotyledons.

FULLY FORMED PLACENTA

- A fully formed placenta is a disc-shaped structure, has a diameter of 15–20 cm and weighs about 500 gm.
- After birth of the baby, the placenta is shed off along with decidua.
- *Maternal surface of placenta,* formed by decidual plate, is rough and divided into various lobes (cotyledons) by the grooves (formed by the bases of placental septa) (Fig. 6.5).

- *Fetal surface of placenta,* formed by chorionic plate lined by amnion, is smooth. Umbilical cord is attached to this surface (Fig. 6.5).

PLACENTAL MEMBRANE: EXCHANGE BETWEEN MATERNAL AND FETAL BLOOD

The maternal and fetal blood do not mix with each other. They are separated by a placental membrane, made up of the layers of the wall of the villus. From the fetal side these are (Fig. 6.6):

- *Endothelium* of fetal blood vessels and its basement membrane;
- *Surrounding mesenchymal tissue* (connective tissue);
- *Cytotrophoblast and its basement membrane*; and
- *Syncytiotrophoblast.*

All interchanges of oxygen, nutrition and waste products between the maternal blood and fetal blood take place through the placental membrane barrier. The total area of the membrane varies from 4 m² to 14 m². Its thickness is 0.025 mm in the beginning and in the later part of pregnancy it is reduced to 0.002 mm, because the cytotrophoblastic layer disappears and also there is considerable thinning of the connective tissue. Thinning of the placental membrane increases its efficiency.

It is important to note that the fetus and the mother are two genetically different individuals and fetus is like a foreign tissue (transplant) in the mother. However, the transplant is well tolerated and not rejected. The possible reasons are:

i. Placental trophoblast which separates maternal and fetal tissues does not express polymorphic MHC class I and II genes, rather it expresses HLA-G (monomorphic) genes. Therefore antibodies against fetal proteins do not develop.

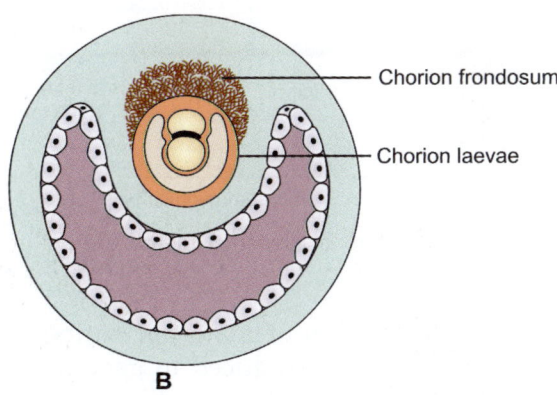

Fig. 6.3: Chorionic villi are initially formed from trophoblast all around (A) but later on chorionic villi in the region of decidua capsularis disappears and that in the region of decidua basalis continue to grow and form chorion frondosum (B).

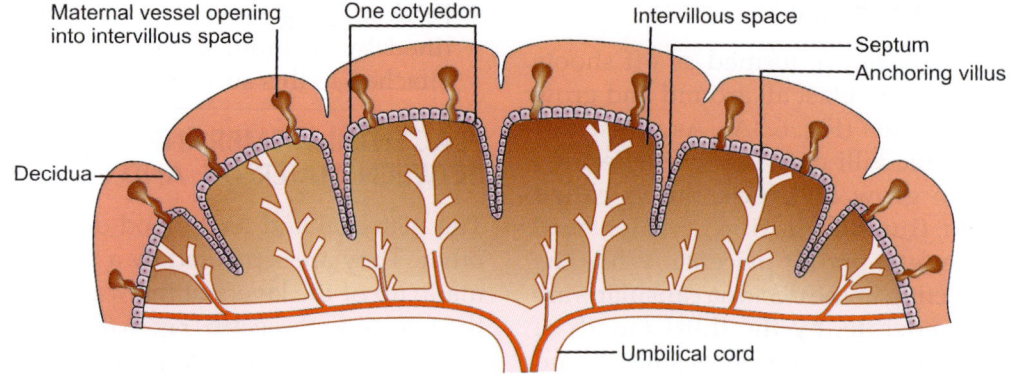

Fig. 6.4: Schematic section of the placenta. Note: placental septa, cotyledons, villi and umbilical cord.

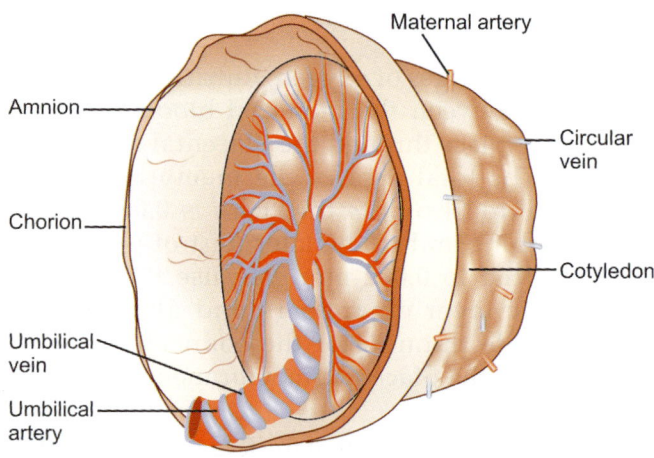

Fig. 6.5: Gross appearance of full term placenta. Note: Maternal surface depicting cotyledons (lobes) separated by grooves (placental fissures) and fetal surface showing attachment of umbilical cord.

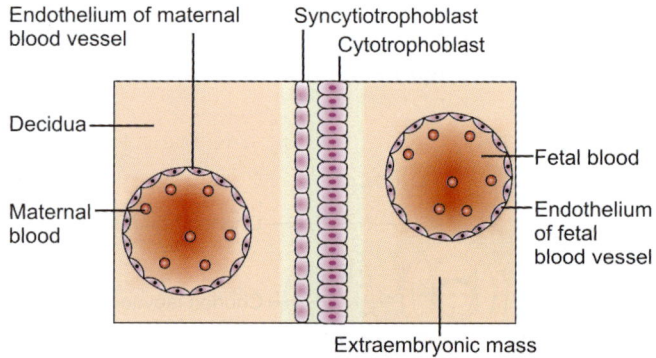

Fig. 6.6: Structure of placental membrane.

ii. Further, production of maternal antibodies during pregnancy is reduced in general. For example, a woman with Graves' disease usually becomes euthyroid during pregnancy and shows decreased level of antithyroid antibodies.

UTERINE CIRCULATION DURING PREGNANCY

The blood supply to uterus comes through uterine arteries and fluctuates cyclically along with the menstrual cycle to fulfil the metabolic demands of myometrium and endometrium. During pregnancy, the uterine blood flow increases parallel to the increase in fetal weight and uterine size (Fig. 6.7A). During early pregnancy, a rise in the levels of oestrogen and progesterone leads to an increase in uterine blood flow which meets the increased O_2 demand. Eventually placenta develops and becomes the circulatory link between the mother and fetus. Owing to increasing demand of O_2 with the progression of pregnancy more and more O_2 is extracted from the uterine blood and consequently in later part of pregnancy the O_2 saturation of uterine blood falls (Fig. 6.7B). As shown in Fig. 6.7A, the uterine blood flow increases tremendously (200–300 ml/min/kg of uterine mass including the fetus) during late pregnancy. To provide for it, the maternal cardiac output increases by 2 to 2.5 L/min near full term. Eighty percent of the uterine blood flow enters the placenta. Just before parturition there occurs a sharp decline in uterine blood flow, but the significance of this is not yet known.

PLACENTAL CIRCULATION

Placental circulation comprises of:
- Circulation of maternal part of placenta, and
- Circulation of fetal part of placenta.

Circulation of maternal part of placenta

Spiral endometrial arteries (80–100 in number) pour oxygenated blood in the intervillous spaces after piercing the decidual plate of maternal part of placenta.

- Blood flows from the spiral arteries is pulsatile and is propelled in jet like fountain at a considerable

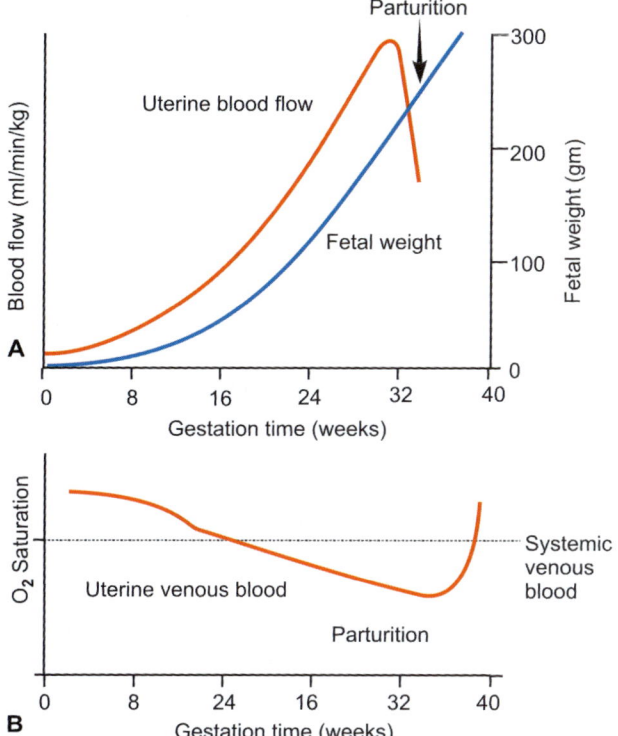

Fig. 6.7: Uterine circulation during pregnancy: A, changes in uterine blood flow; and B, changes in amount of oxygen in venous blood.

high pressure (due to narrow lumen of these arteries).

- The pressure forces the blood deep into the intervillous space and bathes the numerous small villi of the villous tree in oxygenated blood.
- Exchange of metabolic and gaseous products with the fetal blood occurs through placental membrane (described below).

Endometrial veins drains the blood from the intervillous lakes back into the maternal circulation.

Circulation of fetal part of placenta

Umbilical arteries bring poorly oxygenated blood from the fetus to the placenta.

- Umbilical arteries divide into several *chorionic arteries* at attachment with placenta.
- Chorionic arteries branch freely before entering the villi.
- Within the chorionic villi of the placenta exists an extensive *arterio-capillary venous* network which takes part in exchange through placental membrane.
- Well oxygenated blood from the capillaries in the villi pass through thin wall veins. Ultimately this blood reaches the umbilical veins through chorionic veins.

Umbilical veins carry the oxygen rich blood to the fetus. This blood is 80% saturated with O_2 (compared

with 98% saturation in the arterial circulation in adults). The umbilical vein before supplying the blood to liver, bypasses some of the blood to the inferior vena cava through *ductus venosus*.

EXCHANGE BETWEEN MATERNAL AND FETAL BLOOD ACROSS PLACENTAL MEMBRANE

As shown in Fig. 6.8, the placental villi containing fetal blood in capillaries project into and are then bathed by the blood in the maternal sinuses. Hence, in the placenta, the maternal and fetal blood do not mix with each other but are separated by the so-called placental membrane which consists (from fetal side) of following layers (Fig. 6.6):

- Endothelium and basement membrane,
- Surrounding mesenchymal tissue (connective tissue),
- Cytotrophoblast and its basement membrane, and
- Syncytiotrophoblast.

All exchange of O_2, nutrients, and waste products between the maternal and fetal blood takes place through the placental membrane barrier.

1. Gaseous exchange at placenta: placenta as lung (Fig. 6.8)

As shown in Fig. 6.8A, O_2 is taken up by the fetal blood and CO_2 is discharged into the maternal circulation across the placental membrane in a fashion analogous to O_2 and CO_2 exchange in the lungs across the alveolocapillary membrane (Fig. 6.8B). However, it is important to note that placental membrane is much thicker and less permeable than the alveolar membrane, and, therefore, the exchange is much less efficient. Table 6.1 shows the values of gaseous interchange in the placenta.

2. Placental transfer of nutrients: placenta as gut

The major function of placenta is to provide foodstuffs from mother's blood into the fetus.

During first few weeks after implantation the nutrients are derived from the plasma into the oedematous decidua and from endometrial glandular secretions containing glycogen.

Table 6.1: Values of pO_2 and pCO_2 in the maternal and umbilical cord blood

Blood vessel	pO_2 (mmHg)	pCO_2 (mmHg)
Uterine artery	95	36
Uterine vein	50	40
Umbilical artery	20	50
Umbilical vein	35	43

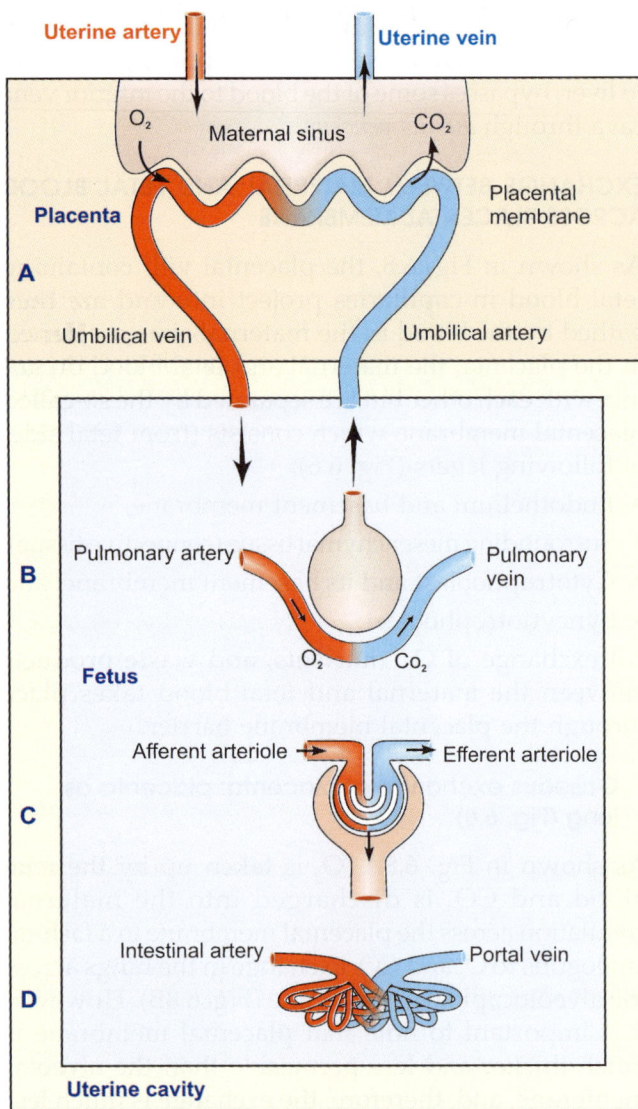

Fig. 6.8: Placental circulation.

By the 4th week of pregnancy the placenta takes up the nutritive functions. The nutritive materials which are transported from mother's blood into the fetus are:

- *Glucose.* Glucose passes by facilitated diffusion through a carrier molecule present on the tropho-blast cells. Glucose level in fetal blood is 20–30% lower than that of maternal blood.

Note. Fructose and sucrose are synthesized in the placenta itself.

- *Fats.* Fetal fat is derived from transfer of free fatty acids and cholesterol across the placenta and is also synthesized from the carbohydrates.

The solubility of fatty acids is high in the cell membranes, therefore, they are transferred by simple diffusion method, but more slowly as compared to glucose.

- *Amino acids*, calcium and inorganic phosphates are actively absorbed by placental membrane.

- *Potassium*, sodium and chloride ions and substances with molecular weight less than 1000 can cross readily by simple diffusion.

3. Excretion of waste products through placenta: Placenta as kidney

Excretory products, especially urea, uric acid and creatinines, etc. formed in the fetus are transported into the mother's blood and then excreted by mother's kidneys. Thus placenta also acts as fetal kidney.

VARIATIONS/ANOMALIES OF PLACENTA

Placenta shows a number of variations and anomalies which can be classified as below:

I. According to the attachment of umbilical cord

1. ***Battle-door placenta.*** In it the umbilical cord is inserted at the margin of the placenta and give it a clublike appearance (Fig. 6.9B).

2. ***Velamentous placenta.*** It is a more extreme type of marginal insertion, the umbilical cord is attached to the chorion and amnion instead of the placenta, and the vessels branch between the membranes before they extend over the placenta (Fig. 6.9C).

3. ***Placenta furcate.*** In it, blood vessels divide before reaching the placenta (Fig. 6.9D).

II. Intrauterine anomalous site of attachment of placenta

Placenta praevia—Normally, the placenta is attached to the upper uterine segment (Fig. 6.10A). When implantation of the blastocyst occurs in the lower part

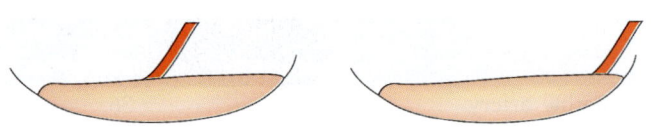
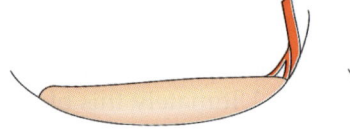
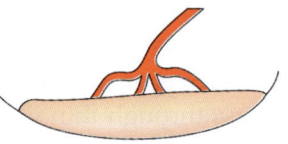

Fig. 6.9: Variations in attachment of umbilical cord to placenta: A, normal attachment of umbilical cord, B, battledoor placenta; C, velamentous placenta; and D, placenta furcate.

of the uterine cavity, the placenta will partially or totally cover the internal os of cervix and is called placenta praevia. It is a common cause of bleeding in later part of gestation and during parturition.

Four degrees of placenta praevia are known:

- *First degree.* Placental attachment extends into the lower uterine segment but does not reach the internal Os (Fig. 6.10B).
- *Second degree.* Placenta praevia is labelled when its margin reaches the internal Os (Fig. 6.10C).
- *Third degree.* Placenta praevia partially covers the internal Os and when cervix dilates during child birth, the placenta does not occlude it (Fig. 6.10D).
- *Fourth degree.* Placenta praevia completely covers the internal Os and occludes it even after full dilatation (Fig. 6.10E).

III. Anomalies in shape of placenta

Normal placenta is disc shaped. Following variations may occur:

1. *Bidiscoidal placenta* consists of two discs (Fig. 6.11A).
2. *Lobed placenta* exhibits two or more lobes (Fig. 6.11B).
3. *Placenta membranous* or a thin diffuse placenta is formed when chorionic villi persist all round the blastocyst cavity (Fig. 6.11C).
4. *Placenta circumvallate:* In it the peripheral edge of the placenta is covered by a circular fold of decidua (Fig. 6.11D).
5. *Placenta succenturiate:* In it an accessory lobe having vascular connection with the main placenta is formed (Fig. 6.11E).
6. *Placenta fenestrated:* When there is hole in the placental disc (Fig. 6.11F).

IV. According to the distribution of umbilical arteries

1. *Disperse type.* In it, the umbilical arteries divide in dichotamatous manner and undergo successive reduction in calibre.

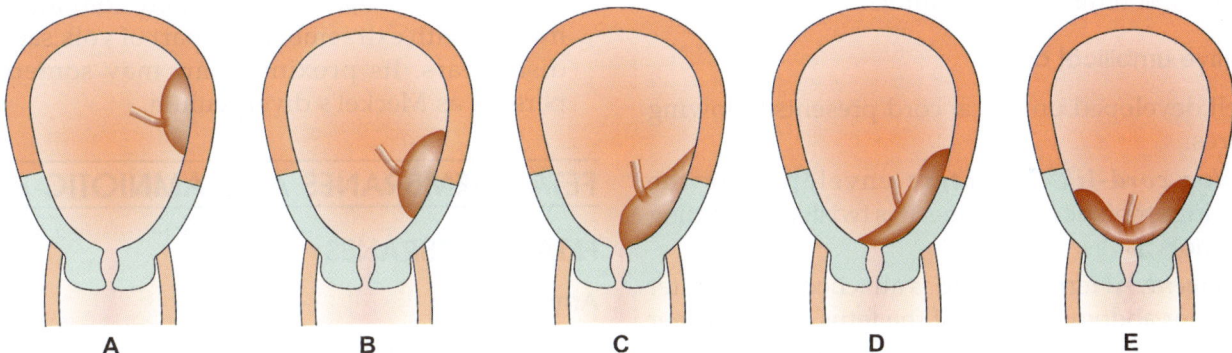

Fig. 6.10: Placenta praevia: A, normal site of attachment of placenta; B, first degree; C, second degree; D, third degree, and E, fourth degree.

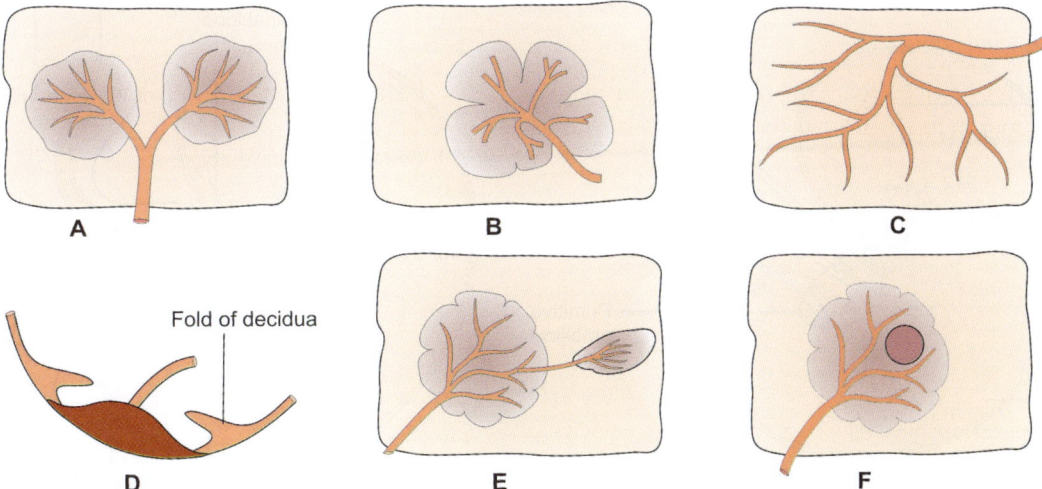

Fold of decidua

Fig. 6.11: Anomalous shapes of placenta: A, bidiscoid placenta; B, lobed placenta; C, placenta membranous; D, placenta circumvallate; E, placenta succenturiate; F, placenta fenestrated.

2. *Magistrol type.* In it, the arteries maintain almost a uniform calibre upto the periphery of the placenta and give off a number of smaller side branches.

UMBILICAL CORD

Primitive umbilical cord

Primitive umbilical cord is formed at about 10 weeks of gestation and consists of (Fig. 6.12):

- *Amnion covering* the primitive umbilical cord is attached to the embryo through *amnioectodermal junctions* known as *primitive umbilical* ring.
- Distally the primitive umbilical cord contains yolk sac and umbilical vessels. Infact yolk sac is found in chorionic cavity and connecting the umbilical cord by its stalk. At the end of 3rd month the chorionic cavity is obliterated and along with it the yolk sac also obliterates.
- Proximally the primitive umbilical cord contains, in addition to umbilical vessels, some intestinal loops and remnants of allantois.

Definitive umbilical cord

A well developed umbilical cord presents following features:

Tubular cord-like structure enveloped by the glistening amniotic membrane. It is twisted presenting false knots.

Attachment. At term, one end is attached to the center of anterior abdominal wall of the fetus and the other end is fixed to the centre of the fetal surface of placenta (Fig. 6.13).

Length at full term is about 50 cm and breadth is about 2 cm. A long cord may encircle the neck of the fetus giving rise to strangulation, or may prolapse into the cervical canal. A too short cord causes difficulty in parturition by pulling the placenta.

Contents of the umbilical cord include (Fig. 6.14):

- *Umbilical arteries,* two in number, derived from the ventral division of the internal iliac arteries convey deoxygenated blood from the fetus to the chorionic villi (for details see page 209, Fig. 14.1).
- *Umbilical vein.* In early pregnancy there are two umbilical veins; but later the right umbilical vein disappears and the left one persists to convey the oxygenated blood to the left branch of portal vein (for details see page 226, Fig. 14.22).
- *Wharton's jelly* protects the umbilical vessels and is formed by mucoid degeneration of the primary mesodermal cells of the connecting stalk.
- *Distal part of the allantoic diverticulum* is fibrosed to form the urachus. Its proximal part forms apex of urinary bladder (for details see page 182).
- *Vitellointestinal duct* which initially communicates midgut with extraembryonic part of yolk sac, later disappears. Its proximal part may sometimes, persists as Meckel's diverticulum.

FETAL MEMBRANES AND AMNIOTIC FLUID

FETAL MEMBRANES

Amnion

Amnion is formed early in the second week by delamination from the cytotrophoblast and encloses

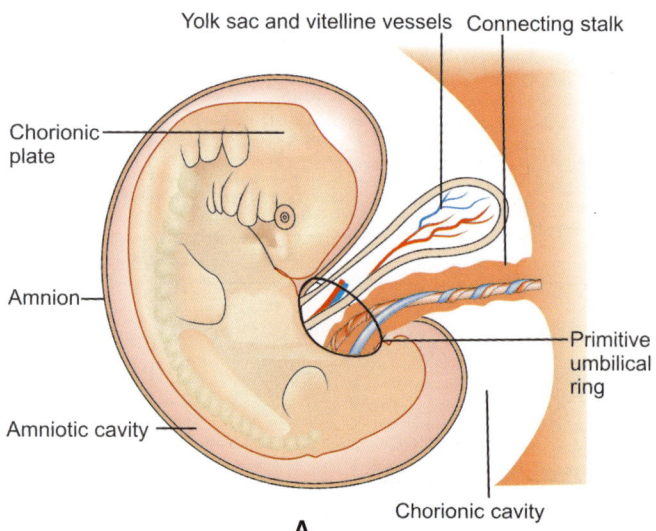

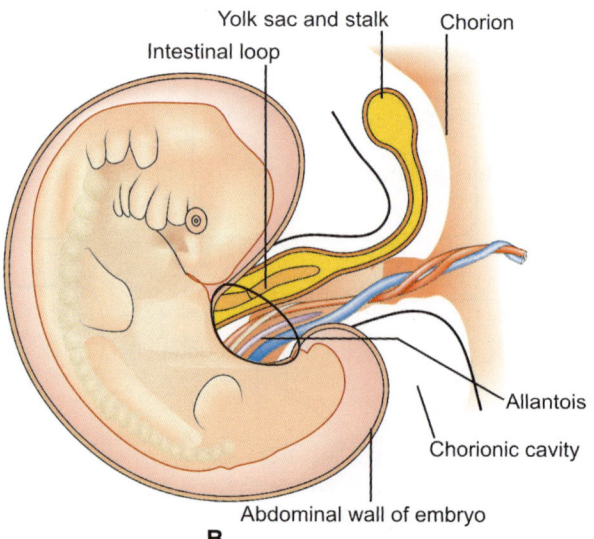

Fig. 6.12: Connective stalk in a 5 week embryo (A) is converted into primitive umbilical cord in a 10 week embryo (B).

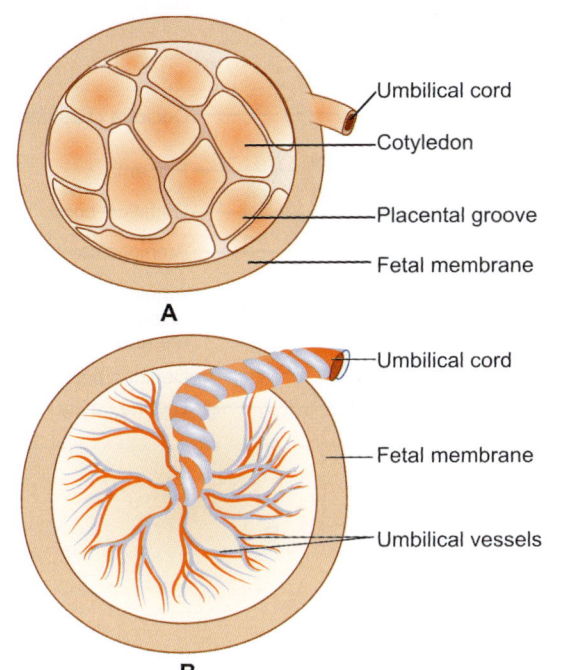

Fig. 6.13: Umbilical cord of near full term fetus seen from placental side (A) and from fetal side (B).

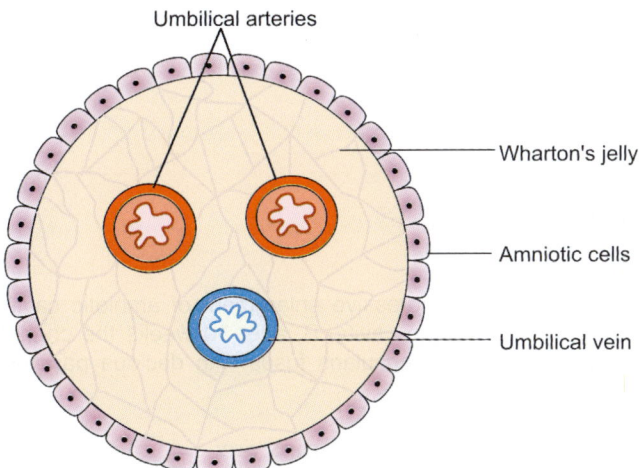

Fig. 6.14: Cross section of the umbilical cord near term umbilical cord depicting the contents.

a cavity called amniotic cavity (for details see page 40, Fig. 6.15A).

After folding of the embryo the amniotic cavity enlarges and comes to surround the embryo on all sides and the amnion also forms the epithelial covering of the umbilical cord (Fig. 6.15B).

Chorion

Chorion is formed in the end of second week by fusion of extraembryonic mesoderm with the overlying cytotrophoblast. It initially encloses the embryo proper and all the other extraembryonic membranes. Later extraembryonic coelom expands and forms a large chorionic cavity (for details see page 41, Fig. 3.5C).

After folding of the embryo the extraembryonic coelom is obliterated (Fig. 6.15B).

Amniochorion membrane

Amniochorion membrane is formed by fusion of aminon with chorion in the 10th week of gestation. It occurs due to marked expansion of the amniotic cavity. At this stage the fetus in the amniotic cavity is thus bounded by amniochorion membrane bounded by decidua capsularis (Fig. 6.15B).

Amnio-chorio-decidual membrane

Further expansion of amniotic cavity leads to obliteration of the uterine cavity by fusion of decidua capsularis with decidua parietalis at 4th month of gestation. From this stage until birth the fetus in the amniotic cavity is bounded by *amnio-chorio-decidual membrane* (Fig. 6.15C). Still further expansion of the amniotic cavity is achieved by enlargement of the uterus. Enlargement of the amniotic cavity is accompanied by an increase in the amount of amniotic fluid.

AMNIOTIC FLUID

Characteristics of amniotic fluid

Amniotic fluid also known as liquor amnii present in the amniotic cavity exhibits following characteristics:

- *Composition.* Amniotic fluid is clear and watery containing about 2% solids which include inorganic salts, urea, proteins and traces of sugar.
- *Produced* in part by amniotic cells, but is derived primarily from the maternal blood.
- *Volume* of amniotic fluid gradually increases upto 6 months from approximately 30 ml at 10 weeks of gestation to 450 ml at 20 weeks to 800 to 1000 ml at 37 weeks.
- *Replacement* of amniotic fluid occurs every 3 months.

Functions of amniotic fluid

- *Provides support* to the delicate tissues of growing embryo and fetus.
- *Protects* the embryo and fetus from external injuries by acting as shock absorber.
- *Allows free movements* of the fetus to take place.
- *Avoids adhesion* of the fetus to amnion.
- *Maintains temperature* of the fetal environment at constant level.

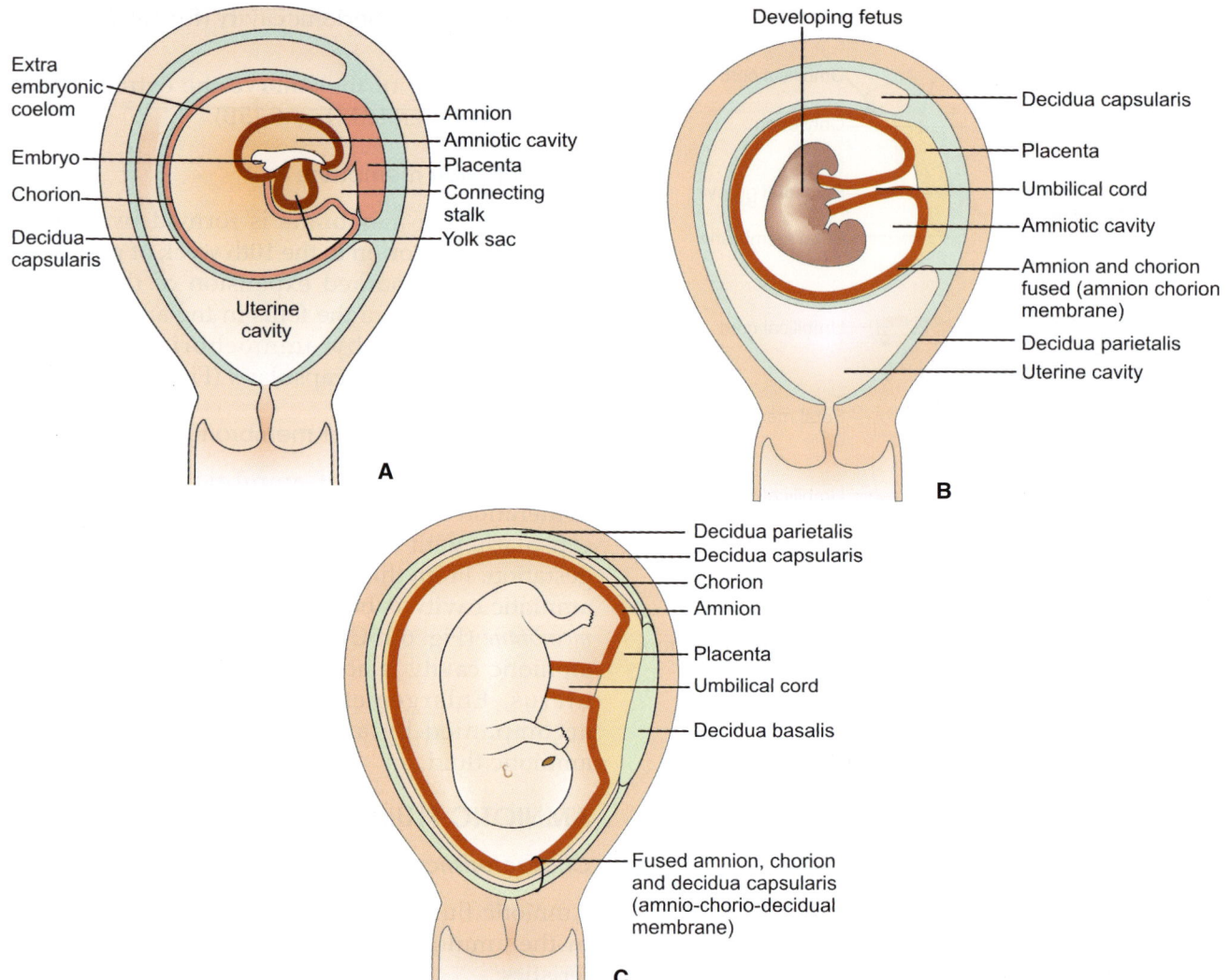

Fig. 6.15: Changing relationship of amnion, chorion and decidua parietalis with progressive enlargment of amniotic cavity: A, before 10 weeks, note three cavities, amniotic, extraembryonic coelom and uterine cavity; B, after 10 weeks the chorion and amnion fuse obliterating extraembryonic coelom; C, at 4 months the decidua capsularis fuses with decidua parietalis obliterating uterine cavity and forming amnio-chorio-decidual membrane.

- *Helps to dilate the cervix* during parturition by making the hydrostastic wedge of amniotic sac.

Regulation of volume of amniotic fluid

It involves following processes:
- *Continuous formation* from maternal blood.
- *Addition of fetal urine* to the amniotic fluid occurs from the 4th month onward, since the metanephric kidneys start functioning from that period.
- *Swallowing of amniotic fluid* is about 400 ml/day occurs from 5th month onward. The swallowed fluid is absorbed through the gut into the blood stream and thence passes into maternal blood through the placenta.

Abnormalities of amniotic fluid

Hydramnios is labelled when the amniotic fluid exceeds 2 liters.

Common causes of hydramnios are:
- 35% cases are idiopathic, 25% cases are due to maternal diabetes, and
- 40% case are due to congenital malformations, which includes anencephaly, and esophageal atresia.

Oligohydramnios, i.e. scanty amniotic fluid, is a rare anomaly associated with congenital agenesis of metanephric kidney, as no urine is added to the amniotic fluid.

FETAL MEMBRANES IN TWINS

Twinning refers to delivery of two fetuses (duplet) during pregnancy very rarely three (triplets), four (quadruplets) and more fetus may be delivered.

Fetal membranes in twins will have different arrangement depending upon the types of twins, which include:

- Dizygotic twins, and
- Monozygotic twins.

DIZYGOTIC TWINS

Definitions and cause: Human are monoovulatory, i.e. shed a single ovum in each cycle thus on fertilization formation of single fetus is the rule. However, twinning and multiple births do occur accidentally and sporadically, due to genetic or environmental factors. In dizygotic twinning two fetuses develops from two zygotes which result from simultaneous shedding of two oocytes and fertilization by separate spermatozoa.

Incidence of dizygotic twinning is 7 to 11 per 1,000 births and increases with maternal age. The dizygotic twinning is more frequent than monozygotic twinning and accounts for 75% of all twins.

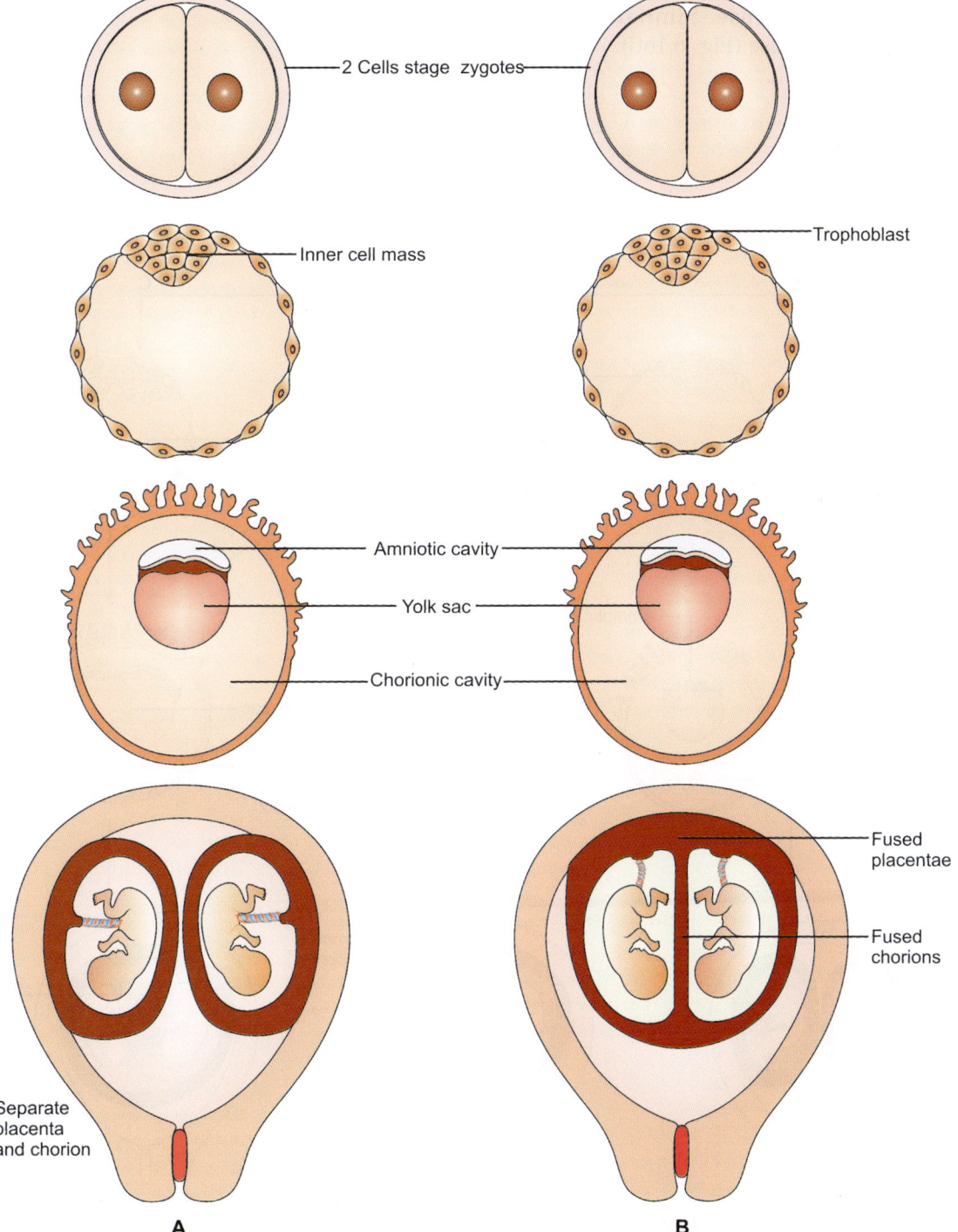

Fig. 6.16: Fetal membranes and placenta in dizygote twinning are usually separate (A); but sometimes they may fuse (B).

Characteristics of dizygotic twins are:

- *Fraternal or unlike* babies conveying different genetic material are formed in dizygotic twinning. So, they do not resemble with each other any more than children of the same parents.
- *Sex* may be same or different.

Placenta and fetal membranes: Since the two zygotes implant individually in the uterus, usually each develops its own placenta, amnion and chorionic sac (Fig. 6.16A). Occasionally the two placentae are so close together that they fuse. Similarly the two chorionic sacs may also fuse (Fig. 6.16B).

MONOZYGOTE TWINS

Definition and causes. In monozygote twinning, two embryos are derived from a single ovum which is fertilized by a single sperm. Monozygote twinning results from splitting of zygote at various stages of development.

Incidence of monozygote twinning is 3 to 4 per 1000 live births. In general monozygote twinning accounts for only 25% the twins borns as compared to 75% dizygote twins.

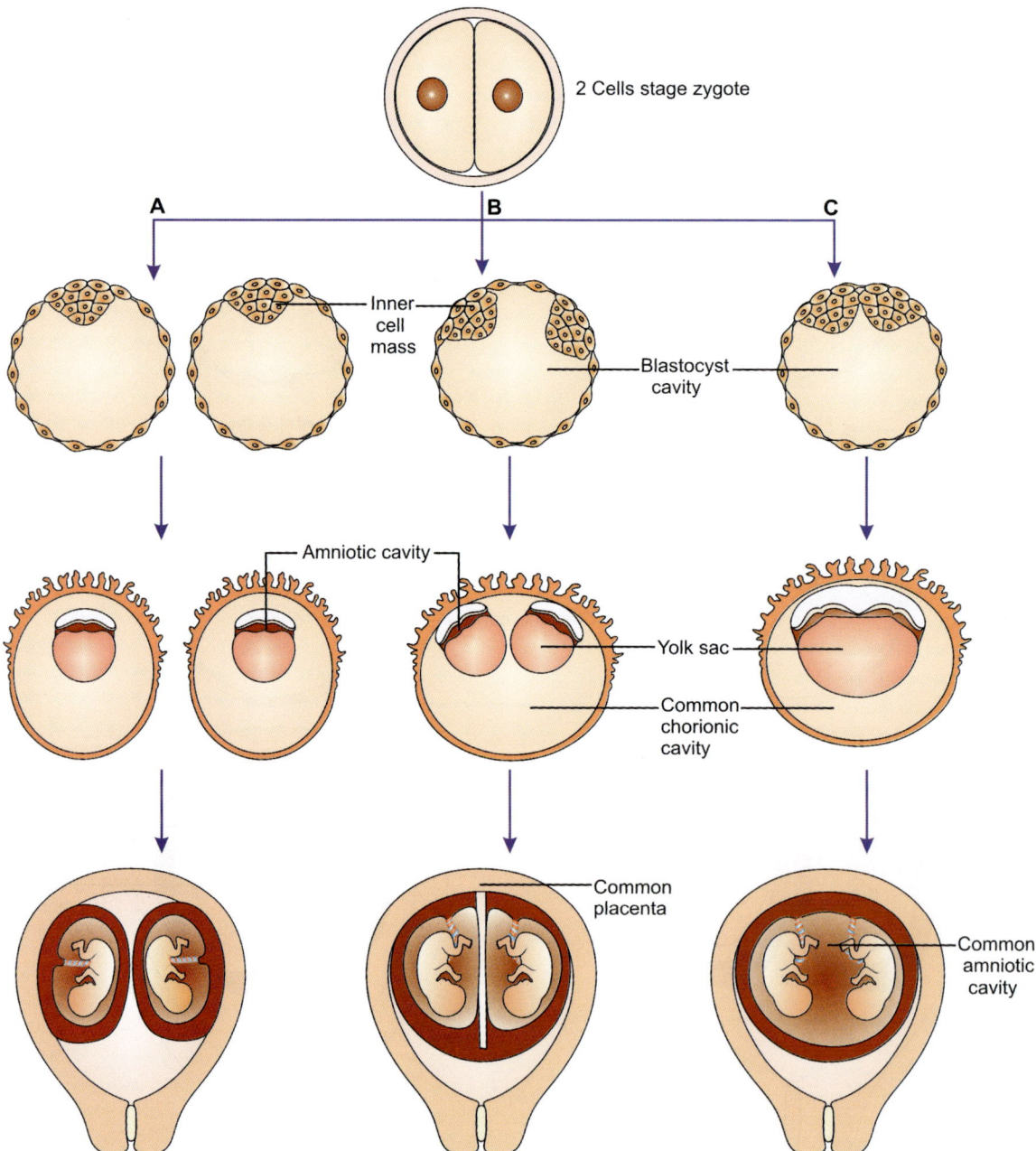

Fig. 6.17: Arrangement of fetal membranes and placenta in monozygote twinning: A, bichorionic twins; B, monochorionic biamniotic twins; C, monochorionic monoamniotic twins.

Characteristics of monozygote twins are:

Identical fetuses possessing similar genetic constitution are formed, i.e. the twins have similar appearance, structures, sex, finger prints and blood groups.

Arrangement of fetal membranes and placenta varies depending upon the stage of development at which splitting occurs. Accordingly the monozygotic twins are classified as below:

- *Monozygotic bichorionic twins.* In 25–30% cases splitting occurs at two-cell stage and two blasto-cysts develop which implant separately like dizygote twinning. Thus, each embryo develops its own placenta, amniotic cavity, and chorionic cavity (Fig. 6.17A).
- *Monochorionic biamniotic twins.* In 70 to 75% of cases the splitting occurs at early blastocyst stage, i.e.

inner cell mass divides into two separate groups forming two embryoblasts in a single blastocyst cavity. Thus, the two embryos have a common placenta and common chorionic cavity, but two different amniotic cavities (Fig. 6.17B).

- *Monochorionic monoamniotic twins.* In 1 to 2% cases, the splitting occurs at the bilaminar germ disc stage, just before the appearance of the primitive streak. Thus, the two embryos have a common placenta, common chorion and common amnion (Fig. 6.17C). Although the twins have a common placenta, blood supply is usually balanced.
- *Conjoint twins or siamese twins* develop due to incomplete separation of two embryos. It occurs due to anomalies of organising center (Fig. 6.18A). According to the site and degree of fusion, the conjoined twins can be classified as below:
  - *Craniopagus:* United by the head (Fig. 6.18B),

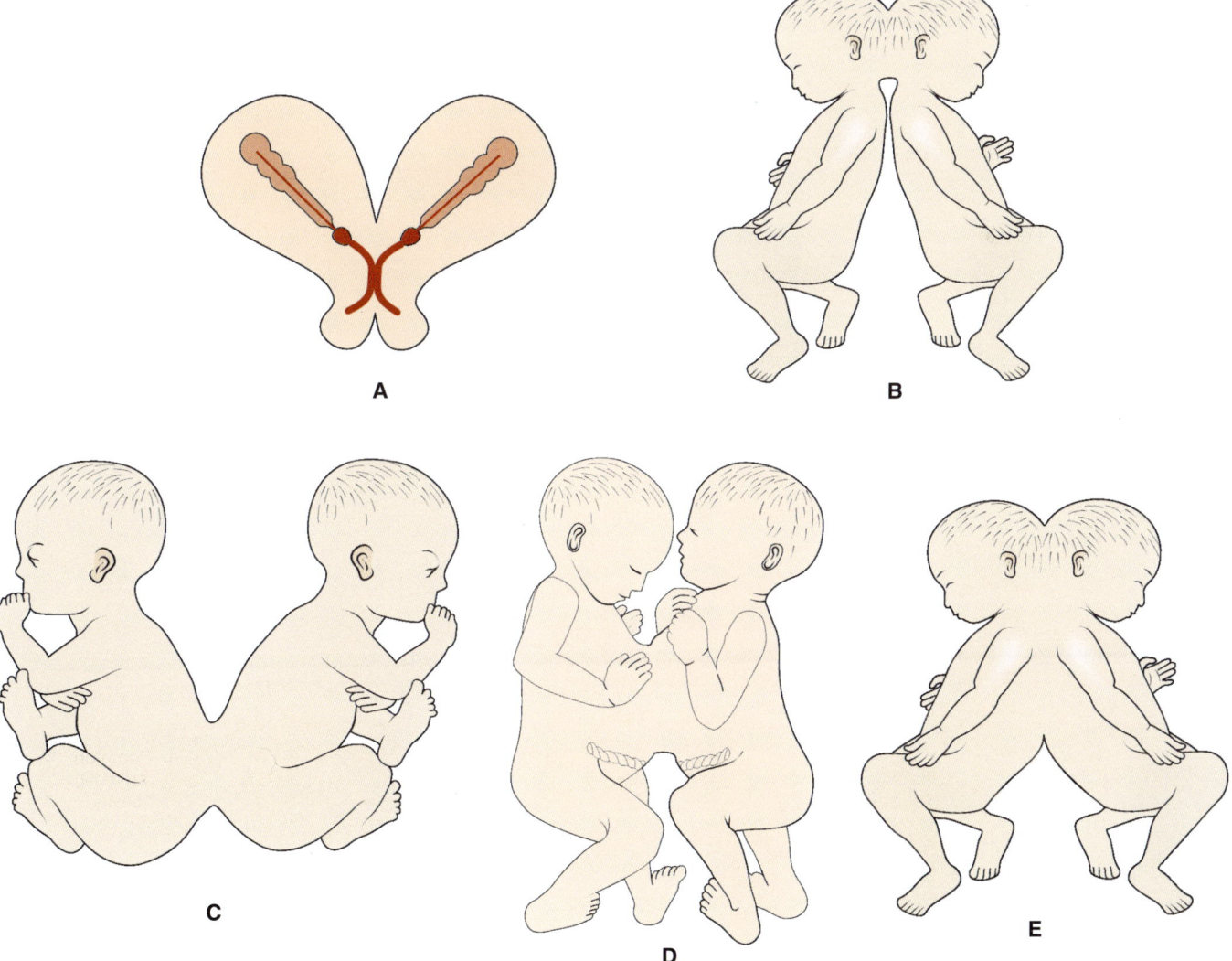

Fig. 6.18: Conjoint twins: A, anomalies of organising center; B, craniopagus; C, pygopagus; D, thoracopagus; E, cephalo-thoracopagus.

– *Pygopagus:* Fused at the sacral region (Fig. 6.18C),
– *Thoracopagus:* Fused at the thoracic region (Fig. 6.18D),
– *Cephalothoracopagus:* Extensive fusion of head and thorax (Fig. 6.18E).

Note: Sometime, it may be possible to completely separate the conjoint twins by surgery.

• *Parasitic twins:* In this situation one partner of the conjoint twins gets markedly diminished blood supply and become rudimentary. It appears to grow like a parasite from the body of well developed co-twin (Fig. 6.19). Very rarely the parasitic twin may be completely enclosed within the body of the co-twin, this condition is called *foetus in foetu.*

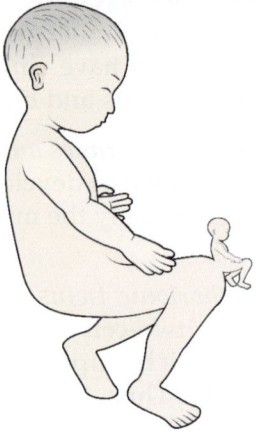

Fig. 6.19: Parasitic twins.

Formation of Body Tissues and Body Cavities

FORMATION OF BODY TISSUES	**Mesenchyme and its derivatives**
Epithelial tissue	▢ Blood
▢ Ectodermal epithelia	▢ Cartilage
▢ Endodermal epithelia	▢ Bone
▢ Mesodermal epithelia	▢ Muscle
Glandular tissue	**FORMATION OF BODY CAVITIES**
▢ Stages in the development of a gland	▢ Overview of body cavities and intraembryonic coelom
▢ Histological types	▢ Development of pericardial cavity
▢ Exocrine and endocrine glands	▢ Development of pleural cavities
	▢ Development of peritoneal cavity and mesentery
	▢ Development of diaphragm

FORMATION OF BODY TISSUES

The various organ systems are formed by various body tissues. Before discussing the development of different organ systems it will be worthwhile to be aware of the formation of the body tissues which are involved in the formation of each organ system.

Mechanisms involved in the formation of body tissues are:

- *Determination,* i.e. the fixation at a definite time in the development of different parts of an embryo.
- *Differentiation,* i.e. creation of new types of substances or cells, or tissues not previously present.
- *Organization,* i.e. the process whereby new elements at every biological level are coordinated into functional units properly sized, spaced, and oriented.

- *Growth,* i.e. process of creating more of a substance or formed elements, such as a cell, which is already present.

Formation of body tissues which include: Epithelial tissues, glandular tissues, connective tissue, blood, muscular tissues, cartilage, and bony tissue is described briefly.

FORMATION OF EPITHELIAL TISSUE

The epithelial tissue or epithelium lines the surfaces and/or cavities of various organs in the body. The epithelium may be derived from any of the three germinal layers viz. ectoderm, endoderm and mesoderm.

Ectoderm gives rise to epithelia covering the external surfaces and some surfaces near the exterior, as below:

- Skin, hair follicles, sweat glands, sebaceous glands and mammary glands.

85

- Cornea and conjunctiva
- External acoustic meatus and outer surface of tympanic membrane.
- Some parts of mouth and lower part of anal canal.
- Terminal part of male urethra and parts of female external genitalia.

Endoderm gives rise to:
- Epithelium lining the entire gut except some part of mouth and lower part of anal canal which develop from ectoderm, as mentioned above.
- Epithelium lining the auditory tube and middle ear.
- Epithelium lining the respiratory tract, and
- Epithelium lining some part of the urinary bladder, urethra and vagina.

Mesoderm gives rise to:
- Epithelium lining most of the urogenital tract, i.e.
  - Tubules of kidney, ureters and trigone of urinary bladder.
  - Uterine tubes, uterus and part of vagina.
  - Testis and its duct system.
- *Endothelium* lining the heart, blood vessels and lymphatics.
- *Mesothelium* lining the pericardial, peritoneal and pleural cavities and cavities of joints.

FORMATION OF GLANDULAR TISSUE

Stages in the Development of a Typical Gland

Almost all glands of the body develop as diverticula from the epithelial lining of the body structures. The stages in the development of a typical gland are (Fig. 7.1):
- *Stage of solid diverticula* (Fig. 7.1A) make the initiation of each gland.
- *Stage of branching.* Each diverticulum branches variously. The branching diverticulae are generally solid to begin with (Fig. 7.1B). The gland may be derived from the elements formed by branching of one diverticulum (e.g. parotid) or by branching of several diverticulae (e.g. lacrimal gland, and prostate).

- *Stage of canalization of duct.* After branching the solid diverticulae are canalized (Fig. 7.1C).
- *Stage of formation of acinar and duct tissue.* The proximal parts of the diverticulae form the duct system and distal parts of the diverticulae form the acini (secretory elements) (Fig. 7.1D).

Histological types of Glands

Depending upon the epithelium from which the glands arise, they may be of following types:

Ectodermal glands are derived from the epithelium which is ectodermal in origin; e.g. for example: sweat glands, and mammary glands.

Endodermal glands are derived from the epithelia which are endodermal in origin, e.g. pancreas and liver.

Mesodermal glands are derived from the epithelia which are mesodermal in origin, e.g. adrenal cortex

Mixed glands are derived from epithelia of different origins, e.g. prostate gland.

Exocrine Versus endocrine Glands

Exocrine glands (e.g. parotid gland) pour their secretions into the cavities through the ducts. The opening of the duct (ducts) is usually situated at the site from which the diverticula originally arise.

Endocrine glands (e.g. thyroid gland) loose their all contacts from the epithelial surface from which they arise. In other words, endocrine glands are ductless glands which pour their secretion into the blood-stream.

MESENCHYME AND ITS DERIVATIVES

Mesenchyme, also known as embryonic connective tissue, consists of loosely arranged mesenchymal cells suspended in a gelatinous matrix. The mesenchymal cells are ameboid and actively phagocytic.

Formation of Mesenchyme

Mesenchyme, the supporting connective tissue of embryo is derived from two sources:

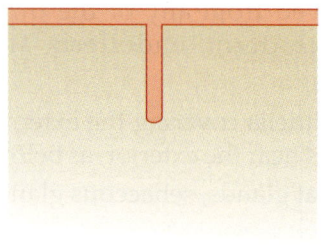 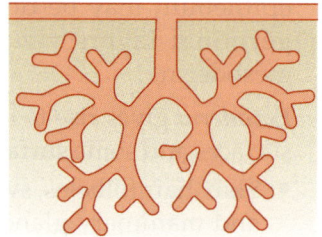 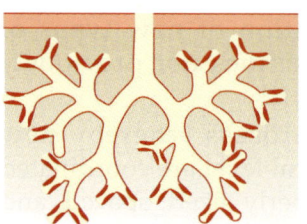 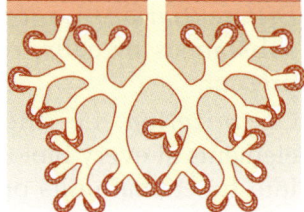

    A   **B**   **C**   **D**

Fig. 7.1: Stages in the development of a typical gland.

1. *Mesoderm cells.* As described earlier the paraxial mesoderm forms a segmented series of tissue blocks on each side of the neural tube, known as *somitomeres* in the head region and *somites* from occipital region caudally. By the beginning of fourth week, cells forming the ventral and medial walls of the somite differentiate into *sclerotome.* By the end of the 4th week the sclerotomes loose their compact organization, become polymorphous, and shift their position to surround the notochord and form the so called mesenchyme.

2. *Neural crest cells.* Considerable mesenchyme in the head region is also derived from the neural crest. The neural crest cells migrate into the pharyngeal arches and form the mesenchyme which forms the bones and connective tissue of craniofacial structures. Homeobox (Hox) genes regulate the migration and subsequent differentiation of the neural crest cells.

Derivatives of Mesenchyme

The mesenchymal cells are characterized by their ability to migrate and differentiate into many different kinds of cells that in turn give rise to various tissues (Fig. 7.2):

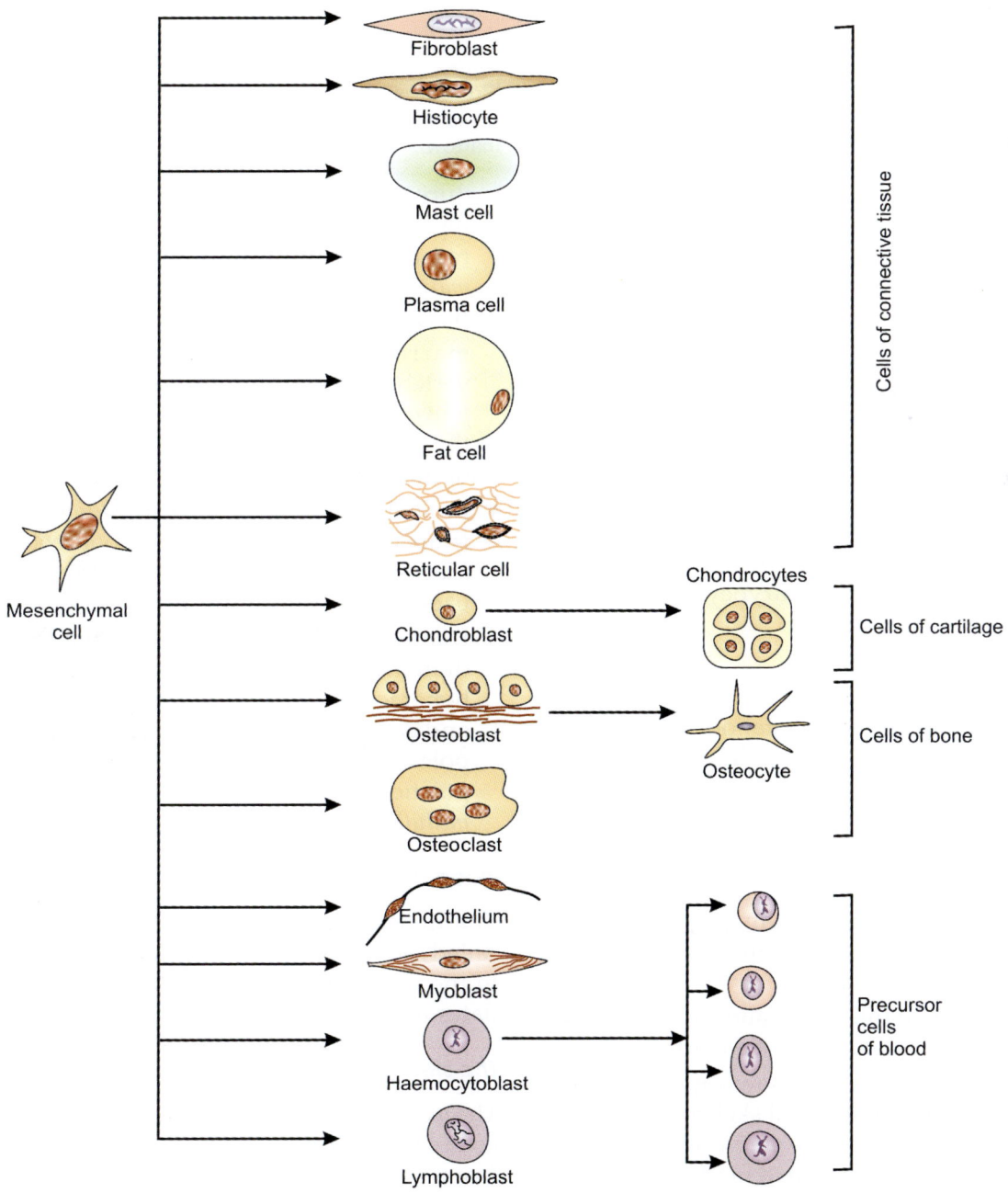

Fig. 7.2: Derivatives of mesenchymal cells.

1. *Chondroblasts.* In areas where cartilage is to be formed the mesenchymal cells proliferate and become rounded and form the cartilage forming cells or chondroblasts.

2. *Osteoblasts.* In areas where bone is to be formed the mesenchymal cells differentiate into osteoblasts (bone-forming cells) which begin to deposit matrix or intercellular substances, the *osteoid tissue* or prebone.

3. *Cells of connective tissue.* The mesenchymal cells also differentiate to form various connective cells such as: fibroblasts, histiocyte, mast cells, plasma cells and fat cells.

4. *Blood forming cells.* Some mesenchymal cells differentiate to form precursors of cells of blood, the *haemocytoblast* and *lymphoblast.*

5. *Vascular endothelial cells.* Some mesenchymal cells differentiate to form vascular endothelial cells from which blood vessels and the primitive heart tubes are formed.

6. *Myoblasts* or muscle forming cells, are also differentiated mesenchymal cells.

Formation of Blood

The process of formation of blood in called *haemopoiesis.* Blood formation begins very early in embryonic life (before somites have appeared) and continues throughout life. The haemopoiesis includes:

• Erythropoiesis, i.e. development of RBCs,
• Leucopoiesis, i.e. development of WBCs, and
• Thrombopoiesis or megakaryocytopoiesis, i.e. development of platelets.

Sites of haemopoiesis

• In the first two months of gestation, the *yolk sac* is the main site of haemopoiesis (Fig. 7.3).

• *From third months of gestation,* liver and spleen become the main sites of blood formation and continue to do so till birth. Spleen makes small contribution as compared to liver.

• *From 20th week of gestation,* haemopoiesis begins in the bone marrow and by seventh or eighth month it becomes the main site.

• *At birth* (in normal full-term), almost whole of the haemopoiesis occurs in the bone marrow.

• *In young children,* active haemopoietic bone marrow is found in both axial skeleton and bones of extremities. The active haemopoietic bone marrow is red in colour due to marked cellularity and hence is called *red bone marrow.* However,

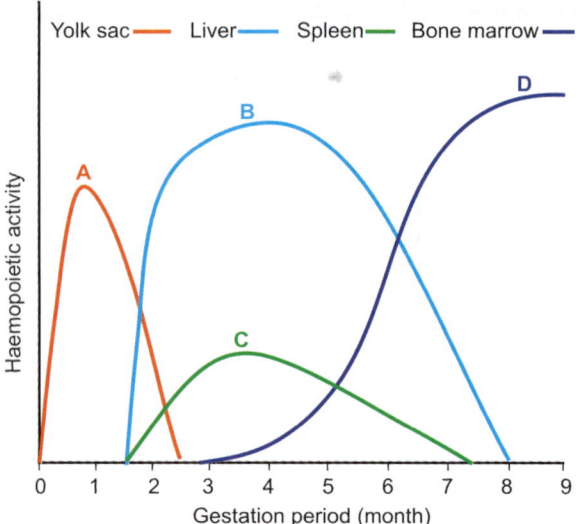

Fig. 7.3: Sites of haemopoiesis during different periods of human life: A, yolk sac; B, liver; C, spleen; and D, bone marrow.

during this period, there occurs a progressive fatty replacement throughout the long bones converting red bone marrow into the so-called *yellow bone marrow.*

• *In adults,* therefore, haemopoietic (red) bone marrow is confined to *axial skeleton* (skull, vertebrae, sternum, ribs, sacrum and pelvis) and *proximal ends of long bones* (humerus, femur and tibia). Even in these haemopoietic areas, about 50% of the bone marrow consists of fat.

• *In adults, during pathological conditions,* when there is an increased demand of blood cells, the *non-haemopoietic (yellow) marrow* is capable of reverting back to active haemopoiesis.

• *During pathological conditions* when the increased demand of blood cells cannot be met by the hyperactivity of bone marrow alone, even the liver and spleen resume there fetal role of haemopoiesis, as the stem cell retains its potential haemopoietic activity. Such a situation is referred as *extra medullary haemopoiesis.*

Blood cell precursors

The first recognizable blood cell in the yolk sac is called *haemocytoblast* (now called *pluripotent stem cell).* In the wall of yolk sac the haemocytoblast differentiates into progenitor cells (Fig. 7.4).

The stem cells

The *monophyletic theory* of haemopoiesis is now widely accepted, according to which all blood cells originate from a single ancestral cell called *pluripotent* or *multipotent stem cell.* The stem cells have the appearance

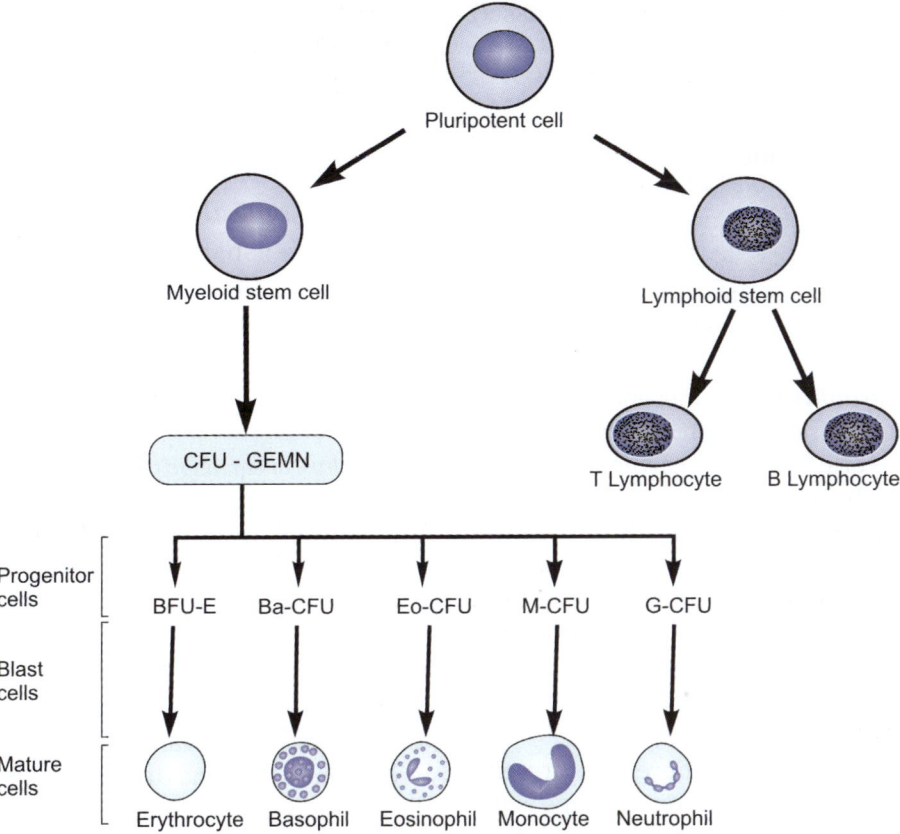

Fig. 7.4: Different blood cells differentiating from the haemocytoblast

of small or intermediate-sized lymphocytes. Stem cells possess two *fundamental properties:*

- *Self-replication,* i.e. stem cells are capable of cell division to give rise to more stem cells, and
- *Differentiation and commitment,* i.e. the stem cells have ability to differentiate into specialized cells called progenitor cells.

Progenitor cells

The stem cells after a series of divisions, differentiate into progenitor cells:

Pluripotent progenitor cells which can give rise to any type of blood cells,

Lymphoid (immune system) stem cells which ultimately develop into lymphocytes, and

Myeloid (trilineage) stem cells which later differentiate into three types of cell lines:

- *Granulocyte-monocyte progenitors* which produce all leucocytes except the lymphocytes,
- *Erythroid progenitors* which produce red blood cells, and
- Megakaryocyte progenitors which produce platelets.

Features of progenitor cells

Morphologically the progenitor cells present in the bone marrow cannot be differentiated from the stem cells, as they both look alike. However, they can be differentiated by immunological techniques, taking advantage of the different types of molecules present on their cell membrane.

Progenitor cells possess ability to give rise to *clones* (group of cells), so they are also called *colony forming cells* (CFC) or *colony forming units* (CFU). The three types of progenitor cells are given:

- *CFU-GEMM* (colony forming unit–granulocyte, erythroid, megakaryocyte, macrophage) refers to a multipotent progenitor cell, i.e. myeloid progenitor cells.
- *BFU-E* (burst forming unit–erythroid) form large colonies of erythroid series.
- *CFU-E* (colony forming unit–erythroid) develop into erythrocytes.
- *Ba–CFU* refers to basophil colony forming units.
- *Eo–CFU* are eosinophil colony forming units.
- *M–CFU* refers to monocyte colony forming units.
- *G–CFU* are neutrophil colony forming units.

The broad outlines of haemopoiesis discussed above are summarized in Fig. 7.4.

FORMATION OF CARTILAGE

The cartilage develops from the mesenchyme. Process of cartilage formation involves following steps:

Formation of chondrification center. In sites where cartilage is to develop, the mesenchymal cells become closely packed, i.e. condense to form the so called *chondrification center* or simply mesenchymal condensation.

Formation of chondroblasts. The mesenchymal cells forming chondrification center proliferate, become round and get converted into the cartilage forming cells, called as chondroblasts.

Formation of cartilage matrix. The chondroblasts secrete collagen fibrils and the ground substance of matrix. Some chondroblasts get imprisoned within the matrix of developing cartilage and are called *chondrocytes.* Depending upon the deposition of collagen and/or elastic fibres in the ground substance of matrix the cartilages are of three types:

- *Hyaline cartilage.* In it, collagen fibres are present, but are not seen easily. The hyaline cartilage is the most widely distributed cartilage (e.g. in joints).
- *Fibrocartilage.* In fibrocartilages the collagen fibres are numerous and obvious. Fibrocartilages are found, e.g. in the intervertebral discs.
- *Elastic cartilages* contain more of the elastic fibres in the intercellular substances or matrix. Example of elastic cartilage includes cartilages present in the auricle of ear.

Formation of perichordium. Perichordium, a fibrous membrane covering the cartilage, is derived from the mesenchymal cells surrounding the surface of the developing cartilage.

FORMATION OF BONE

Before discussing the mechanism and process of formation it will be worthwhile to be familiar with certain other aspects of bone. Therefore, the present discussion will include:

- Types and parts of a bone
- Composition of bone
- Structural considerations
- Cells of bone,
- Mechanism of bone formation, and
- Process of bone formation.

Types and parts of a bone

Types: Bones, depending upon the size and shape, have been classified as:

- *Long bones*, e.g. limb bones.
- *Short bones*, e.g. wrist and ankle bones.
- *Flat bones*, e.g. scapula, skull bones and mandible.
- *Irregular bones*, e.g. vertebrae.
- *Sesamoid bones*, e.g. patella.

Parts of a typical long bone are (Fig. 7.5)

- *Diaphysis* (shaft) is the mid portion of the long bone.
- *Epiphysis* is the widened part on either end of the bone.
- *Metaphysis* is the portion between the diaphysis and epiphysis.
- *Epiphyseal cartilage* or growth plate refers to a layer of cartilage that is present between the epiphysis and metaphysis during growing age. The growth of the bone stops when epiphysis fuses with shaft of the bone.

Composition of bone

Bone, a special form of connective tissue, is composed of a collagenous framework (matrix) impregnated with bone salts. The dry, fat free bone consists of one third organic bone matrix, and two thirds minerals (inorganic).

Bone matrix

Bone matrix also called osteoid, consists of collagen fibres embedded in the gelatinous ground substance.

Collagen fibres are arranged in lamellae. The fibres of one lamellus run parallel to each other, but those of adjoining lamellae run at varying angles to each other. Over 90% of the organic matrix is type I collagen.

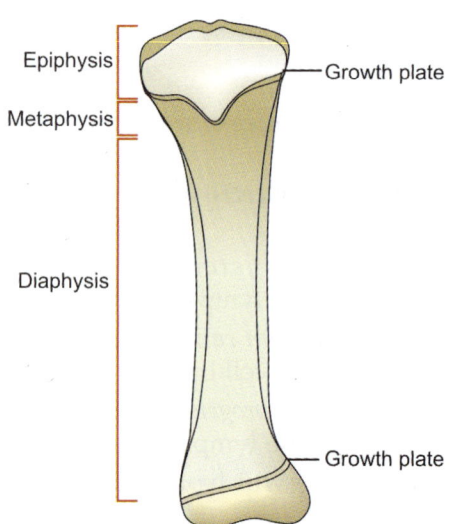

Fig. 7.5: Structure of a long bone as seen in longitudinal cut section.

Ground substance of a lamellus is continuous with that of adjoining lamellae. It is formed by the extracellular fluid and proteoglycans (which include chondroitin sulphate and hyaluronic acid). These substances are concerned with the regulation and deposition of bone salts.

Bone salts

The bone salts constitute the inorganic component of bone which is comprised primarily of calcium and phosphate in the form of hydroxyapatite crystals $[Ca_{10}(PO_4)_6(OH)_2]$. Each crystal measures about 400 Å units in length, 100 Å units in breadth and 10 to 30 Å units in thickness. Adsorbed on the surface of hydroxyapatite crystals are present small amounts of other salts such as sodium, potassium, magnesium and carbonate. The bone salts strengthen the bone matrix.

Structure of bone

Structurally, two types of bones are known: compact or cortical bone, and trabecular or spongy or cancellous bone. In most of the bones, both compact and cancellous forms are present, but thickness of each type varies in different regions of the bone. For example, in long bones, the *epiphyseal region* contains large amount of cancellous bone and outer thin compact bone. While in *diaphyseal regions*, the amount of compact bone is more and cancellous (spongy) bone is very thin (Fig. 7.5).

Structure of compact bone

The compact bone makes the outer layer of most bones and accounts for the 80% of the bone in the body. Histologically, the compact bony tissue is made up of several minute cylindrical structures called *osteons* or *Haversian system* (Fig. 7.6). Each osteon is formed by several layers of collagen lamellae (Haversian lamellae) arranged concentrically around a centrally placed canal called the *Haversian canal* which contains the blood vessels, lymph vessels and nerve fibres. In between the concentric layers of collagen tissue are present many *lacunae* (small cavities) which contain *osteocytes*. The osteocytes send long process called canaliculi all around. The canaliculi from neighbouring osteocytes unite to form tight junctions.

The Haversian canals (and therefore the osteons) run along the longitudinal axis of long bones and branch and anastomose with each other. They also communicate with the external surface of the bone through channels that are called *canals of Volkmann*.

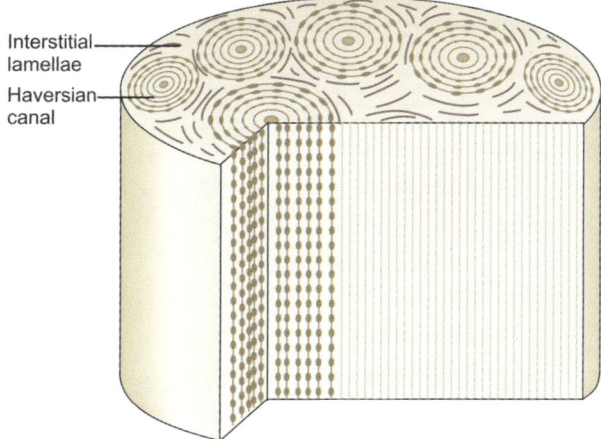

Fig. 7.6: Structure of compact bone.

Blood vessels and nerves pass through all these channels, so that compact bone is permeated by a network of blood vessels that provide nutrition to it. The compact bone is lined externally by periosteum and internally by endosteum. Both periosteum and endosteum of the long bones contain osteoprogenitor cells which can differentiate into osteoblasts or osteoclasts.

Structure of trabecular or spongy bone

The trabecular or spongy or cancellous bone is present inside the compact bone and makes up 20% of bone in the body. It is made up of spicules or plates or trabeculae which are separated by wide spaces that are filled in by bone marrow. Nutrients diffuse from the bone ECF to trabeculae. The surface to volume ratio is much higher in trabecular bone than the compact bone.

The trabeculae are thin and consist of irregular lamellae of bone with lacunae containing osteocytes. The trabeculae are covered by a thin layer of connective tissue called *endosteum* which contains osteoblasts, osteoclasts and osteoprogenitor (stem) cells (Fig. 7.7).

Cells of bone

Osteoprogenitor cells

These are stem cells of mesenchymal origin that can proliferate and convert themselves into osteoblasts whenever there is need for bone formation. They resemble fibroblasts in appearance.

In the fetus, osteoprogenitor cells are numerous at sites where bone formation is to take place.

In the adults, these cells are present over the periosteum as well as endosteum.

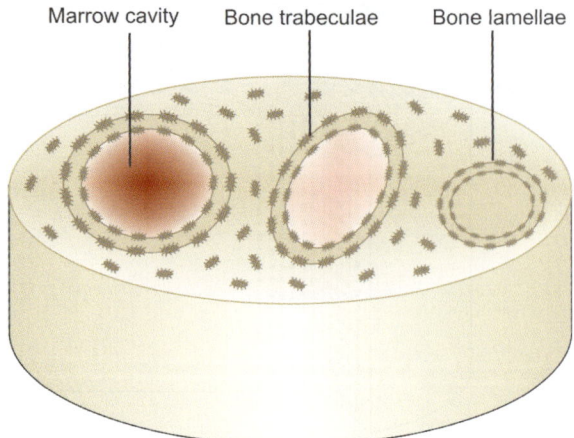

Marrow cavity   Bone trabeculae   Bone lamellae

Fig. 7.7: Structure of trabecular bone.

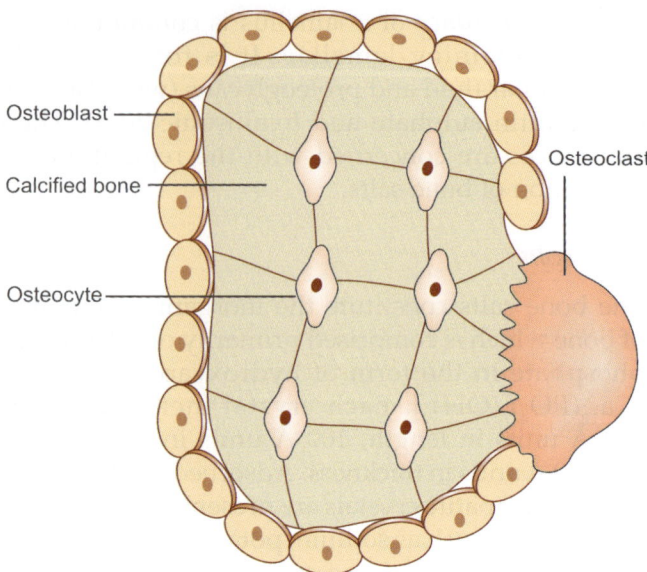

Osteoblast
Calcified bone
Osteocyte
Osteoclast

Fig. 7.8: Location of different types of bone cells.

Osteoblasts

Bone forming cells are called osteoblasts. These are derived from the osteoprogenitor cells. Being concerned with bone formation they are situated in the outer surface of bone (Fig. 7.8), the marrow cavity and epiphyseal plate cells.

Functions of osteoblast cells include:

1. *Role in laying down of the organic matrix of bone.* Osteoblasts are responsible for synthesis of bone matrix by secreting type I collagen and a protein called matrix gla protein (MGP) and other proteins involved in the matrix formation.

2. *Role in calcification.* Enzyme alkaline phosphatase present in the cell membranes of osteoblasts plays important role in the calcification of bone matrix. Osteoblasts are believed to shed off matrix vesicles which possibly serve as points around which formation of hydroxyapatite crystals takes place.

3. *Role in bone resorption.* Osteoblasts may indirectly influence the resorption of bone by inhibiting or stimulating the activity of osteoclasts.

Fate of osteoblasts: After taking part into bone formation the osteoblasts are converted into osteocytes which are trapped inside the lacunae of calcified bone.

Osteocytes

Cells of mature (or developed) bone are called osteocytes. As mentioned above they represent osteoblasts, which during bone formation are 'imprisoned' in the lacunae between the bone lamellae (Fig. 7.8). The cytoplasmic processes from the osteocytes run into canaliculi and ramify throughout the bone matrix. The processes from neighbouring cells have contact with each other forming tight junction.

Functions of osteocytes are:

- Metabolic activity of osteocytes helps to maintain the bone as living tissue.
- Maintain the integrity of lacunae and canaliculi, and thus keep the channels open for diffusion of nutrients through bone.
- Play an important role in maintaining the exchange of calcium between the bone and extracellular fluid.

Osteoclasts

Bone removing cells are called osteoclasts. These are giant multinucleated cells found in relation to surfaces where bone removal is taking place. At such locations these cells occupy pits called *resorption bays* or *lacunae of flowship.* At sites of bone resorption, the surface of an osteoclast shows many folds which are described as a *ruffled membrane* (Fig. 7.8).

Osteoclasts are derived from haemopoietic stem cells via monocytes. Probably they are formed by fusion of many monocytes.

Function. Osteoclasts are responsible for bone resorption during bone remodelling. The lysosomal enzymes required for bone resorption are synthesized and released into the bone resorbing compartment of osteoclasts.

Bone lining cells

Bone lining cells are flattened cells which form a continuous epithelium like layer on bony surfaces where active bone deposition or removal is not taking place. They are present on the periosteal surface as well as endosteal surface.

Mechanism of bone formation

All bone is of mesenchymal origin. The process of bone formation is called ossification. There are two mechanisms of bone formation: endochondral bone formation and intramembranous bone formation.

Endochondral bone formation. During fetal development, formation of most of the bones is preceded by the formation of a cartilaginous model which is subsequently replaced by bone. This kind of ossification is called endochondral bone formation.

Intramembranous bone formation. Formation of some bones, e.g. clavicle, vault of skull and mandibles is not preceded by formation of a cartilage model, but they are formed directly in a fibrous membrane. This kind of ossification is called intramembranous bone formation.

Steps of growth of a long bone

1. *Formation of a cartilage model.* In the region, where a long bone is to be formed the mesenchyme first lay down a cartilaginous model of bone.

2. *Ossification and calcification.* The ossification is carried out by osteoblasts which enter the central part of the cartilaginous model. This area is called *primary centre of ossification* (Fig. 7.9A). Gradually bone formation extends from the primary centre towards the ends of shaft (Fig. 7.9B). Process of formation of bony lamellae from osteoblasts is described separately.

3. *Growth in length and girth.* At about the time of birth developing bone consists of the bony diaphysis formed by extension of primary centre for ossification, and cartilaginous ends. At varying times after birth *secondary centres* of endochondral ossification appear in the cartilages forming the ends of bones. These centres enlarge and convert the cartilaginous ends into bone. The portion of the bone formed from one secondary centre is called *epiphysis*. During growth, the bone of diaphysis and the bone of epiphysis are separated by a plate of actively proliferating cartilage the *epiphyseal plate* (Fig. 7.10). The portion of the diaphysis adjoining the epiphyseal plate is called metaphysis. It is highly vascular and region of active bone formation. The bone increases in length as this plate lays down new bone on the end of shaft. The width of the epiphyseal plate is proportionate to the rate of growth. The width is affected by a number of hormones, but most markedly by the pituitary growth hormone and IGF-1. The bone increases in length as long as the epiphyseal plates remain separated from diaphysis

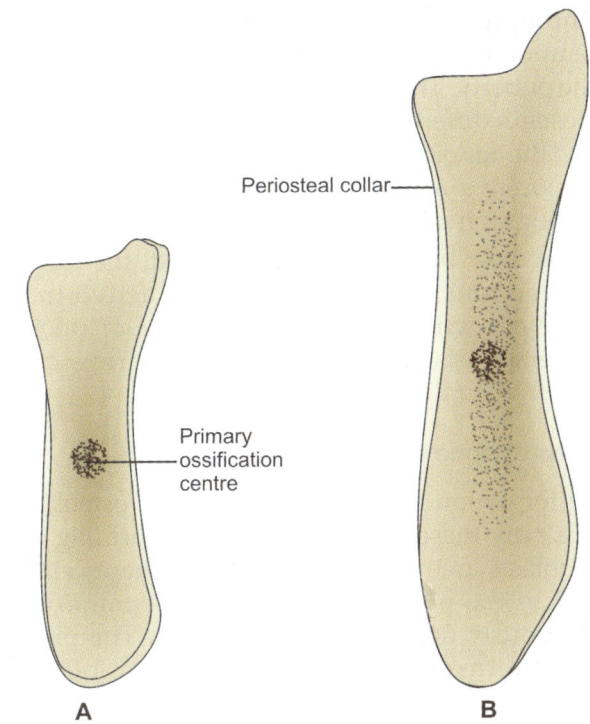

Fig. 7.9: Formation of long bone; A, cartilage model with primary centre for ossification; and B, bone growth by extension of primary centre for ossification.

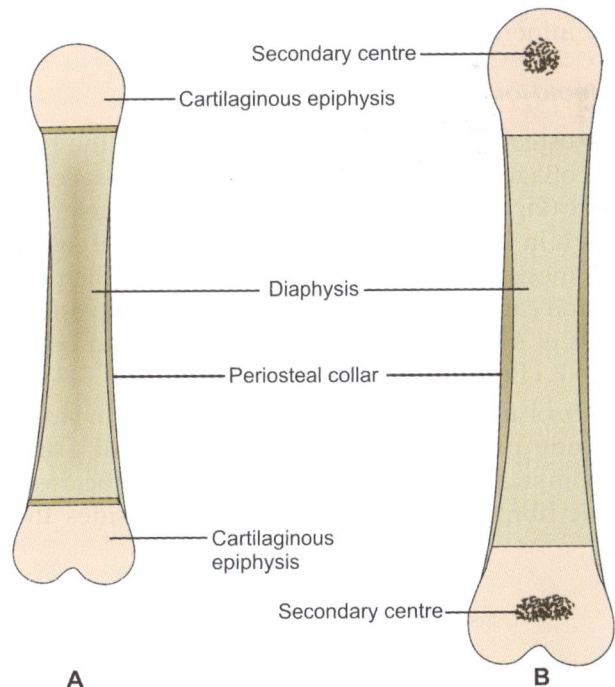

Fig. 7.10: Structure of a typical long bone before (A) and after (B) ossification.

(shaft). The growth of the bone stops when the epiphysis fuses with the diaphysis *(epiphyseal closure).* At this juncture, the cartilage cells stop proliferating, become hypertrophic and secrete VEGF, leading to vascularization and ossification.

The epiphyseal closure occurs in an orderly temporal sequence, the last epiphysis closing after the puberty. The normal age at which the epiphysis closes in different bones of the body is well known, and the age of a young individual can be determined by looking at the open and closed epiphysis in radiograph of the skeleton.

Even after bone growth has ceased, the calcium turnover function of bone is most active in the metaphysis which acts as a storehouse of calcium. The metaphysis does not have a bone marrow cavity and is frequently the site of infection.

Process of bone formation

Bone formation is carried out by active osteoblasts, that is why these are also called bone forming cells. Osteoblasts are modified fibroblasts. These cells are found in the periosteum and endosteum. Bone is continuously deposited by these cells. The process of bone formation can be considered in following steps:

- Formation of bone lamellae,
- Formation of trabecular bone, and
- Formation of compact bone.

It includes two main processes: osteoid formation and mineralization of bone matrix.

Osteoid formation

The osteoblasts synthesize and lay down the type I procollagen molecules into the adjacent extracellular space (Fig. 7.11A). These cells also secrete a gelatinous matrix in which the fibres get embedded. The collagen polymerizes to form collagen fibres which then swell up and can no longer be seen distinctly. The resultant mass of swollen fibres and matrix is called osteoid (Fig. 7.11B).

Factors affecting process of osteoid formation include protein intake and a number of growth factors such as TGF-β, IGF-I, IGF-II, PDGF, acidic and basic fibroblast growth factors, etc. Besides these growth factors, insulin, GH, sex hormones (oestrogens, androgen), thyroid hormones, calcitriol and calcitonin also affect the process of osteoid formation.

Bone matrix mineralization

Soon after formation of osteoid the process of bone matrix mineralization starts. It occurs in two phases: an initial slow process of initiation of mineralization followed by rapid mineralization process.

Initiation of mineralization or nucleation: The bone matrix is surrounded by a metastatic solution of calcium and phosphate ions (solution in which concentration of Ca^{2+} and PO_4^{3-} exceeds the solubility product of the salt but precipitation is inhibited by certain inhibitors like pyrophosphate). For enucleation to take place pyrophosphate has to be cleaved into inorganic phosphate by alkaline phosphatase which also has activity of pyrophosphatase. The process of mineralization greatly depends upon the *calcium × phosphate* ion product in extracellular fluid. This product must be above 30/dl for this process to occur.

Rapid calcification after enucleation: About 10 days elapse between osteoid formation and initiation of mineralization. However, once mineralization is initiated, i.e. after nucleation, most of the calcium phosphate is deposited within 6 to 12 hours. Thereafter, hydroxide and bicarbonate ions are gradually added to the mineral mixture, and mature hydroxyapatite crystals are slowly formed. After the process of mineralization of bone matrix is completed, the osteoid is converted into a bone lamella (Fig. 7.11C).

Formation of a trabecular bone

After the formation of one bone lamella (as described above Fig. 7.11A to C) another layer of osteoid is laid down by osteoblast. The osteoblasts move away from the bone lamella to line the new layer of osteoid. However, some osteoblasts are caught between the lamella and the osteoid (Fig. 7.11D). The osteoid is

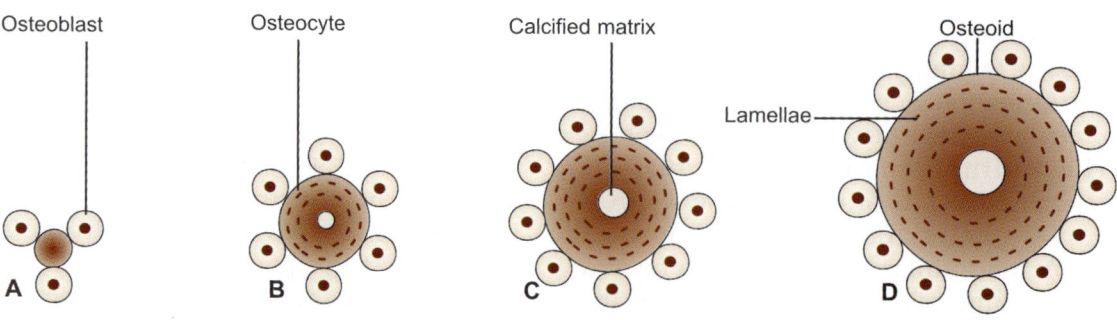

Fig. 7.11: Process of formation of bony lamellae.

now ossified to form another lamella. The cells trapped between the two lamellae become osteocytes. In this way a number of lamellae are laid down one over another and these lamellae together form a trabecula of bone, but many such trabeculae constitute the trabecular or cancellous bone. Within each lamella, mineral fluid containing channels, called *canaliculi*, traverse the mineralized bone. Through these channels, the interior osteocytes remain connected with surface lining cells and with other osteocytes via syncytial cell processes. This system of interconnected cells formed by osteocytes and osteoblasts spreads over all the bone surfaces except small surface area adjacent to osteoclasts. This extensive system of osteocytes and osteoblasts constitutes an osteocystic membrane system which separates bone from ECF. A small amount of fluid called the bone fluid is present between the bone and osteocytic membrane. This arrangement permits transfer of calcium from the enormous surface area of the interior to the exterior of the bone units, and then into the extracellular fluid. This transfer process which is carried out by the osteocytes, is known as *osteocytic osteolysis*. It probably does not actually decrease bone mass, but it simply removes calcium from the most recently formed crystals.

Conversion of trabecular bone to compact bone

All newly formed bone is cancellous. It is converted into compact bone (Fig. 7.12):

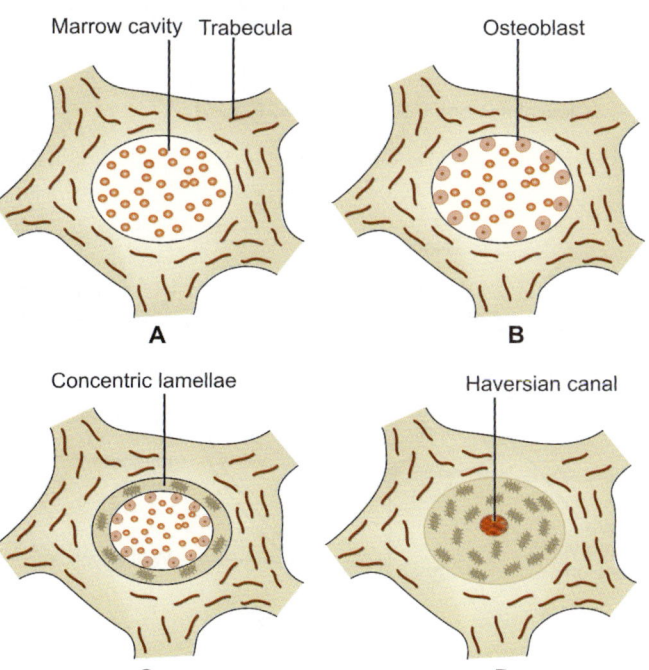

Fig. 7.12: Steps of conversion of trabecular bone into compact bone.

- Each space between the trabeculae of cancellous bone comes to be lined by osteoblasts (Fig. 7.12A and B).
- The osteoblasts lay down lamellae of bone as already described. The first lamella is formed over the inner wall of the original space and is therefore, shaped like a ring (Fig. 7.12C).
- Subsequently, concentric lamellae are laid down inside this ring thus forming an *osteon*. The original space becomes smaller and smaller and persists as a *Haversian canal* (Fig. 7.12D).

Molecular regulation of bone formation

Members of the transforming growth factor-β (TGF-β) family of genes are involved in various stages of bone formation.

Anomalies of bone formation

A few anomalies of bone formation are given below:

1. *Dyschondroplasia* refers to disorderly and excessive proliferation of cartilage cells in the epiphyseal plate or formation of irregular masses of cartilage within metaphysis which occurs after failure of normally formed cartilage to be replaced by bone.

2. *Multiple exostosis* or diaphyseal ectasia occurs as a result of interference with the process of remodelling of bone. It is characterised by formation of abnormal masses of bone in the region of the metaphysis. Such a protusion is called exostosis.

3. *Osteogenesis imperfecta* is a condition of abnormal calcification of bones. Such bones are prone to multiple fractures.

4. *Fibrous dysplasia* refers to a condition in which some parts of a bone are replaced by fibrous tissue.

5. *Achondroplasia* refers to a condition of insufficient, or disorderly formation of bone in the region of the epiphyseal cartilage. It is characterised by restricted growth of long bones resulting in dwarfism.

FORMATION OF MUSCLE TISSUE

The muscle tissue is formed mainly from the *mesoderm* except for the muscles of iris, which develop from the *neuroectoderm*.

- *Skeletal muscles* develop from the mesoderm of myotomes.
- *Cardiac muscles* are derived from the splanchnic mesoderm surrounding the developing endothelial heart tube, and

- *Smooth muscles* develop from the splanchnic mesoderm surrounding the developing gut and its derivatives.

Histogenesis of muscular tissue, i.e. conversion of mesodermal cells into muscular tissue is described on page 112.

Molecular regulation of muscle formation

MYO-D and MYF5, members of the family of myogenic regulatory factors (MRFs), are considered to play important role in the induction of myogenesis in mesenchymal cells.

Signaling molecules involved in the regulation of beginning of myogenesis and induction of myotomes are:

- *Sonic hedgehog (SHH) protein* secreted from the ventral neural tube and notochord.
- *WNTs and BMP4* secreted from the dorsal neural tube and the overlying ectoderm.

FORMATION OF BODY CAVITIES

OVERVIEW OF BODY CAVITIES AND INTRAEMBRYONIC COELOM

It is worthwhile to study the development of various body cavities, before studying the development of various organ systems present in these cavities. The body cavities include:

- Pericardial cavity,
- Pleural cavities, and
- Peritoneal cavity.

All these body cavities develop from the intra-embryonic coelom.

Intraembryonic coelom and visceral mesoderm

As described on page 45, the intraembryonic coelom from which the body cavities are derived, begins to develop near the end of the third week. With the formation of intraembryonic coelom, the lateral plate mesoderm is divided into two layers; parietal and visceral. These layers of mesoderm, ultimately form the parietal and visceral layers of body cavities (Fig. 7.13). During 4th weeks of gestation the intra-embryonic coelom is divided into three body cavities:

- Pericardial cavity,
- Pleural cavity, and
- Peritoneal cavity.

Note: Before studying the detailed development of body cavities (described below), it will be worthwhile to revise the formation of three divisions of mesoderm

and formation of somites, formation of intraembryonic coelom, and effects of folding of embryonic disc on the intraembryonic coelom.

DEVELOPMENT OF PERICARDIAL CAVITY

- *Primordium of pericardial cavity in embryonic disc.* The intraembryonic coelom, early in the fourth week, appears as a horse shoe shaped cavity having a narrow midline portion and two lateral extensions (Fig. 7.14).
- *The midline part,* also known as curve or bend of intraembryonic coelom lies near the cranial end of the embryonic disc and represents the future pericardial cavity.
- *The lateral extensions* of the intraembryonic coelom represent the future pleural and peritoneal cavities. The distal part of each lateral extension of the intraembryonic coelom is continuous with the extraembryonic coelom at the lateral edges of embryonic disc (Fig. 7.13).

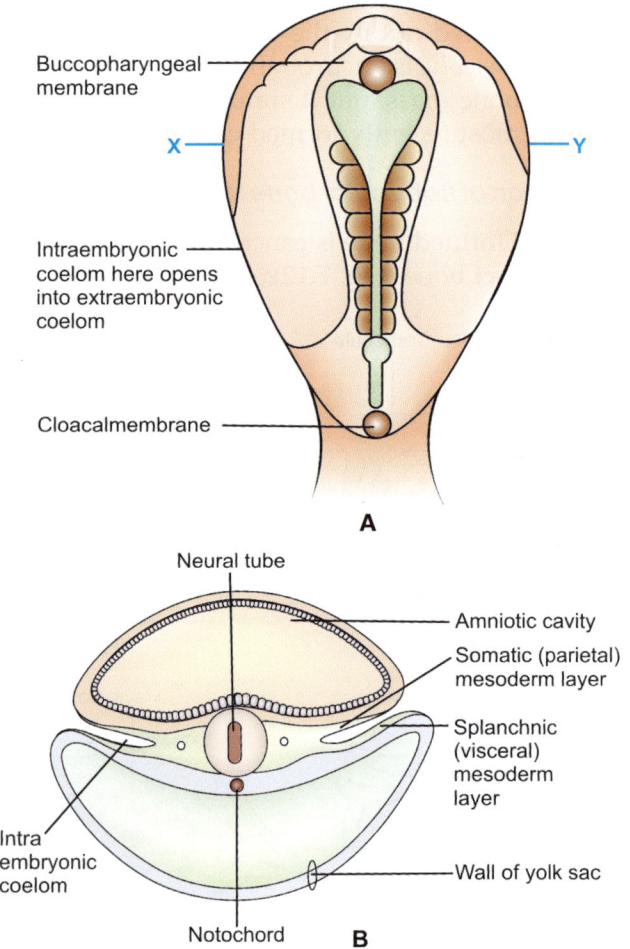

Fig. 7.13: Horseshoe-shaped intraembryonic coelom at about end of third week: A, dorsal view of the embryonic disc; B, transverse section of the embryo at X-Y in A.

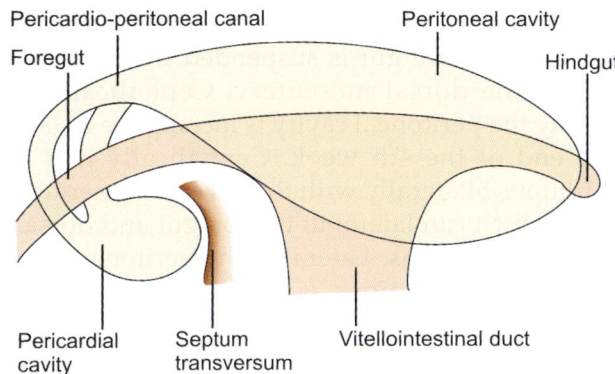

Fig. 7.14: Parts of intraembryonic coelom and their relationship to the developing gut (after folding of the embryo).

Effect of folding of embryo on developing pericardial cavity. With the formation of head fold the developing heart and pericardial cavity come to lie on the ventral aspect of the body of embryo, anterior to the developing foregut.

Further development of pericardial cavity is described along with development of heart.

DEVELOPMENT OF PLEURAL CAVITIES

Pericardio-peritoneal canals. The pericardial and peritoneal cavities are connected to each other, for some time, by the pericardio-peritoneal canal, which pass dorsal to and on either side of the foregut with folding of embryo (Fig. 7.14).

Enlargement of pericardio-peritoneal canal to form pleural cavities: The pericardio-peritoneal canals are invaginated by the lung buds that arise from the foregut (Fig. 7.15). With the growth of lung buds in size the pericardio-peritoneal canals balloon out to form the pleural cavities. As a result of this growth following structural characteristics are noted (Fig. 7.16A):

- *Pericardio-pleural openings* connect the pleural cavities with pericardial cavity.
- *Pleuro-peritoneal openings* connect the pleural cavities with peritoneal cavity.

- *Pleuro-pericardial folds* are formed superior to the developing lung, and
- *Pleuro-peritoneal folds* are formed inferior to the developing lungs.

Pleuropericardial membranes (Fig. 7.16B) are formed by enlargement of the pleuropericardial folds. These close the pericardiopleural openings and thus separate the pericardial cavity from the pleural cavities. These membranes also take part in the formation of fibrous pericardium. The pleuropericardial membranes contain the *common cardinal* veins which drain the primordial venous system into the *sinus venosus* of the primordial heart.

Pleuroperitoneal membranes (Fig. 7.16B) are formed by enlargement of the pleuroperitoneal folds. These membranes close the pleuroperitoneal opening and thus separate the pleural cavities from the peritoneal cavity. These membranes also take part in the formation of diaphragm.

DEVELOPMENT OF PERITONEAL CAVITY AND MESENTERY

Formation of common mesentery and two separate peritoneal cavities

As a result of lateral folding of the embryonic disc the two lateral extensions of the intraembryonic coelom come together ventrally. The same folding process converts endodermal layer into primitive gut. Coincidentally the splanchnic mesoderm of either side envelops the tubular digestive tract to form the primary or common mesentery. The dorsal portion of the common mesentery is called *dorsal mesentery* and its ventral part is called *ventral mesentery* (Fig. 7.17). Thus, from the Fig. 7.17 it can be seen that as a result of folding the lateral extensions of the intraembryonic coelom forms two (right and left) peritoneal cavities separated by the dorsal mesentery, enveloped primitive gut tube and ventral mesentery.

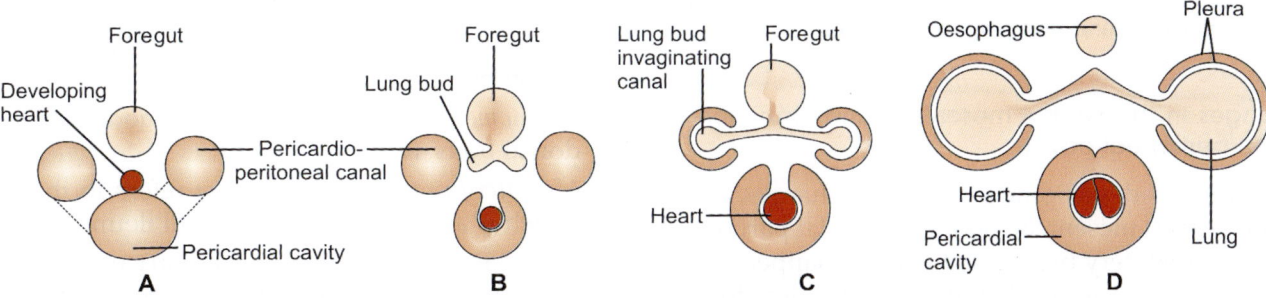

Fig. 7.15: Invagination of pericardio-peritoneal canals by the developing lung buds.

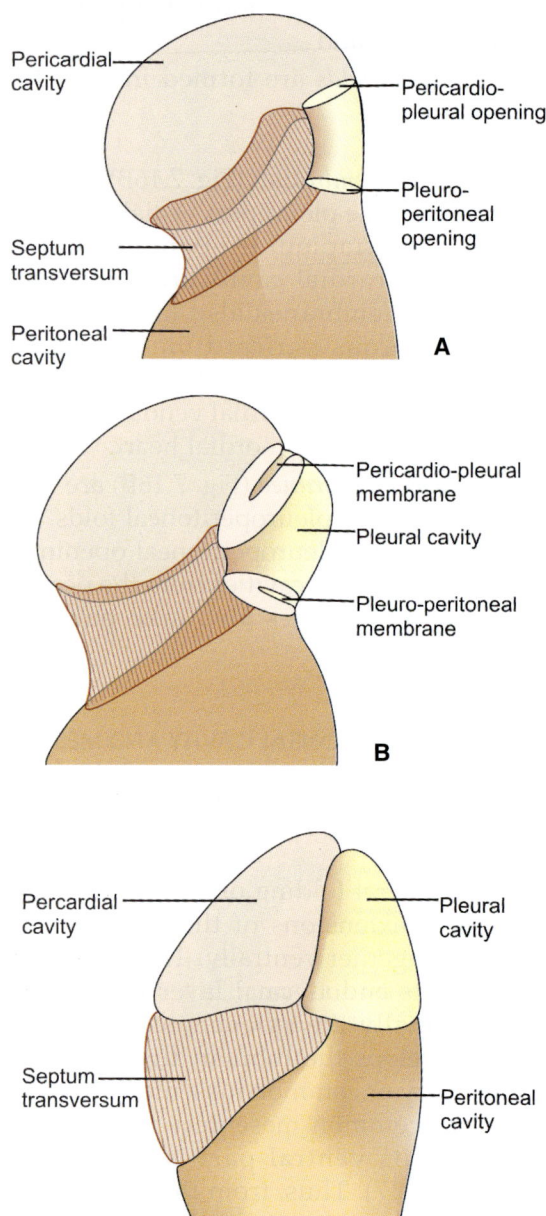

Fig. 7.16: Formation of pleural cavities and their separation from the pericardial and peritoneal cavities: A, depicting position of pericardio-pleural and pleuro-peritoneal openings; B, formation of pericardio-pleural and pleuro-peritoneal membranes separating the pleural cavities from pericardial and peritoneal cavities, respectively; C. completion of separation of pericardial, pleural and peritoneal cavities.

Changes in the ventral mesentery and formation of single peritoneal cavity

With further development following changes occur in the ventral mesentery: soon, the caudal part of the ventral mesentery breaks down and disappear. As a result the right and left halves of the developing peritoneal cavity are united to form a single peritoneal cavity. It is lined with somatic mesoderm and the primitive gut is suspended from its dorsal wall by the dorsal mesentery. Cephalically and laterally the peritoneal cavity is incomplete as late as upto end of the 4th week. Cephalically it is still continuous bilaterally with the pericardio-peritoneal canals which run lateral to the foregut and dorsal to septum transversus. Laterally, the peritoneal cavity maintains connections with the extraembryonic coelom in the region of yolk sac. Later in development as described above these connections are sealed and the peritoneal cavity then becomes a closed sac.

- Some cephalic part of the ventral mesentery that extends from the developing stomach and first part of the duodenum persists. This part of ventral mesentery has a free border caudally, while cephalically it is continuous with the septum transversus. As the liver develops rapidly within the septum transversus, it eventually forces its way between two layers of the ventral mesentery. As a result the ventral mesentery becomes subdivided. The segment of the mesentery between the surface of liver and stomach becomes lesser omentum (ventral mesogastrium) and the segment between the liver and the ventral body wall becomes the falciform ligament of liver. The free edge of this mesentery eventually becomes the margin of the epiploic foramen or foramen of Winslow. The ventral mesentery in association with the septum transversus forms the coronary and left and right triangular ligaments. The ventral mesentery investing the developing liver gives rise to the tunical serosa and fibrosae of the liver.

Dorsal mesentery

In contrast to the ventral mesentery, most of which disappears, almost the entire dorsal mesentery persists as a supporting membrane and as a path for nerves and blood vessels for the gut tissue. It extends from the region of septum transversus to near the termination of the hind gut in the cloaca. Although dorsal mesentery is a continuous sheet, it has been given different names in different regions (Fig. 7.18):

- *Dorsal mesoduogastrium* — attaching stomach to the dorsal body wall.
- *Dorsal mesoduodenum* — attaches duodenum to the dorsal body wall.
- *Mesentery proper or mesentrium* refers to that part which is attached to jejunum and ileum.
- *Dorsal mesocolon* refers to the part of the dorsal mesentery which attaches colon to the posterior body wall.

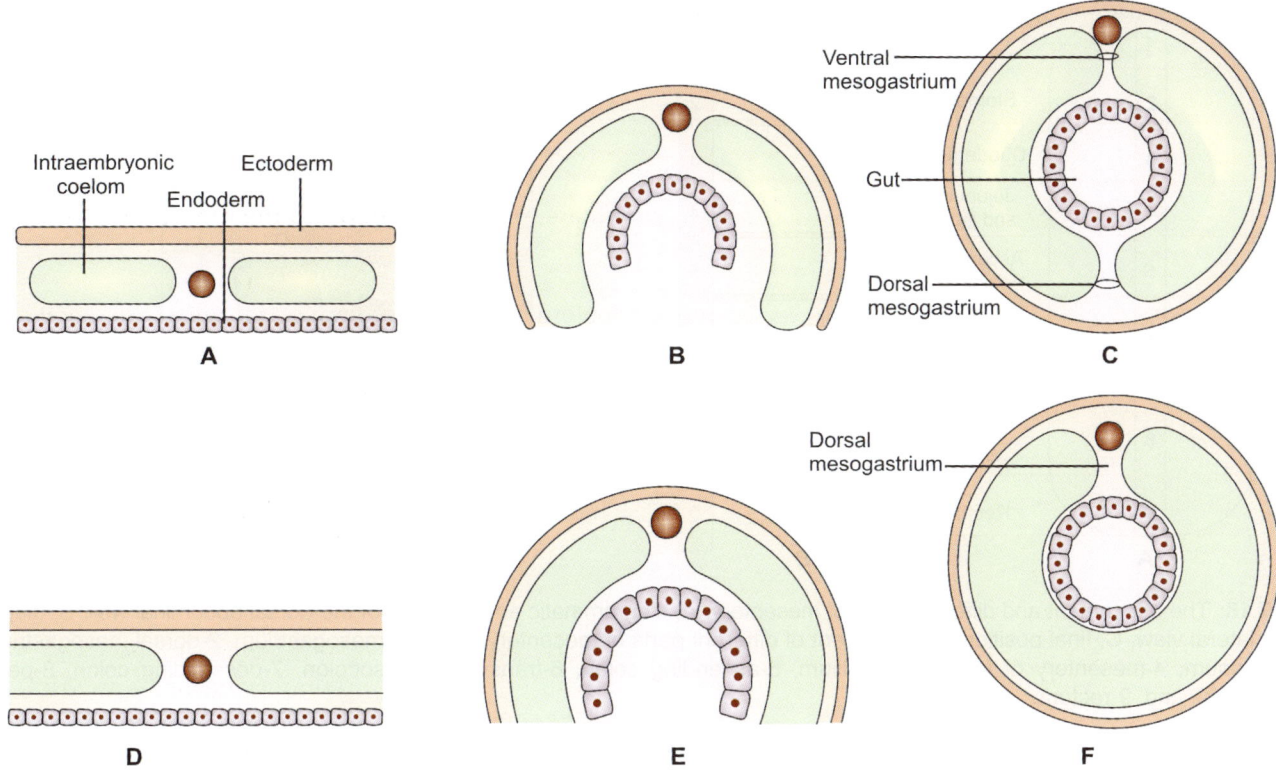

Fig. 7.17: Formation of ventral and dorsal mesentery after lateral folding of embryo.

Later changes in the dorsal mesentery and formation of various folds and sacs in the peritoneal cavity

As shown in Fig. 7.18A and B, initially the attachment of the dorsal mesentery on the posterior abdominal wall is linear and in the midline. However, later in development this primary dorsal mesentery undergoes very complex changes. This results due to involvement of dorsal mesentery in the elongation and folding of the developing digestive tract to which it supports and also as a result of the fat that some parts of the gut become retroperitoneal. The final adult line of attachment of the mesentery is shown in Fig. 7.18C.

As a result of these complex changes in the line of attachment of mesentery and further development, various folds and sacs of peritoneal cavity are formed. The details of their formation is beyond the scope of this book. Some of these peritoneal folds and sac are (Fig. 7.19):

- Lesser sac,
- Lesser omentum,
- Greater omentum,
- Lienorenal ligament, and
- Gastrosplenic ligament.

DEVELOPMENT OF DIAPHRAGM

The diaphragm is a composite structure that separates the pericardial and pleural cavities above it from the peritoneal cavity lying below it. In other words it separates thoracic cavity from the abdominal cavity. It develops from four embryonic structures (Fig. 7.20):

- *Septum transversus*, (which forms ventral unpaired portion, i.e. central tendon of diaphragm.
- *Pleuroperitoneal membrane* (which forms paired dorsolateral portions of diaphragm).
- *Dorsal mesentery of oesophagus*, (which forms an irregular medial dorsal portion of diaphragm), and
- *Muscular in growth from the lateral body* walls (which form the paired peripheral parts of diaphragm).

1. *Septum transversus,* first appears at the end of the third week as a mass of mesodermal tissue cranial to the developing pericardial cavity. After the formation of head fold, during 4th week, the septum transversus comes to lie between the developing pericardial cavity and rest of the intraembryonic coelom (Fig. 7.21). Then it grows dorsally from the ventral body wall and forms a semicircular shelf that separates the heart lying in pericardial cavity above it from the liver developing below it (Fig.

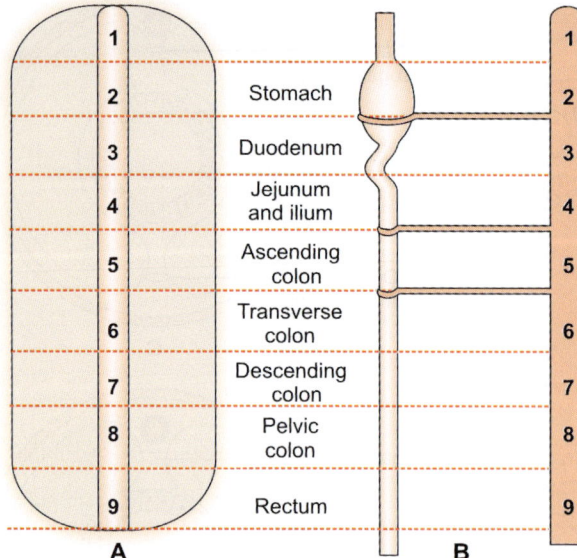
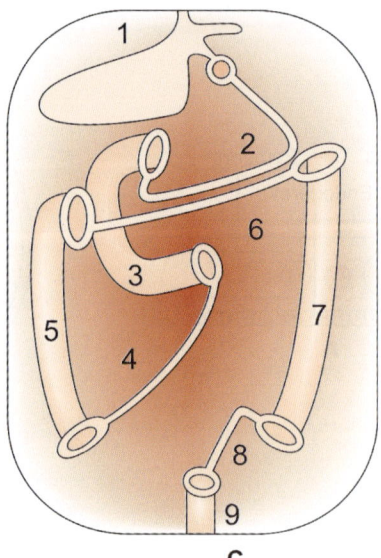

Fig. 7.18: The attachment and different parts of mesentery: A, diagrammatic anterior view of the dorsal abdominal wall; B, diagramatic lateral view, C, final position of attachment of different parts of mesentery: 1-ventromesogastrium, 2-dorsal mesogastrium, 3-duodenum, 4-mesentery of jejunum and ilium, 5-ascending colon, 6-transverse mesocolon, 7-descending colon, 8-pelvic mesocolon, and 9-rectum.

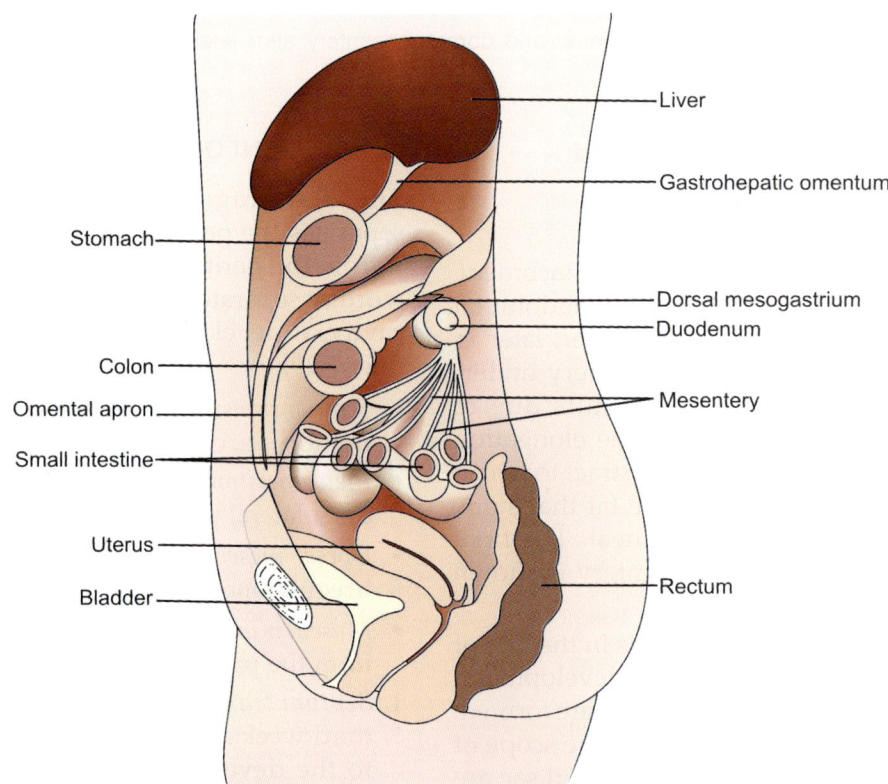

Fig. 7.19: Attachment of mesentery and peritoneal folds and sac in an adult.

7.21B). The septum transversus does not separate the thoracic and abdominal cavities completely. Dorsally the pericardio-peritoneal canals lie on each side of the oesophagus.

The septum transversus forms the *central tendon of the diaphragm* (Fig. 7.20).

2. *Pleuro-peritoneal membranes,* as described earlier, are formed by enlargement of pleuro-peritoneal

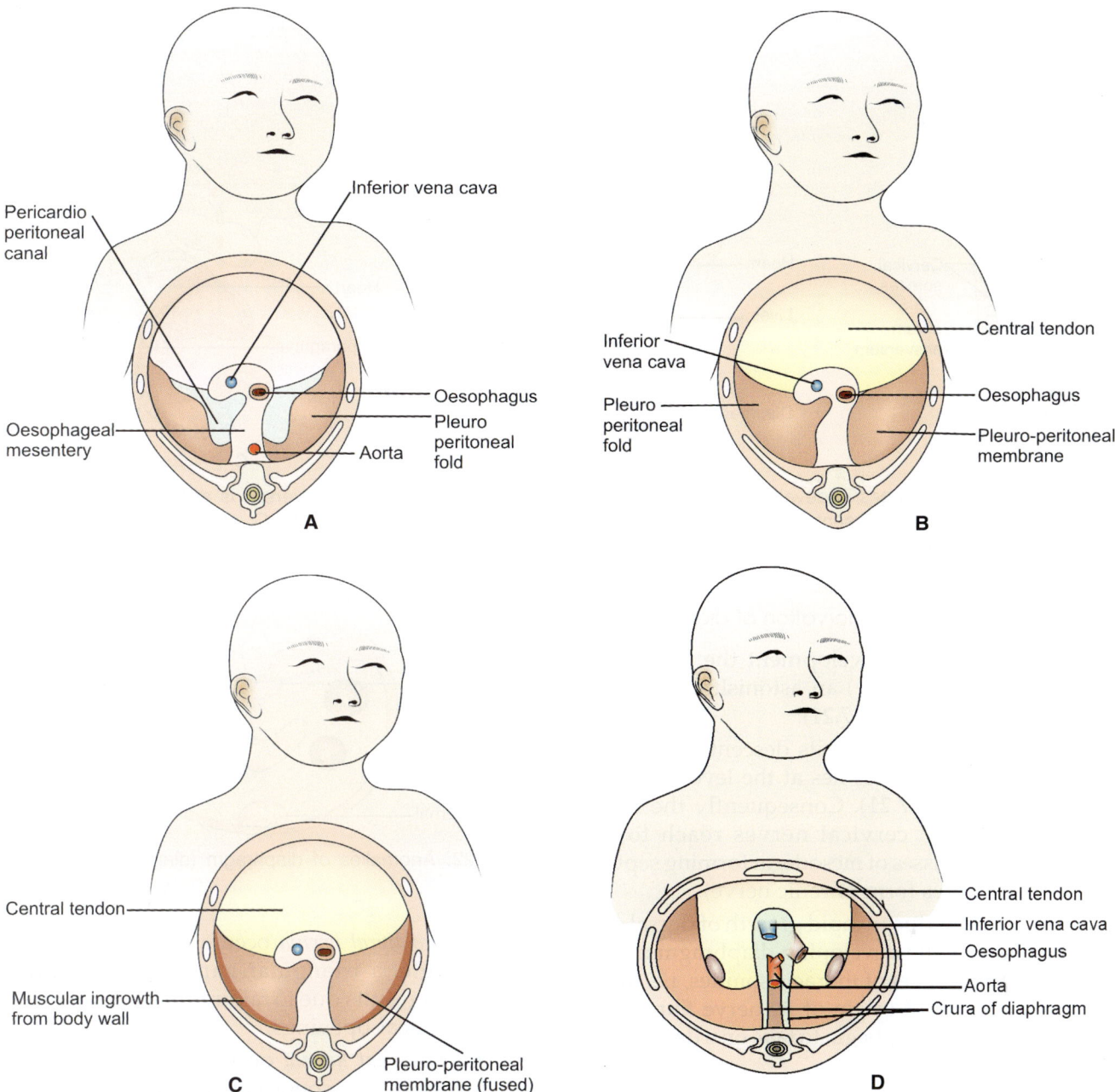

Fig. 7.20: Schematic transverse section depicting inferior view of developing diaphragm: A, showing patent pericardioperitoneal canals and unfused pleuroperitoneal folds at 5th week; B, showing fusion of pleuroperitoneal membrane at end of 6th week; C, showing contribution from lateral body wall at about 12 week; D, showing inferior view of diaphragm of a newborn indicating embryological origin of its components.

folds. These fuse with the dorsal mesentery of oesophagus and the septum transversus and thus complete the separation of thoracic cavity from the abdominal cavity and form the *primordial diaphragm* (Fig. 7.20). As shown in Fig. 7.20B and C the pleuroperitoneal membranes form large portions of fetal diaphragm, however, their contribution in the newborn's diaphragm is comparatively less (Fig. 7.20D).

3. *Dorsal mesentery of esophagus,* forms an irregular median dorsal portion of the diaphragm.
4. *Muscular ingrowth from the lateral body walls* forms the peripheral parts of diaphragm, external to the parts contributed by the pleuroperitoneal membranes (Fig. 7.20). Extension of the growing pleural cavities and lungs into the lateral body walls leads to formation of costodiaphragmatic recesses on each side.

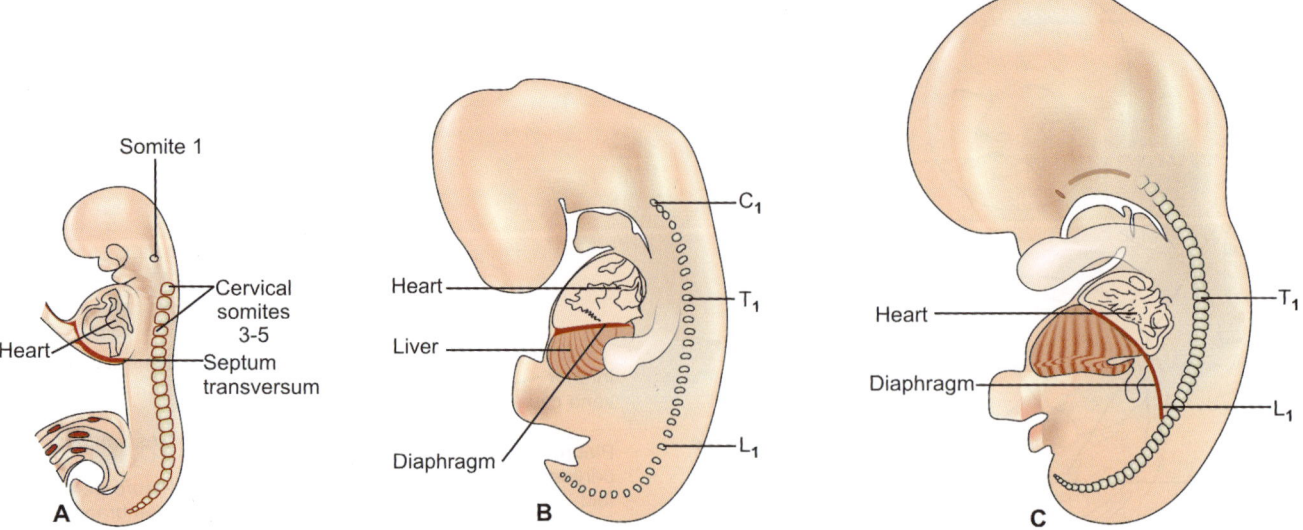

Fig. 7.21: Positional changes in developing diaphragm: A, during 4th week septum transversus is at the level of 3rd to 5th somites; B, during 6th week, septum transversus moves caudally at the mid thoracic level; C, at 8th week the developing diaphragm reaches up to first lumbar segment.

Positional changes and innervation of diaphragm

During the course of development the transverse septum moves (relatively) an astonishing distance caudally in the body (Fig. 7.21).

- *During 4th week,* (prior to its descent with heart) the septum transversus lies at the level of 3rd to 5th somites (Fig. 7.21). Consequently the fibres from 3rd to 5th cervical nerves reach to the premuscular masses of mesoderm forming septum (these new fibres form phrenic nerve).

- *During 6th week,* due to rapid growth of dorsal part of the embryo, the developing diaphragm moves caudally at the level of thoracic somites, i.e. much below the point of origin of its nerve fibres, and so the phrenic nerves begin to take on a descending course (Fig. 7.21B).

- *At eighth week,* the diaphragm moves caudally upto the level of last thoracic or first lumbar segment (Fig. 7.21C). The phrenic nerves are correspondingly lengthened, and in adults they are about 30 cm long. The phrenic nerves supply motor as well as sensory fibres to the diaphragm.

Anomalies of diaphragm

1. *Congenital diaphragmatic hernia* may occur when there are gaps in the diaphragm due to failure of closure of different components of diaphragm. A few gaps in the diaphragm are as follows (Fig. 7.22).

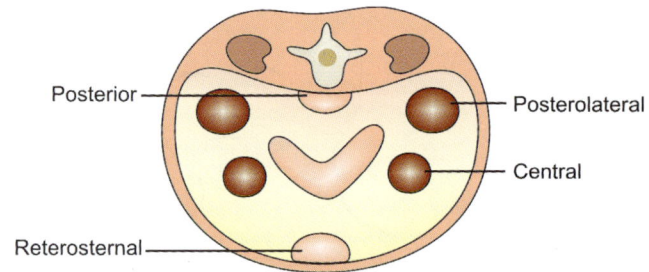

Fig. 7.22: Anomalies of diaphragm (diaphragmatic hernia).

- *Posterolateral hernia* occurs due to Bockdaleh's triangle, a triangular gap in the diaphragm which results due to failure of closure of pleuroperitoneal openings.

- *Retrosternal hernia* occurs due to foramen of Morgagni, an abnormal large gap between the sternal and costal parts of the muscle.

- *Posterior hernia* may occur due to the failure of development of the crura.

- *Central hernia* occurs, rarely when the entire half (usually the left) of diaphragm is absent.

2. *Accessory diaphragm* may be present in the thoracic cavity, very rarely which partially subdivides the lung into two parts.

3. *Congenital eventration of the diaphragm* refers to an upward bulging of diaphragm into the thorax when the muscle is thin, i.e. an aponeurosis. The bulging may be unilateral or confined to small area.

Systemic Embryology

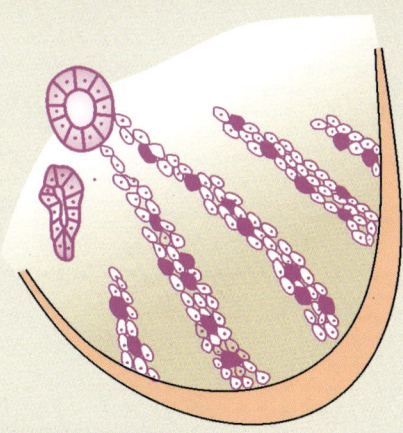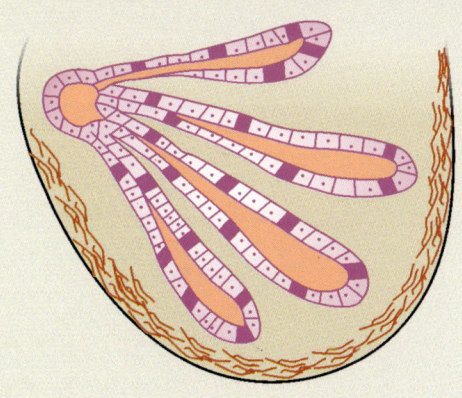

Development of Skin and its Appendages (Integumentary System)

DEVELOPMENT OF SKIN
- Embryonal contributing tissues
- Development of epidermis
- Development of dermis
- Congenital disorders of skin

DEVELOPMENT OF APPENDAGES OF SKIN
- Nails
- Hairs
- Glands of skin including mammary gland

DEVELOPMENT OF SKIN

Skin, the outermost covering of the human body, primarily consists of two layers:
- Epidermis, and
- Dermis or corium.

EMBRYONAL CONTRIBUTING TISSUES

The embryonal tissues contributing for the development of skin are:
- *Surface ectoderm* gives rise to *epidermis,* the superficial layer, of skin.
- *Mesenchyme* derived from dermatomes of somites, form the dermis, the deep layer of skin.
- *Neural crest* contributes melanocytes (pigment cells) which migrate into the dermis.

Induction mechanism. It is important to note that ectodermal (epidermal) and mesenchymal (dermal) interactions involve mutual inductive mechanisms during development of skin.

DEVELOPMENT OF EPIDERMIS

Stages of development of epidermis

Single layered epithelium. The surface ectoderm of the embryo initially (during the first month and in the beginning of 2nd month) is a single layered structure made of simple cuboidal cells (Fig. 8.1A).

Two layered epithelium. About the middle of 2nd month this epithelium divides and forms two layered epithelium (Fig. 8.1B):
- *Periderm* or *epitrichium* is the superficial layer made of flattened squamous cells. These cells are usually cast off at the end of 4th month.
- *Basal layer* or deeper layer is made of germinal cells which form the stratum germinativum.

Three layered epithelium. With further proliferation of cells of basal layer an intermediate layer of cells is formed (Fig. 8.1C).

Multilayered epithelium. During 4th month, due to repeated divisions of cells of basal layer, the epithelium starts becoming multilayered. Finally, by

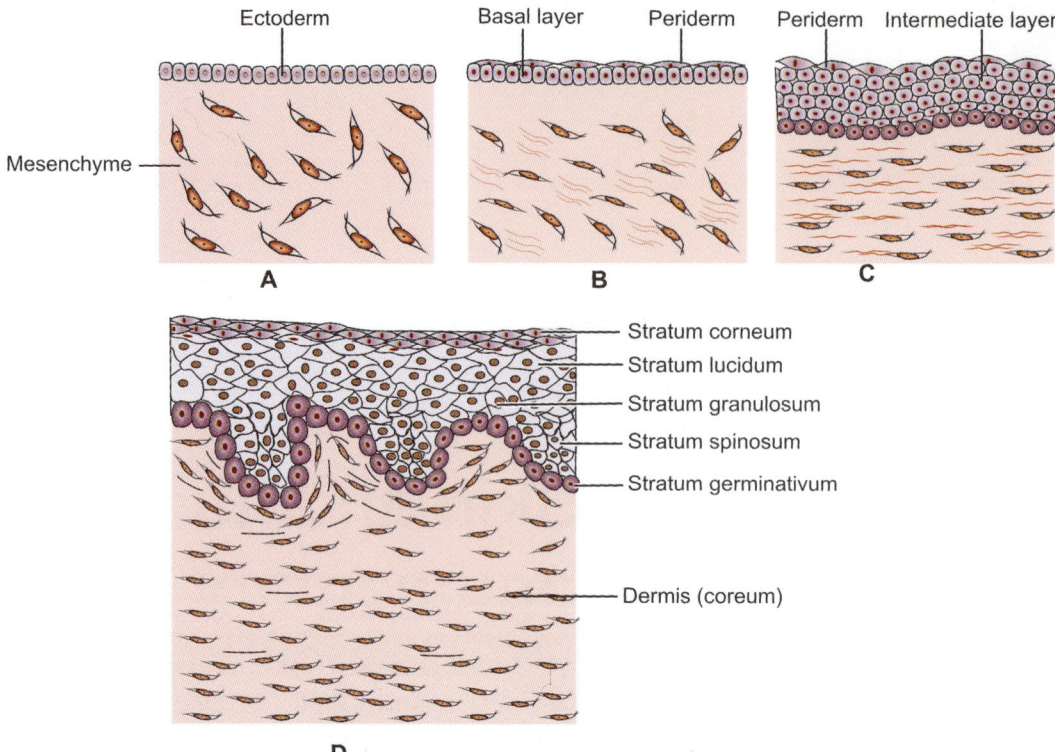

Fig. 8.1: Stages of development of skin: A, stage of single layer epidermis; B, stage of two layered epidermis, C, stage of three layered epidermis and D, stage of multilayered epidermis (definitive structure of skin in a newborn).

the end of 4th month, the epidermis acquires its definitive structure composed of stratified keratinized squamous epithelium (Fig. 8.1D):

- *Stratum basale* or the basal layer, produces new cells throughout life. The new cells are displaced into the layers superficial to it.
- *Stratum spinosum*, refers to the next thick spinous layer consisting of many layers of large polyhedral cells containing fine tonofibrils. The stratum basale and stratum spinosum combinedly form the germinative zone or *stratum germinativum*.
- *Stratum granulosum* is the next layer of cells containing keratohyalin granules (granular layer).
- *Stratum lucidum* is next superficial layer made of clear cells.
- *Stratum corneum*, a thick horny layer, forms the tough scale like surface of the epidermis. It is made of closely packed cells. The cells on the surface are flat, thin, non-nucleated, dead cells or squames in which cytoplasm has been replaced by protein *keratin*. These cells are constantly being rubbed off throughout life and replaced by cells that originate in the germinativum layer and undergo gradual changes as they progress towards the surface.

Formation of ridges. Proliferation of cells in the germinal layer also leads to formation of epidermal ridges which extend into the developing dermis (Fig.

8.1D). The epidermal ridges produce typical grooves on the surface of palm of the hand, finger tips, and soles of the feet. The pattern produced is determined genetically and is different for each individual and therefore, forms the basis of examining fingerprints in criminal investigations (dermatoglyphics).

DEVELOPMENT OF DERMIS

The dermis or corium is formed by condensation and differentiation of mesenchymal cells lying below the surface ectoderm. Most of the mesenchymal cells originate from the somatic layer of lateral mesoderm and only a few of them are derived from the dermatomes of somites. When fully developed, the dermis consists of a closely woven layer of fibroelastic connective tissue, initially the line of junction between the developing epidermis and dermis is straight. However, with the development of epidermal ridges, the dermis is thrown into *dermal papillae* which project upwards and interdigitate with the epidermal ridges. These papillae usually contain a small capillary and sensory nerve end organ. The deeper layer of the dermis the *subcorium* contains large amount of fatty tissue.

Development of pigment cells

Some *neural crest cells*, late in the embryonic period, migrate into the mesenchyme of developing dermis and get converted into *melanoblasts.* These cells migrate to the dermal-epidermal junction and their processes extend into the epidermis. Later, with the formation of pigment granules, these get converted into *melanocytes.* The melanin synthesized by melanocytes is also transferred to the other cells of the epidermis by way of dendritic processes.

Vernix Caseosa

Vernix caseosa refers to white greasy substance covering the fetal skin. It is formed by the desquamated keratinized periderm cells and sebum produced by sebaceous glands.

Functions of vernix caseosa are:
- *Protection of the skin* against macerating action of amniotic fluid mixed with fetal urine.
- *Facilitation of birth of fetus* because of its slippery nature.

CONGENITAL DISORDERS OF SKIN

1. Pigmentary disorders

i. *Albinism* is a disease of abnormal melanin synthesis or processing characterized by globally reduced or absent pigment in skin, hair and eyes (hence also called *oculo-cutaneous albinism (OCA).*

ii. *Vitiligo* refers to patchy loss of pigment from affected areas of skin, overlying hair and oral mucosa. It results from a loss of melanocytes due to an autoimmune disorder.

iii. *Piebaldism* is an abnormality of melanocyte function characterized by patchy absence of hair pigment.

iv. *Waardenburg syndrome (WS)* is also an abnormality of melanocyte dysfunction charac-terized by:
  - White patches of skin,
  - Patches of white hair (usually a forelock),
  - Heterochromia irides, and
  - Deafness.

2. Aplasia and dysplasia of skin

i. *Aplasia* of skin refers to failure of skin to develop in certain area.

ii. *Dysplasia,* i.e. abnormal development of skin may occur alone or in association with mal-development of various ectodermal derivatives including hair, teeth, sweat glands and seba-ceous glands.

DEVELOPMENT OF APPENDAGES OF SKIN

The appendages of skin include:
- Nails,
- Hair and arrector muscles of hair, and
- Glands of skin including mammary gland.

DEVELOPMENT OF NAILS

Nails of the fingers and toes develop from the surface ectoderm of digits.

Milestones in the development of nails are (Fig. 8.2):
- *Formation of nail fields.* The ectoderm at the tip of each digit becomes thickened to form the primordia of nails, the so called *nail fields.* Later these nail fields migrate from the tips of digits on to their dorsal aspects, carrying their innervation from the ventral surface.

- *Formation of nail folds* or epidermal folds soon surround the nail fields laterally and proximally.

- *Formation of nail plate.* The cells from the proximal nail fold proliferate and grow over the nail field and form a thick germinal matrix. Soon the cells covering the nail field are keratinized to form the nail plate.

- *Eponychium, cuticle and hyponychium.* Eponychium refers to superficial layer of epidermis which initially covers the developing nail. Later, the eponychium degenerates, exposing the nail, except at its base, where it persists as cuticle. Hyponychium refers to the skin under the free margin of nail.

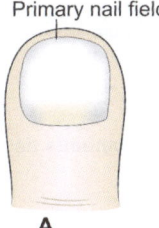
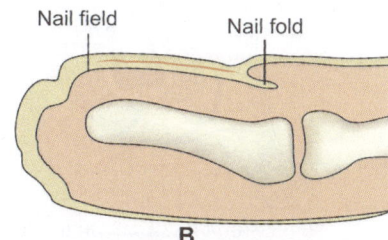
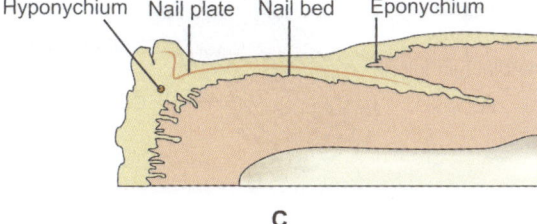

Fig. 8.2: Development of finger nail: A, stage of formation of nail field and nail fold; B, formation of nail plate; C, fully formed nail plate lined by eponychium.

Time schedule of nail development is as below:

- Finger nails start developing at about 10 weeks.
- Toe nails start developing about 4 weeks later than finger nails.
- Finger nails reach upto the tips by about 32 weeks and toe nails by about 36 weeks.

DEVELOPMENT OF HAIR

Hair become recognizable on the eyebrows, eyelids, lips, chin and scalp during the third month. About a month later the hair appear on the skin of the general body.

Stages of development of hair are (Fig. 8.3):

- *Hair bud* is formed by localized proliferation of the epidermal cells of germinal layer which extends into the underlying dermis (Fig. 8.3A).
- *Hair bulb.* By further proliferation of cells the hair bud is converted into a club-shaped hair bulb or primordial hair follicle (Fig. 8.3B).
- *Hair papillae.* The hair bulb soon moulded into a shape suggestive of an inverted cup and is invaginated by a condensation of mesoderm which forms the hair papillae (Fig. 8.3C). The epithelial cells of the hair bulb lying over the hair papillae form the germinal matrix. Melanoblasts migrate into the hair bulb and differentiate into melanocytes. The melanin produced by these cells is transferred to the hair forming cells in the germinal matrix the relative contents of melanin accounts for different hair colour.

- *Formation of hair shaft, epithelial root sheath and dermal root shealth.* Soon, the central germinal cells of the hair bulb (primitive hair follicle) proliferate, become spindle shaped and keratinized forming the *hair shaft.* As it grows the hair shaft is pushed towards the surface by making an opening for it through the center of original cylindrical epithelial ingrowth.

The peripheral cells surrounding the hair shaft form the *epithelial* root sheath. The surrounding mesenchymal cells differentiate into *dermal root sheath.*

- *Arrector pili muscle* is small smooth muscle derived from the mesenchyme. It is usually attached to the dermal root sheath.

Lanugo hair or downy hair refer to the hair that first appears on the fetal skin. These are soft, fine and lightly pigmented and help to hold the vernix caseosa on the skin. The lanugo hairs are shed about the time of birth and are later replaced by coarser hairs arising from the hair follicles. These coarse hairs persist over most of the body, except in the axillary and pubic regions, where they are replaced by even *coarser hairs* at puberty. On the lower side of hair follicle there appear two swellings. The upper one is primordium of sebaceous gland and the lower one called the *epithelial bud,* is a region of activity (cell proliferation).

Congenital anomalies of hair

1. *Hypertrichosis* refers to abnormally excessive growth of hair on any part of the body. It is

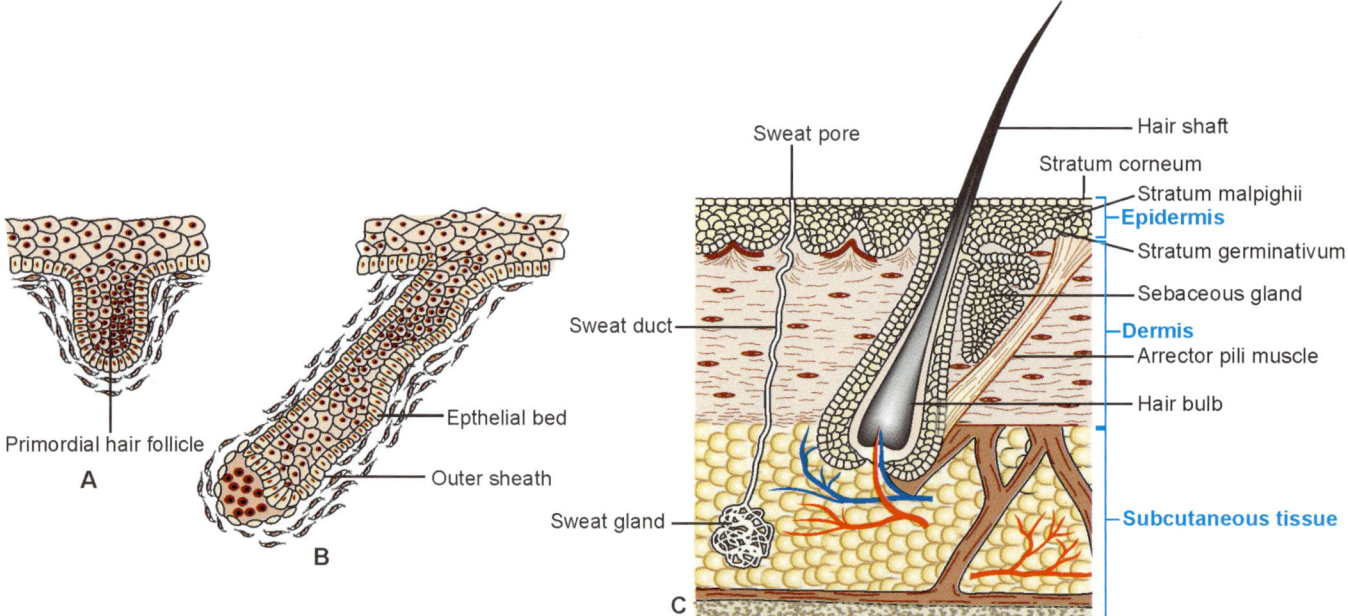

Fig. 8.3: Successive stages of development of hair, sebaceous gland and arrector pili muscle.

commonly seen in association with spina bifida occulta covering the defect in lumbar region.

2. *Atrichia* refers to absence of hair in any part of the body including scalp, eye lashes and eyebrows.
   - *Congenital alopecia* refers to absence of hair from the scalp.
   - *Madarosis* refers to absence of hair from eyelashes or eyebrows.

DEVELOPMENT OF GLANDS OF SKIN

DEVELOPMENT OF SEBACEOUS GLANDS

- *Development of sebaceous* glands associated with the hair follicles begins by formation of *epithelial bud* from the sides of developing hair epithelial root sheaths of hair follicle (Fig. 8.3).
- The epithelial buds then grow into the surrounding connective tissue and rapidly develop into saccular and lobular alveoli and their ducts.
- The central cells of the alveoli start secreting the oil material the sebum, which is poured into the hair follicle.
- Before birth the sebum forms the chief constituent of vernix caseosa (the cheesy material covering fetal skin).
- After birth, the sebum is responsible for the natural oiliness of the hair and skin.

DEVELOPMENT OF SWEAT GLANDS

Sweat glands derived from surface ectoderm, are of two types:
- Eccrine sweat glands, and
- Apocrine sweat glands

Eccerine sweat glands

Eccrine sweat glands are present in most of the skin of the body. They develop as below (Fig. 8.4):

Epithelial bud, a solid cylindrical mass of cells, down grows from the germinative layer of epidermis into the underlying mesenchyme (Fig. 8.4A). These cords continue down, until during the sixth month, their deep ends have reached the subcutaneous connective tissue.

Formation of secretory and ductal parts
- *Coiling of the cell cords* occurs at their distal end to form the primordium of the secretory part of gland (Fig. 8.4B). The peripheral cells of this secretory part of gland differentiate into:
- *Secretory cells* which begin to secrete sweat shortly after birth, and

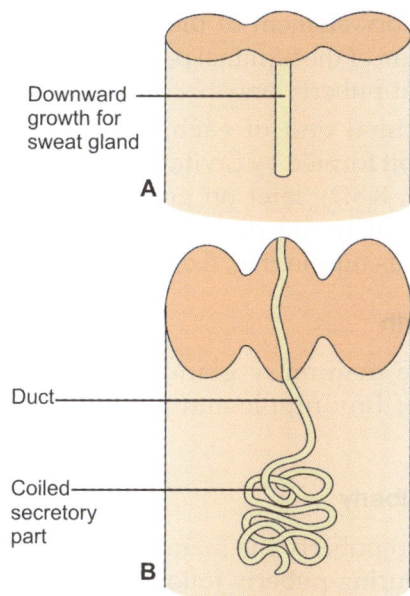

Fig. 8.4: Development of sweat glands: A, epithelial bud formation; B, formation of secretory and ductal parts.

- *Myoepithelial cells* the specialized smooth muscle cells that assist in expelling the sweat from the gland.
- *Primordium of the duct* of these glands is formed by the epithelial attachment of the developing glands to the epidermis. The central cells degenerate to form the lumen of the ducts of the glands.

Apocrine glands

Apocrine glands are mainly found in the axilla, pubic and perineal regions and areolae of the nipples. These develop from the epithelial root sheath of the hair follicles, and thus their ducts open into the upper part of hair follicles unlike eccrine sweat glands, which directly pour on to the skin surface.

DEVELOPMENT OF MAMMARY GLANDS

Mammary glands are present in both the sexes; in males they remain rudimentary but in females they are well developed after puberty. The different phases of its development are described:

Breasts in intrauterine life (embryogenesis)

At 18–19 weeks of gestation mammary glands develop from a thickened mass of epithelium of the epidermis known as mammary bud (Fig. 8.5A).
- From this thickened mass about 16–20 solid outgrowths arise and project into the dermis (Fig. 8.5B).
- Then the thickened mass as well as these outgrowths are canalized (Fig. 8.5C) to form rudimentary duct system.

- The secretory element of the gland is formed by proliferation of the terminal part of the outgrowths. It occurs at puberty only.
- The proximal end of each duct opens into a common pit formed by cavitation of the thickened mass (Fig. 8.5D); later on growth of underlying mesodermal tissue pushes the wall of the pit outwards as nipple (Fig. 8.5E).

Breasts at birth

At birth the mammary glands are rudimentary consisting of tiny nipple and few ducts radiating from it.

Breasts at puberty

From birth to puberty the mammary glands remain quiescent. During puberty following changes occur:

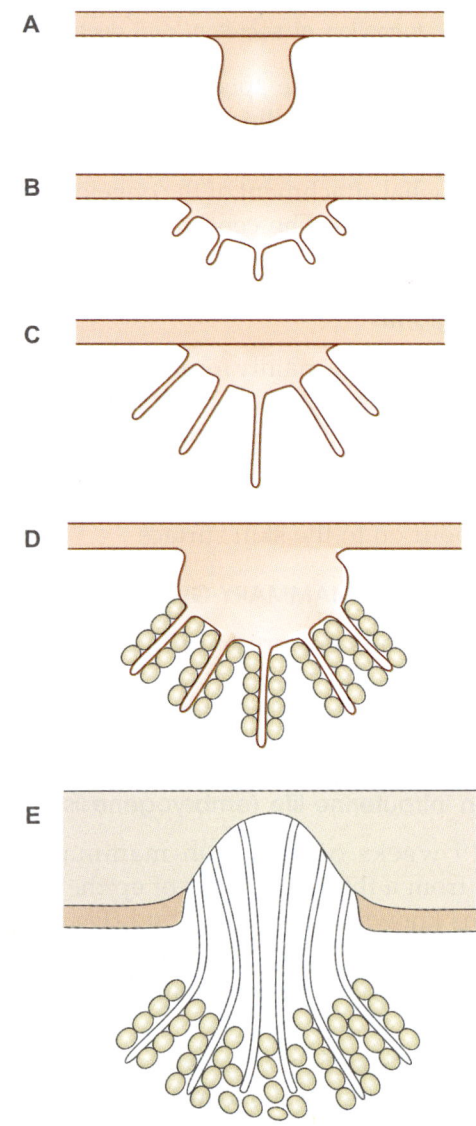

Fig. 8.5: Development of mammary gland.

At thelarche, i.e. at the time of puberty (9–11 years of age), before the start of menses, the breast starts developing and get enlarged. During this stage, only duct system proliferates and shows branching.

At menarche, i.e. after the onset of menses, cyclic growth of mammary glands (period of growth followed by quiescence) occurs in each menstrual cycle. The growth period further corresponds to phases of menstrual cycle.

- *In proliferative phase* (or oestrogen phase), the duct cells proliferate and continue throughout rest of the cycle.
- *In luteal phase* (progestational phase) progesterone stimulates the proliferation of terminal ductules, so there is formation of glandular tissue.
- *At menstruation* (bleeding phase) there occurs no proliferation of duct cells as well as of glandular tissue, because levels of both oestrogen and progesterone are lowered. Hence this period is called quiescence period.

With onset of next menstrual cycle further growth occurs. Thus there is progressive growth of breast in successive cycles, along with modelling of the breast by fat deposition in the adipose tissue. Fig. 8.5F shows the structure of mammary gland in an adult female.

Breasts in pregnancy

During pregnancy remarkable growth of both ductal and glandular systems occurs. It is only during first pregnancy that glandular tissue develops fully.

In first half of pregnancy

The duct system proliferates and shows extensive sprouting and branching along with growth of stroma and deposition of fat.

In second half of pregnancy

There is enormous growth of glandular tissue. The extensive growth of mammary glands during pregnancy is known as *mammogenesis* or preparation of breast for lactation.

Breasts during lactation

After child birth the alveolar cells get enlarged and distended and start forming milk (lactogenesis).

Involution of breast

After a normal period of lactation (7 to 9 months), the alveolar epithelium undergoes apoptosis and glands revert back to prepregnant stage.

CONTROL OF BREAST DEVELOPMENT AND GROWTH

Various hormones necessary for full growth and development of mammary glands at various stages are:

1. *Oestrogen.* It is primarily responsible for ductal growth and fat deposition. It also causes thickening of nipples.

2. *Progesterone.* The development of glandular tissue mainly depends on progesterone. Both oestrogen and progesterone work best with co-operation of hypothalamo-pituitary-adrenal cortex axis.

3. *Other hormones* including growth hormone, thyroxine, cortisol and insulin enhance overall growth and development of mammary glands at all stages.

4. *Corpus luteal and placental hormones*, particularly oestrogen, progesterone, human chorionic somato-mammotropic hormone (HCS, or HPL) are essential for further growth of breast during pregnancy.

5. *Prolactin.* It is another very important hormone for development of breasts during pregnancy and lactation. It acts on mammary gland tissue which has already grown under the influence of oestrogen and progesterone. It needs to be discussed in detail.

DEVELOPMENTAL ANOMALIES OF MAMMARY GLAND

1. *Amastia* refers to absence of breast. It may be unilateral or bilateral.

2. *Micromastia* refers to abnormally small breast.

3. *Macromastia* refers to abnormally large breasts.

4. *Polymastia* refers to development of multiple complete accessory breasts any where along the original mammary line.

5. *Athelia* refers to absence of nipple of the breast.

6. *Polythelia* refers to development of multiple nipples any where along the original mammary line.

7. *Inverted nipple or crater nipple* is a condition in which the nipple fails to develop and the lactiferous ducts open into the original epithelial pit that has failed to evert.

8. *Gynaecomastia* refers to abnormal development of large breasts in the males.

9

Development of Muscular System, Skeletal System and the Limbs

DEVELOPMENT OF MUSCULAR SYSTEM

There are three different types of muscles in the body:
- Skeletal muscles,
- Cardiac muscles, and
- Smooth muscles.

Development of muscles can be studied in two parts:
- Histogenesis of muscles, and
- Morphogenesis of muscles.

HISTOGENESIS OF MUSCLES

Histogenesis of skeletal muscle

The skeletal muscle fibres are mesenchymal in origin and may arise from either the myotome or the regional mesenchyme per se. (see page 55). Steps involved in the histogenesis of a skeletal muscle are (Fig. 9.1):

- *Formation of myoblasts.* The mesenchymal cells destined to form skeletal muscle elongate to form spindle shaped mono-nucleated myoblasts.

- *Formation of multinucleated muscle fibres.* The myoblasts fuse together, the intervening cell membranes disintegrate and form long, multi-nucleated muscle fibres.

- *Myofibrils* appear soon in the elongated muscle fibres, and by the end of 3rd month, cross-striations (because of alternating dark and light bands) characteristic of skeletal muscle appear. These myofibrils first appear in the peripheral part of the fibres, leaving a core of unmodified cytoplasm where nuclei are located.

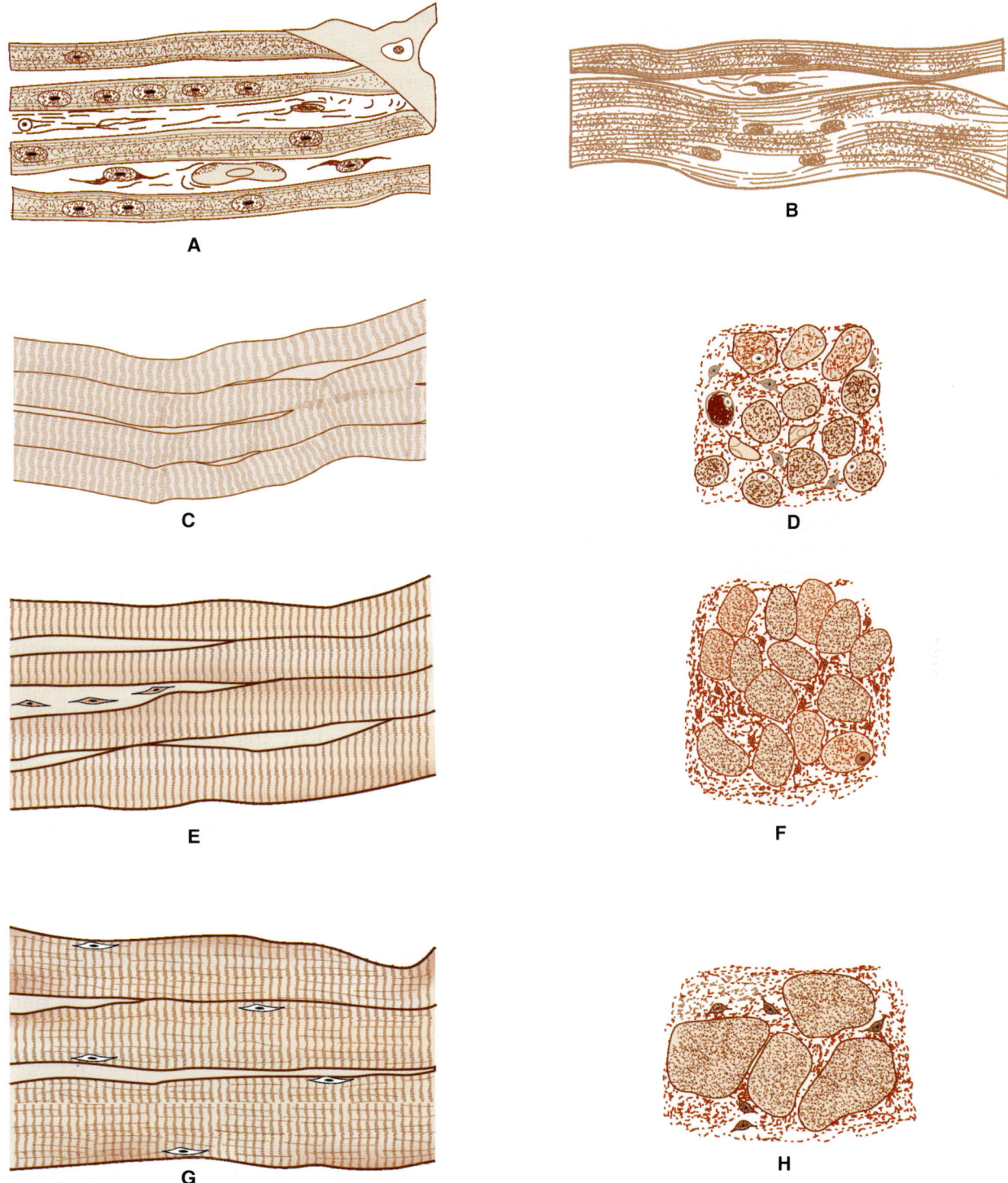

Fig. 9.1: Histogenesis of skeletal muscle; A, in 32 mm embryo; B, in 45 mm embryo; C, in 200 mm embryo; E, in a term fetus; G, in an adult. D, F and H transverse cut sections of C, E and G respectively.

- *Essential histologic characteristics* of adult skeletal muscle are developed in a full term fetus, and need only to elongate later with the body growth.

Histogenesis of cardiac muscle

The cardiac muscle is derived from the *splanchnic mesoderm* surrounding the developing endothelial heart tube. Steps involved in the histogenesis of cardiac muscle are (Fig. 9.2):

Epimyocardial layer, which invests the endocardial heart tube, is first formed from the splanchnic mesodermal cells. The surface cells of the epimyocardium retain their original epithelial nature and form the

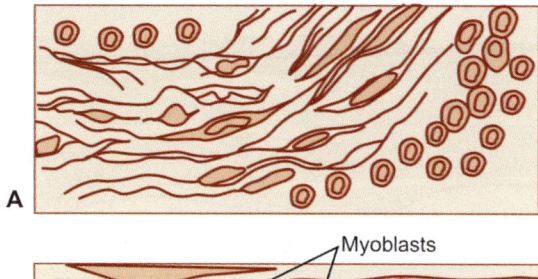

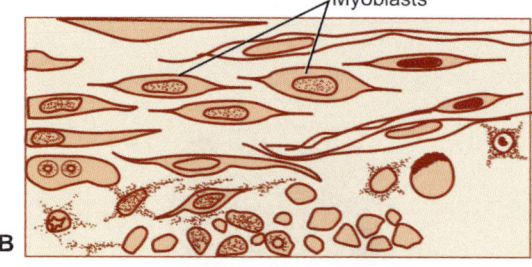

Myoblasts

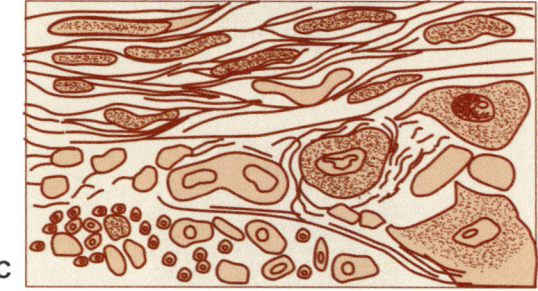

Fig. 9.2: Histogenesis of cardiac muscle.

mesothelial covering of the definitive heart, and the inner layer forms the myocardium.

Myocardium, the musculature of cardiac wall, is developed from the inner layer of the epimyocardium by following steps:

- *Cardiac myoblasts* differentiate from the splanchnic mesodermal cells which elongate and become spindle shaped.

- *Cardiac muscle fibres* arise by differentiation and growth of cardiac myoblasts, unlike striated skeletal muscle fibres, which develop by *fusion of myoblasts.*

- *Myofibrils* then develop inside the muscle fibres producing striations like that of skeletal muscle fibres. Further growth of the cardiac muscle fibres occurs due to formation of new myofilaments.

- *Intercalated discs,* the junctions between the adjacent cardiac muscle fibres develop by adhesion of the cell membranes of developing fibres.

- *Purkinje fibres,* which form the conducting system of the heart, later develop as special bundles of muscle cells with relatively few myofibrils and relatively larger diameter than the typical cardiac muscle fibres.

Histogenesis of smooth muscles

Smooth muscles differentiate from the splanchnic mesoderm surrounding the developing gut and its derivatives; except for the muscles of iris (sphincter and dilator pupillae) which develop from optic cup ectoderm and the peculiar contractile cells in the walls of the sudoriferous (and some other) glands which are also ectodermal in origin. Steps in the histogenesis of smooth muscles are (Fig. 9.3):

Myoblasts are formed by differentiation of splanchnic mesodermal cells which line the developing gut tube, the urogenital ducts, and the large vascular channels. The myoblasts become spindle shaped with elongated nuclei.

- *During early development* new myoblasts continue to differentiate from the mesenchymal cells but not fuse; and remain mononucleated.

- *During later development,* division of existing myoblasts gradually replaces the differentiation of new myoblasts in the production of new smooth muscle tissue.

- *Myofibrils* (filamentous but non-sarcomeric contractile elements) appear, running lengthwise in the cytoplasm of the young smooth muscle cells.

Smooth muscle fibres, typically spindle shaped, are well established by the ninth week of gestation. During the development the external surface of each muscle fibre acquires a surrounding external lamina.

Sheet or bundles of smooth muscle are formed with continued development and acquire autonomic innervation. Fibroblasts and muscle cells synthesize and lay down collagenous, elastic and reticular fibres.

MORPHOGENESIS OF SKELETAL MUSCULATURE

Skeletal muscles are derived from the paraxial mesoderm.

Template for establishment of muscle pattern into which myoblasts migrate to form muscles is provided by the connective tissue derived from:

- *Neural crest cells,* in the head region,
- *Somatic mesoderm* (part of paraxial mesoderm) in the cervical and occipital region, and
- *Somatic mesoderm* (part of lateral plate mesoderm), in the body wall and limbs.

General outlines of morphogenesis of skeletal muscle

Morphogenesis of skeletal muscles from the mesoderm can be traced as below:

Mesoderm first appears between ectodermal and endodermal plates making the embryo a trilaminar

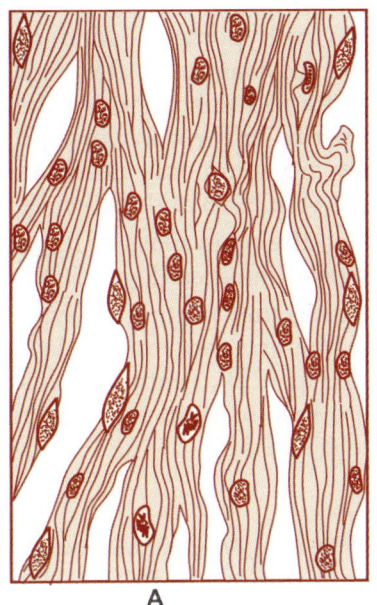
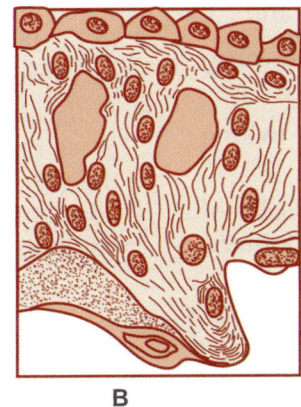
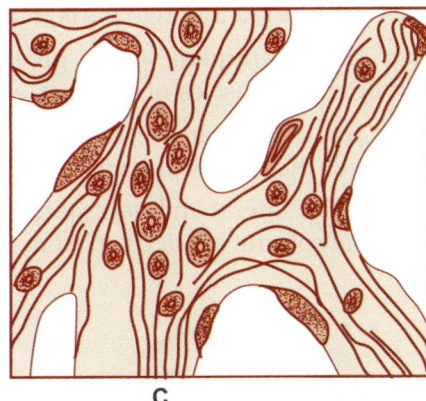

Fig. 9.3: Histogenesis of smooth muscle.

disc by 3rd week of development (see gastrulation) and is divided into following three columns.

- Paraxial mesoderm
- Intermediate mesoderm, and
- Lateral plate mesoderm

Paraxial mesoderm present on both sides of notochord is divided into somitomeres which give rise to mesenchyme of head and are organized into somites which have segmental arrangement along with the associated segmental arrangement of the spinal nerves (8 cervical, 12 thoracic, 5 lumbar, and 5 sacral. Adding to these 30 the usual of 4 occipital and 5 caudal somites make a total of 39 pairs of somites).

Somites give rise to

- *Myotomes,* which give rise to striated muscles of trunk and limbs.
- *Dermatomes,* which give rise to dermis of skin, and
- *Sclerotomes,* which give rise to skeleton except cranium.

Myotomes. The segmental arrangement of somites is maintained in myotomes as well. Figure 9.4 depicts the segmental arrangements of myotomes and their spinal nerves.

By the end of 5th week each myotome and the associated spinal nerve divide into two (Fig. 9.5A):

- *Epimere,* the dorsal smaller part of myotome is supplied by the *dorsal primary ramus* of the spinal nerve, and

- *Hypomere,* the ventral larger part of the myotome is supplied by the *ventral primary ramus.*

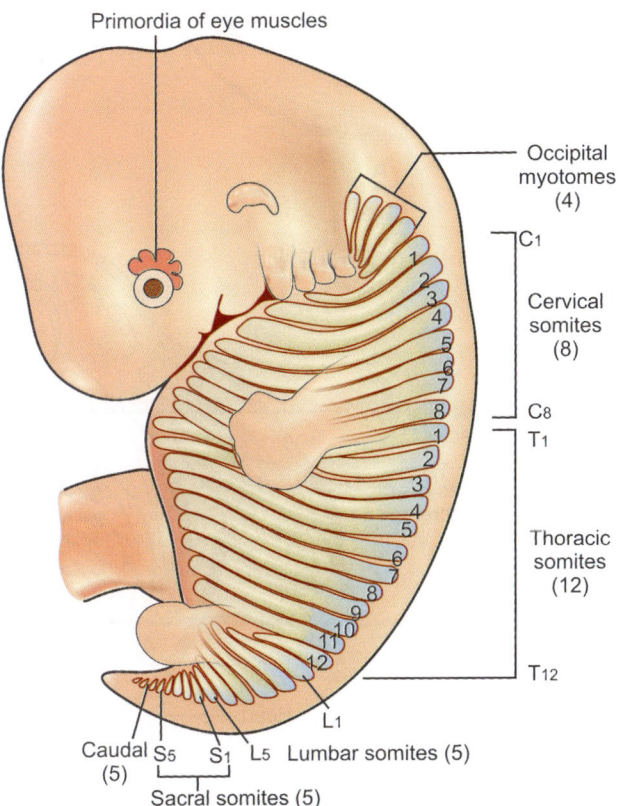

Fig. 9.4: Segmental arrangement of myotomes and their spinal nerves.

The separation between epimere and hypomere occurs at the level of transverse process of the developing vertebrae, and the intermuscular septum developing between them later becomes attached to the transverse process.

Epimere. Extensor muscles of the vertebral column are derived from the epimere. Each epimere shortly becomes subdivided into two parts (Fig. 9.5B and C):

- *Dorsal part* of epimere, which gives rise to deep intervertebral muscles of the neck and back.

- *Ventral part* of the epimere, which gives rise to long muscles of the neck and back.

Hypomere. The lateral and ventral flexor muscles of the vertebral column are derived from the hypomere.

The fate of hypomeres is different at different body levels. At thoracic and abdominal level, the conspicuous outgrowth from the hypomere extends medial to form the long muscles that act as flexors of the trunk (psoas and quadratus lumborum). As they are situated ventral to the ribs or the transverse process of the vertebrae, they are commonly designated as *hypoaxial trunk muscles* (Fig. 9.5B and C).

- *In the thoracic region,* the main mass of hypomere gives rise to intercostal muscles (Fig. 9.5C).

- *In the abdominal region,* the splitting of hypomere gives rise to three characteristic muscle layers of the abdominal wall (Fig. 9.5B): Ventrally, buds from adjacent hypomere fuse to form the long rectus abdominis muscle (Fig. 9.5B).

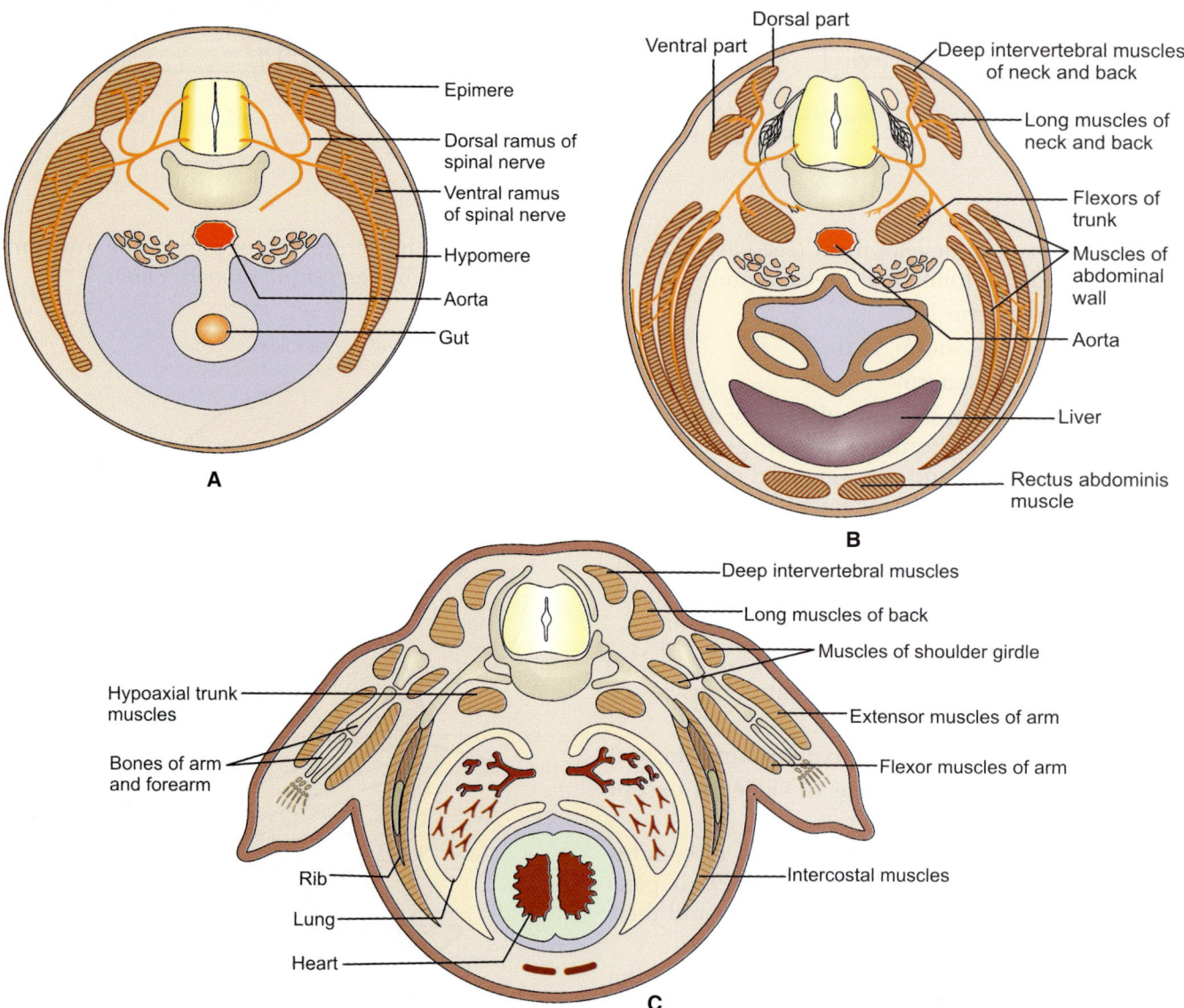

Fig. 9.5: Derivation of skeletal muscles from the myotomes: A, division of myotome into epimere and hypomere; B and C, subdivision of epimere and hypomere and differentiation of muscle primordia at the abdominal level and thoracic level and in the region of arm buds, respectively.

Regional derivation of skeletal muscles

Muscles of trunk and body wall

The derivation of muscles of trunk and body is described in the above discussion.

Muscles of limbs

- The limbs develop from the limb buds. Upper limb buds lie opposite the lower 5 cervical and upper two thoracic segments and the lower limb buds lie opposite the lower four lumbar and two sacral segments (Fig. 9.6).
- The hypomere, parts of myotomes in these segments extend into the limb buds to form the muscles of the limbs, which are supplied by the nerve fibres from the corresponding spinal nerves.
- In general the muscles developing on the original dorsal aspect of the limb become the extensor while those developing ventrally become the flexors (Fig. 9.5C). Later in development, because the arm and leg flex and rotate differently out of their originally similar positions.

Muscles of head region

Muscles of the head region derived from the mesenchymal cells form following mesodermal masses:

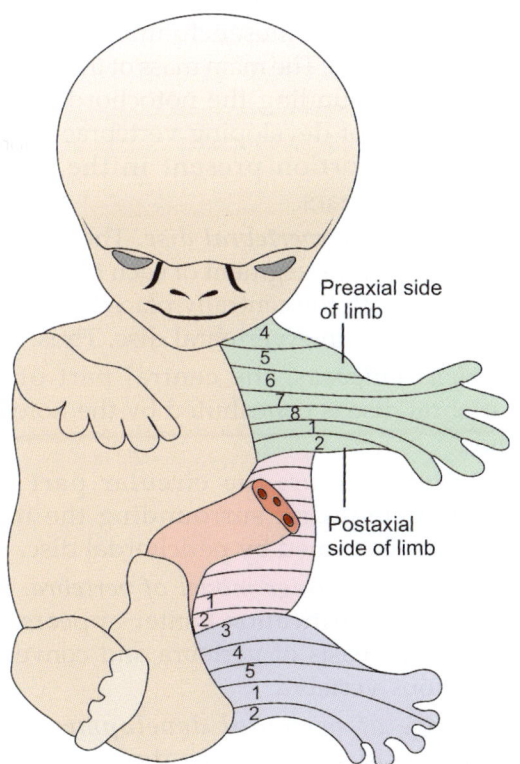

- Head myotomes
- Pharyngeal arches

Head myotomes. As shown in Fig. 9.4 there are four occipital myotomes. One of these, the first completely disappears and the other three differentiate into typical sclerotomes, dermatomes and myotomes.

- *Tongue muscles* arise from the hypoaxial divisions of these three occipital myotomes. The tongue muscles are supplied by the hypoglossal nerve which is formed by the grouping together of segmental nerve bundle which grow out towards these myotomes.
- *Extraocular muscles* are thought to be derived from three pairs of anterior (pre-otic) head myotomes.

Pharyngeal arch muscles. The muscles derived from pharyngeal arch mesoderm and innervated by pharyngeal arch nerves include:

- Muscles of mastication,
- Muscles of facial expression,
- Muscles of pharynx, and
- Muscles of larynx

  (For details see chapter on pharyngeal apparatus page 127).

SKELETAL SYSTEM

GENERAL OUTLINES

Contributing embryonic tissue

The skeletal system develops from the mesenchymal cells which are derived from the mesodermal germ layer and neural crest cells. The contribution of these embryonic tissue in the development of skeletal system is as below:

1. *Paraxial mesoderm,* present on both sides of the notochord, as described earlier is divided into somitomeres. The *somitomeres* give rise to mesenchyme of head and is organized into somites. The somites give rise to myotomes, dermatomes and sclerotomes.

   - Sclerotomes form most of the skeleton mainly vertebrae and ribs
   - Occipital somites and head somitomeres contribute in the formation of a cranial vault and base of skull.

2. *Somatic layer of lateral plate mesoderm* contributes in the formation of:

   - Bones of pelvic girdle,
   - Bones of shoulder girdle, and

Fig. 9.6: Schematic drawing of limb buds at 7 weeks.

- Long bones of the limbs.

3. *Neural crest cells* in the head region differentiate into mesenchyme and migrate into the pharyngeal arches and participate in the formation of bones and connective tissue of the craniofacial structures. Homeobox (Hox) genes regulate the role of neural crest cells.

Process of bone formation

Process of bone formation has been described in detail. It may be recalled that bones are formed by one of the two processes:

1. *Membranous ossification.* In this process mesenchymal cells are directly transformed into *osteoblasts* (bone-forming cells). For example, the flat bones of skull are formed by membranous ossification.
2. *Endochondral ossification.* In this process the mesenchymal cells form *hyaline cartilage models of the bones,* which in turn become ossified by endochondral ossification. Most of the bones, e.g. the long bones of limbs develop by this process.

DEVELOPMENT OF SKELETON

Development of skeleton can be described as:
- Development of vertebral column,
- Development of ribs,
- Development of sternum,
- Development of skull, and
- Development of bones of limbs.

DEVELOPMENT OF VERTEBRAL COLUMN

The vertebrae are developed from the mesenchymal cells derived from the sclerotomes (parts of somites) by process of endochondral ossification, i.e. first a hyaline cartilage model is formed which become later ossified.

Steps in the formation of a vertebrae are summarized below:

1. *Arrangement of mesenchymal cells around the developing spinal cord and notochord.* At the end of 4th week, the sclerotome cells become polymorphases, form loosely woven tissue the mesenchyme, that is arranged around the developing spinal cord and notochord (Fig. 9.7). This mesenchymal arrangement retains traces of the segmental pattern, as the adjacent two mesenchymal blocks are separated by less dense areas containing intersegmental arteries (Fig. 9.8A).
2. *Differentiation of each mesenchymal block into three parts.* Soon each mesenchymal block arranged around the developing spinal cord and notochord differentiates into three distinct regions (Fig. 9.8B):
- Cephalic less condensed region,
- Middle, markedly condensed area, known as *perichordal disc,* and
- Caudal, less condensed region.

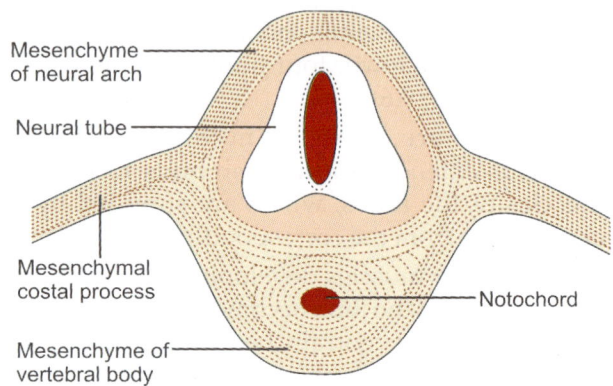

Fig. 9.7: Distribution of mesenchymal cells (derived from the sclerotome) around the developing spinal cord and notochord in the form of a vertebra and mesenchymal costal process (in the thoracic region).

3. *Fusion of less condensed caudal part of upper mesenchymal block with less condensed cephalic part of the adjoining lower mesenchymal block* occurs to form the mesenchymal model of the vertebra (Fig. 9.8C). The main mass of the mesenchymal block surrounding the notochord forms the *centrum* (body of developing vertebrae. Soon the notochordal portion present in the center of centrum disappears.
4. *Formation of intervertebral disc.* The peridermal disc, i.e. the middle segment of each mesenchymal block along with the centrally placed notochordal tissue forms the intervertebral disc. Thus:
- *Nucleus pulposus,* the central part of intervertebral disc is contributed by the notochord, and
- *Annulus fibrosus,* the circular part of the intervertebral disc surrounding the nucleus pulposus is formed by perichordal disc.
5. *Formation of cartilage model of vertebra.* By the 6th week chondrification center appears in the mesenchymal basis of vertebra and convert it in cartilaginous vertebra.
6. *Bony stage of vertebral development.* Endochondral ossification begins during embryonic period by appearance of *primary ossification* centers and is completed by the 25th year of life by the

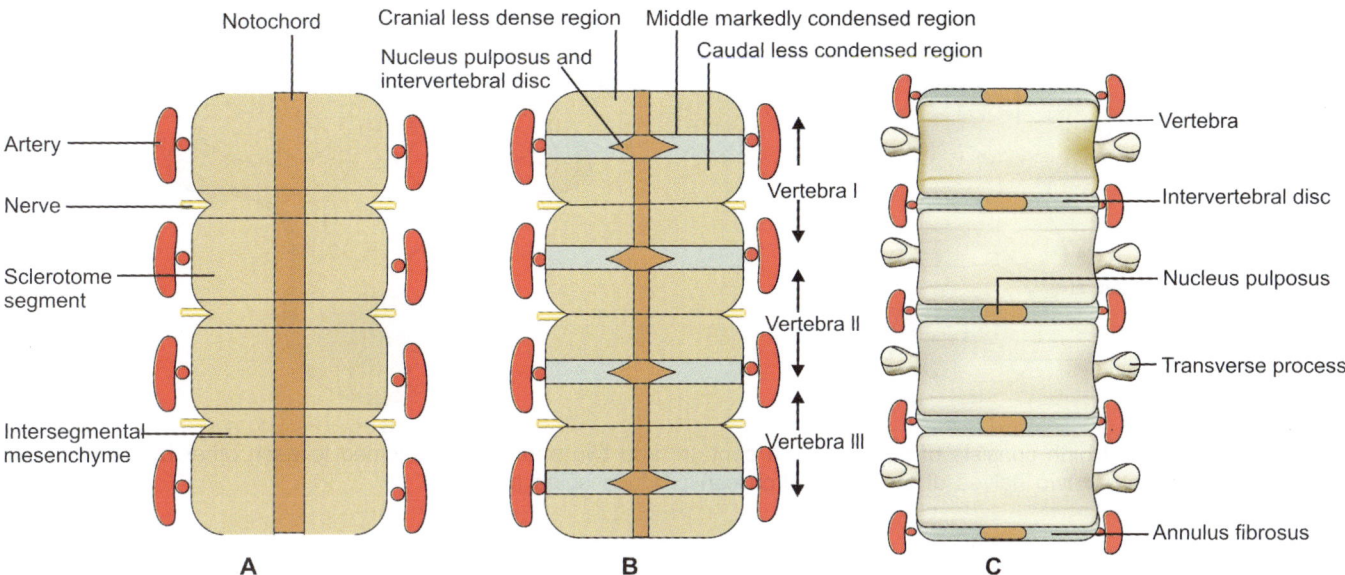

Fig. 9.8: Stages of development of vertebral column: A, segmental arrangement of mesenchyme (derived from the sclerotome) around the notochord, separated by less dense intersegmental tissue. Note the position of segmental nerves, intersegmental arteries and myotomes; B, differentiation of each mesenchymal segment into three parts (central condensed part and, cephalic and caudal less condensed parts); C, fusion of upper and lower less condensed parts of two successive segments form the vertebra. Note the appearance of intervertebral disc, which is derived from the condensed part of each mesenchymal segment.

secondary ossification centers which appear after puberty.

Some important observations to be made from the above method of development of vertebral column are:

- *Vertebra* is an intersegmental structure which develops from two adjacent sclerotomes.
- *Intervertebral disc* represents the position of center of each sclerotome.
- *Transverse processes and ribs* are also intersegmental structures. They separate the muscles derived from adjoining myotomes.
- *Spinal nerves* are segmental structures. They, therefore, emerge between the two adjacent vertebrae and lie between two adjacent ribs.
- *Blood vessels* supplying the structures derived from the myotome are *intersegmental* and lie on each side of vertebral bodies. In the thorax, the dorsal inter-segmental arteries become the intercostal arteries.
- *Myotomes* (are thus the derivatives of the muscles) bridge the intervertebral discs and, therefore, can move the vertebral column.

At birth, a vertebra consists of three separate pieces of bone : a centrum and two neural arches joined to each other by cartilage (Fig. 9.9A).

DEVELOPMENT OF RIBS

- Mesenchymal costal process of the developing thoracic vertebrae give rise to the ribs (Fig. 9.7).

Figure 9.10 depicts the mesenchymal (pre-cartilage) primordia of developing vertebrae and ribs.

- Chondrification of mesenchymal primordia of ribs (during embryonic periods) and later *ossification* (during fetal periods) forms the ribs.
- *Costovertebral joints* represent the original site of union of the costal processes with the vertebrae.
- *True ribs* (seven pairs, (1 to 7) of ribs) attach through their own cartilages to the sternum.
- *False ribs* (five pairs, 8 to 12) attach to the sternum through the cartilage of another rib or ribs.
- *Floating ribs* (last two pairs, 11th and 12th) do not attach to the sternum.

DEVELOPMENT OF STERNUM

Somatic mesoderm in the ventral body wall gives rise to sternum.

Stages of formation of sternum are (Fig. 9.11):

- *Sternal bars or plates* develop on either side of the midline (Fig. 9.11A) during 6th week.
- *Fusion of sternal bars* starts during 8th week at the cranial end (*manubrium*) (Fig. 9.11B), and proceeds caudally towards body of sternum and xiphoid process (Fig. 9.11C) by 9th week.
- *Ossification* of the manubrium and body of sternum occurs by separate ossification center (Fig. 9.11D). The xiphoid process ossifies only late in life form the adult sternum (Fig. 9.11E).

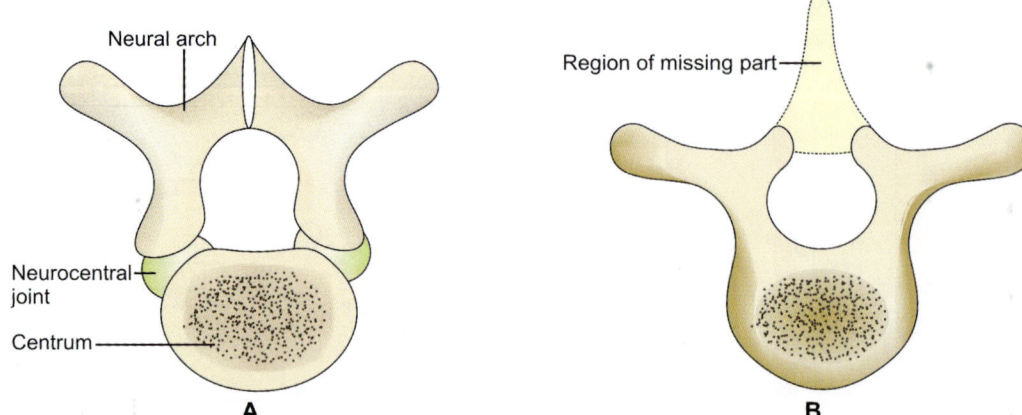

Fig. 9.9: A vertebra at birth consists of three parts, a centrum and two neural arches joined to each other by cartilage (A). Note, how non-fusion of two halves of the neural arch can produce spina bifida (B).

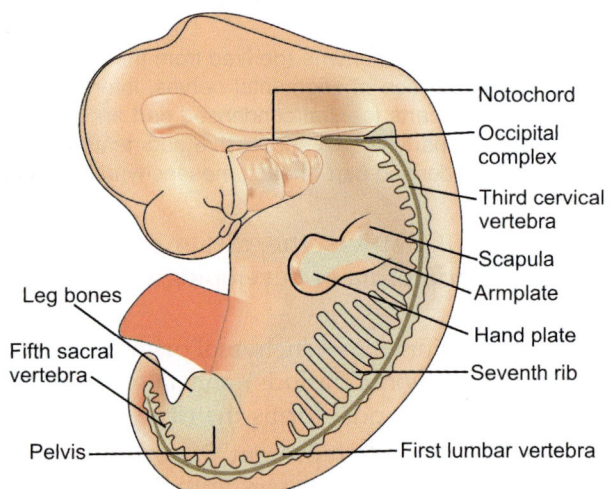

Fig. 9.10: Mesenchymal (pre-cartilage) primordia of developing vertebrae and ribs in 9-mm human embryo.

Anomalies of sternal development include:

- Cleft sternum,
- Perforated sternum, and
- Notched xiphoid process.

These anomalies are all obviously correlated with the paired arrangement of sternal primordia.

DEVELOPMENT OF SKULL

For the purpose of understanding, development of skull can be divided into two parts:

- *Neurocranium,* which forms a protective shell around the brain,
- *Viscerocranium,* which forms the skeleton of face.

Depending upon the type of ossification of bones the neurocranium can be further subdivided into two parts:

- Membranous neurocranium, and
- Chondrocranium or cartilaginous neurocranium.

Contributing embryonic tissue for the development of skull

The skull bones develop from the mesenchyme surrounding the developing brain. The mesenchyme forming skull bones is derived from following sources:

1. *Neural crest cells.* Mesenchymal cells derived from the neural crest cells form:

   - Most of the cranial vault (membranous neurocranium).

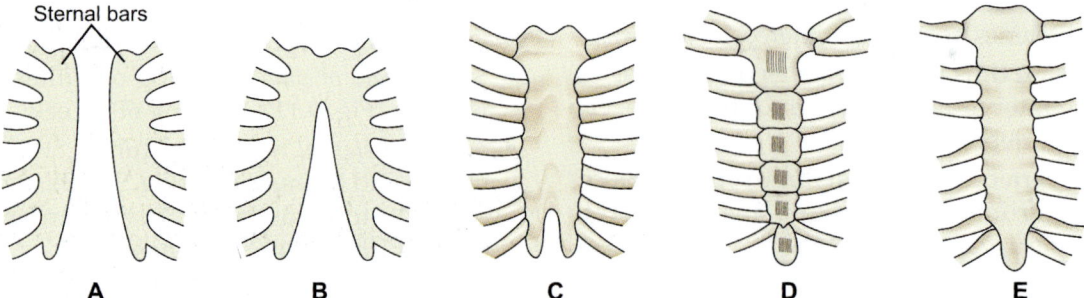

Fig. 9.11: Stages of development of sternum: A, formation of two mesodermal sternal bars; B, fusion of sternal bars at cranial end (manubrium); C, fusion of sternal bars reaches at caudal end by 9th week; D, separate ossification centers in the manubrium and sternal body; and E, an adult sternum.

- Face bones (viscerocranium), and
- Prechordal part of chondrocranium (the part that lies rostral to the notochord).

2. *Paraxial mesoderm* form rest of the skull:
   - *Occipital somites:* The mesenchyme arising from the sclerotomes of these somites help to form part of the base of skull and some part of the vault in the region of occipital bone.
   - *Optic and nasal capsules,* i.e. mesenchyme surrounding the region of developing internal ear and developing nose, respectively, also take part in development of skull.

Development of Neurocranium

Membranous neurocranium

- Membranous neurocranium or protective cranial vault or calvaria develops from the mesenchyme surrounding the upper and outer parts of developing brain.

Sources of mesenchyme, as mentioned above are:
- *Neural crest cells,* which form the roof and most of the sides of cranial vault.
- *Paraxial mesoderm,* which forms only a small part in the occipital region and posterior part of the optic capsule.

Process of bone formation, as the name indicates, is membranous ossification of the mesenchyme without formation of cartilage. Flat bones formed by membranous ossification are characterized by the presence of needle like *bone spicules,* which radiate from primary ossification center towards the periphery (Fig. 9.12).

Bones of skull formed by membranous ossification include:
- Frontal bones,
- Parietal bones,
- Temporal bones (part forming side walls of skull), and
- Intraparietal part of occipital bones

Features of cranial vault in a fetus and in a newborn include (Fig. 9.13):
- *Sutures* or dense connective tissue membrane separate the flat bones from each other.
- *Fontanelle,* i.e. wide areas of sutures where two or more bones meet are present at birth. For example:
  - *Anterior fontanelle,* which is present when two frontal and two parietal bones meet (Fig.13A). It closes about the middle of 2nd year of life.
  - *Posterior fontanelle,* which is present where the two parietal and occipital bone meet. It closes about 3 months after birth.

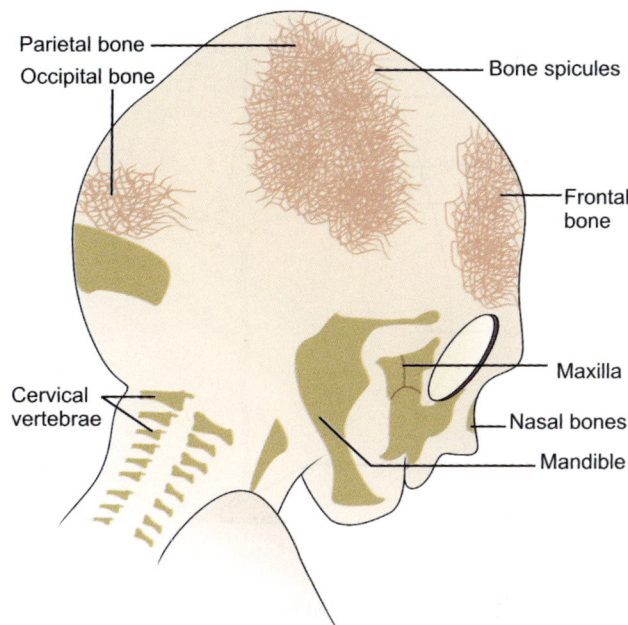

Fig. 9.12: Bones of skull in a 3-month old child. Note bone spicules radiating from the primary ossification center.

Clinical importance of sutures and fontanelles
- *Molding,* i.e. overlapping of the skull bones over each other, which is useful during childbirth, is possible due to presence of sutures and fontanelle.
- *Information about intracranial pressure and process of ossification* in the first few years of life can be obtained by palpating anterior fontanelle.
- *Accommodation of the developing and enlarging brain* after birth is possible because of the several sutures and fontanalle which remain membranous for a considerable time. Usually the full cranial capacity is achieved by 5–7 years of life, some sutures remain open until adulthood.

Cartilaginous neurocranium

Cartilaginous neurocranium as the name indicates, this part of neurocranium develops in two stages:

Cartilaginous model is first formed by the mesenchymal cells derived from the neural crest cells as *walls* and paraxial mesoderm. Name of various cartilages formed is beyond the scope of this book.

Endochondral ossification of the various cartilages then forms the following bones forming base of skull:
- Ethmoid bones,
- Sphenoid bones (body, lesser wing and greater wings)
- Base of occipital bone,
- Petrous part of temporal bone.

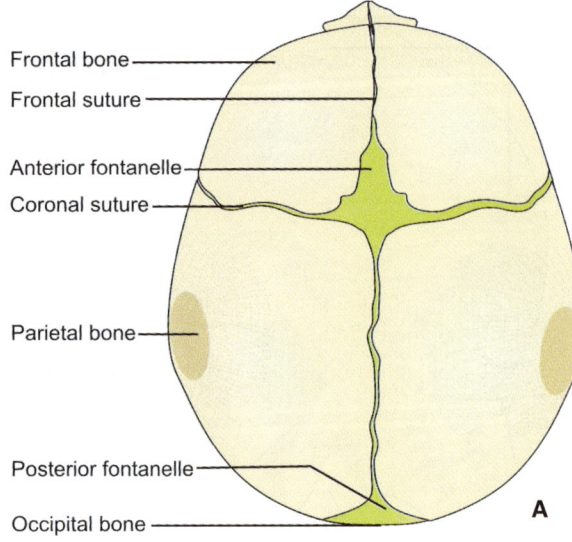

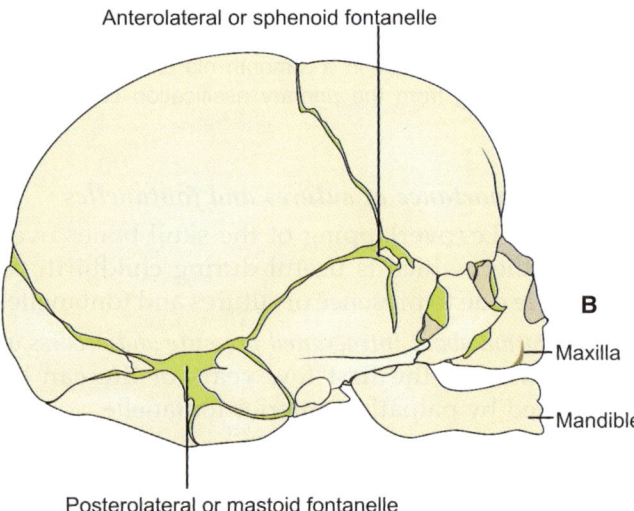

Fig. 9.13: Skull of a newborn; A, as seen from above; and B, right lateral view.

Development of viscerocranium

Viscerocranium includes the bones of face. Some bones of the face are formed by membranous ossification and some by endochondral ossification.

Contributing embryonic tissue and the bones formed by them

1. *First pharyngeal arch cartilage*
   - *Maxillary process* of the first pharyngeal arch gives rise to maxillae, the zygomatic bone, and part of the temporal bone by membranous ossification.
   - *Mandibular process* of the first arch condenses around the cartilage and undergoes intra-membranous ossification to form the mandible.

- *Dorsal end of the first arch cartilage* forms two middle ear bones—the malleus and incus.
2. *Second pharyngeal arch*
   - *Dorsal end of second arch cartilage* forms the stapes of the middle ear and styloid process of the temporal bone.
   - *Ventral end of second arch cartilage* ossifies to form the lesser horn (cornu) and superior part of the body of hyoid bone.

Developmental anomalies of skull (craniofacial anomalies) (Fig. 9.14)

1. **Anencephally** refers to absence of greater part of the vault of skull (Fig. 9.14A).
2. **Craniosynostosis** results from premature closure of one or more cranial sutures. Depending upon the suture involved craniosynostosis may be of following types:

Anomaly	Suture closed prematurely
• Brachycephaly (clover-leaf skull)	All cranial sutures
• Oxycephaly (tower shaped skull)	Coronal suture
• Scaphocephaly (boat shaped skull)	Sagittal suture
• Trigonocephaly (egg-shaped skull)	Frontal suture

3. **Craniofacial dysostosis** (*Crouzon's syndrome*) refers to premature closure of all sutures (brachy-cephaly) associated with maxillary hyperplasia.
   Systemic features are:
   1. Mental retardation,
   2. High-arched palate,
   3. Irregular dentition, and
   4. Hooked (parrot beak) nose.
4. **Mandibulofacial dysostosis** (*Treacher-Collin syndrome*) refers to a condition resulting from hypoplasia of zygoma and mandible.
   Systemic features are:
   1. Macrostomia with high-arched palate,
   2. External ear deformity, and
   3. Bird-like face.

Development of appendicular skeleton

The pectoral girdle, pelvic girdle and the limb bones constitute the appendicular skeleton. The appendicular skeleton is formed from the mesenchyme in the developing limbs.

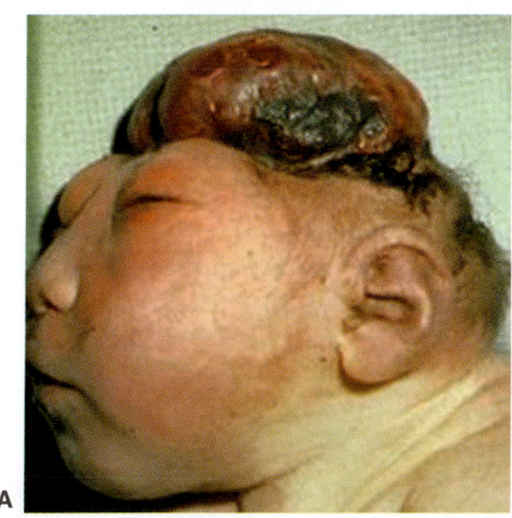
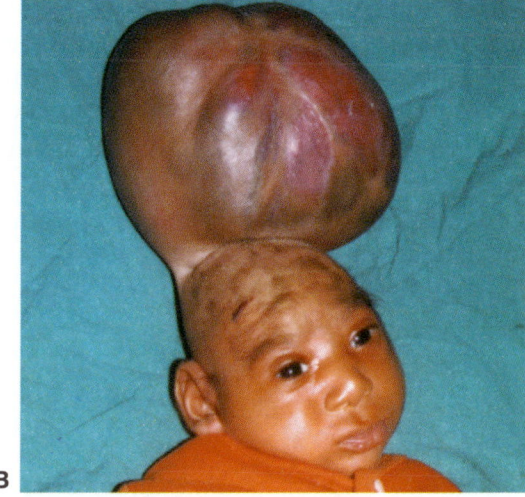

Fig. 9.14: Some congenital anomalies of skull: A, anencephaly; and B. meningocele

Stages of formation of limb bones

1. *Mesenchymal bone models* are formed by condensation of the mesenchyme in the limb buds by 5th week.

2. *Hyaline cartilage bone models* start forming by 6th week and completed by the beginning of 8th week as a result of chondrification of the mesenchymal bone models (Fig. 9.15).

3. *Ossification:* With the exception of clavicle (which is a membranous bone, all other bones are formed by endochondral ossification.

   - *Primary ossification centers* appear in nearly all the limb bones by 12th week. From the primary centers in the shaft (diaphysis) of the bone, the endochondral ossification progresses gradually towards the ends of the cartilagenous models of the developing bones. At birth, the diaphysis (shaft) of the bone is completely ossified but the two extremities, known as the epiphysis, are still cartilagenous.

   - *Secondary ossification centers* appear in epiphysial cartilage at varying times after and cause *growth in length and girth of bone* (For details see page 93).

DEVELOPMENT OF LIMBS

Various stages of development of limbs

Limb buds appear as slight elevations from the ventrolateral body wall towards the end of fourth week (Fig. 9.16 A). The upper limb buds appear 2 days earlier than the lower limb buds.

- Initially, the limb buds are formed by mesenchyme derived from the somatic layer of lateral plate mesoderm covered by a layer of surface ectoderm.

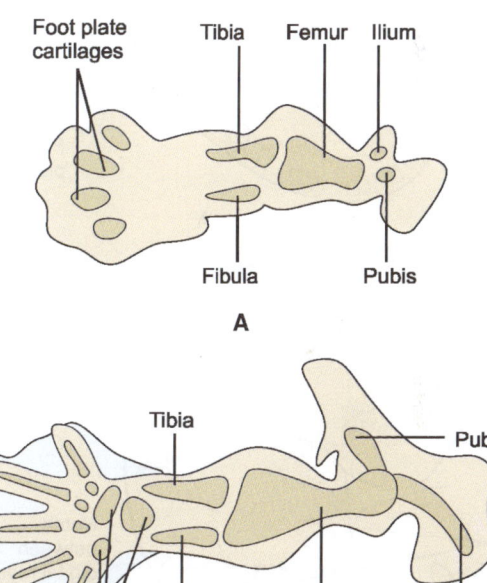
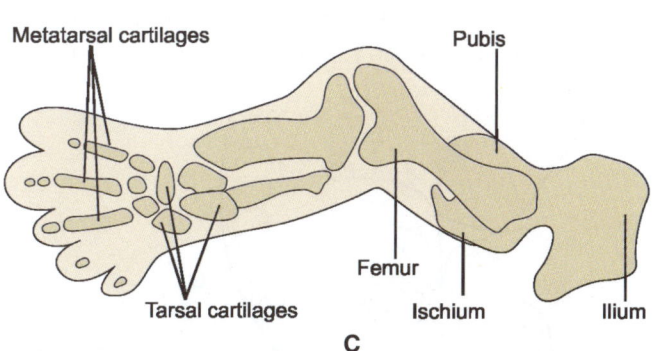

Fig. 9.15: Formation of cartilagenous model of lower limb and pelvic girdle: A, at the beginning of 6th week; B, by the end of 6th week; C, at the beginning of 8th week.

- Mesenchyme will form the bones (see page 93 for details), muscles (page 112) and connective tissue of the limb and surface ectoderm will form skin and its appendages including nails (see page 107).
- *Nerves* grow into the developing limb after muscles masses have formed.
- *Blood vessels* of limb buds arise as buds from aorta and cardinal veins.

- *Apical ectodermal ridge* (AER), appears as thickening of the tip of limb bud, which exerts an inductive influence on the limb mesenchyme promoting growth and development of the limbs. Areas away from the AER undergo differentiation into cartilage muscle, connective tissue, etc.

Hand plates and foot plates are formed, respectively, from the terminal parts of upper limb and lower limb

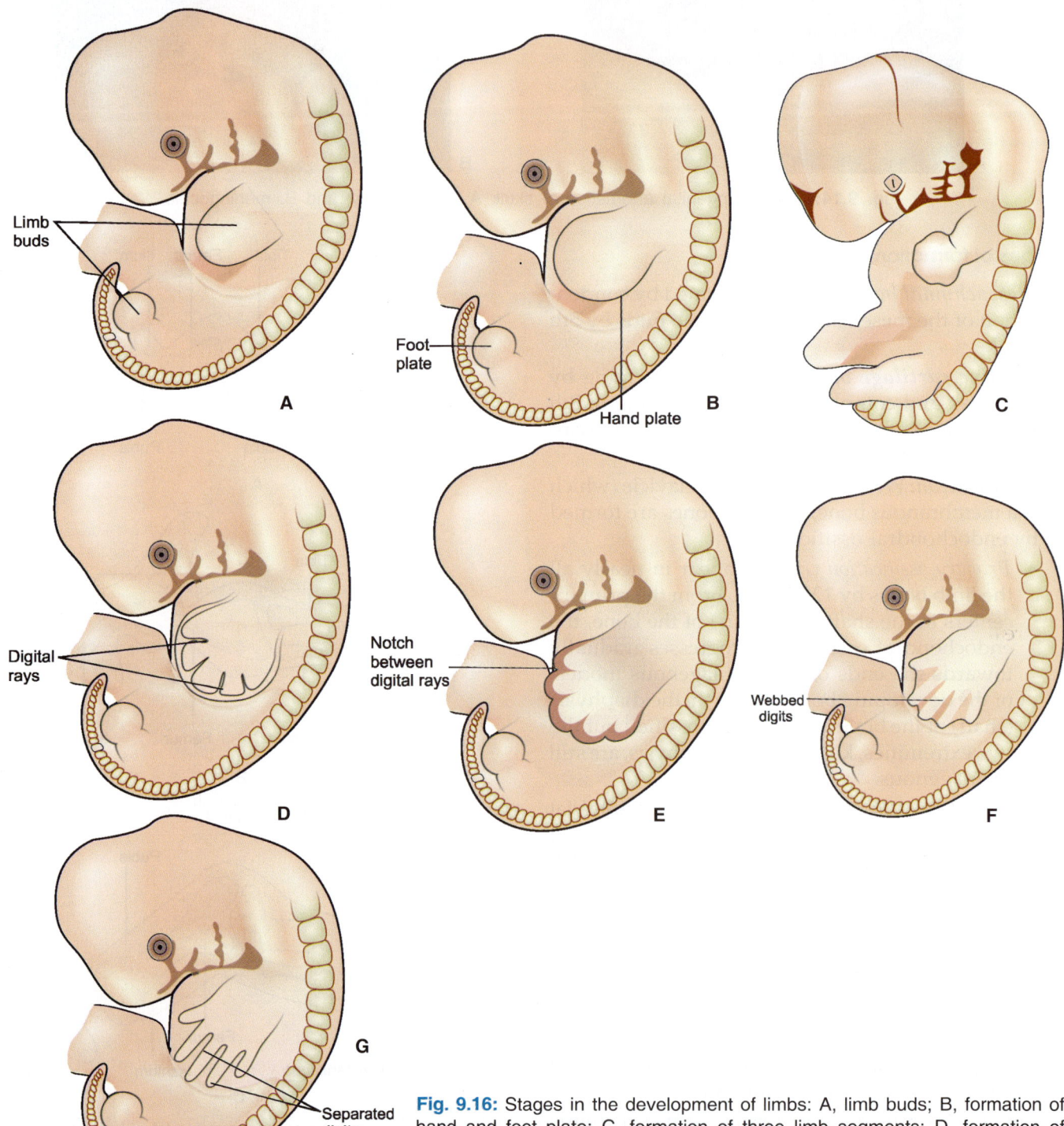

Fig. 9.16: Stages in the development of limbs: A, limb buds; B, formation of hand and foot plate; C, formation of three limb segments; D, formation of digital rays; E, appearance of notches between digital rays; F, formation of webbed digits; and G, fully formed digits.

buds by 6th week. These plates are separated from the proximal parts of the limb buds by a circular constriction (Fig. 9.16B).

- *Formation of three limb segments:* Soon, the proximal parts of the limb buds are divided into two by the appearance of another circular constriction band. In this way the three segments of the limbs can be recognized (Fig. 9.16C):
- Most distal segment, hand and foot plates, will form the hand and foot, respectively.
- Middle segment will form the forearms and legs, and
- Most proximal portion will form the upper arms and thigh regions.

Note: While the external shape is being established, simultaneously the mesenchyme is forming bone and connective tissue. Joints, nerves and blood vessels are also developing simultaneously.

Formation of hand and foot is marked by following events:

- *Digital rays* are formed by condensation of mesenchyme of hand plates into *finger buds* and mesenchyme of foot plates into *toe-buds* (Fig. 9.16D).
- *Formation of digits:* Programmed cell death (Apoptosis) is an important mechanism in formation of digits. Apoptosis in the epical ectoderm ridge (AER) separates this ridge into five parts and *notches* appear between the digital rays (Fig. 9.16E). Digital rays deepen down and the intervals between them are occupied by loose mesenchyme forming *webbed digits* (Fig. 9.16F). As this tissue breakdown progresses, separate digits are formed by the eighth week (Fig. 9.16G).

Note: Patterning of digits is dependent on a group of cells located at the base of limbs on their posterior border known *zone of polarizing activity* (ZPA).

Apoptosis, responsible for formation of digits is probably mediated by *bone morphogenetic proteins (BMP).*

Rotation of the developing limbs is an important event. Initially the developing limbs are directed forward, laterally and caudally (Fig. 9.17) later they project ventrally, and finally, they rotate on their longitudinal axis during 7th week of gestation. The upper and lower limbs rotate in opposite directions:

- Upper limbs rotate 90° laterally, so that the preaxial border becomes the lateral border and the extensor muscles lie on the lateral and posterior surface and the thumbs lie laterally (Fig. 9.18).
- Lower limbs rotate approximately 90° medially, placing the extensor muscles on the anterior surface and big toes lie medially.

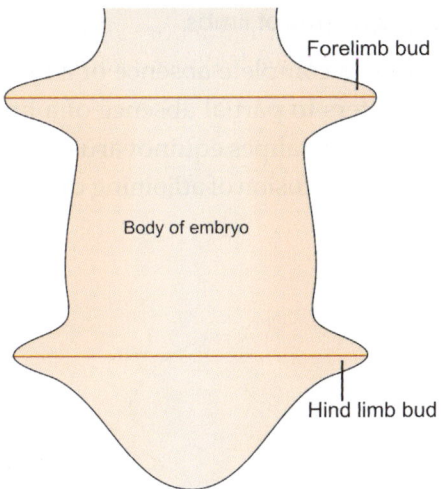

Fig. 9.17: Relation of developing limbs with the embryonic body.

Molecular regulation of limb development

- *Positioning of the limbs* along the cranio-caudal axis in the flank region of embryo is regulated by *Hox genes.*
- *Limb outgrowth* in the forelimb is initiated by TBX5 and FGF10 and in hind limb by TBX4 and FGF10.
- *Formation of apical ectodermal ridge (AER)* is induced by BMPs by signaling through the homeobox gene MSX2.

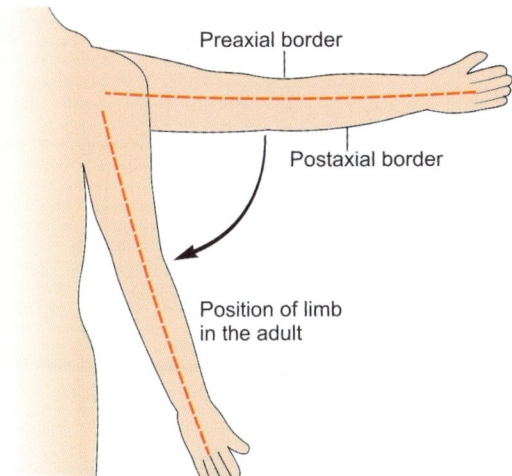

Fig. 9.18: Rotation of upper limbs 90° laterally makes preaxial border as lateral border.

- *Distal growth of the limb* is effected by *progressive zone* which is maintained by FGF4 and FGF8.
- *Patterning of anteroposterior axis* of the limb is controlled by zone of polarizing activity (ZPA) by secreting *retinoic acid* and expression of sonic hedgehog (SHH).

Congenital anomalies of limbs

1. *Amelia* refers to complete absence of a limb
2. *Phocomelia* refers to partial absence of a limb
3. *Deformed foot*, e.g. talipes equinovarus or club foot.
4. *Syndactyl* refers to fusion of adjoining digits of hand.
5. *Macrodactyly*, i.e. abnormally large fingers.
6. *Brachydactyly*, i.e. abnormally small fingers
7. *Polydactyl*, i.e. supernumerary digits.
8. *Lobsterclaw*, i.e. presence of deep longitudinal cleft.

10

Pharyngeal Apparatus and Development of Related Structures of Oral Cavity, Face, Nose, Palate and Neck

PHARYNGEAL APPARATUS

Pharyngeal arches
- Structure
- Derivatives

Pharyngeal pouches
- Derivatives

Pharyngeal clefts
- Fate
- Congenital anomalies

DEVELOPMENT OF STRUCTURES OF ORAL CAVITY AND PHARYNX
- Mouth
- Tongue
- Salivary glands

- Teeth
- Pharynx

DEVELOPMENT OF THYMUS, PARATHYROIDS AND THYROID GLAND
- Thymus
- Parathyroid glands
- Thyroid gland

DEVELOPMENT OF FACE, NOSE, PARANASAL SINUSES AND PALATE
- Face
- Nose (Nasal cavity)
- Paranasal sinuses
- Palate
- Congenital anomalies of face, palate and nasal cavity

PHARYNGEAL APPARATUS

Pharyngeal apparatus includes the structures which form the neck and some structures of the head region. In a 4 week human embryo the head is represented by the bulging caused by the developing brain and below and ventrally the stomodaeum (future mouth) separates it from the developing pericardial cavity (region of future thorax) (Fig. 10.1A). At this stage neck is not present. Soon the pharyngeal apparatus starts developing between the stomodaeum and pericardial cavity which will ultimately form the neck and its structures (Fig. 10.1B, C and D). Since this area resembles formation of gills (branchia) in fishes and amphibia previously it was called *branchial apparatus*. However, in the human embryo real gills (branchia) are never formed.

Pharyngeal apparatus consists of (Fig. 10.2):

- *Pharyngeal arches*, a series of mesodermal thickenings or bars lined on outside by the ectoderm and on inside by the endoderm, which appear in the wall of cranial most part of developing foregut (Fig. 10.2).

- *Pharyngeal pouches* or endodermal pouches refer to the outward bulging area of endoderm which separates the two pharyngeal arches internally (Fig. 10.2).

- *Pharyngeal clefts or grooves* are formed by dipping of ectoderm between two arches. Externally the pharyngeal clefts or ectodermal clefts lie opposite to pharyngeal pouches and thus in this area the ectoderm and endoderm lie close to each other without any intervening mesoderm (Fig. 10.2).

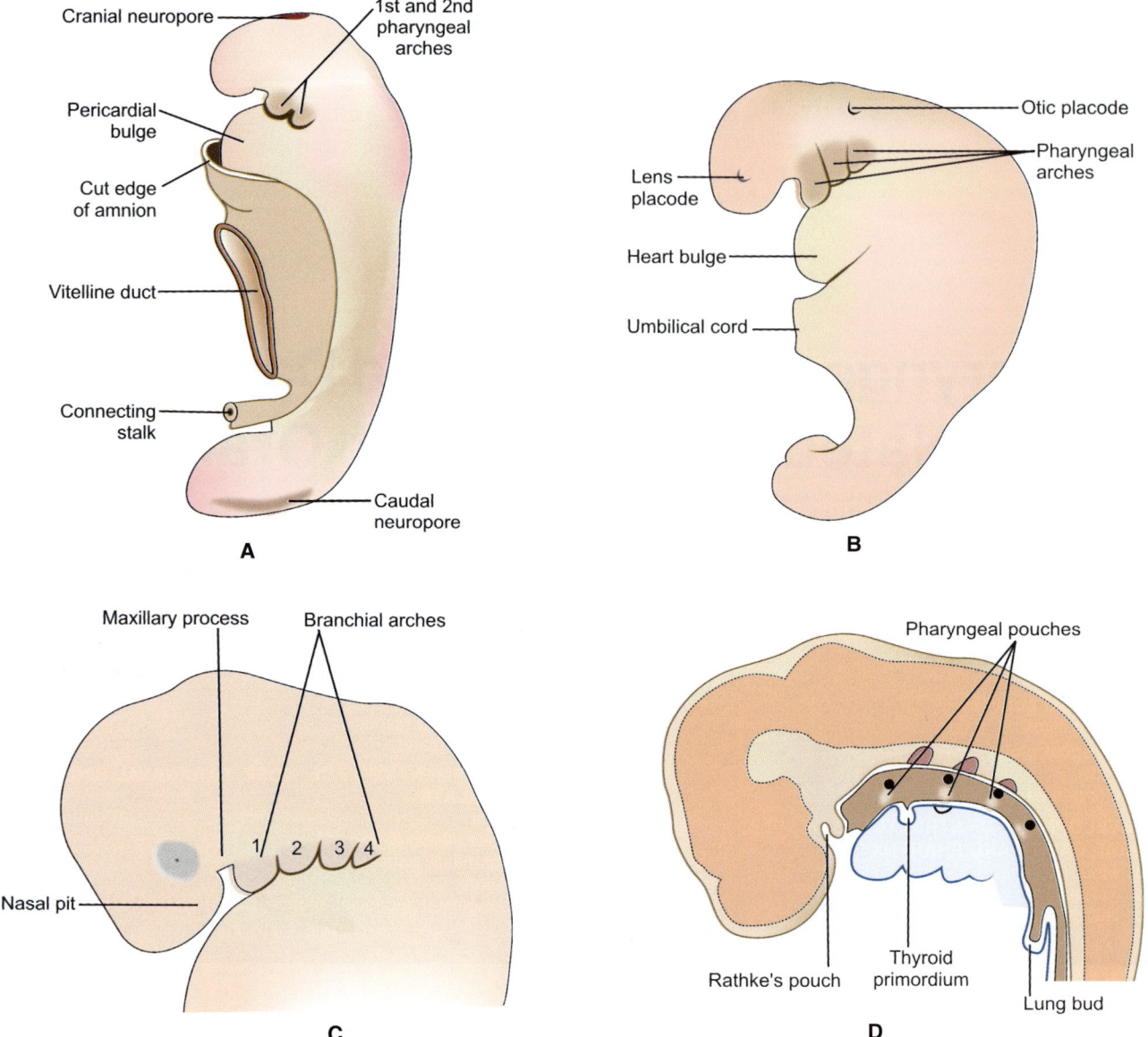

Fig. 10.1: Series of human embryos to show development of pharyngeal arches: A, approximately 25 days; B, 28 days; C, 5 weeks, and D, head opened medially to show pharyngeal pouches.

- *Pharyngeal membranes* are thus formed where the ectoderm of pharyngeal clefts contacts the endoderm of pharyngeal pouches (Fig. 10.2).

PHARYNGEAL ARCHES

As mentioned above, pharyngeal arches are bars of mesodermal tissue which appear in the wall of cranial most part of foregut (destined to form pharynx). The pharyngeal arches of left and right side grow ventrally and fuse with each other in the floor of the developing pharynx. Initially there are six pharyngeal arches, but soon the fifth pharyngeal arch disappears and only five are left (Fig. 10.2).

Structure of a pharyngeal arch

Each pharyngeal arch consists of a core of mesenchyme covered internally by endoderm and externally by ectoderm.

Mesenchyme of pharyngeal arches

- *Original mesenchyme* of the pharyngeal arches is derived from the paraxial and lateral plate mesoderm and gives rise to musculature of face and neck.
- *Neural crest cells* that migrate into pharyngeal arches though neuroectodermal in origin also substantially contribute to this mesenchyme,

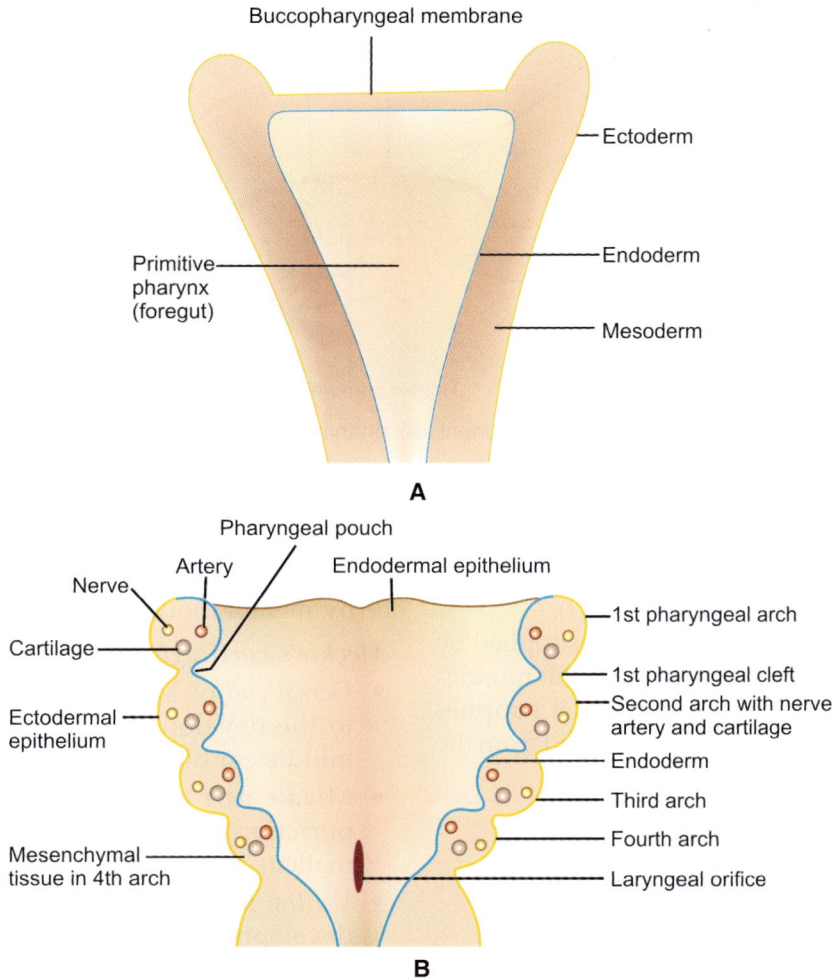

Fig. 10.2: Coronal section through cranial part of foregut : A, before; and B, after formation of pharyngeal arches in the cranial most part of foregut. Note various components of each arch.

which is the major source of connective tissue components, including bone, cartilage, and ligaments in the oral and facial region.

Components of pharyngeal arches

The mesenchyme of each pharyngeal arch forms following components (Fig. 10.2):

1. *Skeletal component* of each arch is *cartilagenous* to begin with. It may:
   - Remain cartilagenous, or
   - Develop into a bone, or
   - Disappear

2. *Muscular components* of the pharyngeal arches form various muscles in the head and neck region. The muscular component of each arch has its own nerve, and wherever the muscle cells migrate, they carry their nerve component with them (Fig. 10.3). Therefore, the derivation of the muscle from any arch can be identified from its nerve supply.

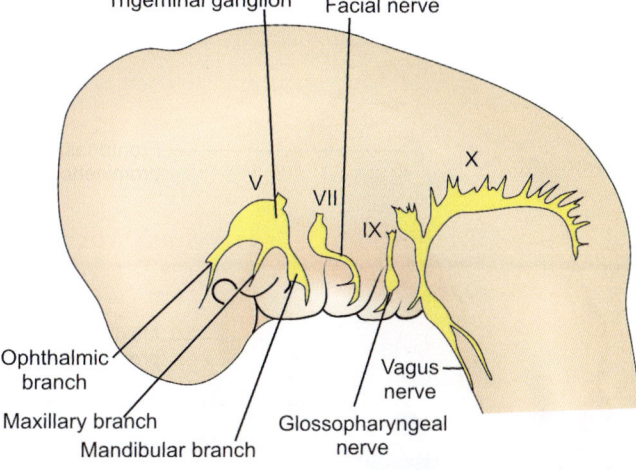

Fig. 10.3: Nerves of pharyngeal arches: location in a 4 week embyro.

3. *Arterial component.* Each pharyngeal arch contains its own arterial component known as *arterial* or *aortic arch*. Each aortic arch extends from the *ventral aorta* (present ventral to the developing

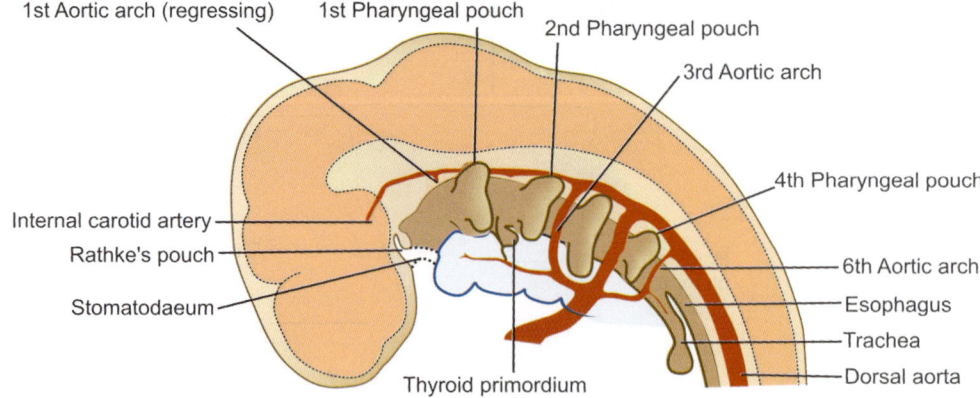

Fig. 10.4: Aortic arches (arterial component of) pharyngeal arches and pharyngeal pouches.

foregut) to the *dorsal aorta* (present dorsal to the developing foregut) (Figs 10.2 and 10.4). The fate of aortic arches is described in chapter on cardiovascular development (page 223).

4. *Nerve supply.* Each pharyngeal arch is supplied by its own nerve (Fig. 10.3) that supplies the muscles derived from each arch. In addition, it supplies sensory nerves to the structures developed from the endoderm and ectoderm of each arch.

Derivatives of pharyngeal arches

First pharyngeal arch or mandibular arch

Skeletal derivatives

First pharyngeal arch also known as mandibular arch develops into two prominences (Fig. 10.5):

- *Maxillary prominence.* Its mesenchyme gives rise to maxilla (upper jaw), zygomatic bone and squamous part of the temporal bone by membranous ossification.

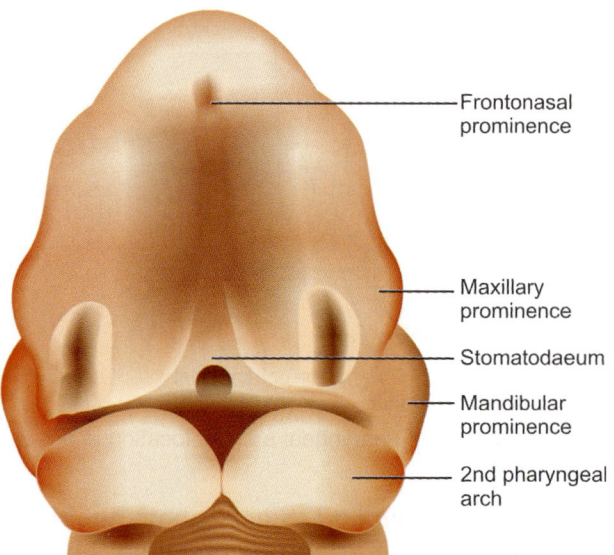

Frontonasal prominence

Maxillary prominence

Stomatodaeum

Mandibular prominence

2nd pharyngeal arch

Fig. 10.5: Frontal view of the embryo depicting maxillary and mandibular prominences of first pharyngeal arch.

- *Mandibular prominence.* It contains the first arch cartilage (Meckel's cartilage) and mesenchyme. Its mesenchyme develops into mandible (lower jaw) by membranous ossification.

Meckle's cartilage. Its fate is (Fig. 10.6):

- *Dorsal end* of Meckel's cartilage is closely related to the developing ear and ossifies to form two middle ear bones, the *malleus* and *incus.*
- *Middle part* of the cartilage regresses, but its perichordium forms the anterior ligament of malleus and sphenomandibular ligament.
- *Ventral part* of the cartilage is surrounded by the developing mandible and disappears.

Muscular derivatives

Muscular derivatives of the first pharyngeal arch are (Fig. 10.7):

- *Muscles of mastication* (temporalis, masseter and pterygoids), and
- *Other muscles include:* Anterior belly of the digastric, mylohyoid, tensor tympani, and tensor palatini.

Nerves of first arch are maxillary and mandibular divisions of trigeminal or 5th cranial nerve. Its :

- *Mandibular division* supplies the muscles derived from 1st arch.
- *Maxillary and mandibular divisions* supply sensory nerves to skin of face.

Note: Ophthalmic division of 5th cranial nerve does not supply the pharyngeal arch components.

Second pharyngeal arch or hyoid arch

Skeletal derivatives

The cartilage of second pharyngeal arch (hyoid arch), also known as Reichert's cartilage contributes as below (Fig. 10.6):

- *Dorsal end* of this cartilage is closely related to the developing ear, and ossifies to form:

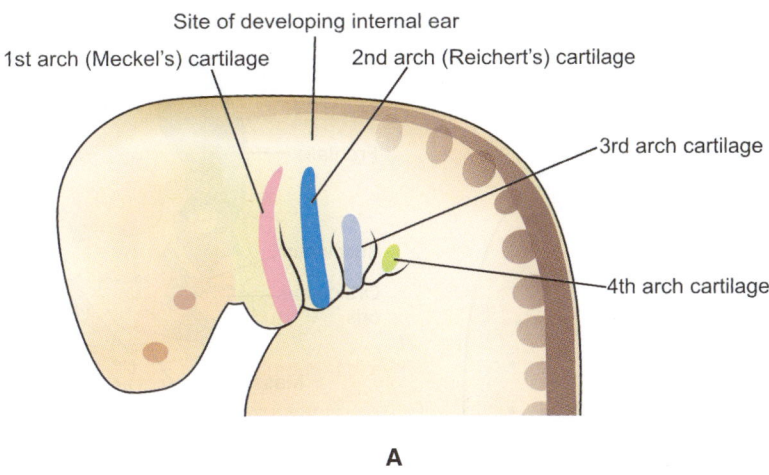

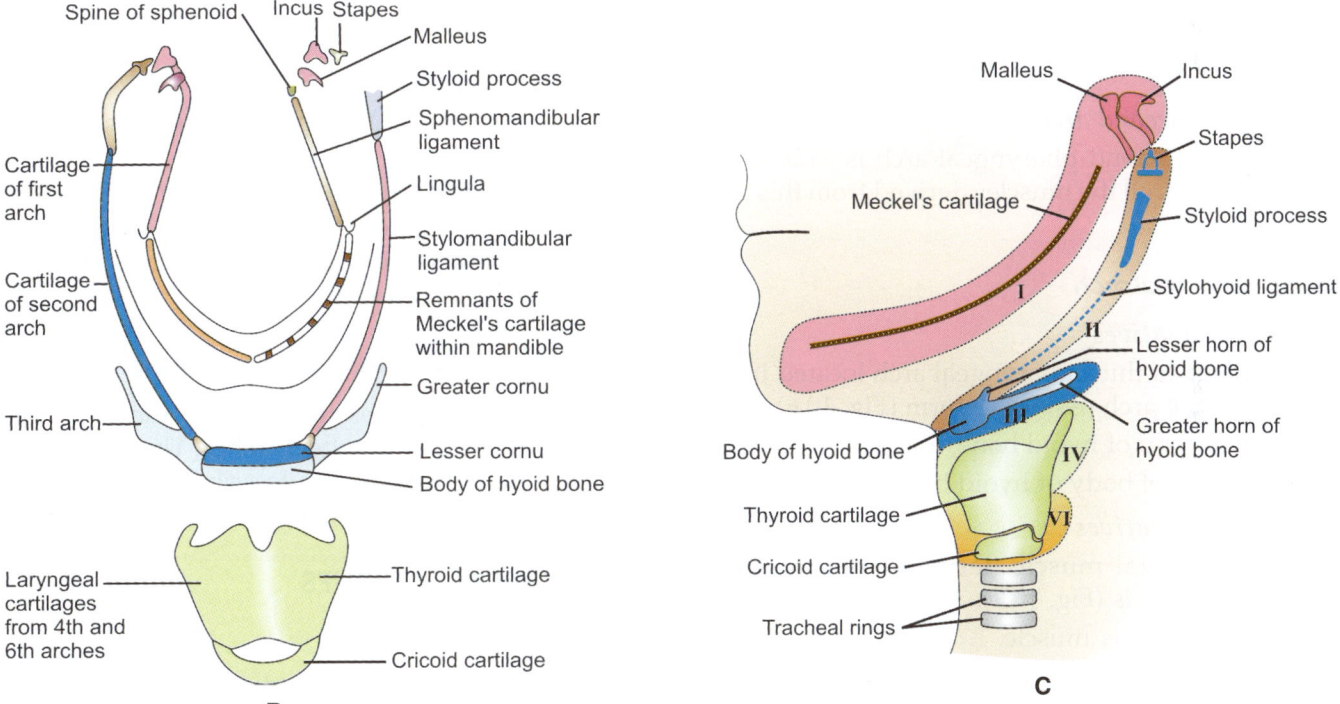

Fig. 10.6: Cartilages of pharyngeal arches and their derivatives: A, location of pharyngeal arch cartilages in a 4 week embryo; B, frontal view of skeletal derivatives, left half of the figure shows an earlier stage of development; C, lateral view of skeletal derivatives.

- – Stapes of the middle ear, and
- – Styloid process of the temporal bone.
- The part of cartilage between the styloid process and hyoid bone regresses; its perichondrium forms the *stylohyoid ligament.*
- *Ventral end* of this cartilage ossifies to form the lesser cornu and the superior part of the body of hyoid bone.

Muscular derivatives

The muscles derived from the second pharyngeal arch include (Fig. 10.7):

- Stapedius
- Stylohyoid,
- Posterior belly of digastric,
- Auricular and
- Muscles of facial expressions.

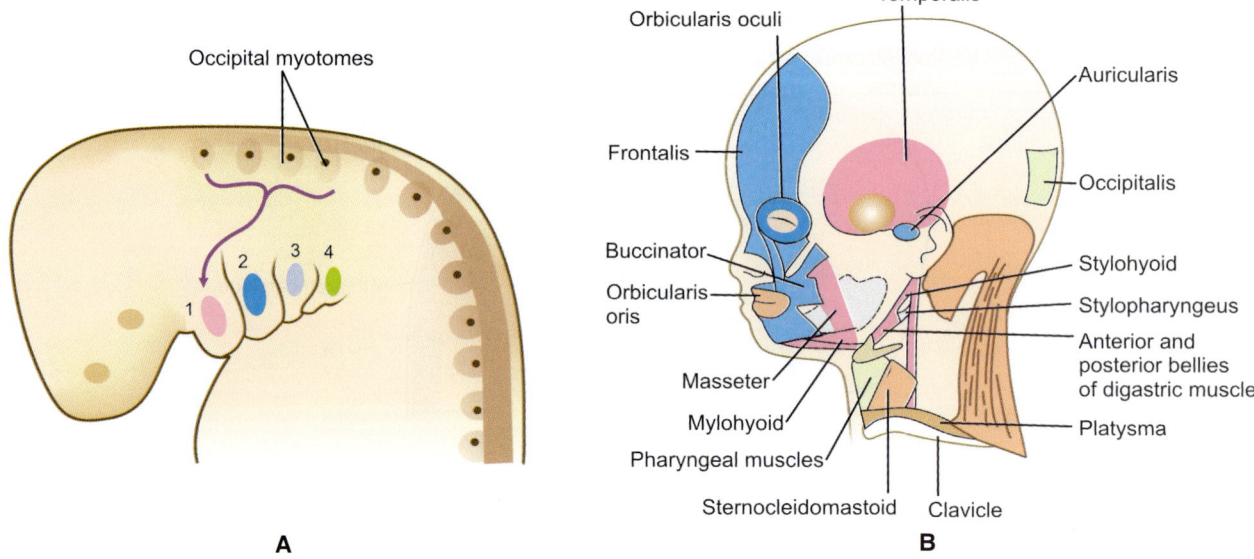

Fig. 10.7: Muscles derived from pharyngeal arches: A, location in a 4 week embryo; B, diagrammatic depiction in a sketch of head and neck region.

Nerve of the second arch

Nerve of the second pharyngeal arch is *facial nerve,* which supplies all the muscles derived from this arch (listed above).

Third pharyngeal arch

Skeletal derivatives

The cartilage of third pharyngeal arch located in the ventral part of arch ossifies to form (Fig. 10.6):

- Greater cornu of hyoid bone, and
- Lower part of body of hyoid bone.

Muscular derivatives

The only skeletal muscle derived from the third pharyngeal arch is (Fig. 10.7):

- Stylopharyngeus muscle.

Nerve of third pharyngeal arch

Nerve of the third pharyngeal arch is *glossopharyngeal nerve,* and supplies the muscles derived from this arch.

Fourth and sixth pharyngeal arches

Skeletal derivatives

The cartilages of fourth and sixth pharyngeal arches fuse to form the cartilages of larynx (except cartilage of epiglottis) which include thyroid, cricoid, arytenoid, corniculate, and cuneiform cartilages (Fig. 10.6).

Muscular derivatives and their nerve supply

- *Muscles derived from fourth pharyngeal arch* include the cricothyroid, levater palatini, and constrictors of the pharynx (Fig. 10.7) superior laryngeal branch

of vagus (nerve of fourth arch) supplies all these muscles.

- *Muscles derived from sixth pharyngeal arch* include the intrinsic muscles of larynx (Fig. 10.7). *Recurrent laryngeal branch of vagus (nerve of the sixth arch)* supplies these muscles.

Summary of derivatives of pharyngeal arches

Table 10.1 summarizes the skeletal and muscular derivatives of the pharyngeal arches. The derivatives of aortic arch arterious are described in chapter on development of cardiovascular system.

PHARYNGEAL POUCHES

Structure

As mentioned above, the endoderm of the developing pharynx lines the internal aspects of the pharyngeal arches and in between the two arches is pushed outward to form the pharyngeal pouches. There are five pouches in the developing human embryo (Figs 10.2 and 10.8).

Derivatives and fate

Derivatives and fate of the pharyngeal pouches is outlined briefly (Figs 10.8 and 10.9).

First pharyngeal pouch

The first pharyngeal pouch expands into an elongated diverticulum, the *tubotympanic recess,* and forms following structures (Figs 10.8 and 10.9):

Table 10.1: Structures derived from skeletal and muscular components of pharyngeal arches

Pharyngeal arch	Nerve of the arch	Muscles derived	Skeletal and ligamentous structures derived
1st (Mandibular arch)	Maxillary and mandibular divisions of trigeminal (5th cranial nerve)	• Muscles of mastication (temporalis, masseter, medial and lateral pterygoids). • Mylohyoid • Anterior belly of digastric • Tensor tympani • Tensor veli palatini	• Malleus • Incus • Anterior ligament of malleus • Sphenomandibular ligament
2nd (Hyoid arch)	Facial (7th cranial nerve)	• Muscles of facial expression (buccinator, auricularis, frontalis, platysma, orbicularis oris, and orbicularis oculi) • Posterior belly of digastric • Stylohyoid • Stapedius	• Stapes • Styloid process • Lesser cornu of hyoid • Upper part of body of hyoid bone • Stylohyoid ligament
3rd	Glossopharyngeal (9th cranial nerve)	• Stylopharyngeus	• Greater cornu of hyoid • Lower part of body of hyoid bone
4th and 6th	Superior laryngeal branch of vagus, and Recurrent laryngeal branch of vagus (10th cranial) nerve.	• Cricothyroid • Levator veli palatini • Constrictor of pharynx • Intrinsic muscles of larynx • Striated muscles of esophagus	• Thyroid cartilage • Cricoid cartilage • Arytenoid cartilage • Corniculate cartilage • Cuneiform cartilage

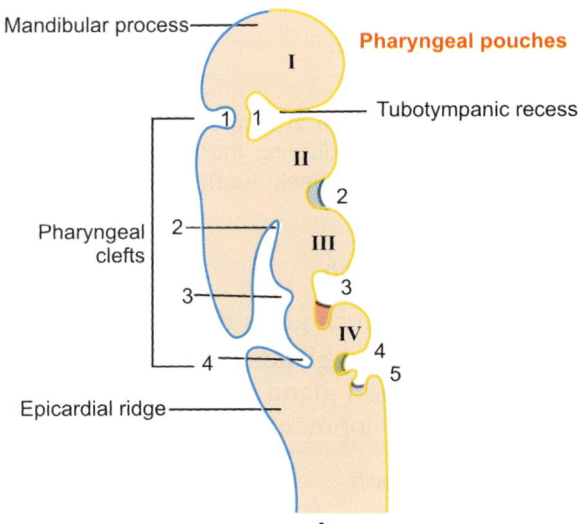

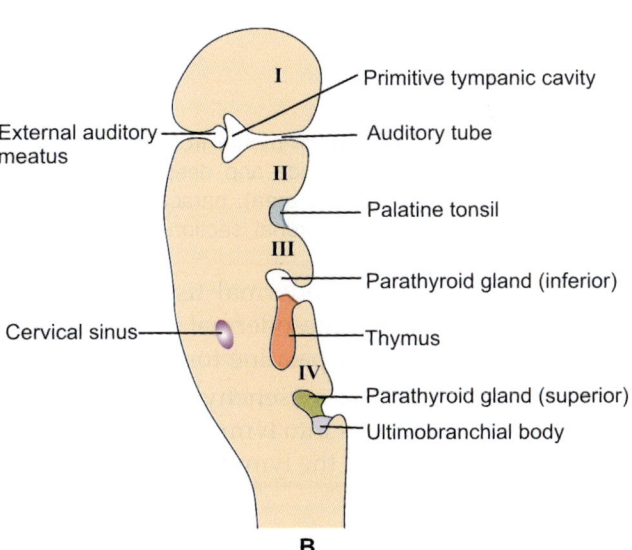

Fig. 10.8: Derivatives of pharyngeal pouches and clefts: A, early stage of development; B, late stage of development.

- *Primitive tympanic or middle ear cavity* is formed by the distal widend portion of the tubotympanic recess.
- *Auditory (eustachian) tube* is formed by the proximal narrow portion of the tubotympanic recess.
- *Tympanic membrane (ear drum)* is formed by the part of endodermal lining which comes in contact with the ectoderm of corresponding pharyngeal cleft.

Second pharyngeal pouch

The second pharyngeal pouch forms palatine tonsils, and tonsillar fossa (Figs 10.8 and 10.9).

1. *Palatine tonsils* are developed by following process:
   - The endoderm of the second pouch proliferates and forms buds that invade the underlying mesenchyme.

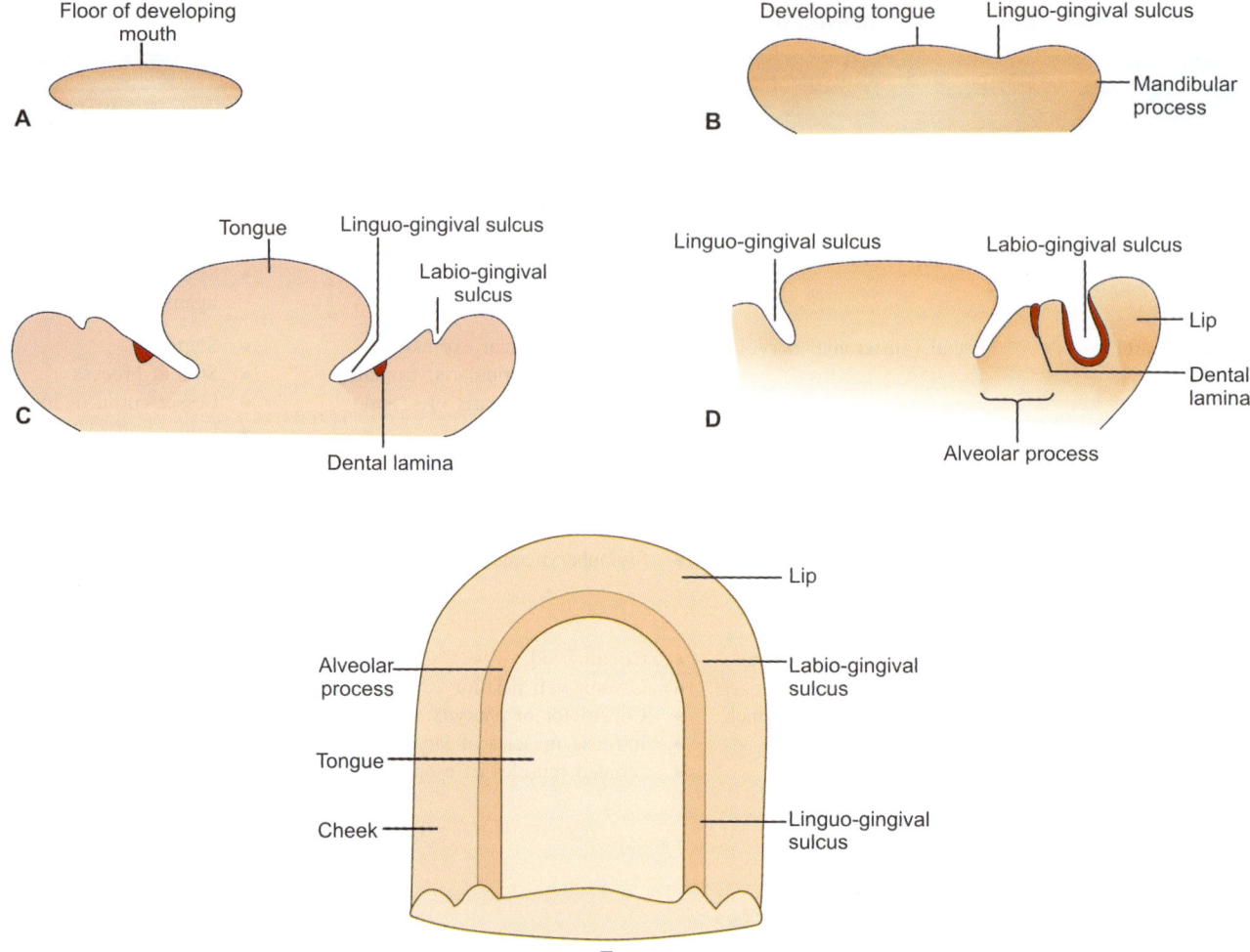

Fig. 10.9: Formation of floor of mouth from the mandibular process: A, B, C and D as seen in coronal section of the oral cavity; the stages of appearance and deepening of linguo-gingival and labio-gingival sulci dividing the mandibular process in three areas: central (tongue area), paracentral (alveolar process), and peripheral (lip and cheek area); E, the view of floor of mouth corresponding to coronal section-D.

- These buds of endodermal tissue are secondarily invaded by mesodermal tissue and form the primordium of palatine tonsils.
- By 20th week the mesenchyme invading the buds differentiates into lymphoid tissue, which soon organize into the lymphatic nodules of the palatine tonsils.

2. *Tonsillar fossa* is formed by the remaining part of the second pharyngeal pouch.

Third pharyngeal pouch

The distal extremity of third pharyngeal pouch is characterized by a dorsal and ventral wing and gives rise to:

- Inferior parathyroid glands, and
- Thymus
  For details of development (See page 141).

Fourth pharyngeal pouch

Fourth pharyngeal pouch gives rise to:

- Superior parathyroid glands, and
- Some part of thyroid gland
  For details of development (See page 142).

Fifth pharyngeal pouch

When it appears as rudimentary pouch for a brief period during development, it fuses with fourth pouch and forms the caudal pharyngeal complex.

PHARYNGEAL CLEFTS

Pharyngeal clefts refer to the four ectodermal grooves present on the external surface of the neck region during the fourth and fifth weeks. As mentioned earlier, these are formed by dipping in of the surface ectoderm in between the pharyngeal arches. These lie opposite the pharyngeal pouches (Fig. 10.2).

Fate of pharyngeal clefts

First pharyngeal cleft penetrates the underlying mesenchyme and gives rise to (Fig. 10.8).

- External auditory meatus, and
- Tympanic membrane (ear drum), which is formed by part of ectoderm of 1st cleft joining the endoderm of first pouch (Fig. 10.8).

Second, third and fourth pharyngeal clefts, soon come to lie in the *cervical sinus* which is formed by downward active proliferation of the mesenchyme of the second arch which comes to overland the 3rd and 4th arches and 2nd, 3rd and 4th pharyngeal clefts. As the neck develops further the 2nd, 3rd and 4th clefts are normally obliterated along with the cervical sinus, and the side of neck (which was marked by grooves) now becomes smooth.

Congenital anomalies related to pharyngeal clefts

- *Branchial sinus,* that open externally on the side of neck results from the failure of obliteration of cervical sinus and 2nd pharyngeal cleft.
- *Branchial fistula,* an abnormal canal, that opens externally on the side of neck and internally into the tonsillar sinus results from persistence of parts of the second pharyngeal cleft and pouch.
- *Branchial cysts* may be formed as spherical or elongated cysts as remnants of parts of the cervical sinus and/or second pharyngeal cleft.

DEVELOPMENT OF STRUCTURES OF ORAL CAVITY AND PHARYNX

DEVELOPMENT OF MOUTH

Mouth is loosely used term to denote the external opening (oral fissure) and the cavity it leads to. The mouth (oral) cavity contains anterior two-third of tongue and the teeth.

Mouth is derived partly from the *stomodaeum* (ectodermal) and partly from the foregut (endodermal). *Buccopharyngeal membrane* separates the stomatodaeum from the foregut (Fig. 10.9). After disappearance of the buccopharyngeal membrane, it is difficult to define the line of junction between the ectoderm and endoderm.

Ectoderm of stomatodaeum contributes epithelial lining inside of the lips, cheeks, palate, gums, and teeth.

Endoderm of foregut gives rise to epithelial lining of the tongue.

Structures of floor of mouth

Mandibular process takes part in the formation of three structures of floor of mouth:

- Lower lip and lower parts of cheek;
- Lower jaw, and
- Tongue

The area of the fused mandibular process which contributes structures of floor of mouth is divided into three parts by appearance and successive deepening of two pairs of sulci the *lingual gingival sulci* and the *labio-gingival sulci* (Fig. 10.9):

- *Central part* between the two lingual-gingival sulci forms the tongue. For details of development of tongue (See page 136).
- *Paracentral parts* between the lingual-gingival and labiogingival sulci on each side form the *alveolar process.* This process forms the lower jaw and teeth develop in relation to it.
- *Peripheral parts* lying lateral to the labio-gingival sulci on each side form the lower lip and the cheek.

Roof of mouth cavity

Roof of the oral cavity is formed by:

- *Palate* (for details of development see page 147), and
- *Alveolar process* of upper jaw which gets separated from the upper lip and cheek by the appearance of a labio-gingival furrow (Fig. 10.10). Because of upward arching of the palate, the medial margins of alveolar process become distinct and defined.

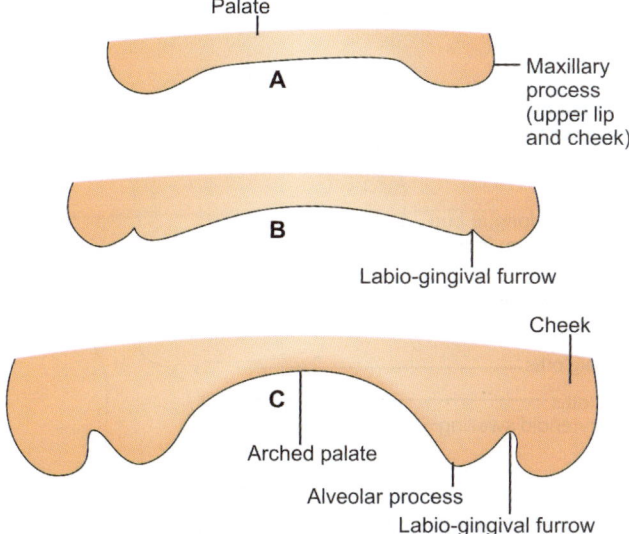

Fig. 10.10: Formation of roof of the oral cavity from the maxillary process and palate.

DEVELOPMENT OF TONGUE

The tongue develops in relation to the ventral portion of the pharyngeal arches in the floor of the developing mouth.

Primordia of developing tongue

Primordia of tongue seen in embryos of 4 weeks include (Fig. 10.11):

Lateral lingual swellings. The medial most parts of the first pharyngeal (mandibular) arches proliferate to form two lateral swellings.

Tuberculum impar. It is a median swelling which partially separates the two lateral lingual swellings. It is also formed by proliferation of medial most parts of the first pharyngeal arches. Immediately behind the tuberculum impar, the epithelium proliferates to form a down growth (*thyroid diverticulum*) from which the thyroid gland develops. The site of down growth is subsequently marked by a depression called *foramen caecum.*

Hypobranchial eminence is another median swelling formed by mesoderm of 2nd, 3rd, and part of 4th pharyngeal arches. This eminence is soon divided into two parts:

- *Cranial part* (known as *copula)* which is related to 2nd and 3rd arches, and
- *Caudal part,* which is related to the 4th arch. It forms the epiglottis. Immediately behind this swelling is the *laryngeal orifice,* which is flanked by the arytenoid swellings (Fig. 10.11A).

Formation of Tongue

Anterior two-thirds of tongue. The two lateral lingual swellings rapidly increase in size, merge with each other, and overgrow the tuberculum impar. The merged lateral lingual buds form the anterior two-thirds (oral part) of the tongue (Figs 10.11B and C). Fusion of the two lateral lingual buds is indicated by a middle groove, the *median sulcus of tongue.*

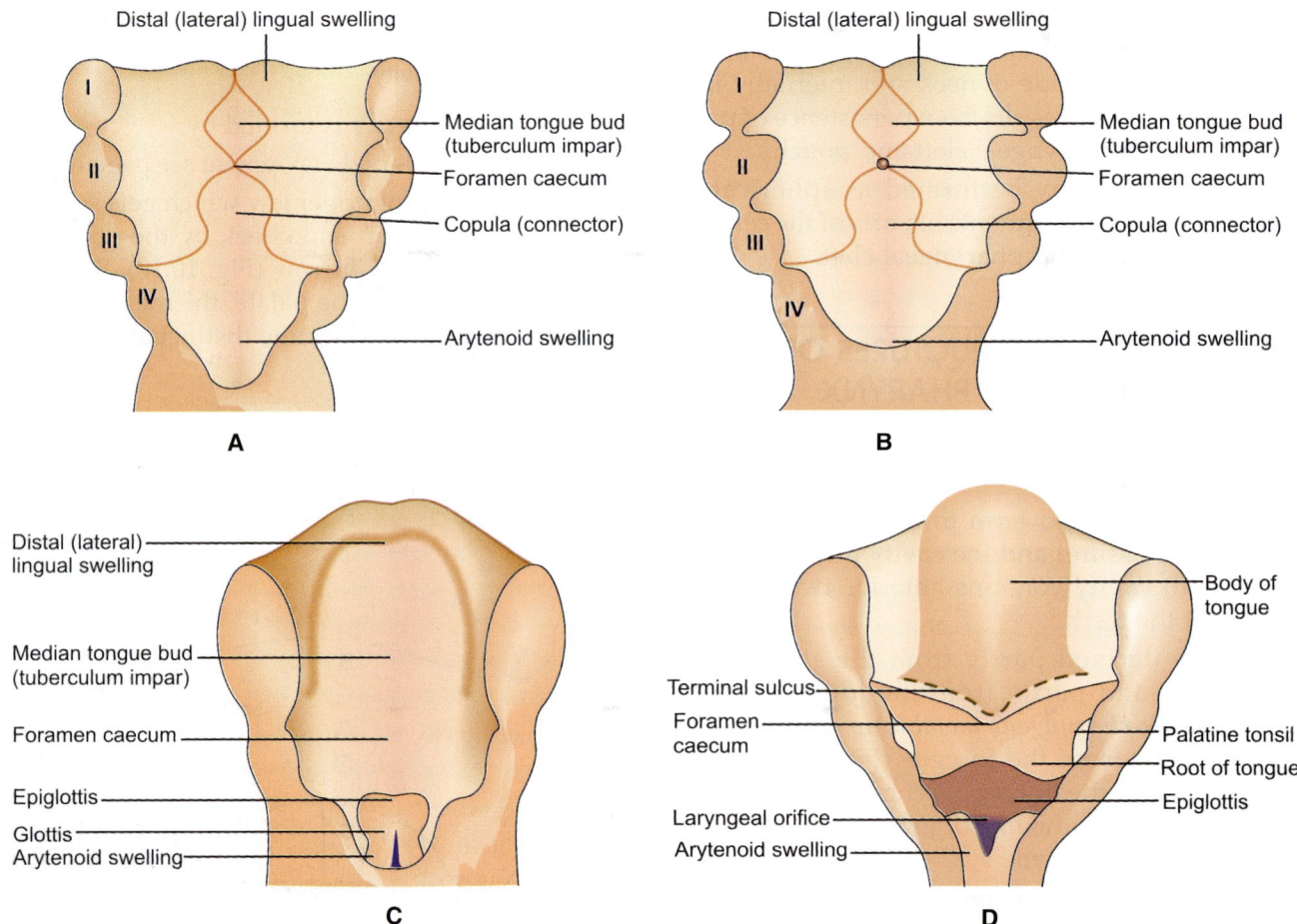

Fig. 10.11: Ventral wall of the developing pharynx to show : A, position of primordia from which tongue is derived and the foramen caecum (between the tuberculum impar and copula) from where the primordium thyroid (diverticulum) arises; B and C, development of tongue from different embryonic structures; D, tongue floor of mouth and pharynx region (pharynx has been cut open from behind).

Nerve supply: Since the anterior two-thirds of tongue is derived from the Ist pharyngeal arch, it is supplied by:

- *Lingual branch* of mandibular nerve, which is post-trematic nerve of the first arch, and
- *Chordatympani,* which is pre-trematic nerve of the Ist arch.

Posterior one-thirds of tongue is formed by copula (the cranial part of hypobranchial eminence). The 3rd arch mesoderm of copula grows over the 2nd arch mesoderm of copula and fuses with the mesoderm of Ist arch (Fig. 10.12). The V-shaped groove (*terminal sulcus)* separates the anterior two-thirds of the tongue from the posterior one third (Figs 10.11B and D).

Nerve supply: Since the posterior 1/3rd of the tongue is mainly derived from the 3rd arch, so it is supplied by *glossopharyngeal nerve,* which is the nerve of 3rd arch.

Most posterior part of tongue and epiglottis are formed by the caudal part of the hypobranchial eminence derived from 4th arch mesoderm.

Nerve supply: The most posterior part of tongue and epiglottis are supplied by the *superior laryngeal nerve* (branch of vagus nerve) which is nerve of the fourth arch.

Musculature of the tongue is mainly derived from myoblasts originating in *occipital somites.* Thus, the tongue musculature is innervated by *hypoglossal nerve.*

Epithelium of the tongue is first made up of a single layer of cells. Later it becomes stratified and papillae become evident. *Taste buds* develop by inductive interaction between the epithelial cells of the tongue and the invading gustatory nerve cells from the chorda tympani, glossopharyngeal, and vagus nerves.

Anomalies of tongue

1. *Macroglossia* refers to a too large tongue.
2. *Microglossia* refers to a too small tongue.
3. *Ankyloglossia* (tongue tie). Normally, extensive cell degeneration occurs and the anterior 2/3rd of the tongue becomes free from the floor except for a small frenulum which ties tongue to the floor of mouth. In ankyloglossia the frenulum is large and the tongue is not freed from the floor of mouth.
4. *Thyroglossal cyst* formed from remnants of thyroglossal duct, may be present in the tongue.

DEVELOPMENT OF SALIVARY GLANDS

General outlines of development of salivary glands

- *Solid epithelial buds* arising from the primordial oral cavity during the 6th and 7th weeks mark the beginning of development of salivary glands. The solid outgrowths grow into the underlying mesenchyme and are later canalized.
- *Duct system* of the glands is formed by repeated branching.
- *Secretory acini* are formed from the terminal parts of the duct system.
- *Connective tissue in the glands* is derived from the neural crest cells.

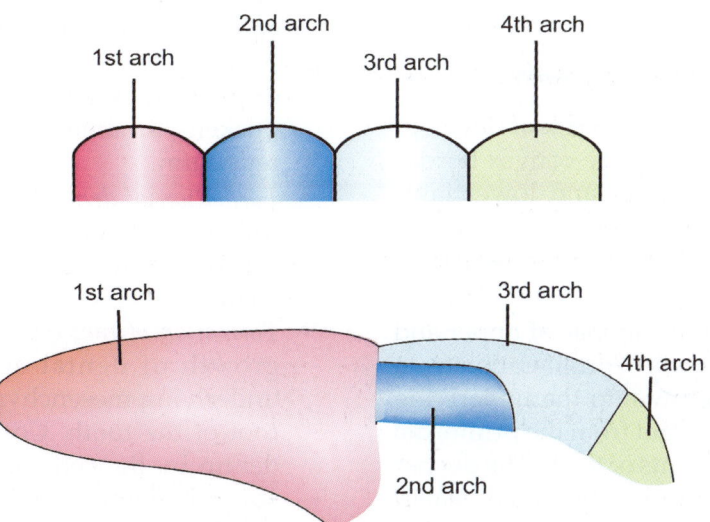

Fig. 10.12: Diagrammatic depiction (in lateral view) of the contribution of 1st to 4th pharyngeal arches in the development of tongue.

Specific outlines of development of salivary glands

Parotid glands: Solid epithelial buds from which parotid glands develop arise from the oral *ectodermal* lining near the angles of stomatodaeum. These grow towards the ears along the line where the maxillary and mandibular processes fuse to form the cheek.

Submandibular glands develop from *endodermal buds* arising from the floor of mouth in relation to the linguo-gingival sulcus.

- *Submandibular duct* is formed by closure of a linear groove that appears lateral to the tongue.
- *Growth of submandibular glands* continues after birth with the formation of mucous acini.

Sublingual glands develop from multiple *endodermal* epithelial buds in the paralingual sulcus. These buds branch and canalize to form 10 to 12 ducts that open independently into the floor of the mouth.

DEVELOPMENT OF TEETH

Teeth are developed in relation to the alveolar processes of upper and lower jaws.

Types of dentition. Two types of dentitions (development of teeth) occur:

- *Primary dentition,* i.e. formation of deciduous teeth and
- *Secondary dentition,* i.e. formation of permanent teeth.

Contributing embryonic tissues from which teeth develop are:

- *Oral ectoderm,* which forms enamel of teeth, and
- *Mesenchyme* (derived from surrounding mesoderm and neural crest) from which all other tissues of teeth develop.

Primary dentition

Stages of development of deciduous teeth

1. *Dental lamina stage.* By the 6th week of development, the epithelium covering the convex border of alveolar processes of upper and lower jaws become thickened to form C-shaped dental lamina, which projects into the underlying mesoderm (Fig. 10.13A and B).

2. *Stage of dental buds.* Dental laminae of upper and lower jaws develop 10 centers of proliferation from which the dental buds grow into the underlying mesenchyme (Fig. 10.13C) and from the primordia of the ectodermal components of teeth. The deeper enlarged parts of the tooth bud is called *enamel organ.*

3. *Cap-stage of tooth development.* Soon the enamel organ of dental bud is invaginated by the mesen-

chyme and it becomes cap-shaped. Various parts and their derivatives during cap-stage of tooth development are (Fig. 10.13D):

- *Dental papilla* is formed by the mesenchyme invaginating the enamel organ. It is the primordium of *dental pulp.*
- *Outer enamel epithelium* is formed by the center cell layer of the cap-shaped enamel.
- *Inner enamel epithelium* is formed by the inner cell layer of the cap-shaped enamel organ.
- *Enamel (stellate) reticulum* refers to the central core of loosely arranged cells between the layers of enamel epithelium.

Tooth germ. The dental papilla and enamel organ combindly form the tooth germ.

Dental sac refers to the vascularized capsular structure formed by condensation of mesenchyme surrounding the developing tooth. It is the primordium of the cement and periodontal ligament.

4. *Bell stage of tooth development.* With further development the indentation of the enamel organ is further deepened and the cup-shaped structure is converted into a bell-shaped structure (Fig. 10.13E).

5. *Further development of tooth.* Various parts of the tooth formed during further development are (Fig. 10.13F):

- *Formation of dentin.* The mesenchymal cells of dental papillae lying adjacent to the inner enamel epithelium differentiate into *odontoblasts* which produce *predentin* and deposit it adjacent to the epithelium. Later the predentin is calcified to become dentin.

- *Formation of dental pulp.* The remaining cells of dental papilla form the tooth pulp.

- *Formation of enamel.* Cells of the inner enamel epithelium differentiate into *ameloblasts,* which produce long enamel prisms (rods) that are deposited over the dentin. When enamel thickens, the ameloblasts retreat into the stellate reticulum.

- *Formation of dental cuticle.* After the enamel is fully formed the ameloblasts disappear leaving a thin membrane (dental cuticle), over the enamel.

- *Formation of root and root canal.* The continued growth of dental epithelial layer into the underlying mesenchyme leads to formation of root of the tooth. Continuous laying down of dentin by the cells of dental papilla, the pulp space becomes progressively narrower and finally is converted into a canal (root canal) containing blood vessels and nerves of tooth (Fig. 10.13G).

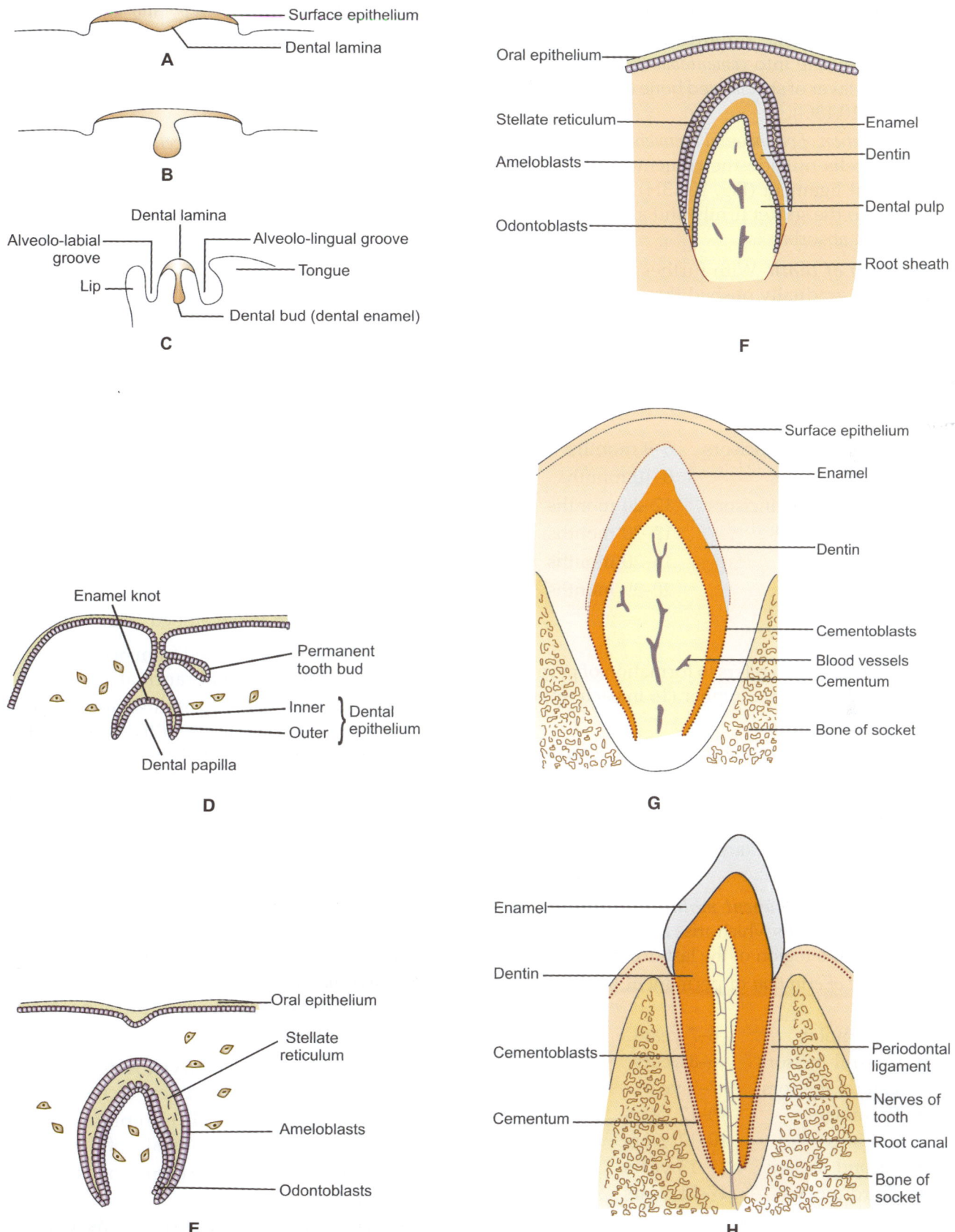

Fig. 10.13: Stages of development of tooth: A and B, dental lamina stage; C, stage of dental bud; D, cap-stage of tooth development; E, bell stage of tooth development; F, stage of formation of dentin, dental bulb, enamel and root; G, formation of root, and cement; and H, eruption of tooth.

- *Formation of cement.* The mesenchymal cells located on the outside of dentin of tooth differentiate into *cementoblasts,* which produce a thin layer of specialized bone called the cement (Fig. 10.13G).
- *Formation of periodontal ligament.* The mesenchymal cells outside the cement form the periodontal ligament (Fig. 10.13H) which holds the root to the socket firmly and also functions as a shock absorber.

6. **Eruption of tooth.** With further development the crown is gradually pushed through the overlying tissue layer into the oral cavity (Fig. 10.13H). This process is called eruption of tooth. The eruption of *deciduous* or *milk teeth* occurs 6 to 39 months after birth as below:

• Lower central incisors	6–9 months
• Upper incisors	8–10 months
• Lower lateral incisors	12–20 months
• First molar	12–20 months
• Canines	16–20 months
• Second molars	20–39 months

Secondary dentition

Secondary dentition refers to formation of permanent teeth, which are 32 in number (16 in each upper and lower jaw).

Formation of permanent incisors, canines and premolars. These teeth develop from the dental buds which arise from the dental lamina and lie on the medial side of each developing milk tooth (Fig. 10.13D) in a manner exactly similar to that described for deciduous teeth.

Formation of permanent molars. These are formed from the dental buds which arise from the dental lamina posterior to the region of the last deciduous tooth.

Average age of eruption of permanent teeth is:

• First molar	6–7 years
• Central incisors	6–8 years
• Lateral incisors	7–9 years
• Premolars	10–12 years
• Canines	10–12 years
• Second molars	11–13 years
• Third molars	17–21 years

Anomalies of teeth

1. *Defective formation of enamel* and dentin, e.g. enamel hypoplasia.

2. *Abnormalities in shape,* e.g. peg shaped incisors, enamel pearls (spherical masses of enamel).
3. *Variation in the number,* e.g. supernumerary, total anodontia (complete absence of teeth), or partial anodontia.
4. *Variation in the position of teeth*
5. *Precocious eruption of teeth,* i.e. too early primary dentition, e.g. lower incisor may be present since birth.
6. *Delayed eruption,* i.e. too late dentition.
7. *Malocclusion,* i.e. misalignment of teeth of upper and lower jaws.
8. *Gemination,* i.e. two or more teeth may be fused with each other.
9. *Dentigerous cyst:* A cyst may develop in the mandible, maxilla or maxillary sinus that contains an unerupted tooth.

DEVELOPMENT OF PHARYNX

Primordium of pharynx. Pharynx is derived from the cephalic (pre-laryngeal) part of the foregut, which extends from the buccopharyngeal membrane to the tracheobronchial diverticulum from which the entire respiratory system is developed (Fig. 10.1.4).

Definitive pharynx is formed from primitive pharynx after the establishment of branchial apparatus. With the establishment of the palate and mouth, the pharynx can be divided into three continuous parts nasopharynx oropharyx and laryngopharynx.

- *Nasopharynx* communicates ventrally with the nasal cavity developed from the cranial part of stomatodaeum after formation of palate. Below it is continuous with the oropharynx.
- *Oropharynx* communicates with the mouth cavity developed from stomatodaeum after rupture of buccopharyngeal membrane. Below, oropharynx continues with laryngopharynx.
- *Laryngopharynx.* It is continuous ventrally with the larynx (developed from the tracheobronchial diverticulum).

Epithelial lining of the pharynx is derived from the endoderm lining the pharyngeal arches:

- Endoderm of first arch is represented by the epithelial lining of lateral walls of the pharynx.
- Endoderm of second arch corresponds with palatoglossal arch.
- Endoderm of third arch corresponds with pharyngoepiglottic fold.
- Endoderm of fourth arch forms epithelial lining of epiglottis.

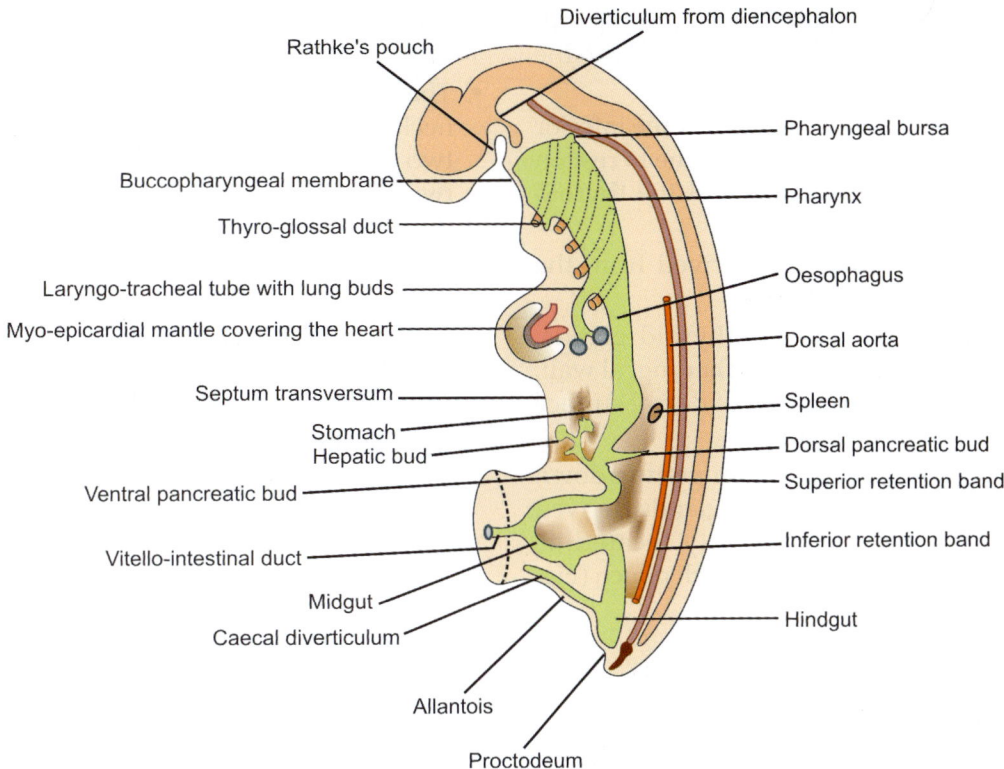

Fig. 10.14: Median section of advanced stage of embryo to show the primordium of pharynx extending from buccopharyngeal membrane to the tracheobronchial diverticulum.

- Endoderm of sixth arch represents the aryepiglottic fold.
- Endoderm of first pouch is represented by the auditory tube.
- Endoderm of 2nd pouch gives rise to tonsils and some part persists as the intratonsilar cleft or tonsillar fossa.

Muscles of pharynx are derived from the 3rd and subsequent pharyngeal arches.

DEVELOPMENT OF THYMUS, PARATHYROIDS AND THYROID GLAND

DEVELOPMENT OF THYMUS

- Thymus develops from the endoderm of the ventral wing of the third pharyngeal pouch (Fig. 10.8) and from the mesenchyme into which the epithelial tubes grow.
- The bilateral primordia of the thymus lose their connections with the pharyngeal wall, come together in the median plane to form bilobed structure which migrates into the superior mediastinum part of the thoracic cavity (Fig. 10.15).
- Thymus continues to grow after birth till puberty, after which it begins to undergo involution.

Consequently, it is difficulty to recognize in old age, as it is atrophied and replaced by fatty tissue.

DEVELOPMENT OF PARATHYROID GLANDS

Inferior parathyroid glands are derived from the dorsal wing of the third pharyngeal pouch.

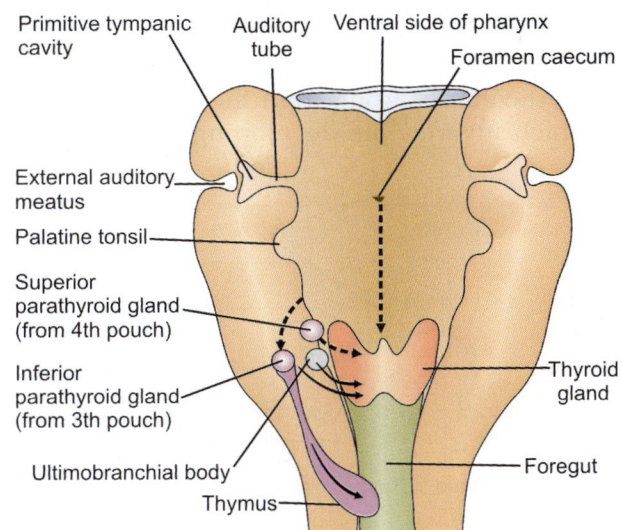

Fig. 10.15: Development of thymus, parathyroids and thyroid gland.

- Primordia of the inferior parathyroids along with primordia of thymus lose their connection with the pharyngeal wall.
- The migrating down thymus also pulls the inferior parathyroids with it, which finally come to rest on the inferior part of dorsal surface of the thyroid gland (Fig. 10.15).

Superior parathyroid glands are derived from the endoderm of 4th pharyngeal pouch.

- The primordia of superior parathyroid glands, after loosing connection with the pharyngeal wall, come to rest on the superior part of dorsal surface of the thyroid gland (Fig. 10.15).
- As mentioned above, because of migration down with the thymus, the parathyroid glands derived from 3rd pouch become inferiorly located as compared to those derived from the 4th pouch (Fig. 10.15).

DEVELOPMENT OF THYROID GLAND

Thyroid gland is derived from:

- An epithelial proliferation in the floor of pharynx, and
- Endoderm of 4th pharyngeal pouch or caudal pharyngeal complex (formed by fusion of 5th rudimentary pouch with 4th pouch).

Thyroid primordium is formed from the epithelial proliferation which grows down as a diverticulum in the floor of the pharynx from a point located between the tubercular impar and copula. This point later develops into foramen caecum (Figs 10.11, 10.15, 10.16).

- The diverticulum descends in the neck passing through the developing tongue and ventral to the developing hyoid bone where it develops into thyroid gland (Fig. 10.16). The part of the diverticulum starting from the foramen caecum (which invades the developing tongue) to the thyroid gland form the *thyroglossal duct* (Fig. 10.16). This duct later becomes solid and finally disappears.
- The tip of the down growing diverticulum in the neck just below the thyroid cartilage divides into two parts, which proliferates and gives rise to the two lobes of thyroid gland connected by isthmus (Fig. 10.17).
- The developing thyroid comes into intimate relationship with the 4th pharyngeal pouch or caudal pharyngeal complex and fuses with it (Fig. 11.17E).
- The *follicular cells* of thyroid gland derived from the thyroid primordium produce colloid that serve as a source of thyroxin, and tri-iodothyronine, by the end of third month. *Parafollicular cells or C-cells* derived from the 4th pharyngeal pouch or caudal pharyngeal complex serve as source of calcitonin.

Anomalies of thyroid gland

I. *Anomalies of shape*

1. *Pyramidal lobe* may be present, which may arise from isthmus, right or left lobe or from remnants of thyroglossal duct.
2. *Agenesis,* i.e. complete absence, or absence of any of the following parts may be there:
   - Absence of isthmus.
   - Absence or hypogenesis of one of the lobes.

II. *Anomalies of position of thyroid gland*

1. *Lingual thyroid,* i.e. presence of thyroid on the dorsum of tongue (Fig. 10.18A).
2. *Intralingual,* i.e. presence of thyroid in the tissues of tongue (Fig. 10.18B).
3. *Suprahyoid thyroid,* i.e. thyroid is present in the midline of neck, above the hyoid bone (Fig. 10.18C).

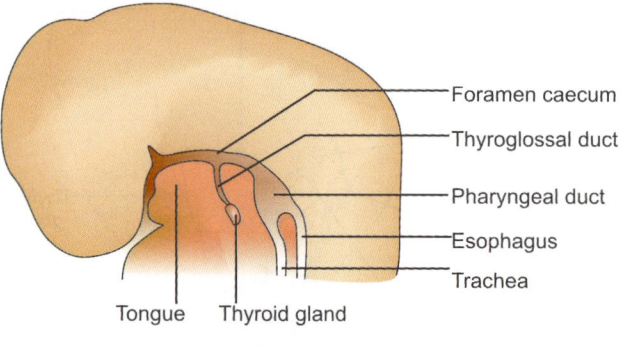

A

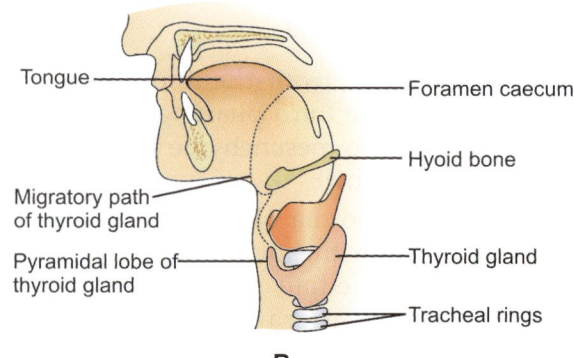

B

Fig. 10.16: A, Thyroid primordium as a diverticulum from the floor of pharynx and invading the developing tongue; and B, position of thyroid gland in adult. Also note path of migration of thyroid primordium.

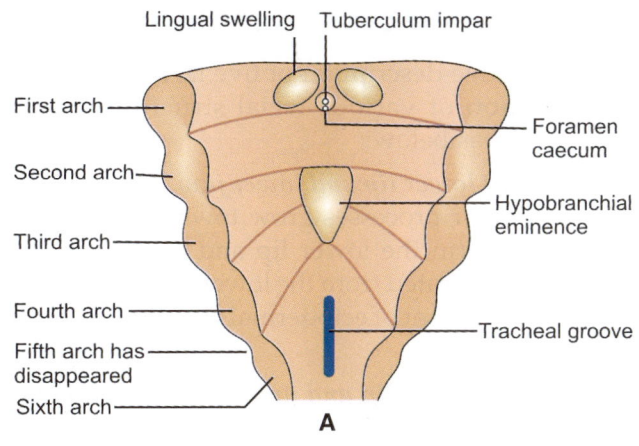

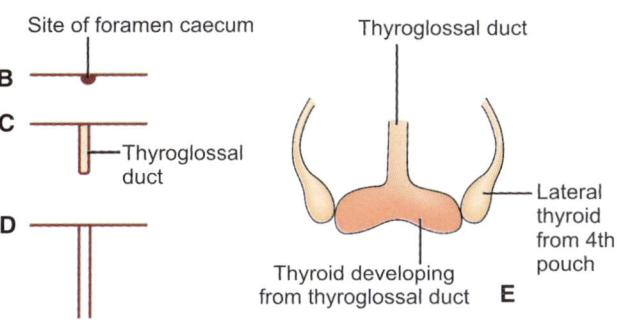

Fig. 10.17: Development of thyroid gland.

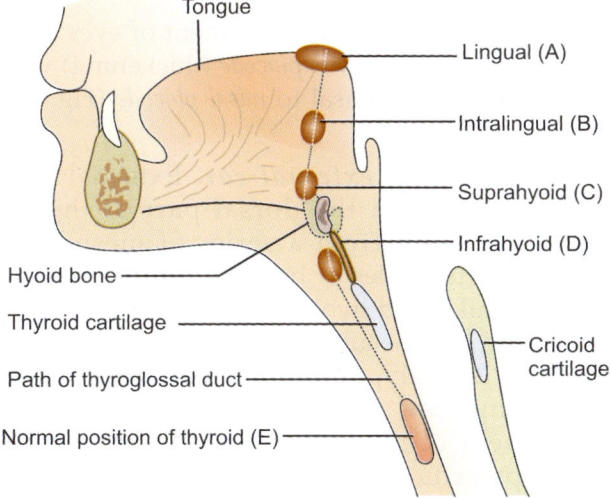

Fig. 10.18: Abnormal locations of thyroid gland and/or locations of thyroglossal cysts: A, lingual; B, intralingual; C, suprahyoid; D, infrahyoid; E, normal thyroid gland.

4. *Infrahyoid thyroid,* i.e. thyroid is present in the midline of neck, below the hyoid bone (Fig. 10.18D).

5. *Intrathoracic thyroid,* i.e. when the entire thyroid gland or a part of it is present in the thoracic cavity.

III. *Ectopic thyroid tissue*

In addition to the normal thyroid in normal position, ectopic thyroid tissue has also been reported in the tongue, larynx, trachea, oesophagus, pleura, pericardium, and ovaries.

IV. *Remnants of thyroglossal duct*

Remnants of thyroglossal duct are not uncommon, and may occur as:

1. *Persistent thyroglossal duct,* i.e. when the duct is present all the way from the foramen caecum to larynx.

2. *Thyroglossal cysts.* These may be present anywhere along the migratory pathway of the thyroid gland (Fig. 10.18).

3. *Thyroglossal fistula,* i.e. when a thyroglossal cyst is connected to the outside by a fistulous canal. Usually, the fistula arises secondarily after rupture of a cyst but, rarely may also be present since birth.

DEVELOPMENT OF FACE, NASAL CAVITY, PARANASAL SINUSES AND PALATE

DEVELOPMENT OF FACE

FACIAL PRIMORDIA

Facial development occurs mainly between 4th and 8th weeks, and is induced by the migration of cells of neural crest, cells that migrate from the lower mesencephalon and upper rhombencephalon regions of the neural folds into the arches during 4th week.

Five facial primordia that appear around the stomatodaeum as prominences of mesenchyme covered by surface ectoderm are (Fig. 10.19A and B):

- Frontonasal process,
- A pair of maxillary processes, and
- A pair of mandibular processes.

Frontonasal process

Boundaries of stomatodaeum. During 6th week the stomatodaeum is separated from the foregut by buccopharyngeal membrane, bounded on the cephalic side by the budding of developing forebrain and caudally by ventral ends of the mandibular arches (Fig. 10.20A).

Formation of frontonasal process. During 5th week, the mesenchyme covering the developing forebrain proliferates and together with the overlying surface of ectoderm forms a downward projection called the *frontonasal process* which overlaps the upper part of stomatodaeum (Fig. 10.19A).

Appearance of nasal placodes and formation of nasal and lateral nasal processes. The *nasal cofactors placodes* the two ectodermal elevations appear on each side of the median plane on the frontonasal process (Fig.10.5). Soon the surface depression of the placodes, by the overgrowth of surrounding mesenchyme, convert them into nasal (olfactory) pits, which are thrown into open communication with the roof of the stomatodaeum. The edges of the each nasal pits are much raised above the surface and form the medial nasal process on the medial side, and lateral nasal process on the lateral side (Fig. 10.19C and D).

- *Lateral nasal processes* are more prominent and form the alae of nose.
- *Medial nasal processes* merge with each other (as a result of medial growth of maxillary prominence) to form the *intermaxillary segment* which gives rise to (Fig. 10.19E and F):
  - Philtrum or middle part of the upper lip,
  - Premaxillary part of the maxilla (upper jaw), which carries the four incisor teeth, and
  - Primary palate.

Cranially the intermaxillary segment is continuous with the rostral portion of the nasal septum, which is formed by frontal prominence.

Maxillary processes

- During the period of differentiation of frontonasal process, each mandibular arch (forming lateral wall of stomatodaeum) gives rise to a *maxillary process.*
- Each maxillary process grows ventromedially below the developing eye, meets and fuses with the lateral nasal processes.
- Initially, the maxillary process and lateral nasal process are separated by a deep furrow, the *nasolacrimal groove* (Fig. 10.19C). Ectoderm in this groove is buried into the underlying mesenchyme as a *solid epithelial cord,* which is subsequently canalized to form *nasolacrimal duct.* The upper end of the developing nasolacrimal duct widens to form the *lacrimal sac.*
- The maxillary processes grow further medially below the nasal pits and push the medial nasal processes medially which fuse to form the intermaxillary segment (as described above). The maxillary process of each side also fuses with the intermaxillary segment and takes part in the formation of cheek, upper lip and the maxilla (Fig. 10.19E and F).

Mandibular process

Caudal to the maxillary process, the mandibular arch grows as a *mandibular process* on each side.

FORMATION OF VARIOUS FACIAL STRUCTURES

From the above description of five facial primordia, the formation of various facial structures can be summarized as below:

Formation of lower lip and lower jaw. The right and left mandibular processes grow towards each other and fuse to form the lower lip and lower jaw. The lower lip is separated from the lower alveolar process by the development of ectodermal *alveolo-labial groove* (Fig. 10.19).

Formation of upper lip and upper jaw. As described above in differentiation of frontonasal process and maxillary processes:

- The philtrum or middle part of the upper lip is derived from the intermaxillary segment of frontonasal process.
- Lateral parts of the upper lip are derived from the maxillary processes.

Maxilla (upper jaw) is derived from the maxillary process. The upper lip is separated from the upper alveolar process by the development of ectodermal *alveolo-labial groove.*

Formation of cheeks. The cheeks are formed by progressive fusion of maxillary process and mandibular process with each other on each side (Fig. 10.19E and F).

Formation of eyes. The development of eyes begins with the formation of *lens placode* (thickening) which appears lateral and nasal to *nasal placode* (Fig. 10.19 G).

Formation of the external ear. External ear is developed around the dorsal part of the first ectodermal cleft, from a series of mesodermal thickenings (tubercles or hillocks) which appear on the mandibular and hyoid arches adjoining the first cleft. Fusion of these tubercles results in the formation of pinna. Initially, the pinna lies caudal to the developing jaw (Fig. 10.19G and H). Later enlargement of mandibular process pushes the pinna upwards and backwards to its definitive position.

MOLECULAR REGULATION OF FACIAL DEVELOPMENT

Face develops from the pharyngeal arches. Facial skeleton develops from the neural crest cells that migrate into the pharyngeal arches. From hindbrain region, crest cells migrate from segments called *rhombomeres.*

Genes regulating facial development from neural crest cells of different pharyngeal arches are:

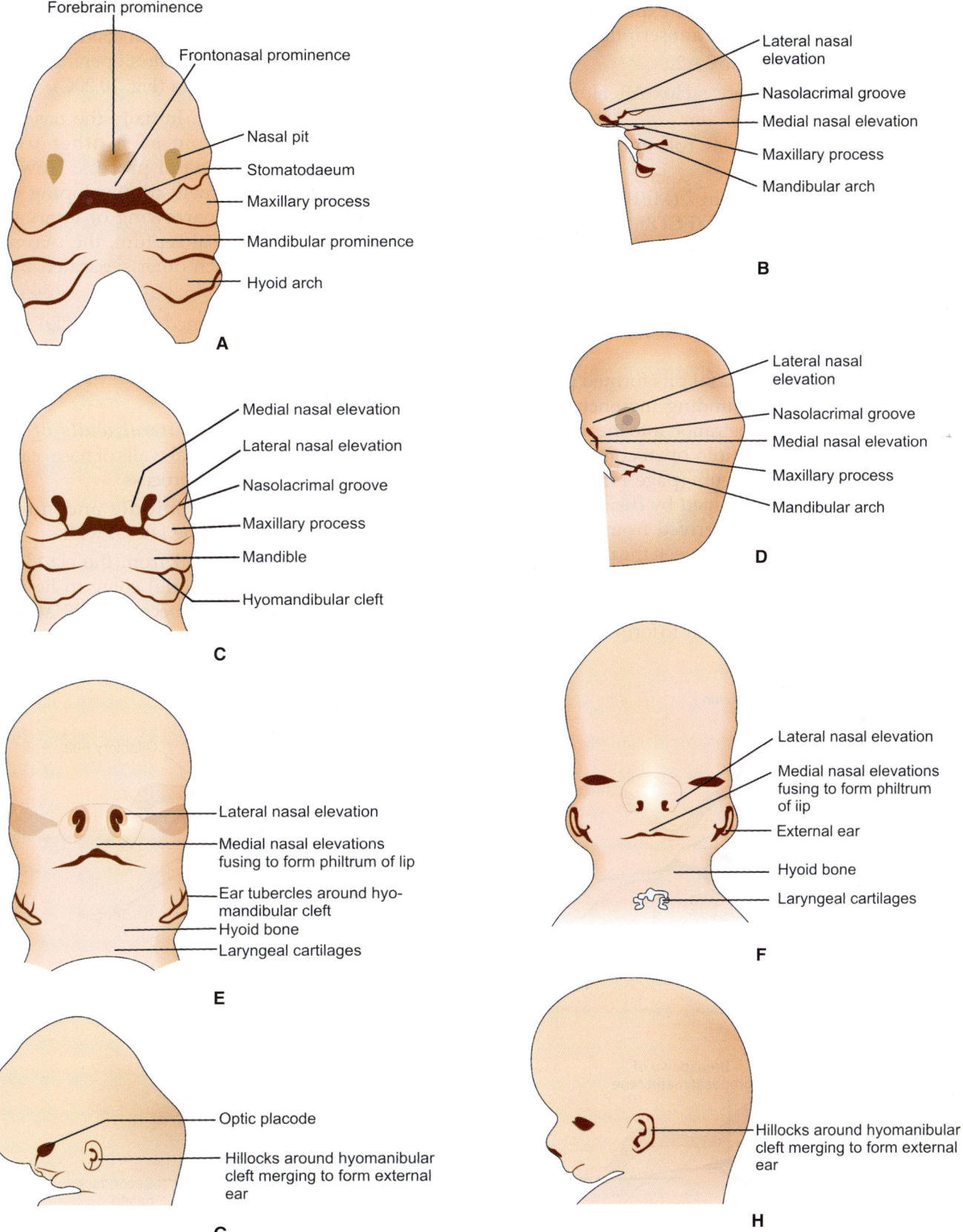

Fig. 10.19: Formation of the face: A and B, frontal aspect and lateral view of the embryo depicting facial primordia (frontonasal process, paired maxillary and mandibular processes); C and D, formation of medial and nasal processes, intermaxillary segment; E, F, G, and H, formation of lower and upper lips, cheeks, eyes, external ear, upper and lower jaws.

- *First arch* is Hox negative. It expresses OTX2, a homeodomain containing transcription factor.
- *Second arch* expresses Hox-A2.
- *Third to sixth arches* express Hox-A3, Hox-B3, and Hox-D3.

Signaling molecules that play role in facial development are:

- Bone morphogenic protein 7 (MBP7),
- Fibroblast growth factor 8 (FGF8), and
- Sonic hedgehog (SHH) proteins.

DEVELOPMENT OF NASAL CAVITY

Main steps in the development of nasal cavities are (Fig. 10.20):

Formation of nasal pits. Nasal pits formed partly by over growth of the surrounding mesenchyme and partly because of their penetration into the underlying mesenchyme, are thrown into open communication with the roof of stomatodaeum (page 145, Fig. 10.19). Soon the *primitive palate* formed by fusion of medial and lateral nasal process (derived from frontonasal process) creates a partition between the nasal pits and stomatodaeum (Fig. 10.20).

Formation of nasal sacs. Soon, the nasal pits deepen and enlarge dorsally and caudally to form the nasal sacs.

The dorsal part of each nasal sac is initially separated from the *bucconasal membrane,* which soon disappears, forming the primitive *posterior nares* opening into the posterior part of stomatodaeum (Fig. 10.20C).

Formation of nasal septum. Initially the nasal sacs are widely separated from each other by the intervening part of frontonasal process. However, with progressive enlargement of developing nasal cavities and progressive narrowing of intervening tissue which form the nasal septum, the two nasal cavities come closer to each other separated by the *nasal septum* (Fig. 10.21).

Secondary palate, once formed (Fig. 10.20D) finally separates the nasal cavities from the mouth cavity (formed from stomatodaeum after disappearance of buccopharyngeal membrane).

Formation of structures of lateral walls of nasal cavity. The structures on lateral walls of nasal cavities are derived from the lateral process.

- *Nasal conchae,* superior, middle and inferior, develop as elevations of the lateral wall.
- *Olfactory epithelium* derived from the ectodermal thickening (olfactory placode) come to lie in the roof of nasal cavities and become specialized to form the olfactory epithelium.

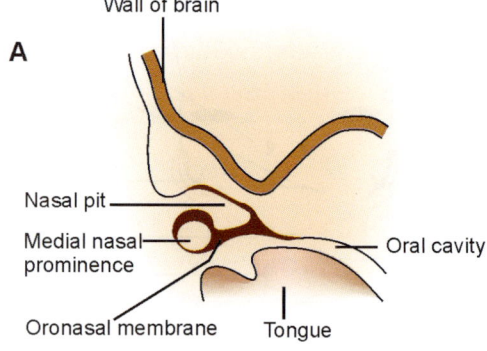

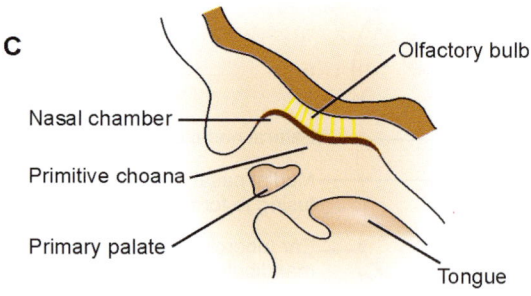

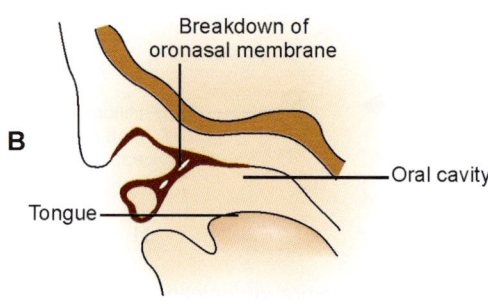

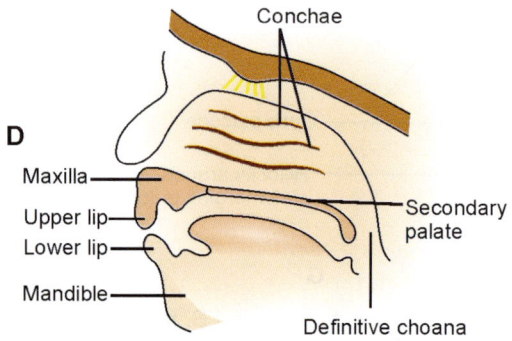

Fig. 10.20: Formation of nasal cavities.

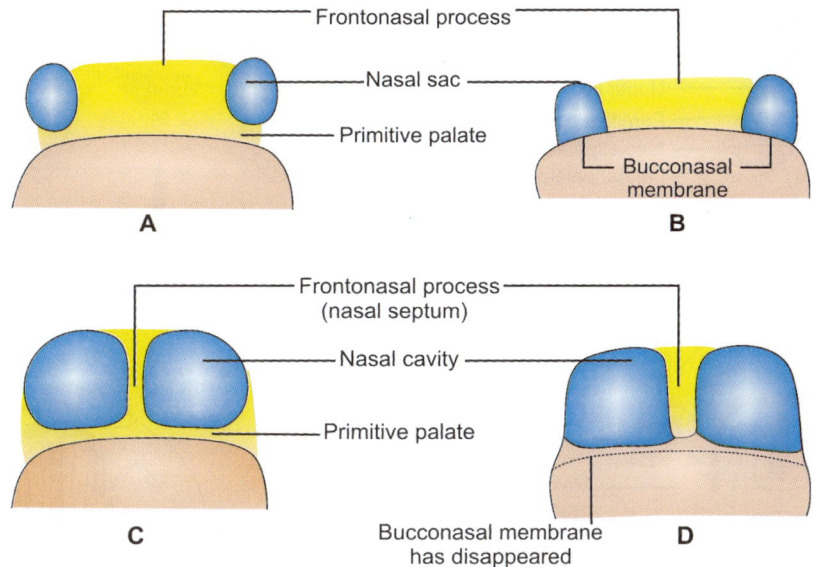

Fig. 10.21: Formation of nasal septum.

DEVELOPMENT OF PARANASAL SINUSES

Maxillary and sphenoidal sinuses begin to develop during late fetal life, other sinuses develop after birth.

Main steps in development of paranasal sinuses are:

- *Diverticulae,* from which paranasal sinuses develop arise from the walls of nasal cavity.
- *Invasions of the bones* (after which they are named), occurs gradually by these diverticulae; these then take the shape of pneumatic (air-filled) extension of nasal cavities in the bones involved.
- *Original opening* of the diverticulae persist as orifices of the adult sinuses.
- *Enlargement of paranasal sinuses* is associated with over all enlargement of the facial skeleton including the jaws.

DEVELOPMENT OF PALATE

Primordia from which the definitive palate develops are:

- Primitive palate, and
- Secondary palate

Primitive palate

Primitive palate, a triangular wedge shaped structure, is formed by *intermaxillary segment* (derived from frontonasal processes (Fig. 10.22A). It forms the premaxillary part of maxilla. In the adult hard palate is represented by a small part which lies anterior to the incisive fossa and is associated with central four incisors.

Secondary palate

Secondary palate begins to develop in the 6th week from the maxillary processes.

Main steps in the development of secondary palate are:

- *Formation of lateral palatine processes.* During 6th week, the lateral palatine processes start developing as shelf-like projection from the inner surface of each maxillary process (Fig. 10.22)
- *Initial growth of lateral palatine processes* is directed obliquely downward along the side of developing tongue (Fig. 10.22C). This prevents the two processes to meet and fuse with each other.
- *In later growth the palatine processes* are directed horizontally (superior to the tongue) and lead to formation of secondary palate by fusion with each other (Fig. 10.22D).

At the same time, the nasal septum also grows down and fuses with the medial edges of the palatine processes in the ventral 3/4th area. This fusion of palatine processes with each other and the down growing nasal septum begins anteriorly and proceeds backward. It is completed by eighth week.

Definitive palate

Definitive palate is thus formed by fusion of secondary palate with the primitive palate ventrally in a Y-shaped manner. This junction is represented in adult by the *incisive fossa* (Fig. 10.22E).

Definitive palate, in further development, consists of two parts (Fig. 10.22E):

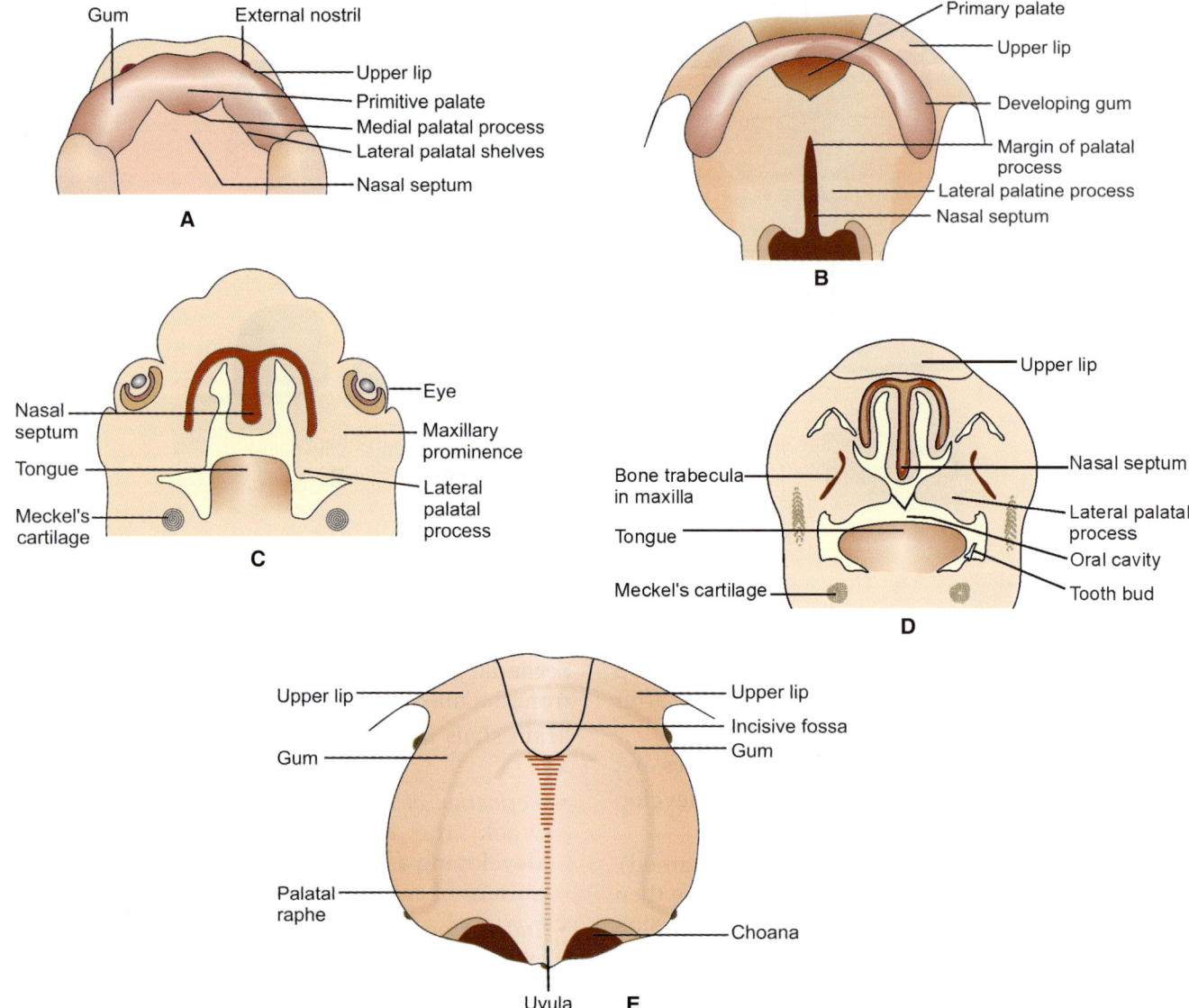

Fig. 10.22: Development of the palate: A, horizontal section through the maxillary process showing the position of intermaxillary segment (which forms primitive palate in later development); B, vertical section depicting relationship of the developing nasal cavities and nasal septum with the maxillary processes; C, formation of lateral palatine process from maxillary processes. Note: In initial growth palatine process is obliquely downward along the tongue; D, in later development the palatine process grows horizontally superior to the tongue, meet and fuse with each other and with the down crossing nasal septum; E, components of adult definitive palate.

- *Hard palate.* Ventral 3/4th part of the developing definite palate is converted into bone by membranous ossification and forms the hard palate.
- *Soft palate.* Dorsal 1/4th part of the developing definitive palate, which is not fused with nasal septum, hangs as a curtain and forms the soft palate.

CONGENITAL ANOMALIES OF FACE, PALATE AND NASAL CAVITIES

CONGENITAL ANOMALIES OF FACE

1. *Hare lip* (cleft lip) of following types may occur due to failure in proper fusion of various primordia forming the upper and the lower lips:

- *Central cleft upper lip* (Fig. 10.23A) occurs due to failure of fusion of intermaxillary segment.
- *Lateral cleft upper lip* may occur due to failure of fusion of maxillary process with the intermaxillary segment on one side (unilateral cleft lip) or both sides (bilateral cleft lip) (Fig. 10.23B and C).
- *Central cleft lower lip* (Fig. 10.23D) may occur due to failure of fusion of mandibular processes with each other.

2. *Facial cleft.* A rare anomaly, which occurs due to failure of fusion of maxillary process with the lateral nasal process. In it the nasolacrimal duct is

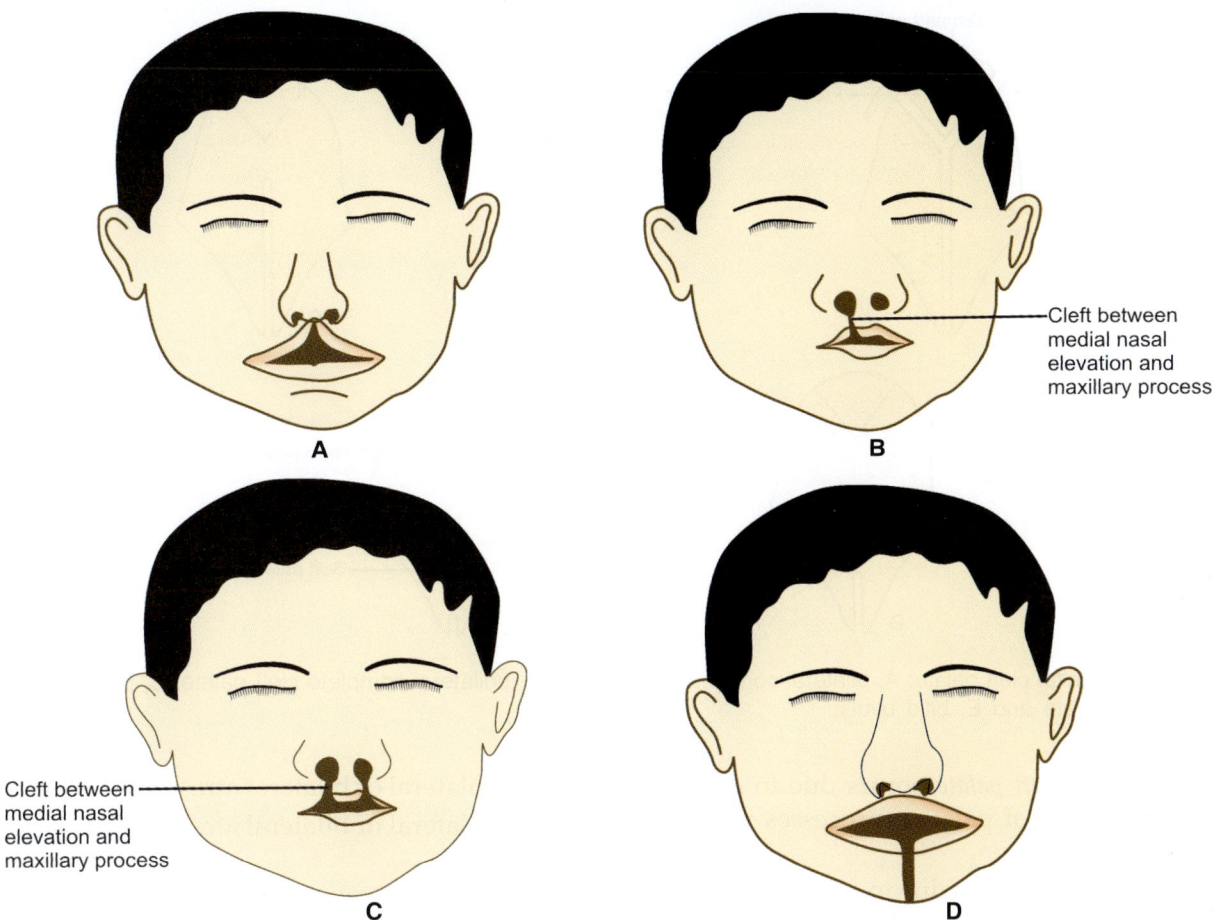

Fig. 10.23: Congenital hare (cleft) lip: A, central cleft upper lip; B, unilateral cleft upper lip; C, bilateral cleft upper lip; and D, central cleft lower lip.

exposed to the exterior. Also there is associated lateral cleft lip on the same side (Fig. 10.24).

3. *Macrostomia,* i.e. large sized oral fissure may occur due to unilateral or bilateral failure of fusion of maxillary process with mandibular arches.

4. *Microstomia,* i.e. small sized oral fissure occurs due to excessive fusion between the maxillary processes and the mandibular arches.

5. *Mandibulofacial dysostosis* or first arch syndrome occur due to underdevelopment of first pharyngeal arch and is characterised by maldevelopment of lower eyelid, maxilla, mandible, cheeks and external ear.

6. *Retroganthic* or receding chin is the result of congenitally small mandible in relation to the face.

7. *Hypertelorism,* i.e. abnormally wide separation of the two eyes.

CONGENITAL ANOMALIES OF PALATE

Cleft palate. Following varieties of cleft palate may occur due to failure of proper fusion of various primordia forming palate:

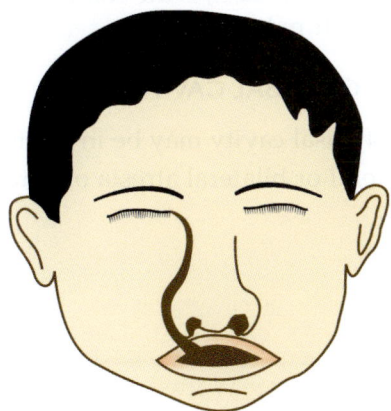

Fig. 10.24: Facial cleft with lateral cleft of the upper lip of same side.

• *Bilateral complete cleft palate* occurs due to complete non fusion giving rise to a Y-shaped cleft, accompanied by bilateral cleft lip (Fig. 10.25A).

• *Unilateral complete cleft palate* occurs due to complete arrest of fusion of palatine process of one side with the primitive palate and nasal septum (Fig. 10.25B). It is usually associated with unilateral hare lip.

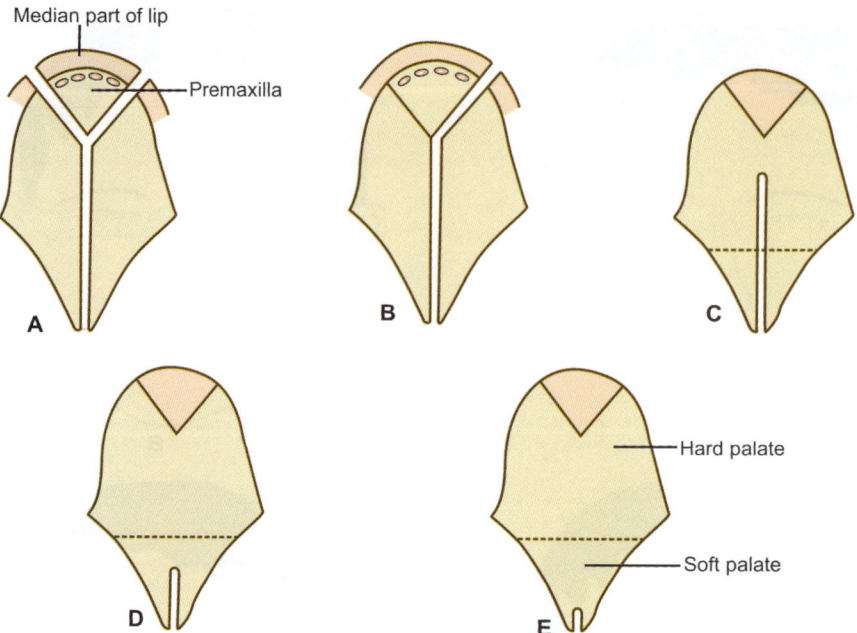

Fig. 10.25: Congenital cleft palate: A, bilateral complete cleft palate; B, unilateral complete cleft palate; C, partial midline cleft; D, cleft of soft palate and E, bifid uvula.

- *Partial midline cleft palate* occurs due to complete failure of fusion of palatine processes with each other (Fig. 10.25C).
- *Cleft of soft palate* occurs due to failure of fusion of palatine processes with each other in the dorsal 1/4th area (Fig. 10.25D).
- *Bifid uvula* (Fig. 10.25E) is the commonest example of partial cleft palate.

ANOMALIES OF NASAL CAVITY

1. *Atresia* of nasal cavity may be in the form of:
   - Unilateral or bilateral atresia of external nares.
   - Unilateral or bilateral atresia of posterior nares.
   - Unilateral or bilateral atresia of the nasal cavity proper.
   - Total absence of nasal passages.
2. *Abnormal communication of nasal cavity and cranial cavity* may occur due to congenital defects in the cribriform plate of ethmoid bone.
3. *Anomalies of nasal septum* include:
   - Deflected nasal septum (DNS), and
   - Absence of nasal septum.
4. *Abnormal communication of nasal cavity with mouth cavity* occurs due to cleft palate.

11

Development of Alimentary System

GENERAL CONSIDERATIONS

Primordia and histogenesis of alimentary system

Primordia of alimentary system: The alimentary system develops from:

- Pharyngeal arches, and
- Primitive gut.

Histogenesis of alimentary system organs occurs as below:

- *Epithelial lining* of most of the alimentary system and parenchyma of the related glands is derived from the endoderm of primitive gut, except in the region of mouth and anal canal, where some of the epithelium is derived from the ectoderm of the stomatodaeum and proctodaeum, respectively.

- *Muscular*, connective, peritoneal and other layers of walls of the gut are derived from the splanchnic mesenchyme surrounding the primitive gut.

Formation of primitive gut

The primitive gut is formed during 4th week from that part of the endoderm lined yolk sac cavity which is incorporated into the embryo as a result of cephalo-caudal and lateral folding of the embryo.

Note. It will be prudent to revise the formation of primitive gut (described on page 51), before proceeding further.

151

Divisions of primitive gut

The primitive gut extends in the median plane from the buccopharyngeal membrane at its cephalic end to the cloacal membrane at its caudal end. For descriptive purposes the primitive gut is divided into three parts (Fig. 11.1):

1. **Foregut.** It extends from the buccopharyngeal membrane to its junction with the midgut, known as anterior intestinal portal. In adults this junction roughly corresponds with the termination of bile duct in the second part of duodenum. The foregut can be subdivided into two parts:

   - *Pre-laryngeal or cephalic part of foregut* also known as *pharyngeal gut*, extends from the buccopharyngeal membrane to the tracheobronchial diverticulum (Fig. 11.1B).
   - *Post-laryngeal or caudal part of foregut* extends from the tracheobronchial diverticulum to its junction with the midgut.

2. **Midgut** extends from the anterior intestinal portal to the posterior intestinal portal (which corres-

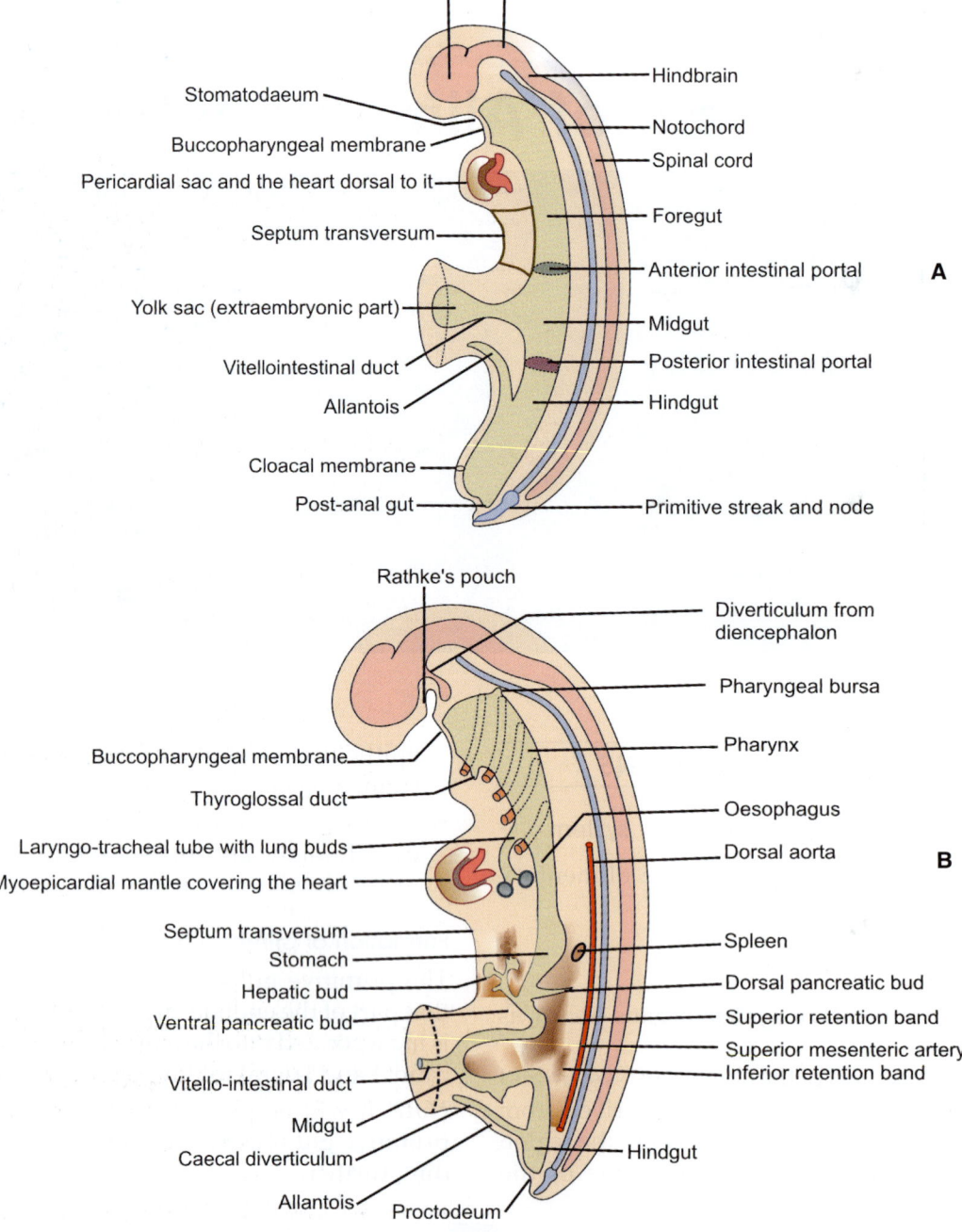

Fig. 11.1: Median section of the human embryo to depict primitive gut: A, early stage; and B, advanced stage.

ponds in adults with the junction of right two-thirds and left one-third of transverse colon). The midgut can be subdivided into two parts with the development of caecal diverticulum:

- Pre-caecal segment, and
- Post-caecal segment.

3. *Hindgut* extends from the posterior intestinal portal to the cloacal membrane. The attachment of the allantoic diverticulum subdivides the hind gut into two parts:

- Pre-allantoic hindgut, and
- Post-allantoic hindgut.

Derivatives of primitive gut

Derivatives of pre-laryngeal foregut. Pre-laryngeal foregut also known as pharyngeal gut gives rise to:

- Part of floor of definitive mouth,
- Pharynx, and
- With the development of pharyngeal arches and pharyngeal pouches the pre-laryngeal foregut becomes the place for development of tongue, palatine tonsils, submandibular and sublingual glands, auditory tubes and the middle ear, and lower respiratory passages (which develop from tracheobronchial diverticulum).

Note. Development of all derivatives has been described in Chapter 10, except that of lower respiratory passages which has been described in Chapter 12.

Derivatives of post-laryngeal or caudal part of the foregut are:

- Oesophagus,
- Stomach,
- Proximal part of duodenum upto the termination of hepatopancreatic ampulla,
- Liver and extra-hepatic biliary system, and
- Pancreas.

Derivatives of midgut

Pre-caecal segment gives rise to:

- Distal part of the duodenum below the hepato-pancreatic ampulla,
- Jejunum, and
- Ileus.

Post-caecal segment gives rise to:

- Caecum,
- Appendix,
- Ascending colon, and
- Proximal two-thirds of transverse colon.

Derivatives of hindgut

Pre-allantoic part gives rise to:

- Distal one-third of transverse colon,
- Descending colon, and
- Sigmoid colon.

Post-allantoic part is dilated to form the endodermal cloaca which is divided into two parts by urorectal septum:

- Dorsal part — primitive rectum, which forms
  - Rectum, and
  - Upper part of anal canal
- Ventral part — primitive urogenital sinus, which forms parts of urogenital system
- Mesenteries

Molecular regulation of gut tube development

Molecular studies suggest that *Hox* and *Para Hox* genes, as well as *hedgehog signals* (SHH) regulate the regional differentiation of the primordial gut to form the different parts. As a matter of fact the SHH is secreted by the gut endoderm and induces a nested expression of Hox genes in surrounding mesoderm. Hox expression then initiates a cascade of genes that instruct gut endoderm to differentiate into its regional identities. Signaling between the two tissues is an example of the epithelial mesenchymal interaction.

DEVELOPMENT OF DERIVATIVES OF POST-LARYNGEAL OR CAUDAL PART OF FOREGUT

OESOPHAGUS

Primitive oesophagus. As mentioned earlier, in a 4 week embryo, a *tracheobronchial diverticulum* (Fig. 11.1B) appears in the ventral aspect of the foregut at the caudal end of pharyngeal foregut. Soon the *oesophagotracheal septum* develops and divides this region of foregut into two parts (Fig. 11.2):

- *Respiratory primordium* is formed by the ventral part, and
- *Primitive oesophagus* is formed by the dorsal part, which extends down upto the dilatation marking the beginning of the stomach.

Elongation of oesophagus. Primitive oesophagus at first is very short, but with the descent of heart and lungs, it elongates rapidly.

Histogenesis of the oesophagus occurs as follows:

- *Epithelial lining* of oesophagus is derived from the endoderm forming the gut tube. Initially this lining

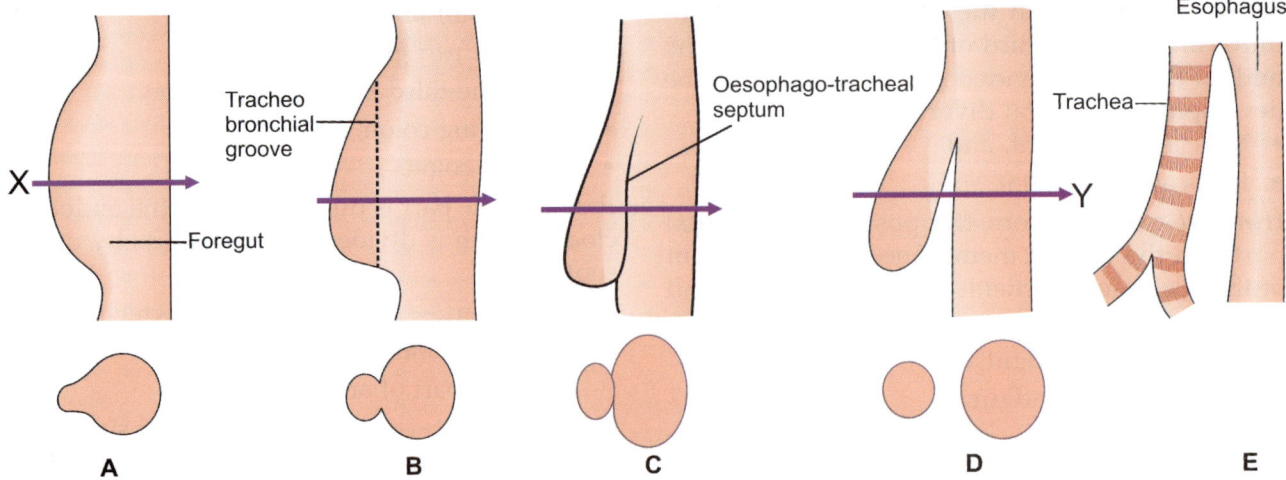

Fig. 11.2: Successive stages of development of respiratory primordium and primitive oesophagus through partitioning of part of foregut by oesophago-tracheal septum.

is simple columnar, then it becomes ciliated and finally is transformed into stratified squamous epithelium by the process of metaplasia.

- *Muscular and connective tissue coats* of oesophagus are derived from the surrounding splanchnic mesoderm. Muscular coat of oesophagus is formed by striated muscles in the upper two-thirds (innervated by vagus nerve) and by smooth muscles in the lower one-third (innervated by the splanchnic plexus).

Anomalies of oesophagus

1. *Tracheoesophageal fistula* (anomalous communication of oesophagus with trachea) of various types may develop due to anomalous partitioning of the oesophagus from the trachea (Fig. 11.3).
2. *Oesophageal atresia,* i.e. narrowing of oesophagus may occur alone or in association with the tracheoesophageal fistula. Due to atresia of the oesophagus the fetus is unable to swallow amniotic fluid leading to hydramnios.

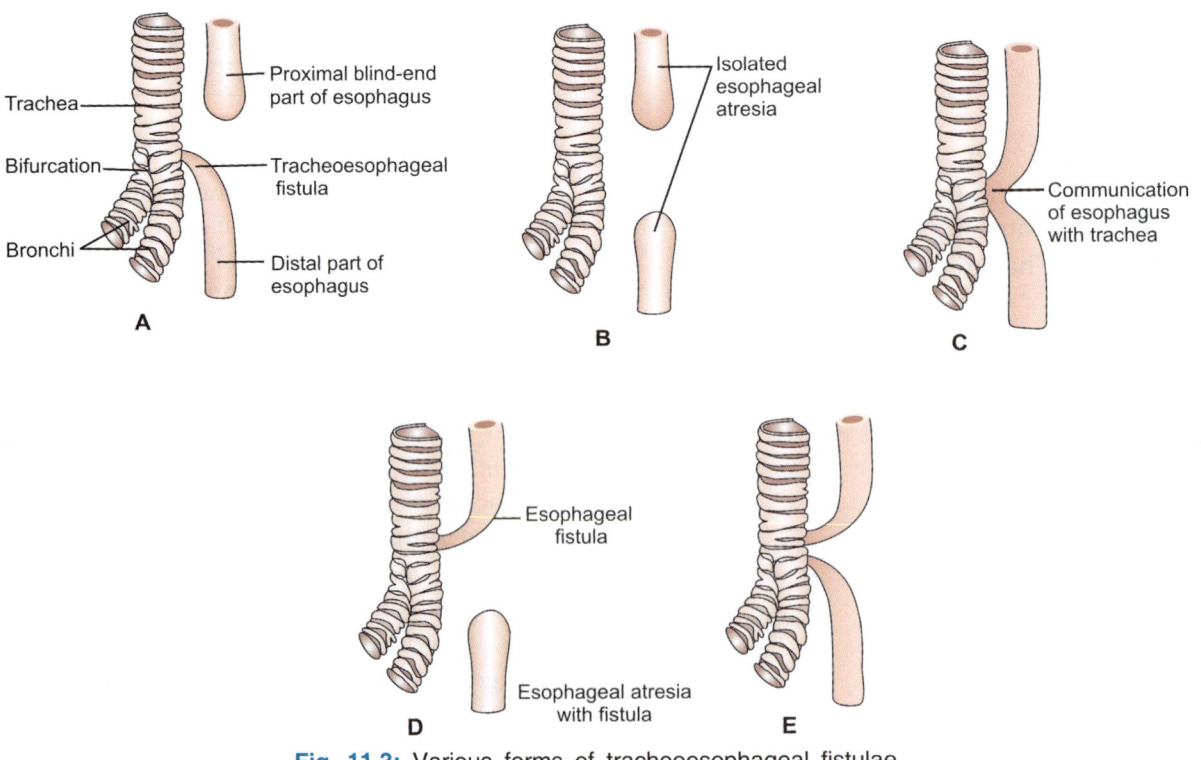

Fig. 11.3: Various forms of tracheoesophageal fistulae.

3. *Oesophageal stenosis* may occur at the lower end of oesophagus due to incomplete canalization or vascular abnormalities.

STOMACH

Though the stomach and its mesenteries are developing simultaneously, but for the purpose of understanding their development is described separately.

Milestones in the development of stomach

Various milestones in the development of stomach can be summarized as below (Fig. 11.4):

Stage of fusiform dilatation. During 4th to 5th week, the stomach develops as a fusiform dilatation from the caudal part of foregut and is placed in the median plane (Fig. 11.4A and B).

Stage of differential growth. Later on the stomach undergoes differential growth, its dorsal border grows more rapidly than the ventral border showing the formation of the rudimentary fundus and greater curvature. Eventually the ventral border becomes concave which form the future lesser curvature (Fig. 11.4C).

Rotation of the stomach. As the stomach enlarges and acquires its adult shape, it undergoes rotation along its longitudinal axis as well as antero-posterior axis.

Rotation along longitudinal axis by 90° clockwise converts the original:

- Left surface into ventral surface, and
- Right surface into dorsal surface (Fig. 11.4D). This explains why left vagus nerve supplies the anterior wall and the right vagus nerve innervates the posterior wall of the stomach.

Rotation along antero-posterior axis causes the original:

- *Caudal or pyloric part* of the stomach to move to the right and upward, and
- *Cephalic or cardiac portion* to the left and slightly downward (Fig. 11.4E).

Mesenteries of stomach

Mesogastrium. Initially the developing stomach is placed in the median plane and attached to the dorsal body wall by *dorsal mesogastrium* and ventral body wall by *ventral mesogastrium* (Fig. 11.4A and B).

Formation of lesser omentum, falciform ligament and coronary ligament of the liver. The hepatic buds enter the ventral mesogastrium and divide into two partitions (Fig. 11.4F):

- *Lesser omentum* refers to the part between the stomach and liver, and
- *Falciform ligament and coronary ligament* of the liver are formed by the part of ventral mesogastrium which persists between the liver and ventral body wall (Fig. 11.4D).

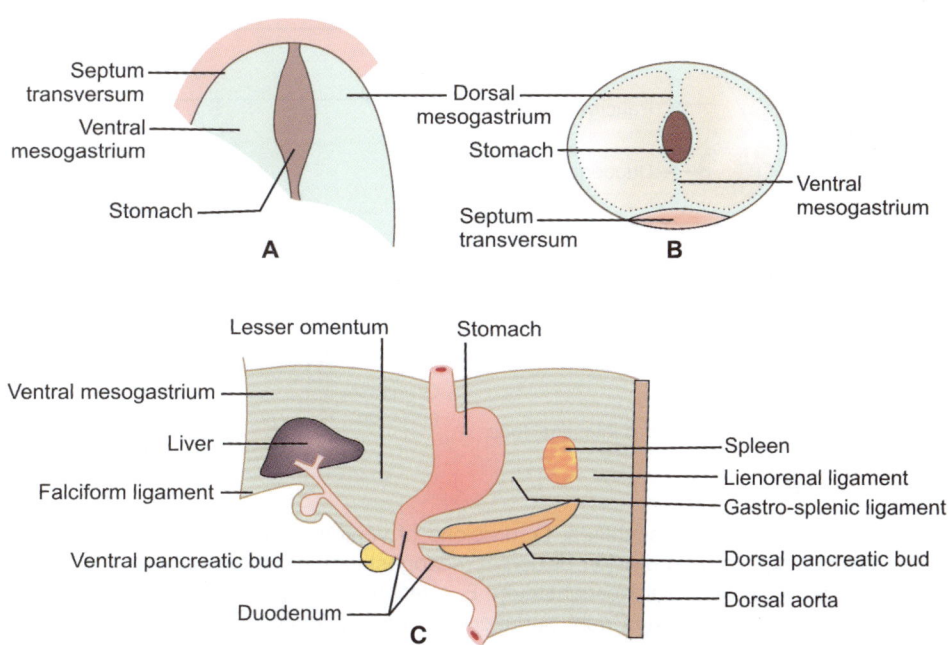

Fig. 11.4: Formation of stomach and its mesenteries: A and B, side view and transverse section to depict fusiform stomach placed in the midline and attached to the ventral body wall by ventral mesogastrium and dorsal body wall by dorsal mesogastrium; C, side view depicting formation of lesser and greater curvatures.

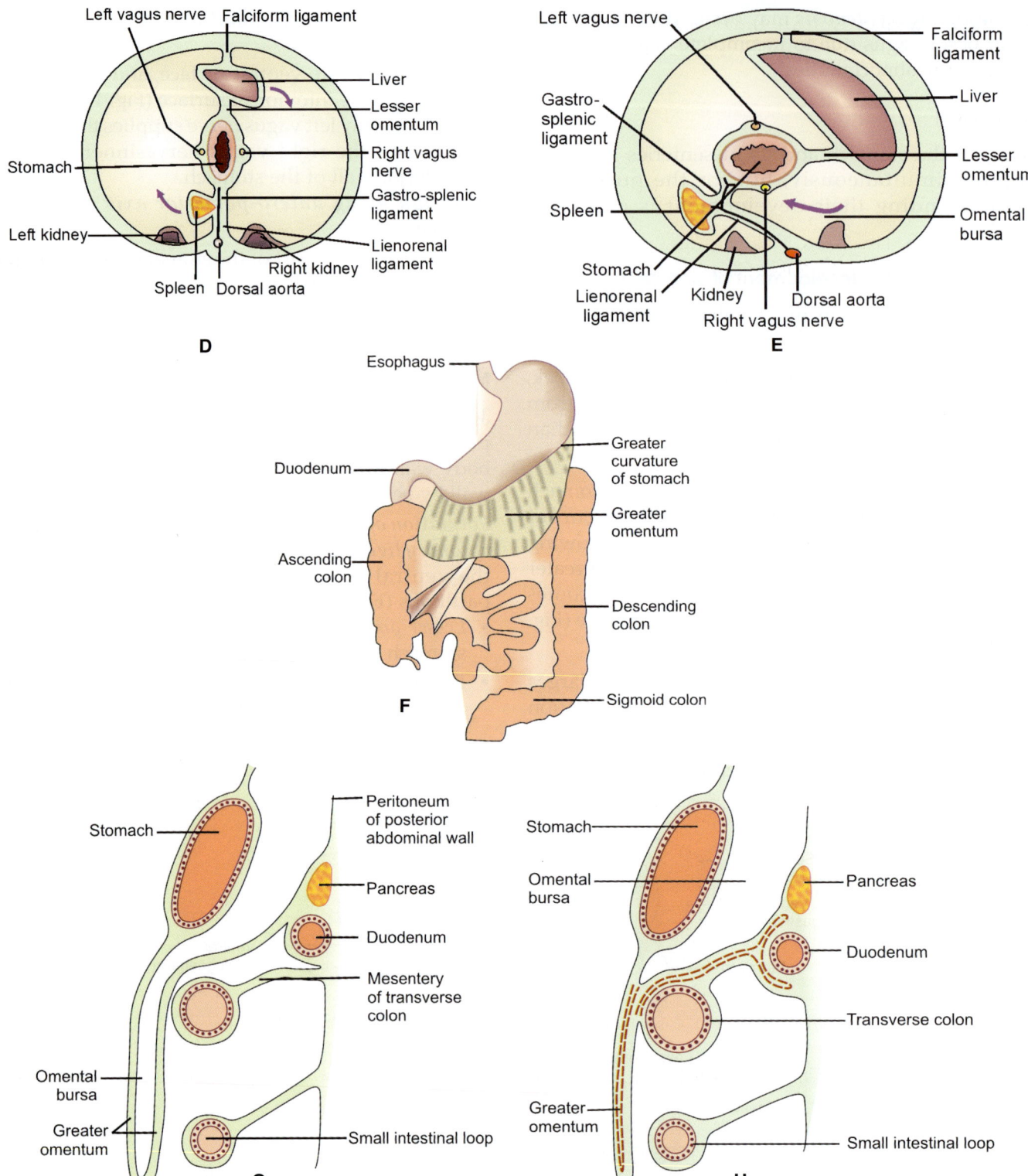

Fig. 11.4: Formation of stomach and its mesenteries: D, divisions of ventral mesogastrium into lesser omentum, and falciform ligament of liver by the developing liver and division of dorsal mesogastrium into gastrosplenic and lieno-renal ligaments by the developing spleen under the left layer of dorsal mesogastrium; E, rotation of stomach around longitudinal axis converts the original left surface of stomach into ventral surface and right surface into dorsal surface, and leads to formation of omental bursa; F, rotation of the stomach around anteroposterior axis, the greater curvature of stomach is diverted downwards and the dorsal mesogastrium hangs down; G, downward growth of hanging dorsal mesogastrium leads to formation of four layers of greater omentum; H, four layers of greater omentum fuse to form a single hanging sheet over the transverse colon and loops of intestines; and posterior layer of greater omentum fuses with the human mesentery of transverse colon.

Formation of gastrosplenic and lienorenal ligaments. The spleen develops from the mesenchyme under cover of left layer of dorsal mesogastrium and divides the dorsal mesogastrium into two portions (Fig. 11.4D):

- *Gastro-splenic ligament* is formed by the part between the developing stomach and spleen, and

- *Lienorenal ligament* is formed by the part between the spleen and region of the dorsal body wall where kidney is developing as a retroperitoneal structure.

Formation of omental bursa. The omental bursa a space behind the stomach, is formed when dorsal mesogastrium is pulled to the left as a result of rotation of stomach around longitudinal axis (Fig. 11.4D).

Formation of greater omentum. With the rotation of stomach around antero-posterior axis, the dorsal mesogastrium attached to the original dorsal border of the stomach hangs in a downward direction and grows further downward to form a double-layered sac which is continuous with the omental bursa above and extends below over the transverse colon and small intestine loop like an apron (Fig. 11.4G). This four layered apron is called *greater omentum.* Subsequently its four layers too form a single sheet which hangs down from the greater curvature of the stomach. The posterior most layer of greater omentum fuses with the mesentery, of transverse colon (Fig. 11.4H).

Anomalies of stomach

1. *Pyloric stenosis* occurs due to hypertrophy of the circular muscles of the pyloric sphincter. It is more common in males than females, and is characterised by progressive vomiting between 2nd week to 2nd month of life.

2. *Duplication of stomach* is a rare anomaly of stomach.

3. *Presence of prepyloric septum* is another rare congenital anomaly of stomach.

DUODENUM

Primordia from which duodenum is derived are (Fig. 11.5):

- *Terminal part of foregut* gives rise to the superior (or first) part and upper half of the descending (or second) part of duodenum.

- *Most proximal part of midgut* gives rise to rest of the duodenum. The dual development of duodenum explains its blood supply being derived from the

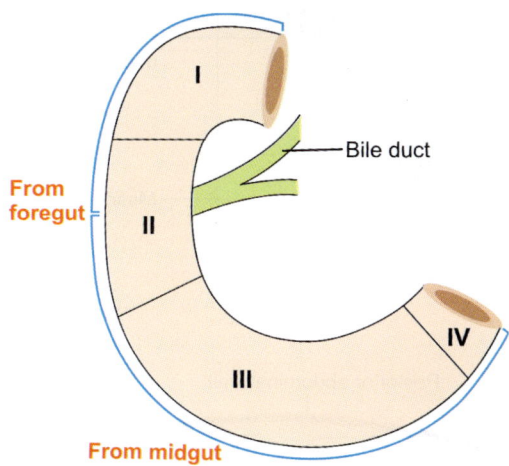

Fig. 11.5: Parts of the adult duodenum derived from foregut (I and upper half of II part) and midgut (lower half of II, III and IV parts).

branches of coeliac artery (artery of the foregut) and branch of superior mesenteric artery (artery of midgut).

Note. From the endodermal lining of junction of the embryonic foregut and midgut arises *hepato-pancreatic bud.* In the adult duodenum it corresponds with the termination of the hepatopancreatic ampulla at the major duodenal papilla.

Major events in the development of duodenum can be summarized as:

- *Primitive duodenum* is in the form of a loop with a ventral convexity placed in the median plane. It is attached to the posterior abdominal wall by a mesentery (mesoduodenum) (Figs 11.6A and B).

- *Dextrorotation:* Later in development the loop of primitive duodenum is pushed to the right and against the dorsal body wall by the gut returning into the abdominal wall (form physiological umbilical hernia) (Fig. 11.6C). As a result of this:

- Ventral convex margin forms the lateral border, and

- Original right surface becomes posterior and the left surface becomes anterior (Fig. 11.6C).

- *Retroperitonisation and posterior fixation.* As a result of dextro rotation the peritoneum covering the posterior surface of rotated duodenum comes in contact with the parietal peritoneum of the dorsal abdominal wall (Fig. 11.6C). Later in development, these posterior layers of peritoneum disappear by zygosis and the duodenum a retroperitoneal structure fixed to the posterior abdominal wall (Fig. 11.6D), except near the pylorus of the stomach, where a small portion of the duodenum (*duodenal cap*) remains intraperitoneal.

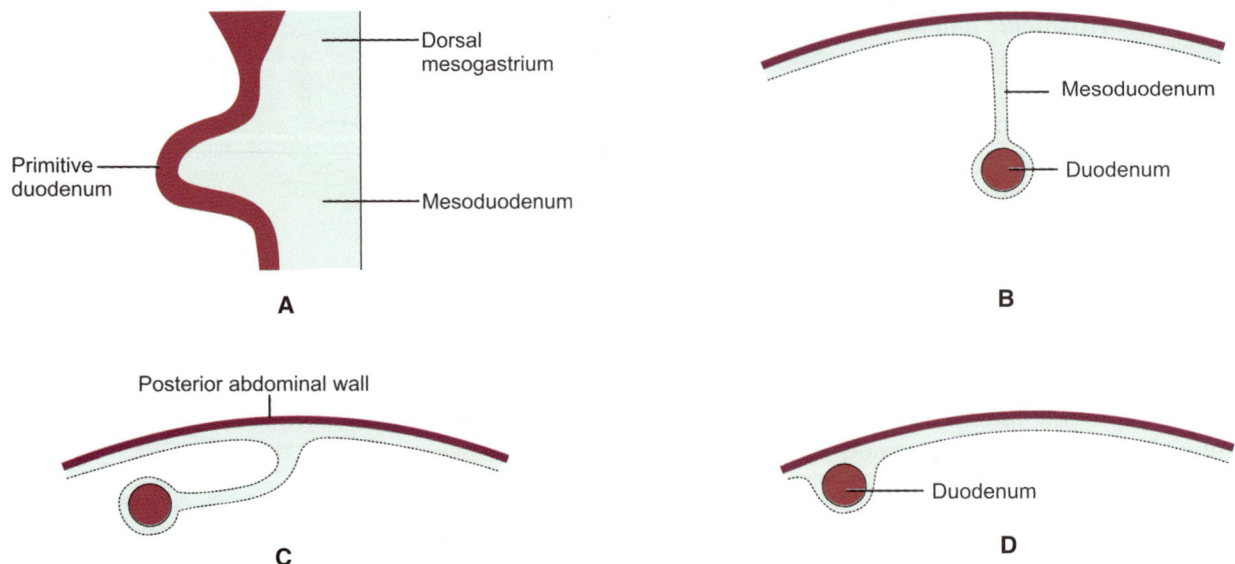

Fig. 11.6: Phases of development of duodenum: A and B, primitive duodenum with mesoduodenum as seen in side view and transverse section, respectively; C, dextrorotation of duodenal loop against the dorsal abdominal wall; D, retro-peritonisation of duodenum.

- *Axial rotation:* Due to differential growth of the wall of duodenum there occurs axial rotation; as a result of it (Fig. 11.7):
  - Ventral pancreatic duct comes toward the dorsal bud, and
  - Bile duct which is initially attached to the ventral aspect of duodenum is carried around the dorsal aspect.
- *Lumen changes:* During the 5th and 6th weeks, the lumen of duodenum becomes progressively narrow and is temporarily obliterated by the proliferation of the lining endodermal cells. Normally by the end of the third month the lumen is recanalized by degeneration of the epithelial cells.

Anomalies of the duodenum

1. ***Duodenal atresia,*** i.e. complete occlusion of the lumen of duodenum, may affect any part of duodenum, but is more frequently below the hepato-pancreatic ampulla (Fig. 11.7A). It may occur as an isolated anomaly or in association with Down syndrome, annular pancreas (Fig. 11.11A) and cardiovascular anomalies. Infants with duodenal atresia develop vomiting a few hour after birth.
2. ***Duodenal stenosis,*** i.e. partial occlusion of the duodenal lumen, usually results from incomplete recanalization of the duodenum resulting from defective vacuolization. It manifests as vomiting often containing bile.

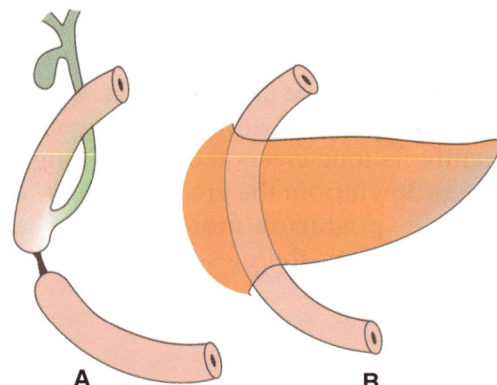

Fig. 11.7: Duodenal atresia below the hepato-pancreatic ampulla (A), and duodenal stenosis (B).

LIVER, GALLBLADDER AND BILIARY APPARATUS

Major events in the development of liver, gallbladder and biliary apparatus can be summarized as below:

Endodermal diverticulum

Liver, gallbladder and biliary apparatus develop from an *endodermal diverticulum* that arises from the ventral aspect of terminal part of the foregut during the 4th week. This diverticulum grows into the ventral mesogastrium and reaches the septum transversum and divides into two parts:

- *Pars hepatica,* the larger cranial part which will form the liver and
- *Pars cystica,* the smaller caudal part which will form the gallbladder.

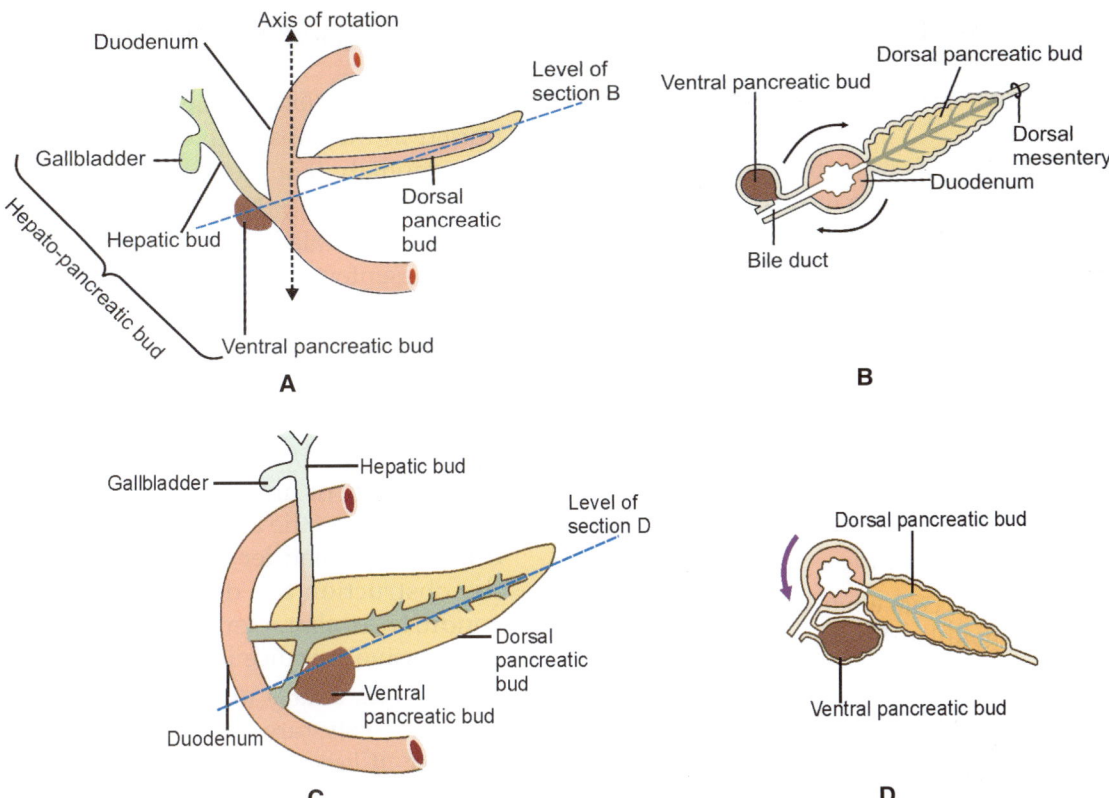

Fig. 11.8: Relationship of bile duct, ventral pancreatic bud and dorsal pancreatic bud seen in front view and transverse section, respectively: A and B, before axial rotation; and C and D, after axial rotation.

Development of liver

Liver parenchyma is developed from the endoderm of pars hepatica. The pars hepatica grows into the septum transversum and divides into right and left branches which form the right and left lobes of the liver.

- *Liver cells and biliary capillaries.* Each branch of pars hepatica gives rise to clusters of cells, the *hepatic cylinders,* which eventually form two solid masses. The cells of these masses differentiate into plates of liver cells which form the liver parenchyma and the lining of biliary capillaries.
- *Hepatic capillaries and liver sinusoids.* During development of plates of liver cells, the umbilical and vitelline veins which lie in the septum transversum break up into the capillary network and joins secondarily with hepatic sinusoids which develop *in situ* between the plates of liver cells from the mesenchyme of septum transversum.
- *Haematopoietic cells and Kuffer cells* are derived from the mesoderm of septum transversum.
- *Capsule and fibro-areolar stroma of liver* is also formed by the mesenchyme of the septum trans versum.

Peritoneum covering of liver. Mesoderm on the surface of liver differentiates into visceral peritoneum except on its cranial surface where the liver remain in contact with the developing diaphragm. This area is called *bare area of the liver.*

Molecular regulation of liver formation

- *Fibroblast growth factor 2 (FGF2)* secreted by the cardiac mesoderm interact with the prospective liver forming endoderm and induce formation of the hepatic diverticulum.
- *BMPs* secreted by septum transversum appear to enhance the competence of prospective liver endoderm to respond to FGF2.
- *Hepatocyte nuclear transcription factors (HNF3 and 4)* partially regulate the differentiation of prospective liver endoderm into hepatocytes and biliary cell lineages.

Development of gallbladder and biliary apparatus

Gallbladder and its duct, the *cystic duct* develop from the pars cystica.

Bile duct. The original stalk of the endodermal diverticulum connected to the foregut (duodenum) forms the bile duct. Parts of the right and left branches of pars hepatica form the right and left *hepatic ducts* which are continuous with the intrahepatic part of the biliary passages on the side and join to form the common hepatic duct on other side. The common hepatic duct and the cystic duct seem to join to form the bile duct.

Initially the bile duct opens on the ventral aspect of the developing duodenum. As a result of axial rotation of duodenum (due to differential growth of the walls of the duodenum), the bile duct comes to open on the dorsomedial aspect of the duodenum along with the ventral pancreatic bud (Fig. 11.8A and C).

Congenital anomalies of liver, gallbladder and biliary apparatus

Liver anomalies may occur in the form of variations in lobulation, but are not significant clinically.

Gallbladder anomalies include:

1. *Antretic gallbladder* occurs when the cystic duct fails to canalize. The gallbladder may be rudimentary or even absent (agenesis).

2. *Septate gallbladder* is formed when a transverse or longitudinal fold of mucous membrane subdivides the interior of the gallbladder (Fig. 11.9A).

3. *Duplication of gallbladder,* i.e. two gallbladders are connected by a cystic duct (Fig. 11.9B). This condi-

tion is not uncommon and is usually asymptomatic.

4. *Intra-hepatic gallbladder,* i.e. gallbladder completely buried in the substance of liver is comparatively rare anomaly (Fig. 11.9C).

5. *Mobile or floating gallbladder* refers to a condition in which the gallbladder is suspended from the liver by a mesentery.

6. *Absence of cystic duct* may occur rarely. In this condition the gallbladder neck directly opens into the bile duct.

Bile duct anomalies include:

1. *Extrahepatic biliary atresia (EHBA),* i.e. non-canalization of any part of extrahepatic biliary passage. When the atresia affects the common bile duct, the gallbladder and the bile passages above the obstruction are distended (Fig. 11.9D). The condition is characterized by the persistent and progressive jaundice in a new born.

2. *Intrahepatic biliary duct atresia and hypoplasia* is comparatively rare anomaly.

3. *Absence of hepatopancreatic ampulla of vater* may occur sometimes. In this condition the bile duct and main pancreatic duct open separately into the duodenum.

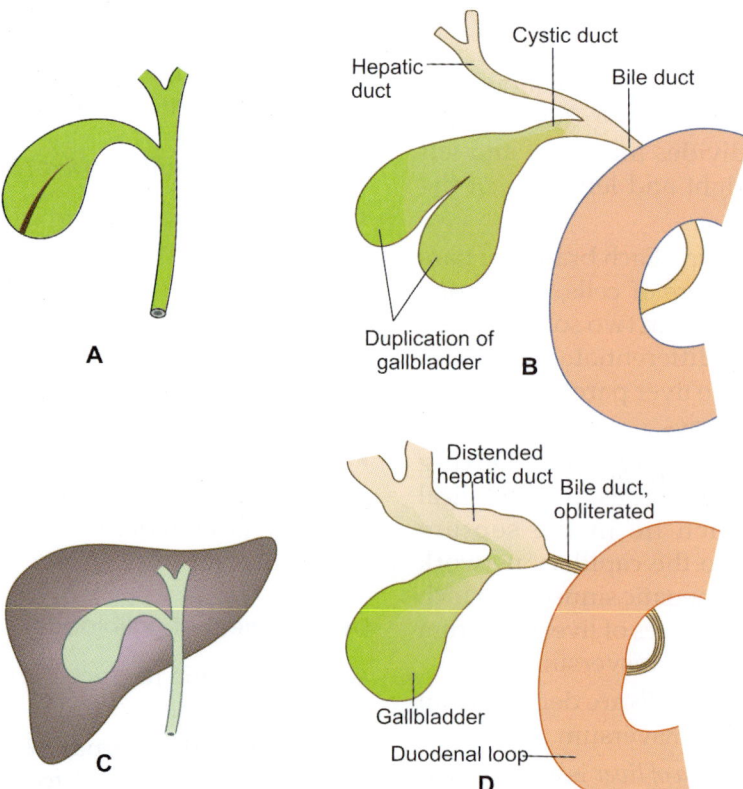

Fig. 11.9: Anomalies of gallbladder and biliary apparatus: A, septate gallbladder; B, duplication of gallbladder; C, intrahepatic gallbladder; D, bile duct atresia resulting in distention of the gallbladder and hepatic ducts distal to the obliteration.

PANCREAS

Major events in the development of pancreas

Major events in the development of pancreas can be summarized as below:

Pancreatic buds and their derivatives. The pancreas is developed from the two pancreatic buds that arise from the duodenal segment of foregut:

- *Dorsal pancreatic bud* is larger and most of the pancreas is derived from it. It is located in the dorsal mesentery (Fig. 11.10A and B).
- *Ventral pancreatic bud* arises as a diverticulum near the entry of the bile duct into the duodenum. It is smaller bilobed structure that forms the lower part of the head of the pancreas including the uncinate process.

Changes in the position of the pancreatic buds

- *Initially,* as the name indicates, the dorsal duct is located dorsally and ventral duct is located ventrally (Fig. 11.10A and B).
- *With the dextrorotation of the duodenal loop,* the ventral bud comes to lie on the right side and the dorsal bud on the left side of the developing duodenum (Fig. 11.10C and D).
- *With the axial rotation of the duodenum* (due to differential growth of its wall) the attachment of ventral pancreatic duct along with that of bile duct wind round the posterior surface of the duodenum and comes to lie on the postero-medial aspect, where it meets with the dorsal pancreatic duct (Fig. 11.10E and F).

Formation of the pancreatic mass. During 7th week of development the ventral and dorsal pancreatic buds fuse to form the single pancreatic mass. As mentioned above the dorsal bud forms most of the pancreas (upper part of the head, body and tail), and the ventral bud forms the lower part of the head and uncinate process.

Formation of duct system, acini, parenchyma and connective tissue of pancreas. After the fusion of ventral and dorsal pancreatic buds, their ducts develop cross communications. Final duct system of pancreas is formed as below (Fig. 11.10G and H):

- *Main pancreatic duct* (duct of Wirsung) is formed by the duct of ventral bud, distal part of the duct of dorsal bud, and a oblique communication between the two. The main pancreatic duct, together with the bile duct, enters the duodenum at the site of *major papilla.*
- *Accessory pancreatic duct* (duct of Santorini) is formed by the proximal part of the duct of dorsal

bud. It opens into the minor duodenal papilla, located about 2 cm cranial to the main duct.

- *Smaller ductules and acini* of the pancreas are formed by the repeated sprouting of the ducts of the dorsal and ventral pancreatic buds.
- *Islet cells of Langerhans* are derived from groups of cells that separate from the ductules and come to lie between the acini. Insulin secretion begins during early fetal period.
- *Glucagon and somatostatin secreting cells* also develop from the parenchymal cells.
- *Connective tissue* of the pancreatic gland develops from the splanchnic mesoderm surrounding the pancreatic buds.

Peritoneal relation of pancreas can be summarized as below:

- *Initially,* when the pancreas grows in the dorsal mesentery it is lined by peritoneum on right and left side.
- *Later,* with the dextrorotation of the duodenum and subsequent development, the pancreas along with duodenum becomes a retroperitoneal structure (see page 157), except its tail.

Molecular regulation of development of pancreas

Formation of ventral pancreatic bud is controlled by fibroblast growth factor 2 (FGF2) secreted by the cardiac mesoderm.

Formation of dorsal pancreatic bud is controlled by fibroblast growth factor 2 *(FGF2)* and *activin* secreted by the notochord.

Specification of endocrine cell lineage is controlled by paired homeobox genes PAX4 and 6. Cells expressing both genes become β (insulin secreting), δ (somatostatin secreting) and γ (pancreatic poly-peptide secreting) cells; whereas those expressing only PAX 6 become α (glucagon secreting) cells.

Anomalies of pancreas

1. *Annular pancreas* an uncommon anomaly, warrants description as it may produce duodenal obstruction. It results when the two components of the ventral bud fail to fuse and grow in opposite direction around the duodenum and meet the dorsal pancreatic bud (Fig. 11.11A).
2. *Accessory pancreatic tissue* may be found:
   - In the wall of stomach or duodenum,
   - In an ileal diverticulum, e.g. Meckel's diverti-culum.

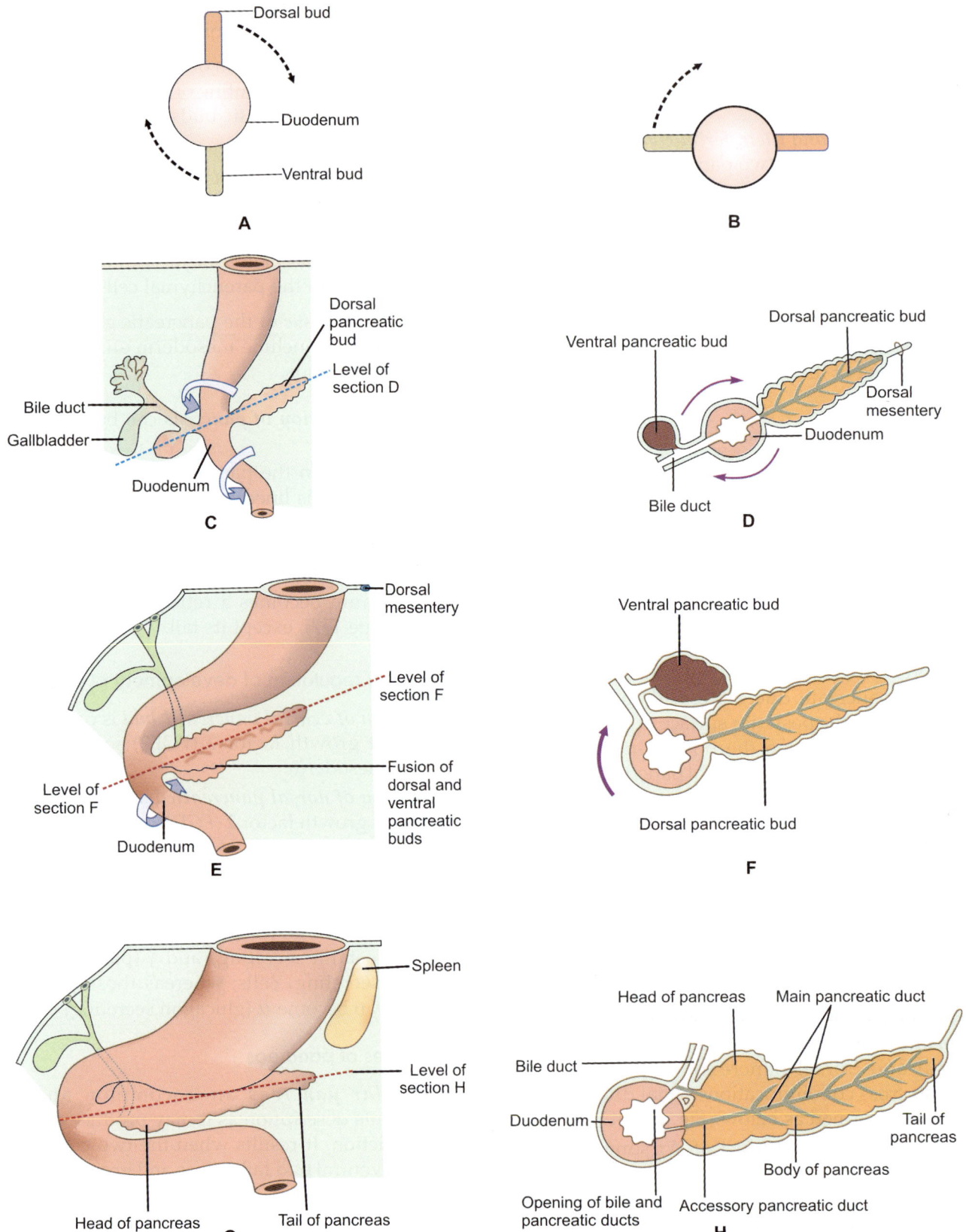

Fig. 11.10: Development of pancreas. Note position of dorsal and ventral pancreatic buds: A and B before axial rotation of duodenum; C and D. after dextrorotation of duodenum; E and F, after axial rotation of the duodenum; G and H, formation of pancreatic mass and duct system.

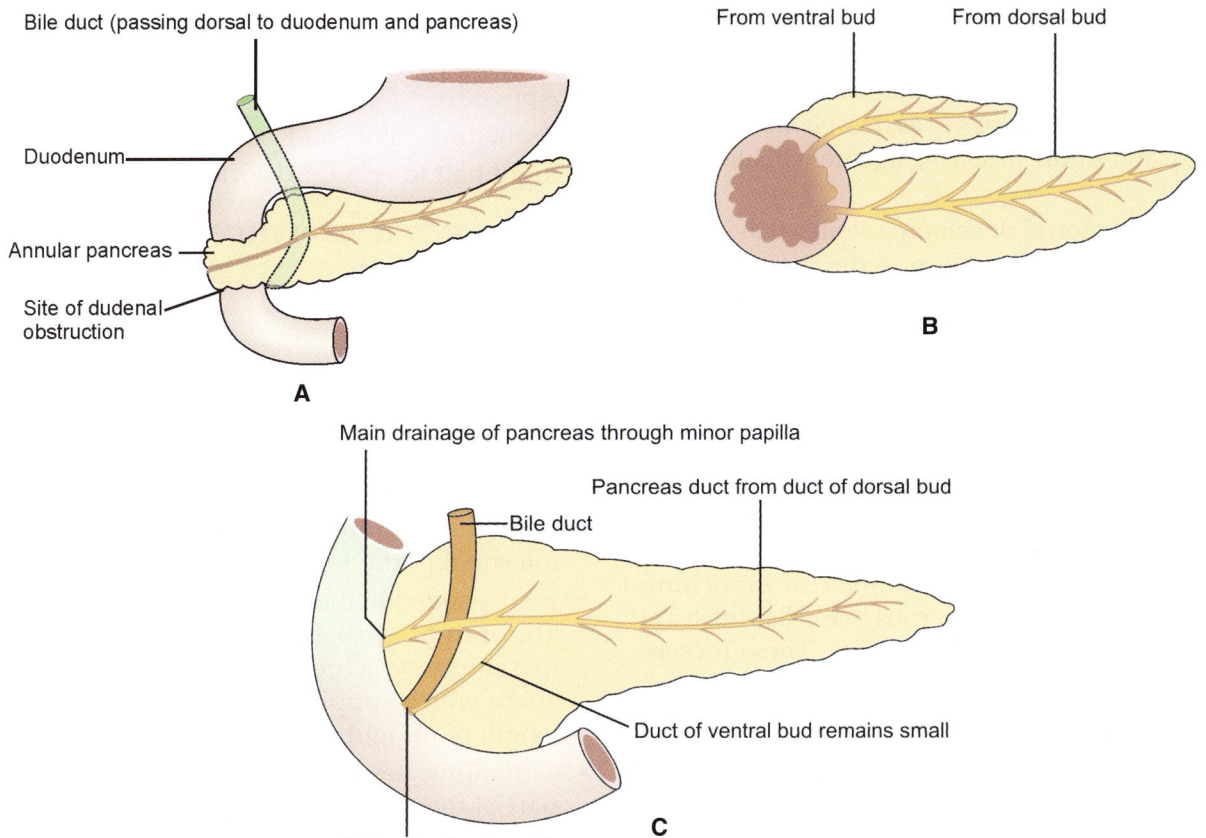

Fig. 11.11: Anomalies of pancreas: A, annular; B, divided pancreas; C, inversion of pancreatic ducts.

3. *Divided pancreas* is formed when the ventral and dorsal pancreatic buds fail to fuse with each other (Fig. 11.11B).

4. *Inversion of pancreatic ducts.* The embryonic arrangement of the ducts persists, i.e. the main pancreatic duct is entirely formed by the duct of dorsal bud, and opens at the minor duodenal papilla. The duct of the ventral bud remains small (Fig. 11.11C).

SPLEEN

Spleen, though not a derivative of foregut, is described here because it develops in association with mesogastrium. Major events in the development of spleen are:

Formation of mesenchymal mass. The spleen develops from the mesenchymal cells which proliferate to form a mesenchymal mass in the dorsal mesogastrium (Fig. 11.12A).

Formation of lobules and single mass of splenic tissue. Initially the splenic tissue is arranged as number of *lobules* which later join together to form a single splenic mass. The notches in the superior border of the adult spleen are representatives of the growth that separated the lobules during fetal period.

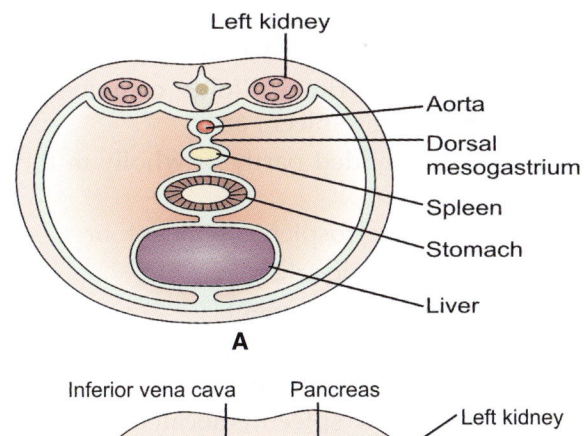

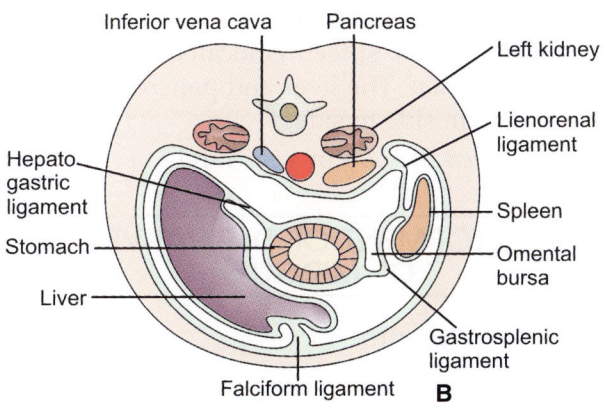

Fig. 11.12: Development of spleen: A, mesenchymal mass (forming spleen) in the dorsal mesogastrium; B, relationship with developing peritoneum after rotation of stomach.

Relationship of spleen with developing peritoneum can be summarized as below:

- *Dorsal mesogastrium* is divided into two parts by the developing spleen—*gastrosplenic ligament* infront, and future *lienorenal* ligament behind (Fig. 11.12A).
- With the rotation of developing stomach the spleen shift to left and the surface of the mesogastrium fuses with the peritoneum over the left kidney (Fig. 11.12B). This explains the attachments of lienorenal ligament in the region of left kidney.

Histogenesis of spleen. The mesenchymal cells in the splenic primordium differentiate to form:

- *Capsule* of the spleen outside,
- *Connective tissue* which forms framework of the spleen.
- *Parenchyma* is formed as number of branching trabecular cords and numerous free cells which are entangled between the trabeculae. These mesenchymal cells differentiate into lymphoblasts and other blood forming cells. The haemopoietic function of the spleen continues during fetal life, and regresses after birth. However, it retains its potential for blood cell formation even in adult life.

Anomalies of spleen

1. *Accessory spleen* is formed in about 10% individuals. It may be located:
   - In one of the peritoneal folds, commonly near the hilum of the spleen, or
   - May be embedded partly or wholly in the tail of pancreas, or
   - Within the gastrosplenic ligament, or
   - Along the splenic artery, or
   - In the lienorenal ligament
2. *Lobulated spleen* may be formed rarely due to persistence of fetal pattern.
3. *Sites inversus,* i.e. spleen is located on the right side of abdomen. The liver and pancreas are also reversed from side to side.
4. *Absent spleen* may occur very rarely.

DEVELOPMENT OF DERIVATIVES OF MIDGUT

DERIVATIVES OF MIDGUT

Derivatives of midgut supplied by its artery (the superior mesenteric) include:

- Most of the duodenum,
- Jejunum,
- Ileum,
- Caecum,
- Appendix,
- Ascending colon, and
- Right half to two-thirds of transverse colon.

MAJOR EVENTS IN THE DEVELOPMENT OF MIDGUT DERIVATIVES

Major events in the development of midgut derivatives can be summarized as below:

Primitive midgut

The primitive midgut, in a 5 week embryo, has following features (Fig. 11.1A):

- Is a straight tube extending from the anterior intestinal portal to posterior intestinal portal.
- Is suspended in the median plane from the dorsal abdominal wall by a short *primitive* dorsal mesentery which convey the *superior mesenteric artery* which supplies the midgut over the entire length of midgut.
- Communicates ventrally with the extraembryonic part of the yolk sac by the *vitellointestinal duct.*

Formation of primary intestinal loop

The rapid ventral elongation of the midgut results in formation of primary intestinal loop having following characteristics (Fig. 11.1B):

- It is a U-shaped loop having a cephalic limb or pre-arterial segment and a caudal limb or post-arterial segment.
- The superior mesenteric artery runs forward in the elongated dorsal mesentery in between the cephalic and caudal limbs.
- The narrow vitelline duct attached at the apex of the loop connects it with the yolk sac.
- Cephalic limb of the loop develops into the lower part of duodenum distal to the entrance of the bile duct, jejunum and part of the ileum.
- Caudal limb forms the lower portion of the ileum, the caecum, the appendix, the ascending colon and proximal two-thirds of the transverse colon.

Occurrence of physiological umbilical hernia and first rotation of the midgut loop (by 90°)

During the beginning of 6th week, along with the appearance of the caecal diverticulum there occur rapid elongation of the primary intestinal loop, particularly the cephalic limb forming coils of jejunum and ileum. Soon these intestinal loops herniate into the remains of extraembryonic coelom in the proximal part of umbilical cord (physiological umbilical hernia) (Fig. 11.13A and B).

Factors responsible for physiological umbilical hernia seem to be the shortage of space in abdomen caused by:

- Relatively massive growth of liver and the mesonephric kidneys, and
- Rapid elongation of midgut loop.

Period of physiological hernia extends from 6th to 10th week. The midgut loop communicates with yolk sac through the narrow vitelline duct until the 10th week.

First rotation of the midgut loop by 90°. Simultaneous with the rapid growth and physiological herniation. The primary intestinal loop rotates counter clockwise by 90° around the axis formed by the superior mesenteric artery. As a result (Fig. 11.13 C and D):

- The cephalic limb moves downward and to the right, and
- The caudal limb moves upward and to the left.

Continued growth of intestinal loop during this period leads to formation of a number of loops of jejunum and ileum.

The caecal diverticulum develops from the anti-mesenteric border of the caudal limb of intestinal loop near its apex during 6th week. Over the period of growth it will form the caecum and appendix.

Retraction of the herniated midgut to the abdomen and second rotation (by 180°)

During 10th week the herniated midgut loop start retracting back into the abdomen.

Factors thought to be responsible for reduction of physiological hernia (though not known exactly) include:

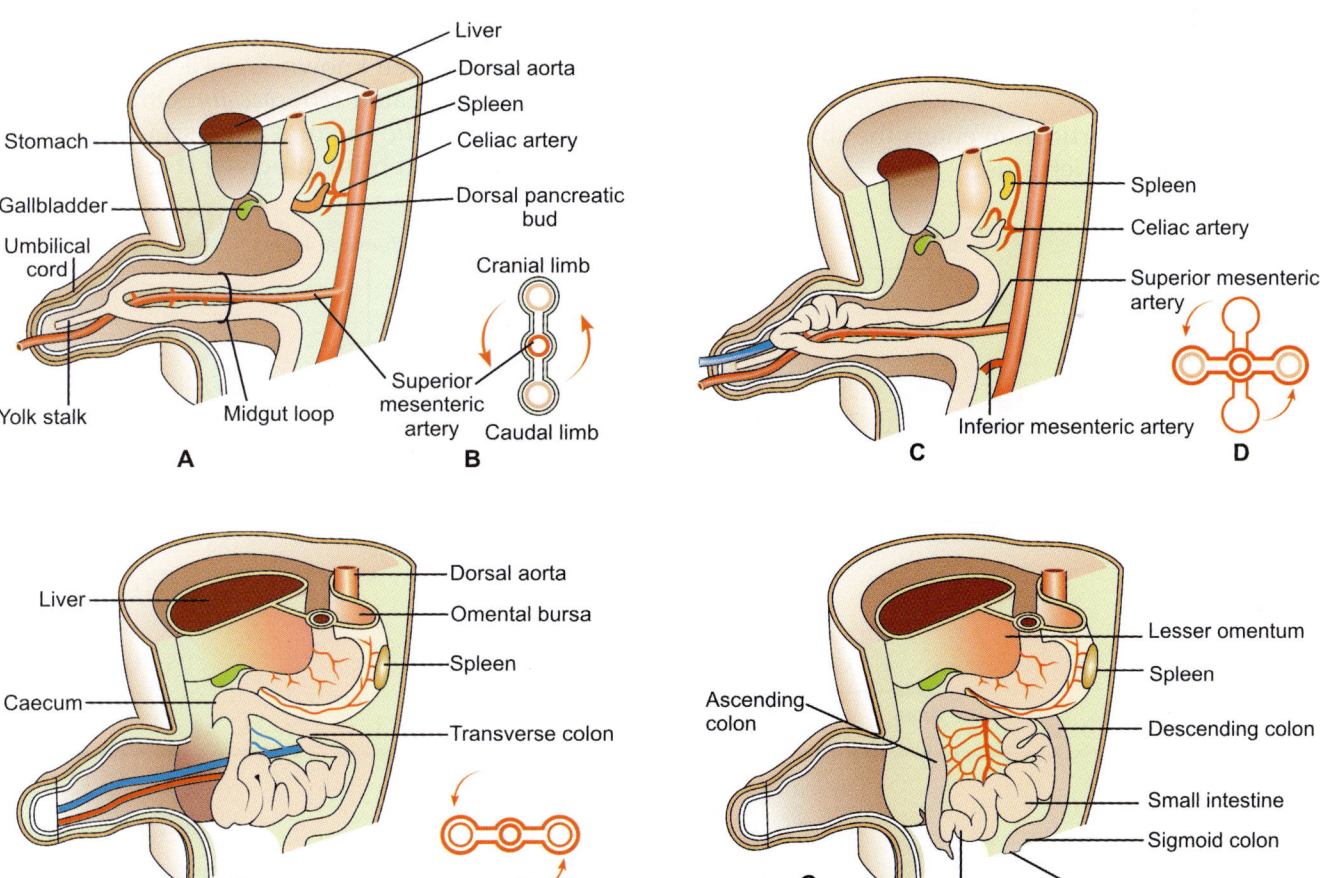

Fig. 11.13: Major events in the development of midgut derivatives: A and B, occurence of physiological hernia as seen in sagittal section and coronal section of midgut, respectively; C and D, first rotation of the midgut loop by 90° as seen in schematic drawing of sagittal view and coronal section of midgut, respectively; E and F, reduction of midgut hernia and second rotation of intestinal loops by another 180°, respectively. Note; the third part of duodenum is pushed to the left behind superior mesenteric artery, proximal loops of jejunum occupies left and rest of the jejunal and ileal loops occupy the right and dorsal part of the abdomen. Also note the position of caecal bud in the right upper quadrant of the abdomen; G, final position of the intestinal loops after descent of caecum and appendix into the right iliac fossa.

- Decrease in the size of liver and kidney, and
- Enlargement of the abdominal cavity.

Definite order of withdrawal of the herniated gut.
The herniated intestinal loops do not reduce en mass, because the umbilical ring is much smaller than the mass of intestinal loops. The reduction occurs stepwise in following definite order:

- *Proximal portion of the jejunum* is the first part to enter the abdominal cavity. Cord comes to lie on the left side. Because of the presence of the great pressure of the intestinal loops entering the abdomen, the proximal (duodenal) part of the midgut passes dorsal to the origin of the superior mesenteric artery and pushes the dorsal mesentery of the hindgut to the left side (Fig. 11.13E).
- *Remaining loops of the jejunum and ileum* follow the proximal part of jejunum and come to lie on the dorsal and right side of the abdominal cavity (Fig. 11.13E).
- *Left limb* of the midgut (from which develops caecum and associated colon) returns last in the abdomen.
- The caecum diverticulum enters the abdomen last and occupies the left side.

- Soon the caecum and transverse colon rotate counter clockwise by 180° to the right infront of superior mesenteric artery (Fig. 11.13E and F). Thus, the total range of rotation executed by the caecum and appendix around the axis of the superior mesenteric artery is about 270°.
- Then temporarily, the caecum comes to lie below the right lobe of liver (Fig. 11.13E).
- Thereafter, the *caecal diverticulum* descends into the right iliac fossa, thereby placing the ascending colon and hepatic flexure on the right side of abdominal cavity (Fig. 11.13G).
- Meanwhile the enlarged proximal part of caecal diverticulum forms the caecum and the narrow distal part forms the appendix. At birth, the appendix is a long tube arising from the distal end of caecum (Fig. 11.14A). After birth, the appendix is attached at the medial side of the caecum (Fig. 11.14B) because of the unequal growth of the caecal walls. However, variations in the position of appendix are well known. In 64% individuals the appendix is located *retrocaecally*. Other positions include *retrocolic* (behind the ascending colon), *pelvic* (located at brim of pelvis) (Fig. 11.14C).

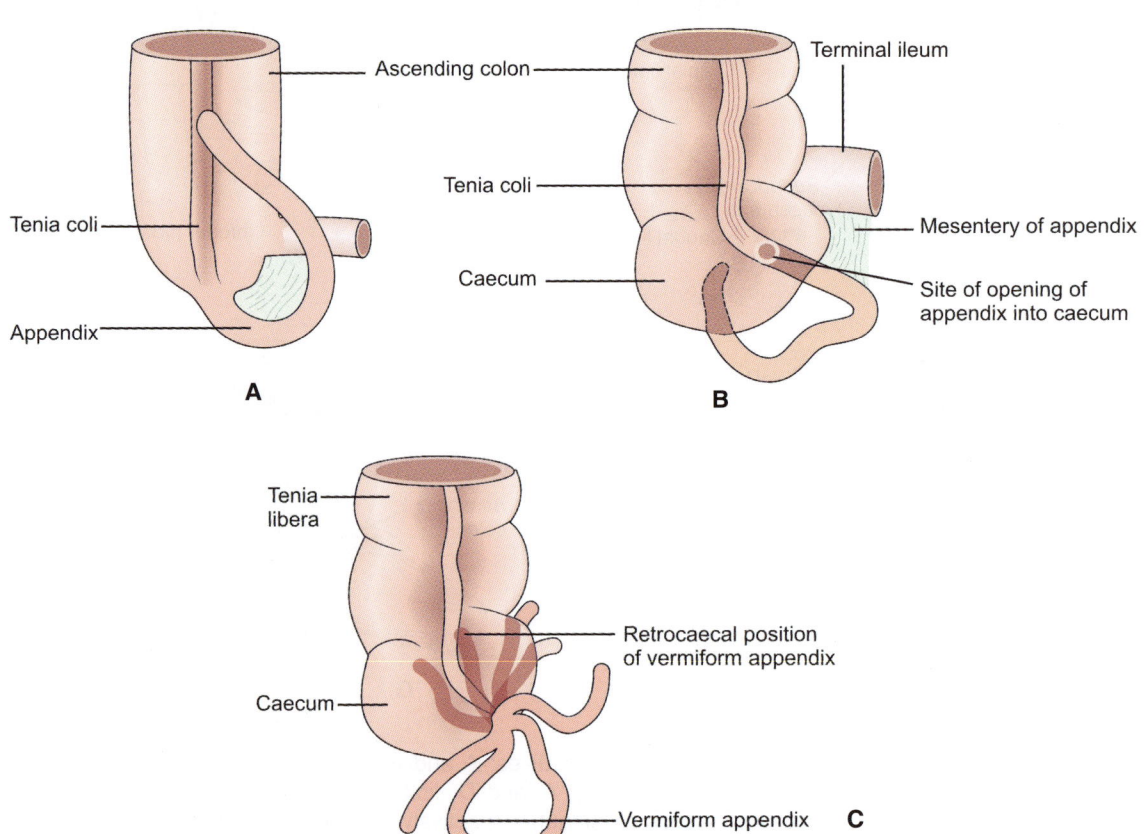

Fig. 11.14: Last stages of development of caecum and appendix: A, at birth (note appendix is long and attached to distal end of caecum; B, in adults appendix is relatively short and lies on the medial side of caecum; and C, schematic drawing depicting normal variations in position of appendix.

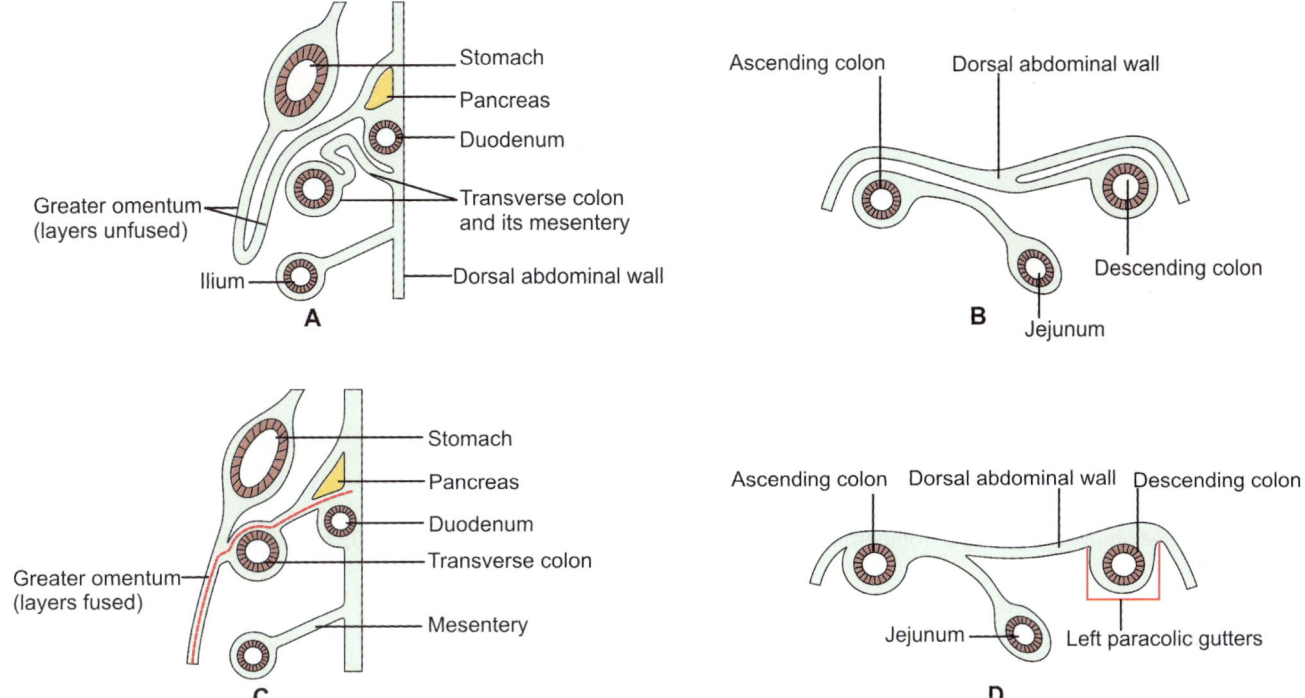

Fig. 11.15: Mesentery of intestinal loops and process of fixation as depicted in sagittal and coronal sections, respectively: A and B, before fixation; C and D after fixation.

Mesenteries of the intestinal loops and process of fixation of gut

Initially the primary intestinal loops and their derivatives have dorsal mesentery (*mesentery proper*) with the rotation the mesentery proper undergoes profound changes and the derivatives of midgut undergo *process of fixation* as below:

- *Twisting of dorsal mesentery* around the origin of superior mesenteric artery occurs during first rotation when the caudal limb of the primary intestinal loop moves to the right side of abdomen (Fig. 11.13C).
- *Dorsal mesentery of ascending colon,* fuses with the peritoneum of the posterior abdominal wall and as a result it becomes retroperitoneal (Fig. 11.15). The appendix and lower end of the caecum retain their free mesentery.
- *Dorsal mesentery of the cephalic limb of the primary intestinal loop* persists as the fan-shaped mesentery of jejunoileal loops. After retroperitonisation of ascending colon, the mesentery of jejunoileal loops obtains a new line of attachment that passes from the duodenojejunal junction inferolaterally to the ileocaecal junction (Fig. 11.15).
- *Dorsal mesentery of transverse colon* (transverse mesocolon) fuses with the posterior wall of the greater omentum (Fig. 11.15) but maintains its mobility.

ANOMALIES OF MIDGUT DERIVATIVES

1. *Errors of midgut rotation.* These include (Fig. 11.16):
   - *Non-rotation of midgut loops* occurs when the umbilical ring is large and leads to en mass reduction of umbilical hernia. In this condition the small intestine occupies the right side of abdomen and the large intestine including caecum lie on the left side (Fig. 11.16A).
   - *Reversed rotation of midgut loops.* In this condition the caecum enters the abdomen first during reduction of umbilical hernia and rotates upwards and to the right behind the origin of the superior mesenteric artery. As a result the transverse colon crosses behind the superior mesenteric artery and third part of duodenum comes to lie in front of the vessels (Fig. 11.16B).
   - *Mixed rotation and volvulus.* This occurs due to failure of the midgut loop to complete the final 90° of rotation. In this condition, the caecum lies just inferior to the pylorus of the stomach and is fixed to the posterior abdominal wall by peritoneal bands that pass over the duodenum (Fig. 11.16C).
2. *Congenital omphalocele* refers to a condition in which the intestine fail to return to the abdomen from physiological umbilical hernia during the 10th week. The contents of the hernial sac are lined

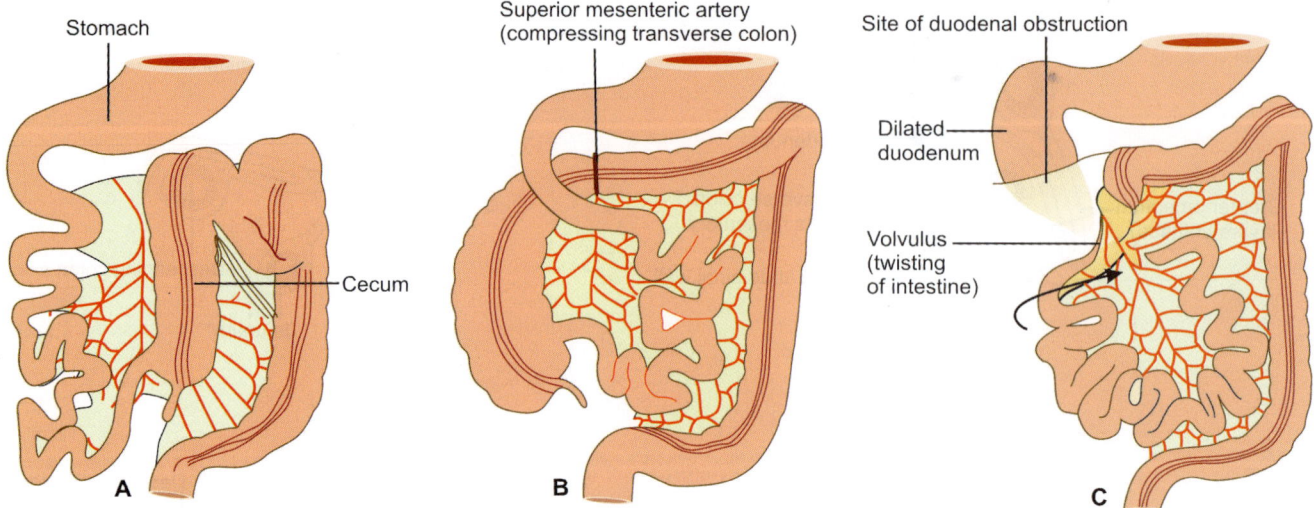

Fig. 11.16: Anomalies of midgut rotation: A, non-rotation; B, reversed rotation, and C, mixed rotation and volvulus.

by the epithelium of the umbilical cord which is derived from amnion. Therefore, in newborn with congenital omphalocele a bulky mass is found in the umbilical cord at birth.

3. **Umbilical hernia.** Unlike the omphalocele the physiological umbilical hernia is reduced completely, but later contents of the abdomen (usually the greater omentum and some small intestine) herniate through an imperfectly closed umbilicus. Therefore, the coverings of this hernia are subcutaneous tissue and skin (amnion derived epithelium in omphalocele).

4. **Umbilical faecal fistula occurs** when the vitello intestinal duct remains completely patent, through which the contents of small intestine are discharged at the umbilicus (Fig. 11.17A).

   • *Meckel's diverticulum* refers to persistent proximal part of the vitellointestinal duct (Fig. 11.17B). It typically appears as a finger-like pouch about two inches long attached to the antimesenteric border of ileum about 2 ft proximal to the ileocaecal junction. It is seen in 2–4% of people and can develop following complications:

      – *Peptic ulceration* and even perforation when the acid secreting oxyntic cells are present in its mucosa.

      – *Inflammation of diverticulum,* may mimic appendicitis.

      – *Intestinal obstruction* may occur when a loop of small gut happens to encircle the fibrous band attached to the diverticulum.

   • *Enterocystoma* refers to small cystic remnant of vitellointestinal duct, on both sides of which the duct is closed (Fig. 11.17C).

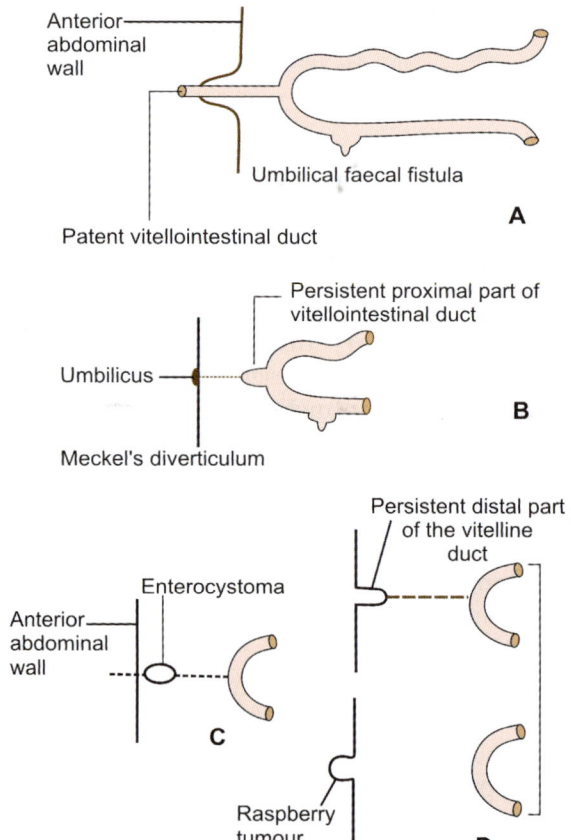

Fig. 11.17: Anomalies of vitellointestinal duct: A, umbilical faecal fistula; B, Meckel's diverticulum; C, enterocystoma; and D, raspberry tumour at the umbilicus.

   • *Raspberry tumour of the umbilicus* is produced when the remnant of distal part of vitellointestinal duct attached to umbilicus invaginate (Fig. 11.17D).

5. **Errors of fixation of gut** include:

   • *Persistence of mesentery,* in those structures which normally become retroperitoneal (e.g. duodenum, ascending, and descending colon), leads to their abnormal mobility. This may result in the twisting of the involved gut (*volvulus*).

- *Abnormal adhesion of peritoneum* may lead to fixation of that part of the intestine which normally have mesentery.

6. *Duplication of intestine* may occur as a localized cystic protrusion of the gut or as a separate segment of tubular gut formation (Fig. 11.18).

7. *Anomalies of caecum* include:

- *Subhepatic caecum and appendix* result due to failure of its descent into the right iliac fossa.

- *Pelvic caecum* results when the caecum moves to pelvis during its descent from the subhepatic region.

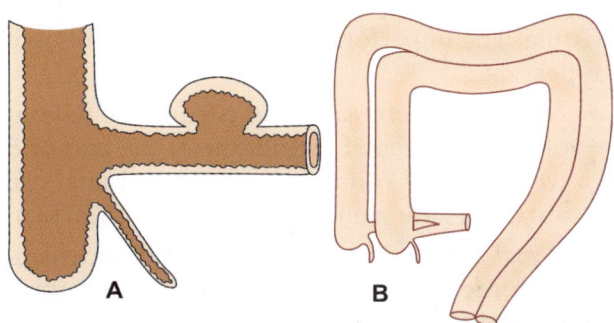

Fig. 11.18: Duplication of duct : A, cystic protrusion; B, tubular segment of duplicate gut present on the mesenteric side of gut.

DEVELOPMENT OF DERIVATIVES OF HINDGUT

DERIVATIVES OF HINDGUT

Derivatives of hindgut, supplied by its artery (inferior mesenteric artery) include:

Pre-allantoic part of hindgut gives rise to:

- Distal one-third of transverse colon,
- Descending colon, and
- Sigmoid colon

Post-allantoic part of hindgut

Dorsal part: primitive rectum forms:

- Rectum, and
- Upper part of anal canal

Ventral part: primitive urogenital sinus forms part of urogenital system (see page 173).

MAJOR EVENTS IN THE DEVELOPMENT OF HINDGUT DERIVATIVES

Primitive hindgut

The primitive hindgut, an endodermal structure, in a 5 week embryo has following features (Fig. 11.1A):

- Contained within the tail fold, it extends from the posterior intestinal portal to the cloacal membrane.
- Suspended in the median plane from the dorsal abdominal wall by a short primitive dorsal mesentery which also carries the inferior mesenteric artery.
- Ventrally, a diverticulum from the primitive hindgut extends upto the fetal part of umbilical cord, and divides the hindgut into two parts the pre-allantoic part and post-allantoic part.

Development of derivatives of pre-allantoic part of hindgut

Pre-allantoic part of the hindgut is narrow and tubular. During further development it forms:

- Distal third of transverse colon,
- Descending colon, and
- Sigmoid colon.

Dorsal mesentery of the descending colon disappears, and it becomes a retroperitoneal structure while that of sigmoid colon persists as pelvic mesocolon.

Development of derivatives of post-allantoic part of the hindgut

Endodermal cloaca refers to dilated post-allantoic part of hindgut, which early in the development is joined on each side by the mesonephric duct. The ventral wall of cloaca is formed by *cloacal membrane* which consists of opposing layers of ectoderm and endoderm without intervening mesoderm. Due to differential growth soon the cloacal membrane comes to lie at the bottom of cloaca and forms an ectodermal depression called the *external cloaca or proctodaeum*

Urorectal septum, a coronally oriented partition arises in the angle between the allantois and the hindgut and grows caudally towards the cloacal membrane. It divides the cloaca, incompletely at first, into two parts:

- Primitive rectum (dorsal part), and
- Primitive urogenital sinus (ventral part) connected to each other by *cloacal duct* (Fig. 11.19A). Soon the septum reaches and fuses with the dorsal membrane and the cloacal duct is closed. Now, the part of cloacal membrane anterior to the attachment of urorectal septum is called *urogenital membrane* and posterior to it is called *anal membrane* (Fig. 11.19B). The area of fusion of urogenital septum with the cloacal membrane forms the future *perineal body*.

Rectum is formed by the proximal part of the primitive rectum (dorsal part of endodermal cloaca).

Anal canal is developed from two sources the distal part of primitive rectum (dorsal part of endodermal

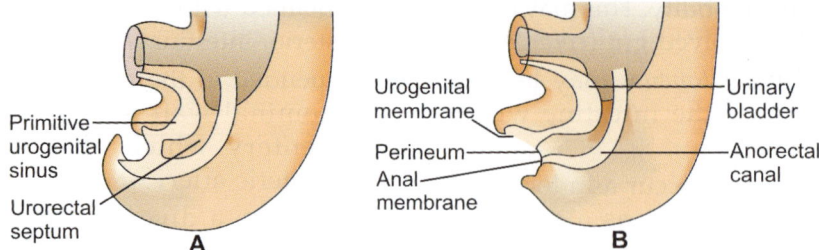

Fig. 11.19: Partitioning of cloaca into rectum and urogenital sinus by urorectal membrane: A, at 4 weeks; and B, at 7 weeks.

cloaca) and the external or ectodermal cloaca separated from each by the anal membrane (Fig 11.20). In the later development the anal membrane ruptures and the rectum now communicates with the exterior through the *anal canal*. In adult anal canal the *pectinate line* represents the line of attachment of anal membrane. Musculature and other coats of rectum and anal canal are derived from the surrounding splanchnic mesoderm.

ANOMALIES OF HINDGUT

1. *Persistent cloaca or undivided cloaca.* This rare condition occurs when the urorectal septum fails to develop completely. In this condition there is a common outlet for intestinal, urinary and reproductive tracts (Fig. 11.21A).
2. *Rectal fistulas* occurs due to incomplete closure of the urorectal septum. These include:
   - *Rectovesical fistula* (high fistula). The rectum communicates with the bladder usually in the region of internal trigone (Fig. 11.21B).
   - *Rectourethal and rectovaginal fistula* (low fistula). These conditions occur due to failure to development of lateral folds of Rathke of urorectal septum.
   - *Vertical element:* Though the vertical element of the septum is well developed, it is characterised

by communication of rectum with the urethra in males (rectourethral fistula) (Fig. 11.21C) and with vagina in female (rectovaginal fistula), (Fig. 11.21D).

3. *Imperforate anus* may occur with or without rectal fistula. The imperforate anus may be of following types:
   - *Membranous atresia of anus* occurs due to failure of rupture of anal membrane at the end of 8th week. In this condition rectum and anal canal are otherwise well developed (Fig. 11.21E).
   - *Rectal atresia,* in which anal canal and rectum both are formed but are separated by imperforated tissue (Fig. 11.21F).
   - *Anorectal agenesis,* in which the anal canal is not developed. Usually it is associated with rectourethral (Fig. 11.21C) or rectovaginal fistula (Fig. 11.21D).

4. *Anal agenesis,* i.e. non-formation of normal anal opening. It may be following types:
   - *Ectopic anus:* In females the anal and vaginal orifices may open into vestibule (cleft between labia minora. In males the anal opening may be present at the base of scrotum (Fig. 11.21G).
   - *Anoperineal fistula:* The anus opens into the perineum (Fig. 11.21H).

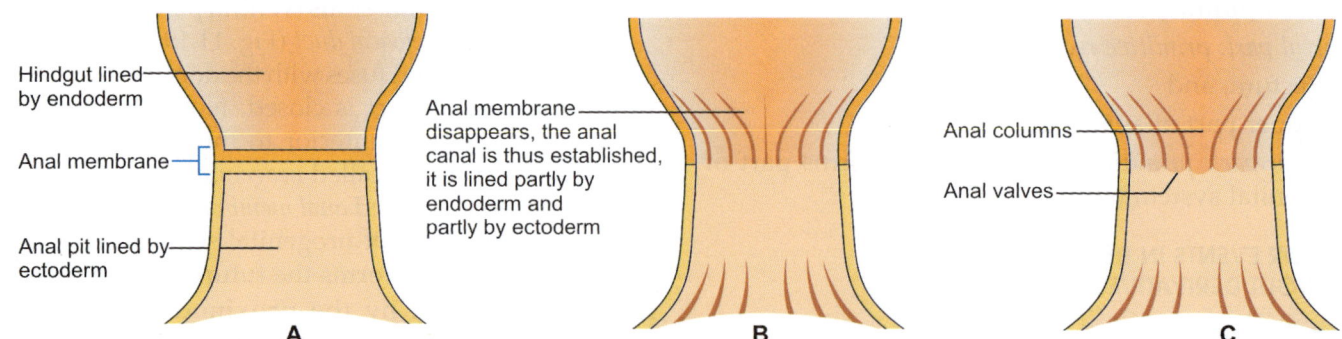

Fig. 11.20: Development of anal canal: A, anal membrane separating endodermal cloaca (primitive rectum) from ectodermal cloaca (anal pit); B, anal membrane disappears; and C, anal canal after birth.

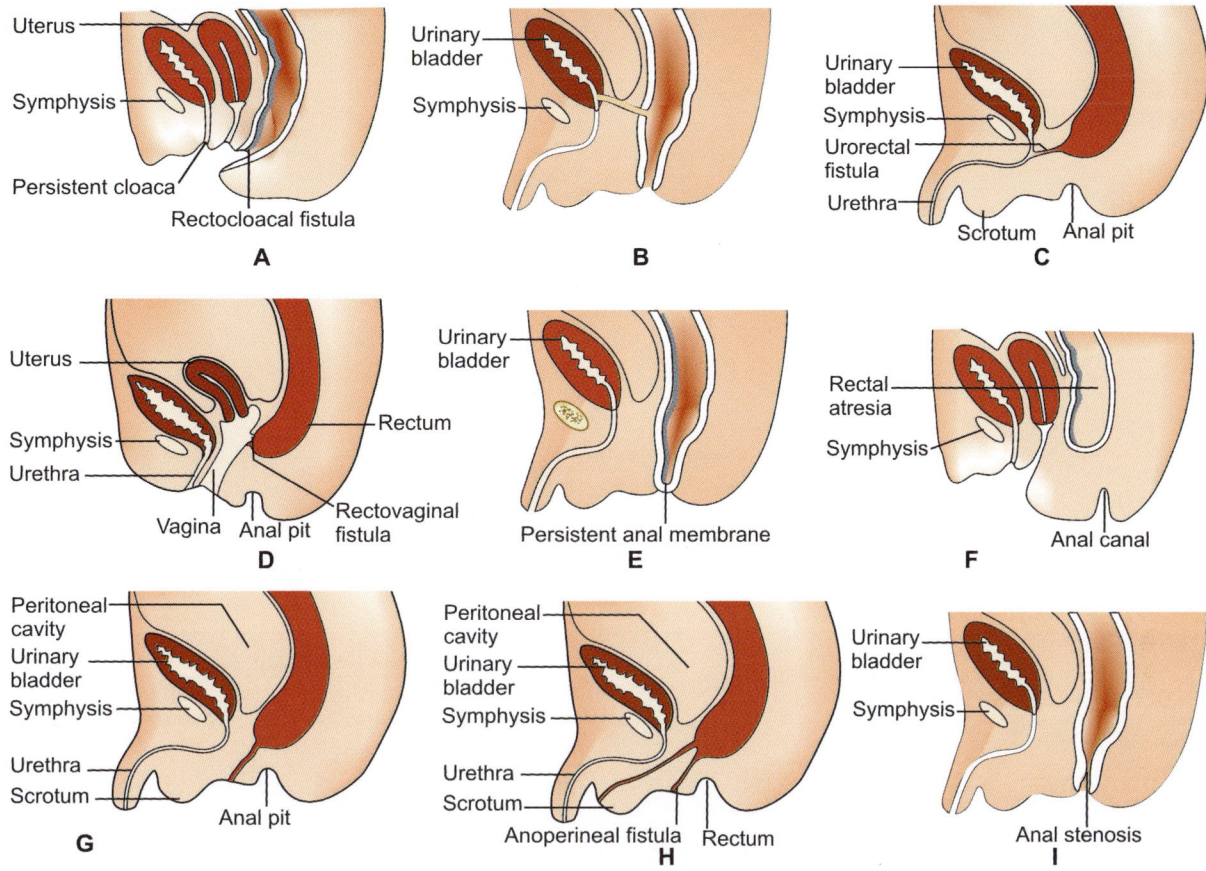

Fig. 11.21: Some anomalies of hindgut: A, persistent cloaca; B, rectovesical fistula; C, rectourethral fistula; D, rectovaginal fistula; E, imperforate anus: membraneous atresia; F, rectal atresia; G, ectopic anus (in male); H, anal agenesis: anoperineal fistula; and I, anal stenosis.

- *Anal agenesis with low rectal fistula (Fig. 11.21C and Fig. 11.21D).*

5. ***Anal stenosis.*** Anus and anal canal are developed in their normal position but their lumen is very narrow (Fig. 11.21I). This anomaly is caused by dorsal deviation of urorectal septum.

6. ***Congenital megacolon*** or Hirschsprung disease occurs due to absence of autonomic ganglion cells in the myenteric plexus in a segment of the colon, which becomes narrow, i.e. fails to respond to the waves of peristalsis. Consequently, the segment of colon proximal to the site of anomaly is dilated and enlarged.

Development of Urogenital System

PRIMORDIA OF UROGENITAL SYSTEM

The urogenital system includes two entirely different functional units, the *urinary system* and the *genital system*. However, embryologically and anatomically they are closely related. The primordia (embryonic structures) from which these systems develop are described here briefly. These include:

- Intermediate mesoderm,

- Cloaca, and

- Coelomic mesothelium.

INTERMEDIATE MESODERM

As described earlier (page 45), the intraembryonic mesoderm of each side of the embryo is divided into three parts (Fig. 12.1):

- *Paraxial mesoderm,* lying on either side of the notochord, in the course of later development becomes segmented to form the somites.

- *Lateral plate mesoderm,* in which appear the intraembryonic coelom, and

- *Intermediate mesoderm,* a longitudinal strip, lying between and connecting the above two parts. It plays an important role in the development of urogenital system.

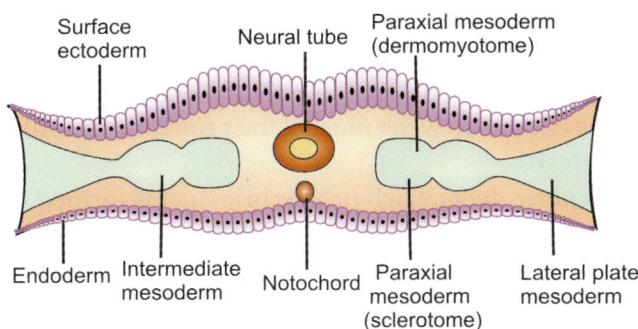

Fig. 12.1: Transverse section of 18 days embryo showing three divisions of intraembryonic mesoderm: paraxial, intermediate and lateral plate.

Developmental changes in intermediate mesoderm

Important developmental changes in the intermediate mesoderm are as below:

Positional changes. During folding of the embryo in the horizontal plane, the intermediate mesoderm is carried somewhat ventrally and loses its original connection with the somites. Somewhat later it loses its connection with the coelomic mesoderm except for sporadic strands.

After the folding of embryonic disc the intermediate mesoderm is arranged on each side of the primitive dorsal aorta and projects into the dorsal wall of the coelomic cavity. It can be divided into two parts (Figs 12.2 and 12.3):

Nephrotomes. These refer to the segments of intermediate mesoderm seen in the cervical and thoracic regions, which take part in the formation of non-functioning kidneys.

Urogenital ridge. Caudal to the segmental nephrotomes the intermediate mesoderm forms a continuous column of cells called the *urogenital ridge.* It gives rise to parts of urinary and genital system. The urogenital ridge can be divided into two:

* *Nephrogenic cord* or ridge refers to the part of urogenital ridge that takes part in the formation of permanent urinary system, and
* *Gonadal ridge,* the part which gives rise to the genital system.

CLOACA

As described earlier, the endodermal cloaca refers to the dilated post-allantoic part of hindgut which early in the development on each side by the mesonephric duct. It is divided by the urogenital septum into two parts (Figs 12.3 and 12.4):

* *Primitive rectum,* the dorsal part of the cloaca, forms the rectum and part of anal canal, and
* *Primitive urogenital sinus* (UGS), the ventral part of the cloaca which plays important role in the development of urogenital system.

COELOMIC MESOTHELIUM

At about 8th week the coelomic mesothelium covering the medial side of the mesonephric ridge proliferates to form an elongated *genital ridge* from which develops male and female *gonads.*

Note. In spite of close embryological and anatomical relationships between the urinary and the genital systems, it is worthwhile for the purpose of understanding to describe the major events of the developments of the two systems separately, as:

* Development of urinary system, and
* Development of genital system.

DEVELOPMENT OF URINARY SYSTEM

The urinary system begins to develop about 3 weeks earlier than the genital system. It consists of:

* Kidney,
* Ureters,
* Urinary bladder, and
* Urethra

DEVELOPMENT OF KIDNEYS AND URETERS

Development of kidneys evolves through formation of three successive kidney systems, which include (Fig. 12.3):

* Pronephroi, the rudimentary and non-functional set of kidney,

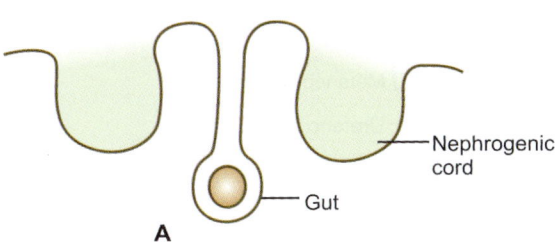

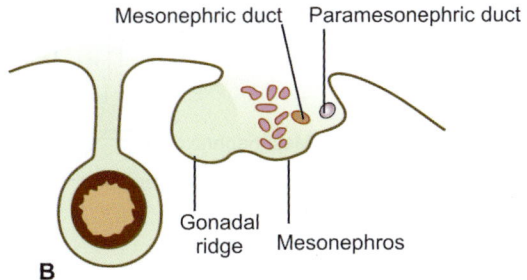

Fig. 12.2: The nephrogenic cord (A) and urogenital ridge (B).

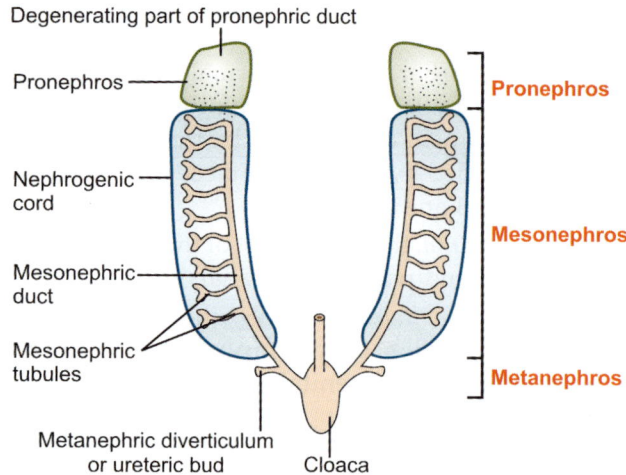

Fig. 12.3: The nephrotome, nephrogenic cord and the position of pronephric, mesonephric and metanephric sets of kidney.

- Mesonephroi, the second set of kidney which acts as temporary organ of excretion, and
- Metanephroi, which forms the permanent kidney.

Pronephroi

In human embryos, pronephroi, the first set of kidneys are exceedingly transitory structures. These are vestigial, nonfunctional, rudimentry kidneys. The pronephric kidneys are analogous to the permanent kidneys in cyclostomes and some telecost fishes. In human embryos these are represented by the pronephric tubules and pronephric ducts (Fig. 12.4).

Pronephric tubules. About 7 pairs of poorly developed pronephric tubules appear in the cervical region opposite somites 7 to 14 late in the 3rd week of gestation. The most cephalic tubule, the first to be formed regresses before more caudal ones are formed. By the end of 4th week most of the pronephric tubules disappear.

Pronephric ducts. Each pronephric duct is formed by fusion of distal ends of pronephric tubules, grows caudally and opens into the ventral part of cloaca (Figs 12.4 and 12.5).

Fate of pronephroi. As mentioned above, the pronephric tubules, disappear, but the pronephric duct persist and are utilized by the next set of kidneys (mesonephroi) (Fig. 12.5).

Mesonephroi

Mesonephroi, the second set of kidneys, serve as temporary organ of excretion in human embryos. These are analogues to the permanent kidneys in amphibians and most of the fishes. In young mammalian embryos, the mesonephroi attains a considerable degree of development and are represented by the mesonephric tubules and mesonephric ducts (Fig. 12.4):

Mesonephric tubules. The mesonephric tubules (about 70 to 80) are formed from the nephrogenic cord in the lower thoracic and lumbar region caudal to the rudimentary pronephroi late in the 4th week of gestation. The mesonephric kidneys are represented by highly differentiated tubules and glomeruli and serve as temporary organ of excretion for about 4 weeks, until the permanent kidneys develop.

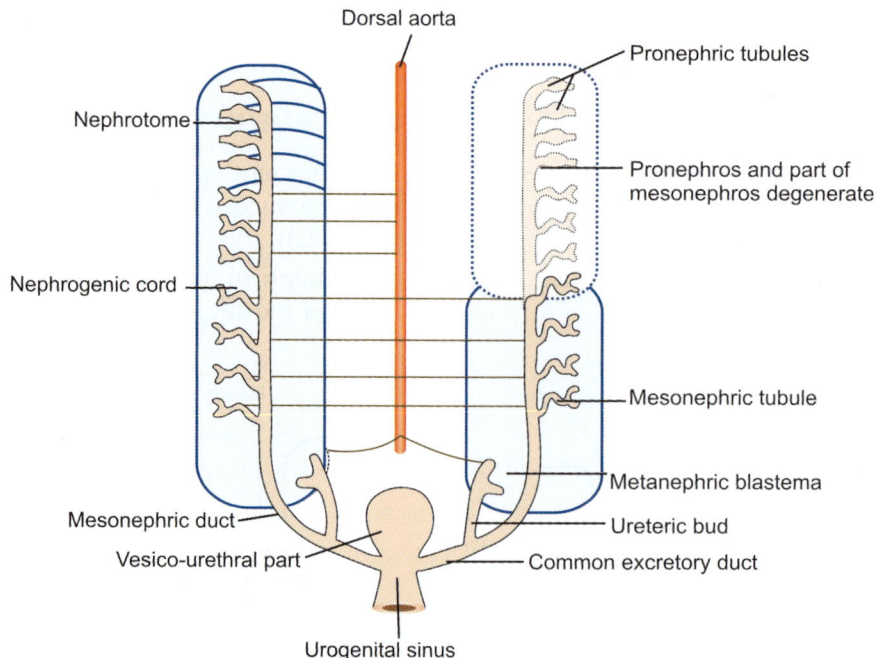

Fig. 12.4: The developing pronephroi, mesonephroi and metanephroi.

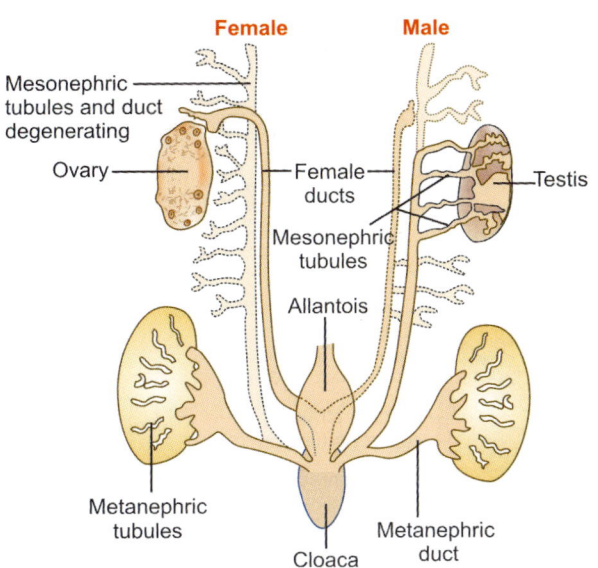

Fig. 12.5: Fate of pronephroi, mesonephroi and metanephroi.

Mesonephric ducts. As mentioned above, the pronephric tubules disappear, but the pronephric ducts persist and are utilized by the mesonephroi and hence forth they are called *mesonephric ducts* or *Wolffian ducts.* The mesonephric tubules open into these ducts.

Urogenital ridge. Somewhere in the middle of 2nd month, each mesonephroi forms an ovoid organ which projects into the coelomic cavity as *mesonephric ridge.* At the same time the coelomic mesothelium covering the medial side of the mesonephric ridge proliferate to form an elongated *genital ridge* which will give rise to the male and female gonads. Because of the close proximity of the mesonephric ridge and genital ridges, the two combinedly are termed as urogenital ridge (Fig. 12.2B).

Fate of mesonephroi. By the 5th week the mesonephric tubules begin to show progressive degenerative changes in a cranio-caudal pattern, i.e. while caudal tubules are still differentiating, cranial tubules and glomeruli show degenerative changes. By the end of 8th week most of the mesonephric tubules disappear and the few which are left take part in the formation of genital system as below (Fig. 12.5).

Fate of mesonephroi in males

Mesonephric tubules, which persist form:
- *Ductus aberrant superior* is formed by one or two proximal mesonephric tubules.
- *Efferent ductules of testis* are formed by the next successive six to twelve tubules.
- *Ductus aberrant inferior* and paradidymis is formed by the distal tubules.

Mesonephric duct forms the:
- Canal of epididymis,
- Vas deferens,
- Seminal vesicles and
- Ejaculatory duct
- Ureteric buds arising from the mesonephric duct take part in the formation of collecting system of permanent kidneys.

Fate of mesonephroi in females

- *Mesonephric tubules,* most of them disappear, and some persist in rudimentary forms as the tubules of:
  - Epoophoron, and
  - Paroophoron
- *Mesonephric ducts,* mostly degenerate *except:*
  - *Duct of epoophoron* (duct of Gartner), a vestigial part present in the broad ligament is the remnant of mesonephric duct, and
  - *Ureteric buds* arising from the caudal parts of mesonephric duct take part in the formation of collecting system of permanent kidney as in males.

Metanephroi

Metanephroi, the third set of kidneys, are the primordia, from which develop the permanent kidneys in higher forms of vertebrates including the human (Fig. 12.4). The metanephroi start developing in the 5th week and begin to function about 4 weeks later. The two systems of the metanephroi develop from two separate primordia which induce each other (reciprocal induction):
- *Collecting system* develops from the ureteric buds, (metanephric diverticuli), and
- *Excretory system* develops from the metanephric blastema (the metanephric mass of intermediate mesoderm).

Development of collecting system

Ureteric buds or the metanephric diverticulae arise from the mesonephric ducts close to their entrance into the cloaca (Fig. 12.6A). The part of mesonephric duct caudal to the origin of the ureteric bud is called the *common excretory duct.*

Each ureteric bud grows dorsally and penetrates the metanephric tissue, which as a cap, is moulded over its distal end (Fig. 12.6B). Subsequently the elongated ureteric bud forms the following structures (Figs 12.6C to E):

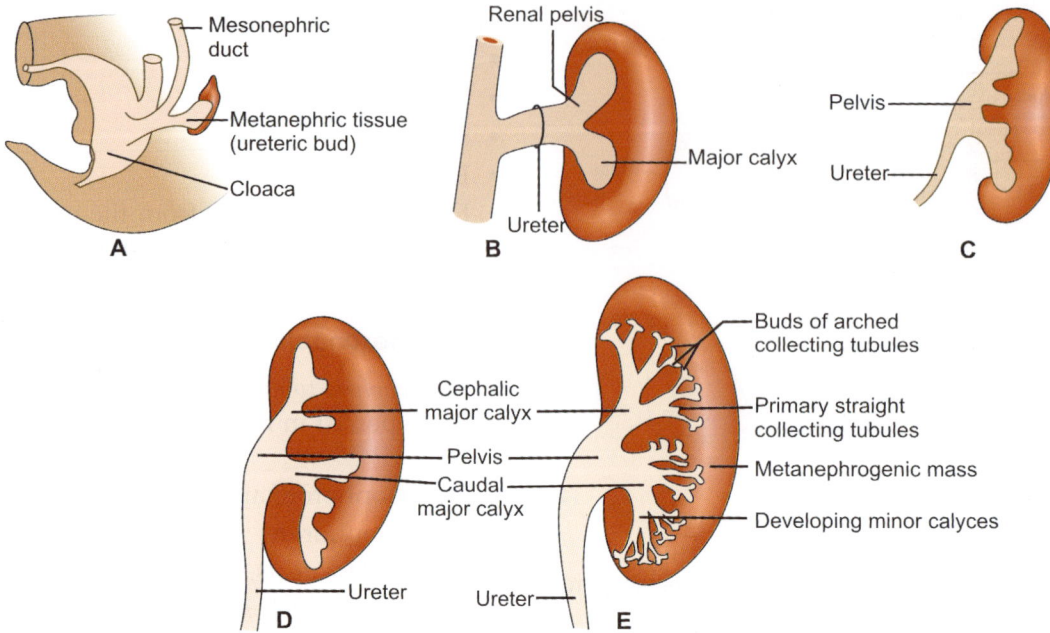

Fig. 12.6: Development of collecting system of permanent kidney: A, formation of ureteric buds, B, penetration of metanephric mesoderm by ureteric buds; C to E, formation of ureter, renal pelvis, major calyces, minor calyces and collecting tubules.

- *Ureter* is formed by the elongated stalk of ureteric bud which extends from the cloaca to the metanephric cap.
- *Renal pelvis* is formed by the distal dilated end of the ureteric bud.
- *Major calyces* are formed by the division of renal pelvis into cranial and caudal portion. Each calyx subdivides repeatedly into successive orders of branches until 13 or more generations of collecting tubules of different orders are formed.
- *Minor calyces* are formed when the second generation of the tubules (described above) enlarge and absorb the branch of 3rd and 4th order of the tubules.
- *Collecting tubules* of the permanent kidney are thus formed by all branches from the 5th and subsequent order of branches. About 1 to 3 million collecting tubules are formed in each permanent kidney.

Development of excretory system

Nephrons, which form the excretory system of permanent kidney are developed from the metanephric mass of intermediate mesoderm after induction by the metanephric tubules. The major events in the formation of nephrons can be summarized as below (Fig. 12.7):

- *Metanephric blastema* refers to the cells of metanephric intermediate mesoderm which covers the distal dilated end of each newly formed collecting tubule as metanephric tissue cap (Fig. 12.7A).

- *Renal vesicles* are clusters of cells formed from the cells of metanephric tissue caps under the inductive influence of the collecting tubules (Fig. 12.7B). These vesicles are the precursors of the nephrons of the kidney.

- *Nephron* is then formed from each renal vesicle as below:
  - Each vesicle becomes an S-shaped tube (Fig. 12.7C).
  - Distal end of each S-shaped tube forms *Bowman's capsule*, which is deeply indented by a glomerulus (tuft of capillaries derived from the angiogenic mesenchyme of the nephrogenic cord) (Fig. 12.7D).
  - Distal end of each S-shaped tube forms an open connection with one of the collecting tubule, thus establishing a passageway from Bowman's capsule to the collecting unit.
  - On further growth the middle segment of each S-shaped tube extends towards the future medulla as the *loops of Henle* and the associated part of the tubule forms the *proximal* and *distal convoluted tubules* (Fig. 12.7E).

Note. Between the 10th and 18th weeks of gestation, the number of nephrons increase gradually, then they increase rapidly until 32nd week, when an upper limit is reached. Thus the new nephrons are formed throughout life; the earlier evolved nephrons (juxtamedullary) occupy the depth of the kidney at the cortico-medullary junction.

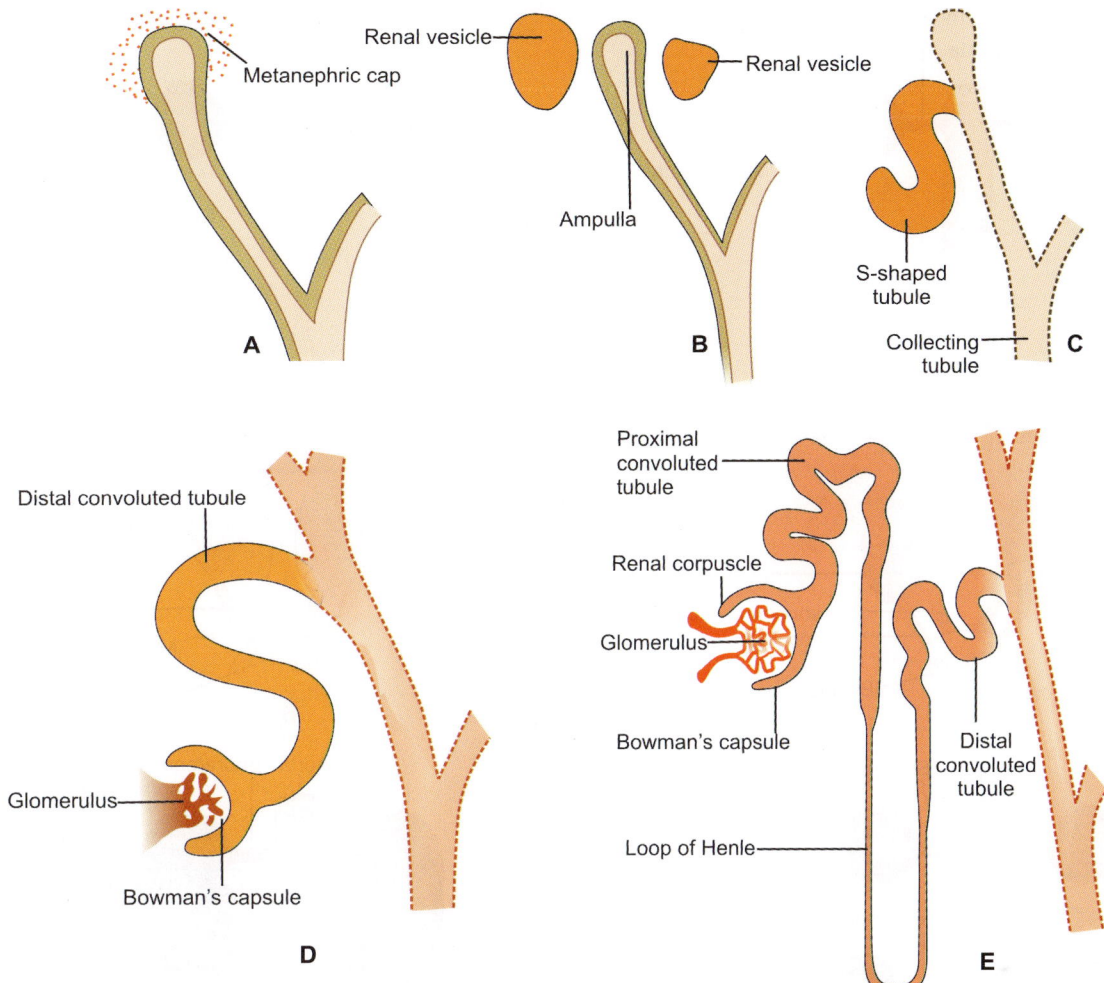

Fig. 12.7: Development of excretory system of permanent kidney: A, metanephric cap; B, renal vesicles; C, s-shaped tubule; D, bowman's capsule and glomerulus; E, differentiation and growth of different parts of nephron, loop of Henle, proximal and distal convoluted tubules.

Functioning of the permanent kidney

Urine formation by the permanent kidney begins at the end of 3 months of gestation and is passed into the amniotic cavity. The urine mixed in amniotic fluid is than swallowed by the fetus and enters the systemic blood after getting absorbed from the intestinal tract. From the systemic blood the urine is again excreted into the amniotic fluid.

Note. Since during fetal life the placenta also acts as main organ of excretion of waste products, so kidneys are not much involved in this function.

Positional changes in permanent kidneys

The initial position. The metanephroi (primordia of permanent kidneys) develop during 5th week in the *pelvis* ventral to the sacrum (Fig. 12.8A).

Adult position, i.e. lumbar region of abdomen is attained by the developing permanent kidneys in 9th

week. Thus the positional changes in the kidneys include:

- *Progressive ascent of kidneys* from pelvis to abdomen (Figs 12.8B to D), and
- *Medial rotation of the kidneys:* As a result of medial rotation the hilum of kidney which initially faces ventrally, rotates by 90° and faces medially. The nerves and vessels of the kidney enter and leave the kidneys through the hilum.

Changes in the blood supply of the kidneys

Due to ascent of kidneys the blood supply of the kidneys also changes as below (Fig. 12.8):

- *Initially* when the kidneys are in pelvis the renal arteries are the branches of common iliac arteries (Fig. 12.8A).
- *With progressive ascent,* the arteries to kidneys are derived from different levels of aorta (Fig. 12.8B and C).

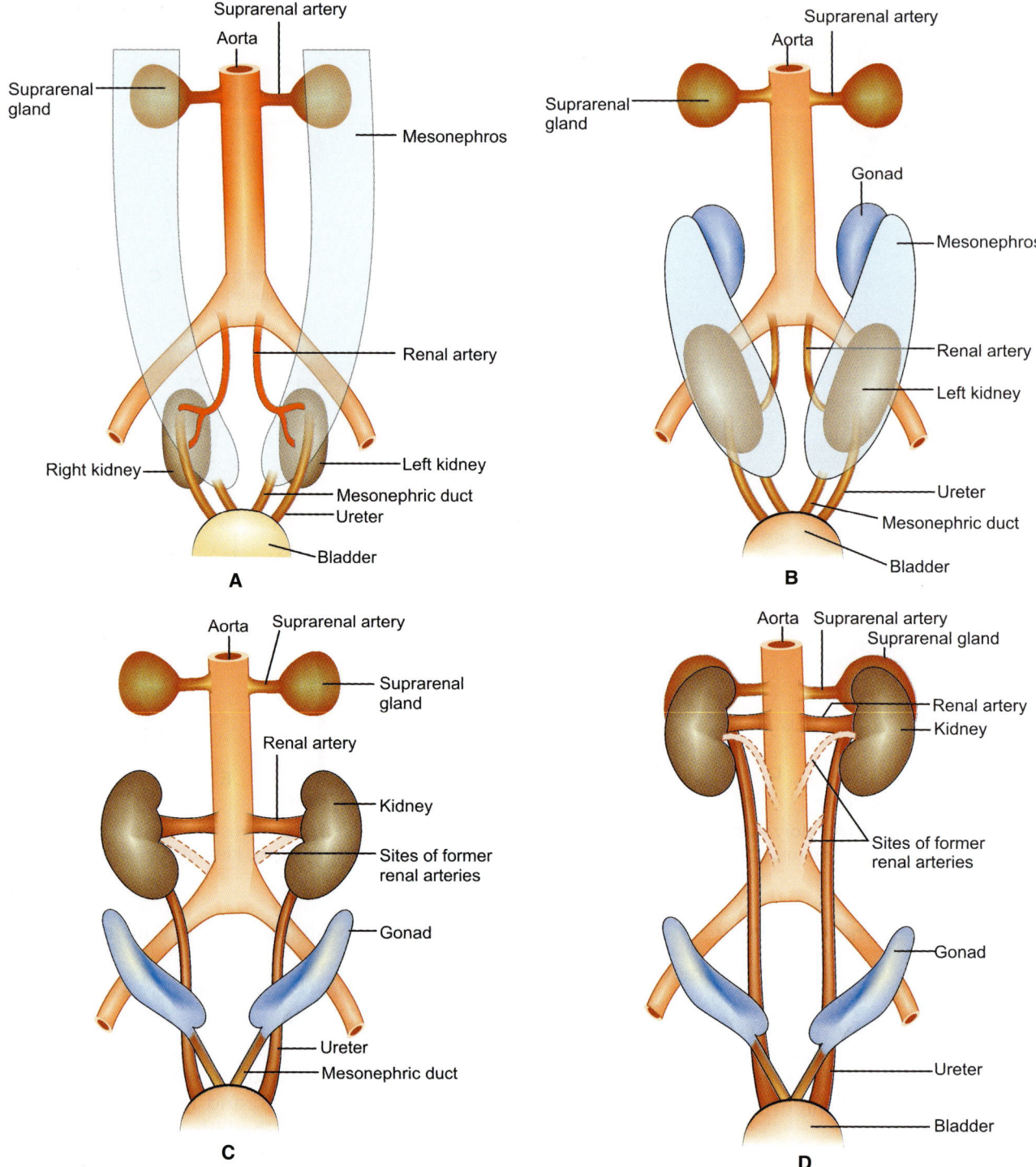

Fig. 12.8: Changes in position and blood supply of permanent kidneys: A, initial position and vessels; B and C, intermediate position and vessels; and D, final position and vessels.

- *Permanent renal arteries* are the most cranial branches from the abdominal aorta. The caudal branches from the aorta to the kidney undergo involution and disappear (Fig. 12.8D).

Kidneys at and after birth

At birth the kidneys have somewhat lobulated appearance indicating the division of fetal kidney into lobes (which disappear at the end of fetal period). At term kidneys usually contain about 8 to 10 lakh nephrons.

During infancy the lobulation disappear due to increase in size of the nephrons and increase in the amount of interstitial tissue. It is believed that usually number of nephrons do not increase after birth.

Molecular regulation of renal development

Molecular regulation of renal development can be summarized as below:

- *Transcription factor WT1 expressed by the mesen-chyme of metanephric blastema,* enables this tissue to respond to induction by the epithelium of ureteric bud from the mesonephros.
- *Glial-derived neurotrophic factor (GDNF) and hepatocyte growth factor (HGF)* also produced by the mesenchyme of metanephric blastema interact through their receptors in the ureteric bud to stimulate growth of the bud and maintain the interactions. Production of GDNF and HGF is regulated by WTI.
- *Growth factor (FGF2) and BMP7* stimulate prolifera-tion of mesenchyme and maintain WT1 expression.
- *PAX2 and WNT4,* produced by the ureteric bud cause the mesenchyme to epithelize in preparation for excretory tubule differentiation.

ANOMALIES OF KIDNEYS AND URETERS

A. Anomalies of number of kidneys

1. **Unilateral agenesis of kidney,** i.e. non-formation of one kidney occurs due to failure of one of the ureteric bud to develop. Sometimes one kidney is underdeveloped (*hypogenesis*).
2. **Bilateral agenesis of kidneys,** i.e. non-formation of both kidneys may occur rarely. Bilateral absence of the kidneys is incompatible with postnatal life.
3. **Multiple kidneys.** Due to early splitting of ureteric bud, rarely, more than one kidney may be present on one or both sides separately or as fused kidneys.

B. Anomalies of position of (ectopic) kidneys

Unilateral or bilateral ectopic kidneys may occur due to anomalous ascent of the kidneys.

1. **Pelvic kidney** results due to complete failure of ascent of the kidney (Fig. 12.9A). Such a kidney has normal function and does not warrant any surgical interference.
2. **Lumbar kidney,** lying opposite the lower lumbar vertebrae, may occur due to incomplete ascent (Fig. 12.9A).
3. **Thoracic kidney** may occur rarely due to anomalous excessive ascent of a kidney (12.9A).
4. **Crossed renal ectopia** may occur in two forms:
   - *Unilateral crossed renal ectopia,* i.e. both kidneys lie on one side of the midline separately or fused

to each other. The ureter of the displaced kidney crosses to the opposite side to open in the bladder (Fig. 12.9B).

- *Bilateral crossed renal ectopia,* i.e. both kidneys exchange their positions with each other. In such cases ureters cross each other in the midline (Fig. 12.9C).

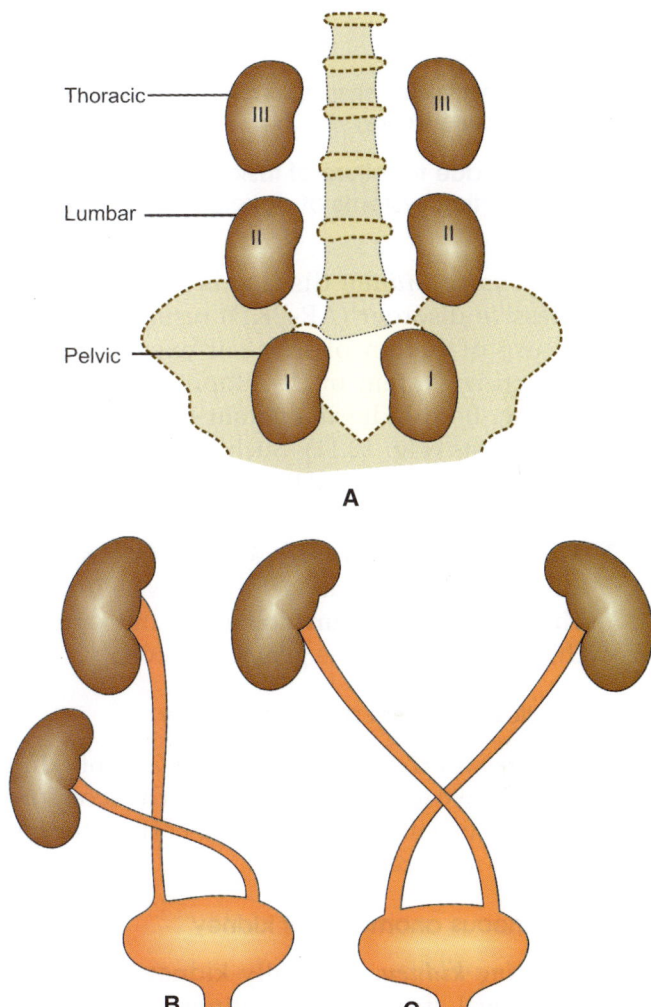

Fig. 12.9: Anomalies of kidney: A, ectopic kidney (I Pelvic, II Lumbar, and III thoracic kidney), B. unilateral crossed renal ectopia; and C, bilateral crossed renal ectopia.

C. Anomalies of shape of kidneys

1. **Horseshoe kidneys** occur when either the lower poles or upper poles (comparative rare) of the kidneys are connected by an isthmus of kidney tissue which lies in front of aorta and vena cava (Fig. 12.10A). Such kidneys are located lower than their normal position, because the ascent is blocked by the inferior mesenteric arteries.
2. **Pancake kidney** also known as *discoid* kidney is formed by fusion of two kidneys across the mid line (Fig. 12.10B).

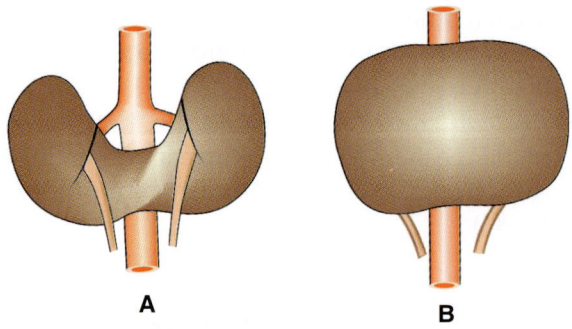

Fig. 12.10: Anomalous shapes of kidney: A, horseshoe kidney; B, pancake kidney.

D. Anomalies due to failure of fusion of excretory and collecting systems of developing permanent kidney

1. *Polycystic kidney* disease is an autosomal recessive disorder (AR-PKD) resulting due to failure of fusion of most of excretory and collecting system of developing permanent kidney. Both kidneys contain many hundred small cysts (Fig. 12.11). Such kidneys are non-functional and death of the infant usually occurs shortly after birth.

2. *Multicystic dysplastic kidney (MDK)* is a milder form of disease with few cysts formed. These kidneys are functional and outcome for children with MDK is generally good.

E. Anomalies of arterial supply of kidney

Accessory renal artery/arteries: About 25% of adult kidneys have two to four renal arteries. The accessory renal arteries usually arise from the aorta, superior or inferior to main renal artery.

F. Miscellaneous anomalies of kidney

1. *Floating kidney.* Normally kidney is a retro-peritoneal structure. Sometimes it may have mesentery and float in the abdomen. In such case, downward tilting of the upper pole of kidney may lead to twisting of renal vessels and

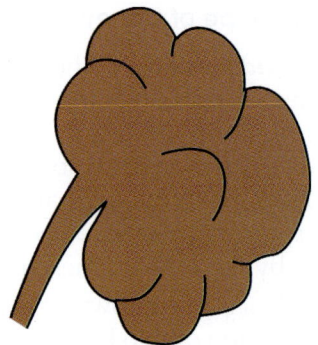

Fig. 12.11: Polycystic kidney disease.

ureters. This leads to severe pain in the loin with suppression of urine (Diert's crisis).

2. *Abnormal rotation of kidney* include:
   - *Non-rotation,* i.e. hilum faces venterally
   - *Incomplete rotation,* i.e. hilum faces antero-medially
   - *Reverse rotation,* i.e. hilum faces antero-laterally.

3. *Multiple kidney anomalies,* i.e. two or more of the above described anomalies may co-exist. For example, anomalies of position are frequently associated with those of rotation.

G. Anomalies of ureters of kidney

1. *Double ureters.* Sometimes there are two ureters connected to a single kidney which open in the bladder either by a common orifice (Fig. 12.12A) or by separate orifices (Fig. 12.12B).

2. *Ectopic termination of ureter.* Instead of opening into the urinary bladder, ectopically the ureter may terminate in the prostatic urethra, ductus deferens, seminal vesicles, or rectum, in the male (Fig. 12.12C) and in the urethra, vagina, vestibule, or rectum in the female (Fig. 12.12D).

3. *Hydroureter,* i.e. dilated ureter, may occur because of obstruction to the urine flow.

4. *Diverticuli or valves* may be present in the ureter.

DEVELOPMENT OF URINARY BLADDER AND URETHRA

Primordia of urinary bladder and urethra

Primordia from which the urinary bladder and urethra develop are:
- Primitive urogenital sinus (endodermal),
- Lower end of mesonephric ducts (mesodermal), and
- Splanchnic mesoderm.

Primitive urogenital sinus

As described earlier, the endodermal cloaca is divided by the urorectal septum into two parts: primitive rectum (dorsal part) and primitive urogenital sinus (ventral part) (Fig. 12.13). By the opening of mesonephric ducts the primitive urogenital sinus is divided into two parts: vesicourethral canal and definitive urogenital sinus.

Vesicourethral canal. It is the cranial part of the primitive urogenital sinus which communicates with the allantoic diverticulum. In further development it gives rise to urinary bladder.

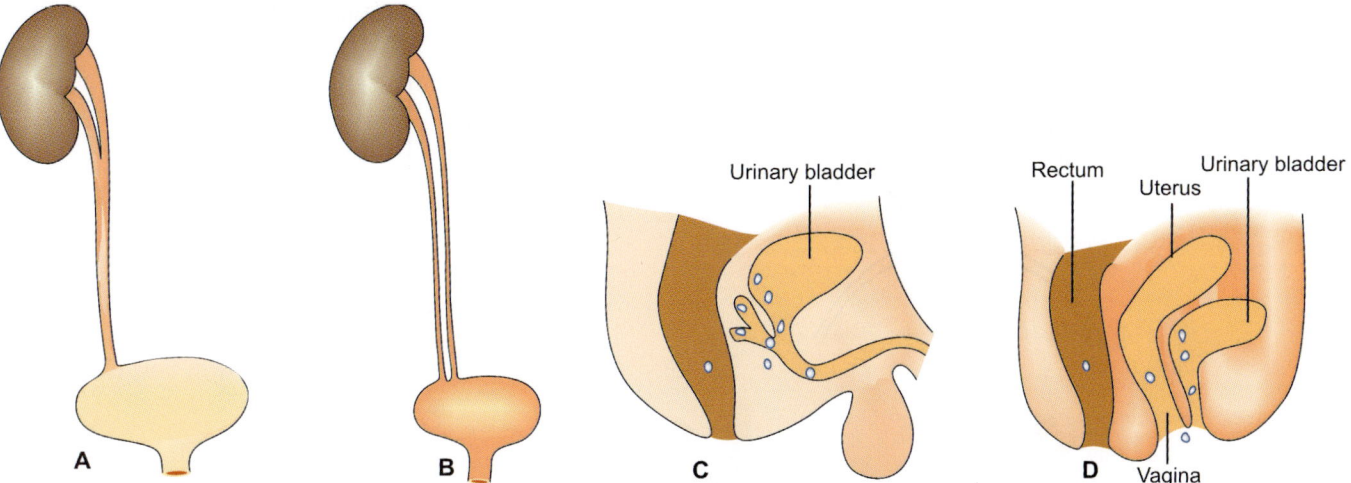

Fig. 12.12: Anomalies of ureter: double ureter opening in the bladder by a common orifice (A) and by two separate orifices (B), Ectopic sites of termination of ureter in male (C) and in female (D).

Definitive urogenital sinus (UGS) refers to the part caudal to the opening of mesonephric ducts. It can be subdivided into two parts:

- *Pelvic part of UGS* is a narrow canal which in the males gives rise to prostatic and membranous part of urethra and in females the entire urethra. In its dorsal wall open the mesonephric ducts, which in females, disappear, but in males persist as ejaculatory ducts.
- *Phallic part of UGS* is the caudal dilated part which is bounded below by the urogenital membrane. It grows towards the genital tubercle.

Lower parts of mesonephric ducts

Lower parts of mesonephric ducts are the other primordia which take part in the development of urinary bladder. As described earlier the lower part of mesonephric duct caudal to the origin of ureteric bud is called *common excretory duct* (Fig. 12.14A). During further development this part of mesonephric ducts is absorbed into the vesicourethral part of UGS,

as a consequence the mesonephric ducts and ureteric buds come to open in this part of UGS by separate opening (Fig. 12.14B). The openings of mesonephric ducts and ureteric buds, which are initially close to each other (Fig. 12.14C) soon are separated due to cranial and lateral movement of the *ureteric opening* (Fig. 12.14D). Thus the triangular area of dorsal wall of vesicourethral canal between the openings of ureteric buds and mesonephric duct is derived from the absorbed part of mesonephric ducts mesodermal in origin (Fig. 12.14D).

Development of urinary bladder

Mucous membrane of urinary bladder is derived from following sources (Fig. 12.14):

- *Vesico-urethral canal (endodermal),* the cranial part of urogenital sinus (Figs 12.13 and 12.14), forms the epithelium of the entire urinary bladder, except the area of internal trigone.
- *Absorbed lower part of mesonephric ducts (mesodermal)* form the epithelium of the internal trigone area of

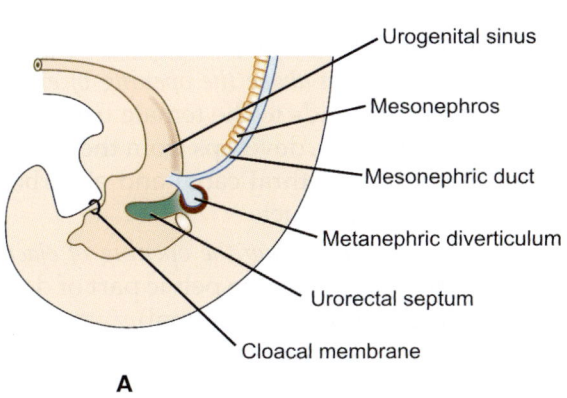

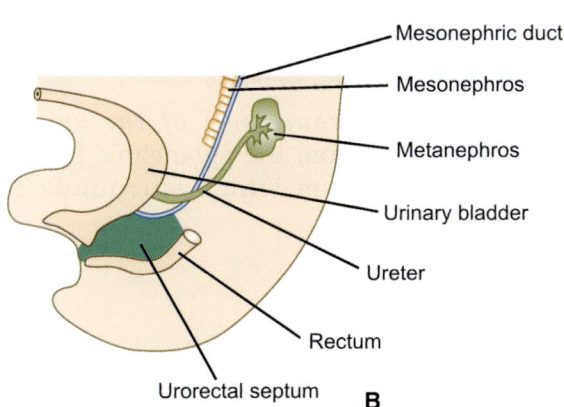

Fig. 12.13: Schematic sagittal section through primitive urogenital sinus: early (A) and late (B) stage of development.

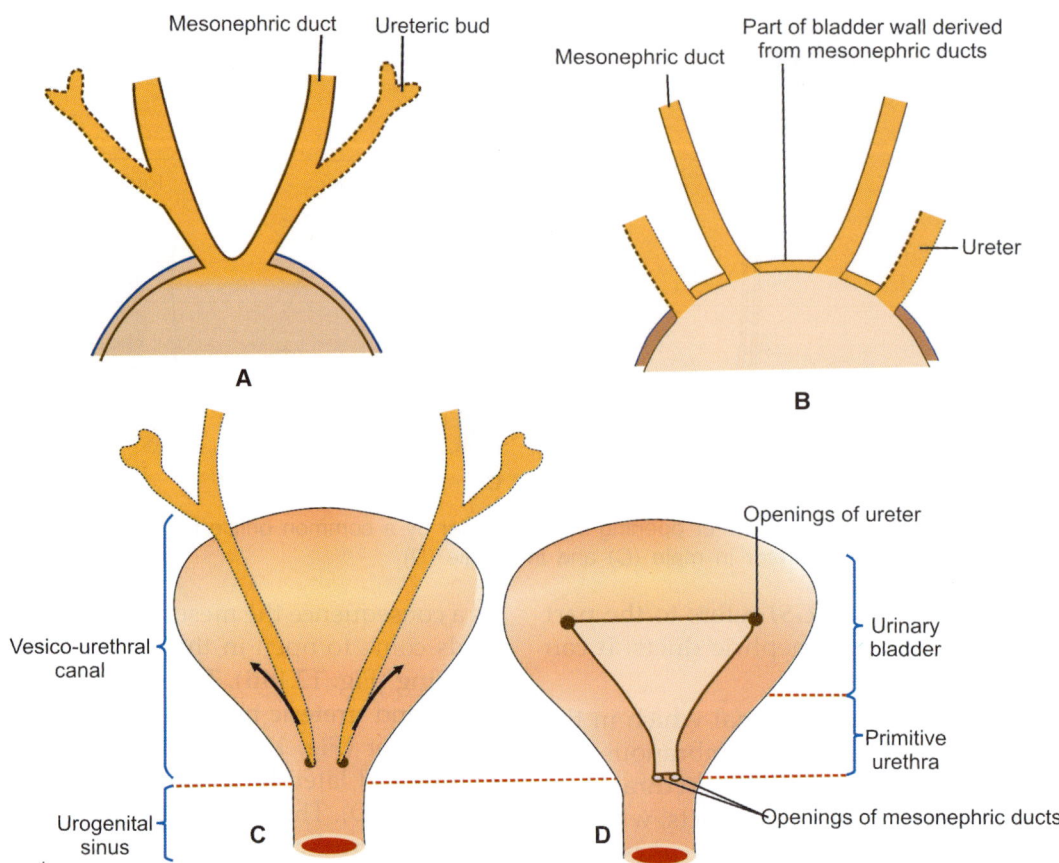

Fig. 12.14: Primitive urogenital sinus depicting: A, ureteric buds arising from lower part of mesonephric ducts; B, absorption of lower part of mesonephric duct into urogenital sinus leading to separate openings of ureteric buds and mesonephric ducts; C and D internal location of openings of ureteric buds and mesonephric ducts on the dorsal wall of vesicourethral canal initial stage and later stage, respectively.

the urinary bladder. However, recently it is believed that, this area is later over grown by the surrounding endodermal cells.

- *Allantois,* a vestigial structure and initially bladder is continuous with it. The most proximal small part of allantois is absorbed to form the mucosa of apex of the bladder. Most of the allantois soon constricts to form a thick fibrous cord called the *urachus,* which extends from the apex of bladder to the umbilicus. In the adult, the *median umbilical ligament* represents the urachus.

Musculature and serous wall of the urinary bladder are derived from the splanchnic layer of lateral plate mesoderm which surrounds the endodermal cloaca.

Development of urethra

Female urethra

Female urethra is mainly developed from the caudal part of vesico-urethral canal (endodermal). The absorbed mesonephric ducts (mesoderm) forms its posterior wall (Fig. 12.15A). In general, development of female urethra corresponds with the development of prostatic part of male urethra above the level of colliculus seminalis (Figs 12.15 A and B).

Male urethra

Three parts of male urethra, prostatic, membranous, and penile (spongy) part are developed as below (Fig. 12.15):

1. ***Prostatic urethra*** develops as below:
   - *Prostatic urethra above the opening of ejaculatory ducts,* corresponds to the female urethra and as described above, develops from the caudal part of the vesico-urethral canal and absorbed part of mesonephric ducts.
   - *Prostatic urethra below the opening of ejaculatory ducts* develops from the pelvic part of definitive urogenital sinus (endodermal).

2. ***Membraneous urethra,*** like lower part of prostatic urethra, develops from the pelvic part of the definitive urogenital sinus (endodermal).

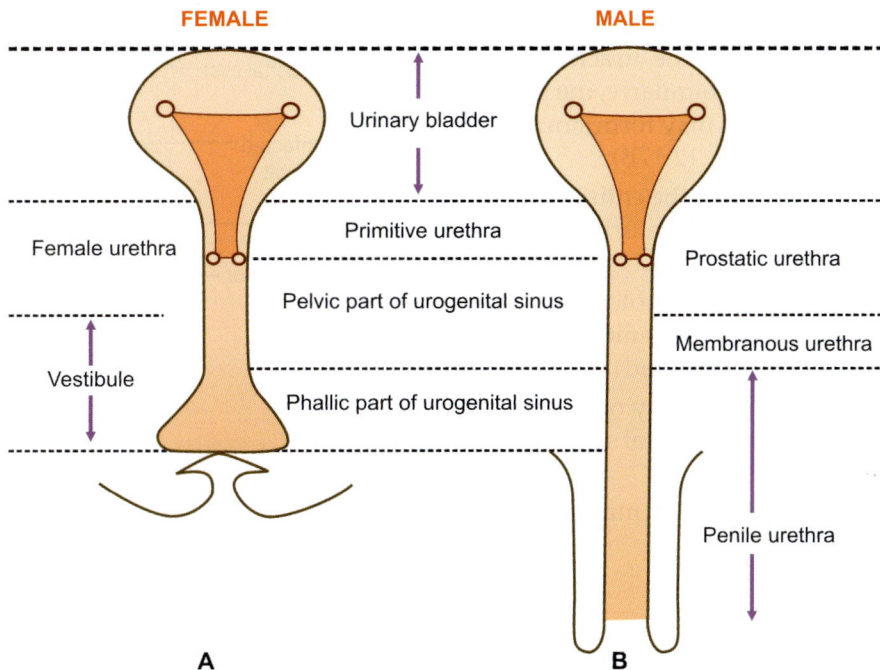

Fig. 12.15: Development of female (A) and male (B) urethra.

3. *Penile (spongy) urethra* develops from two sources:
   - *Penile urethra except the terminal part* develops from the phallic part of definitive urogenital sinus (endodermal). For details see development of penis (page 199).
   - *Terminal part of penile urethra,* that lies in the glans of the penis, is derived from a solid cord of *ectodermal cells* that grows from the glans and joins rest of the penile (spongy) urethra.

Connective tissue and smooth muscles of urethra

Connective tissue and smooth muscles of urethra, both in males and females, are derived from splanchnic mesoderm.

Anomalies of urinary bladder and urethra

Anomalies of urinary bladder

1. *Agenesis,* i.e. urinary bladder may be completely absent.
2. *Duplicated,* i.e. double urinary bladder may be present.
3. *Hour glass bladder,* i.e. the bladder is divided into two compartments because of a constriction in the middle (Fig. 12.16A).
4. *Ectopia vesicae* also known as *exstrophy of bladder* is characterised by deficient anterior wall and exposure and protusion of the posterior wall of the bladder with a ventral body wall defect (Fig. 12.16B). It occurs due to lack of mesodermal migration into the region between the umbilicus

and genital tubercle, followed by rupture of the thin layer of ectoderm. The anomaly is rare, occurring about once in 10,000 to 40,000 births. It chiefly occurs in males and may be associated with:
- Epispadias,
- Wide separation of pubic bones,
- Penis may be divided into two parts, and
- Two halves of the scrotum may be widely separated.

5. *Urachal anomalies,* which may develop from the remnants of the epithelial lining of urachus include:
   - *Urachal cyst* is formed when the proximal and distal parts of allantoic diverticulum obliterate and the middle part remain patent (Fig. 12.17A).

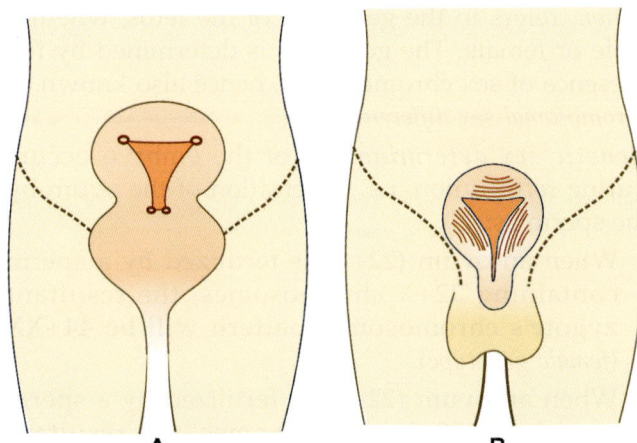

Fig. 12.16: Anomalies of urinary bladder: A, hour-glass bladder; and B, ectopia vesicae.

- *Urachal sinus.* The patent inferior end of the urachus may dilate to form the urachal sinus that opens into the bladder. Similarly, the patent superior end of the urachus may form sinus that opens at the umbilicus (Fig. 12.17B).
- *Urachal fistula* is formed when the entire urachus remains patent. In this condition urine escapes from the umbilicus (Fig. 12.17C).

6. *Congenital megacystis,* i.e. a pathological large bladder, which results from a congenital disorder of the metanephric bud (ureteric bud).
7. *Congenital recto-vesical fistula* may occur due to incomplete development of uro-rectal septum (see page 170).
8. *Congenital vesico-vaginal fistula* may occur in females (see page 197).

Congenital anomalies of urethra

1. *Urethral stenosis* may occur at its junction with the bladder.
2. *Diverticulae* may be present in the urethra
3. *Duplicated urethra* (partial or complete) may occur
4. *Urethral fistulae,* e.g. recto-urethral, (see page 170) and vagino-urethral (see page 197),
5. *Hypospadias* and *epispadias* (see page 200).

DEVELOPMENT OF GENITAL SYSTEM

In human embryo development of genital system involves two processes:
- Sex determination, and
- Sex differentiation

SEX DETERMINATION

Sex determination also known as *genetic differentiation,* refers to the genotype of the fetus, whether male or female. The genotype is determined by the presence of sex chromosomes, hence also known as *chromosomal sex differentiation.*

Genetic sex determination of the embryo occurs during fertilization, i.e. penetration of the ovum by the sperm as:

- When an ovum (22+X) is fertilized by a sperm containing 22+X chromosomes, the resultant zygote's chromosomal pattern will be 44+XX (*female genotype*).
- When an ovum (22+X) is fertilized by a sperm containing 22+Y chromosomes, the resultant zygote's chromosomal pattern will be 44+XY (male genotype).

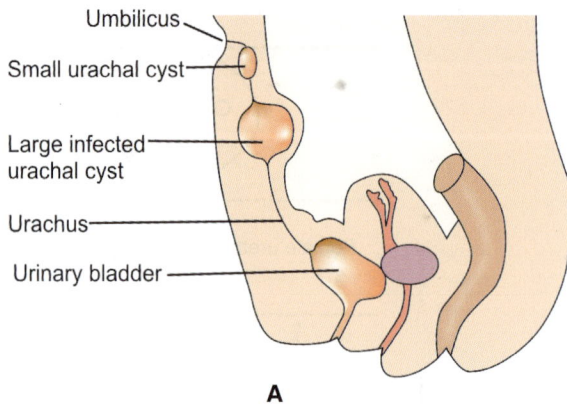

A

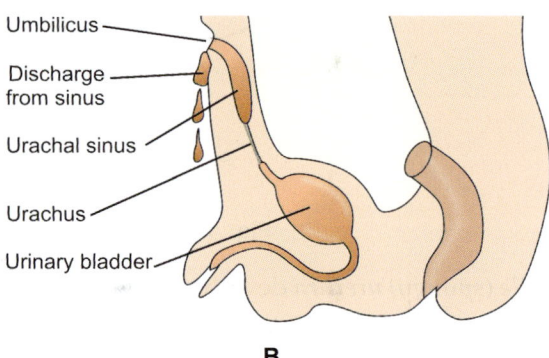

B

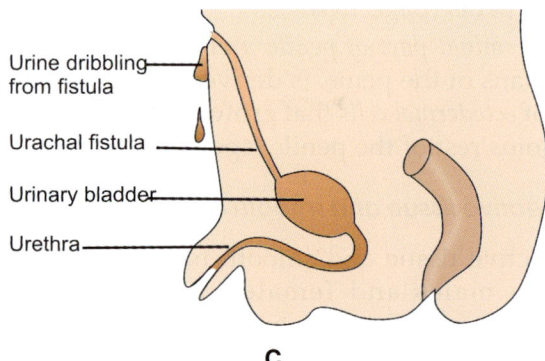

C

Fig. 12.17: Urachal anomalies: A, urachal cyst; B, urachal sinus; and C, urachal fistula.

- The human Y-chromosome is smaller than the X chromosomes. The sperms containing the Y chromosomes are lighter and able to swim faster up in the female genital tract, thus reaching the ovum rapidly. This probably accounts for the fact that the number of males born is slightly greater than the number of females.

SEX DIFFERENTIATION

After the sex determination (genotype sex) during fertilization, the normal sex differentiation in the embryo proceeds sequentially. The stages of sex differentiation are:

- Gonadal differentiation (development), and
- Genital differentiation (development).

DEVELOPMENT OF GONADS AND GENITAL DUCT SYSTEM

INDIFFERENT GONADS

Gonadal differentiation or *gonadogenesis* refers to formation of gonads, i.e. testes in males and ovaries in females. Gonadal sex differentiation is dependent on the genotype of the embryo.

Genital ridge or the urogenital ridge (the condensation of mesenchymal tissue present on each side near the adrenal glands) is the site where gonads develop.

Primordial germ cells are developed in the 4th week by proliferation of endodermal cells of the dorsal wall of *hindgut*. These cells are initially bipotential and migrate dorsocranially through the dorsal mesentery of the gut (Fig. 12.18).

The primordial germ cells migrate into the genital ridge, where proliferation of both germinal and nongerminal cells leads to formation of bipotential gonads.

Bipotential gonads. Bipotential gonads are also known as primordial or primitive or indifferent or ambisexual gonads. In human embryo these can be identified after 30 days of fertilization. Upto 6 weeks of gestation the bipotential gonads are identical in both sexes and have the rudiments of both male and female gonads.

Structure: The bipotential gonad consists of a medulla, a cortex and primordial germ cells. The germ cells are embedded in the layer of cortical epithelium surrounding a core of medullary mesenchymal tissue (Fig. 12.19).

Fate of indifferent gonds. Depending upon the genotype of human embryo, the indifferent gonads give rise to either testis or ovary.

INDIFFERENT GENITAL DUCT SYSTEM

During 5th and 6th weeks, the genital system in the human embryo is in indifferent state. In this stage, both male and female embryos have two pairs of genital ducts:

- Mesonephric ducts, and
- Paramesonephric ducts.

Mesonephric ducts

As described earlier (see page 175) the mesonephric ducts, also known as Wolffian ducts as the urine draining ducts of the mesonephric kidney, which are later incorporated into the genital system.

Fate of mesonephric ducts

- *In male embryo,* the mesonephric ducts and the remaining mesonephric tubules play an essential role in the development of male reproductive system (see page 175).
- *In female embryo,* the mesonephric ducts mostly degenerate, the only remnant being the duct of epoophoron (duct of Gartner), a vestigial part present in the broad ligament.

Paramesonephric ducts

Paramesonephric ducts (Müllerian ducts) develop in both male and female human embryo as a longitu-

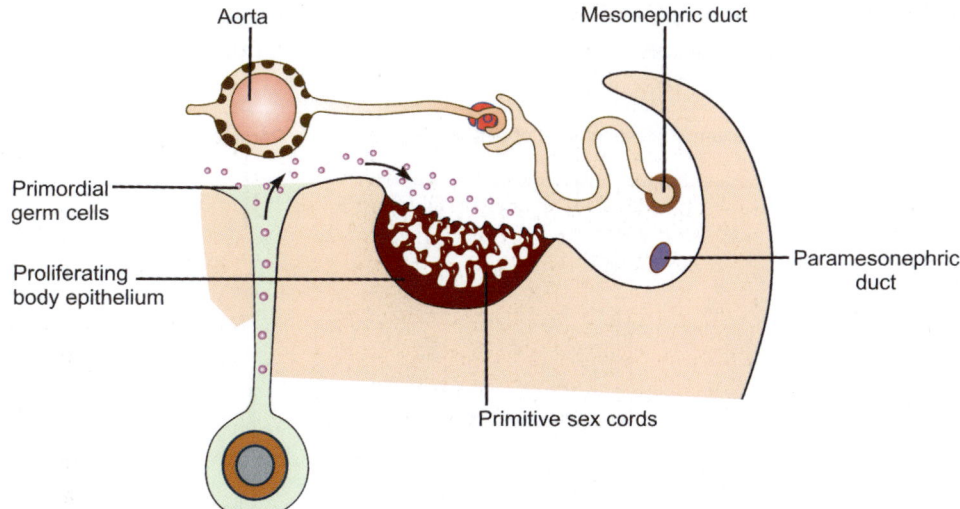

Fig. 12.18: Migration of primordial germ cells from the dorsal wall of hindgut through its dorsal mesentery into the genital ridge.

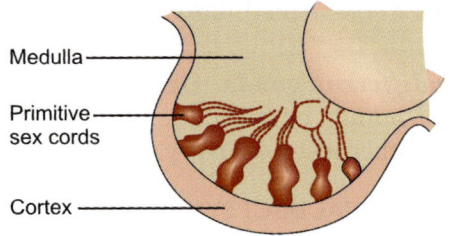

Fig. 12.19: Diagrammatic structure of human bipotential gonad.

dinal groove-like invagination of the coelomic epithelium during 6th week (Fig. 12.20). The margins of the groove fuse and convert it into a duct.

Parts of paramesonephric duct. A fully developed paramesonephric duct can be divided into three parts (Fig. 12.21):

- *Cephalic vertical part* which lies lateral to the mesonephric duct and its cranial end opens into the coelomic cavity with a funnel-like structure.
- *Intermedial horizontal part* of the paramesonephric duct runs horizontally medial wards ventral to the mesonephric ducts and enter into the urorectal septum.
- *Caudal vertical parts* of the ducts of two sides meet in the midline. Initially the two ducts are separated by a septum to form the *uterovaginal canal* (or uterine canal). The caudal end of this canal comes in contact with the dorsal wall of the phallic part of the definitive urogenital sinus and bulges as *Müllerian tubercle*.

DEVELOPMENT OF TESTES AND MALE DUCT SYSTEM

Development of testes

In genetic male (44+XY) embryo, the bipotential gonads begin to differentiate into testes at approximately 6th week. The Y-chromosome plays key role in the process of testicular differentiation.

Role of Y-chromosome in testicular differentiation

- Two transcription genes, one for testicular differentiation and another for formation of Müllerian duct inhibitory substance (MIS) are present on the Y-chromosome.
- The gene responsible for testicular differentiation is located near the tip of the short arm of Y-chromosome and is called SRY gene (SRY= Sex-determining region of the Y-chromosome).
- The SRY gene encodes the *testis determining factor* (TDF) which triggers the testicular differentiation.
- The TDF gene product causes Sertoli cell differentiation. Sertoli cell activity is critically important for all subsequent events in male sexual differentiation.

Process of testicular differentiation

At about 6th week of gestation, the testicular differentiation begins with the appearance of primitive seminiferous cords (sex cords) from the germinal epithelium covering the medulla of bipotential gonad (Fig. 12.19).

At about 7th week of gestation

- The solid sex cords are canalized to form seminiferous tubules,
- Meanwhile, a large number of Sertoli cells appear and get organized along the seminiferous tubules.
- The cortical region (from which female gonad develop) undergoes regression.

At about 8th week of gestation, Leydig (interstitial) cells appear in the interstitial spaces of seminiferous tubules and continue to proliferate. The Leydig cells are derived from the sex cords that are not canalized. The membrane of Leydig cells has receptors for human chorionic gonadotropins (HCG) and for luteinizing hormone (LH).

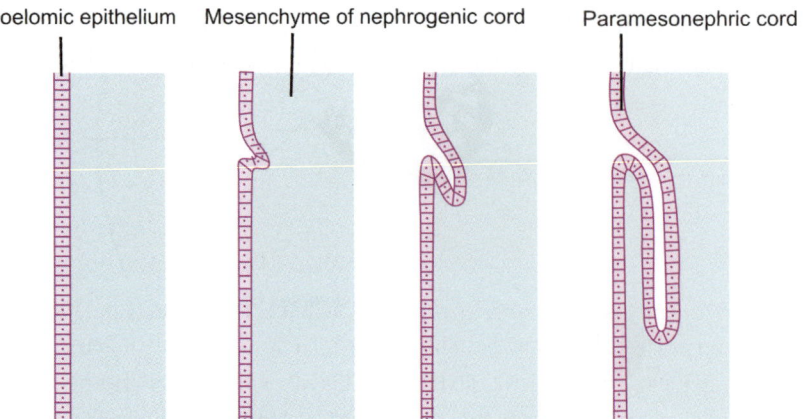

Fig. 12.20: Formation of paramesonephric ducts by invagination of coelomic epithelium.

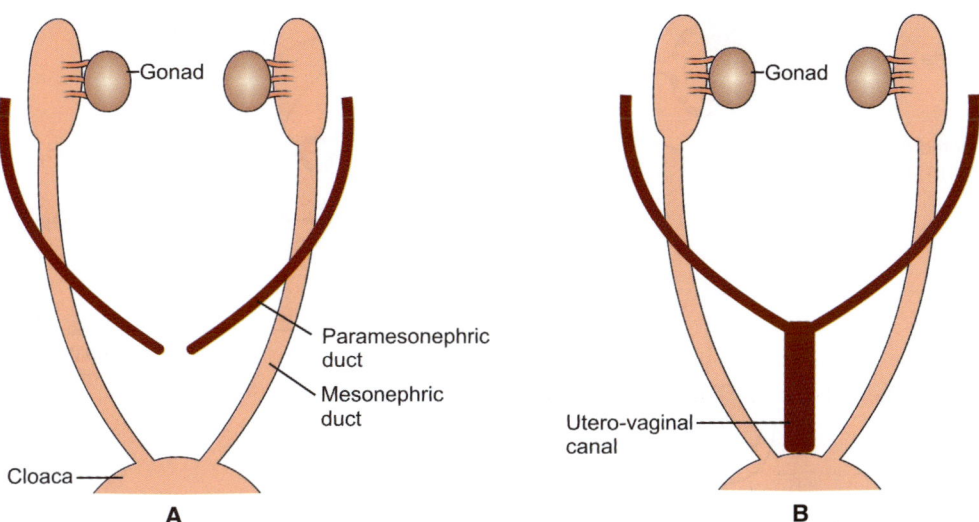

Fig. 12.21: Parts of paramesonephric ducts and their relationship with mesonephric ducts before (A) and after (B) fusion of their caudal vertical parts to form uterovaginal canal.

At about 9th week of gestation, the Leydig cells synthesize and secrete testosterone in response to HCG secreted by placenta.

At about 14th week of gestation, the number of Leydig cells is so much increased that they form more than half of the volume of the testes.

At the end of 16th week (4 months), the number of fetal Leydig cells decreases and at term only a few are present.

At about the 35th week of gestation, there occurs descent of testes through inguinal canal into scrotum. This marks the final stage of testicular differentiation.

Development of testicular tissue

Testis develops from the medulla of undifferen-tiated genital ridge, (bipotential gonad) while its cortex atrophies. Steps involved in the differentiation of testicular tissue are (Fig. 12.22):

Sex cords (primitive seminiferous cords) are formed by proliferation of the germinal epithelium covering the medulla of bipotential gonad at about 6th week.

Seminiferous tubules are formed by canalization of the sex cords which get detached from the surface of genital ridge.

- The primitive germ cells (sex cells) in the walls of tubules persist as the *spermatogonia.*
- *Seroli cells* differentiate from the medullary cells and get organized along the seminiferous tubules.

Rete-testes. The ends of the seminiferous tubules anastomose with one another to form the rete-testes.

Interstitial (Leydig) cells appear in the interstitial spaces around the seminiferous tubules. The leydig cells are derived from the sex cords that are not canalized.

Tunica albuginea, a dense layer of fibrous tissue is formed from the mesenchymal cells surrounding the developing testes. It completely separates the sex cords from the germinal epithelium, and there after the epithelium can make no further contribution to testicular tissue.

Development of duct system of testes

As described earlier (See page 175), some of the mesonephric tubules and mesonephric ducts take part in the formation of duct system of testes as below (Fig. 12.23):

Vasa efferentia is formed by the persisting meso-nephric tubules. The rete-testis establishes contact with these vasa efferentia.

Epididymis. The cranial part of mesonephric duct becomes highly coiled on itself and form the epididymis.

Ductus deferens is formed by the remaining distal part of the mesonephric duct.

Seminal vesicles arise as diverticulae from the lower end of mesonephric duct.

Ejaculatory ducts are formed by the part of meso-nephric ducts between the origin of seminal vesicle diverticulae and their openings, into the prostatic urethra.

Descent of testes

Journey of the testes from the site of their develop-ment to the final destination is as below (Fig. 12.24):

Lumbar region of the posterior abdominal wall is the area where the testes develop as retroperitoneal structures (Fig. 12.22A).

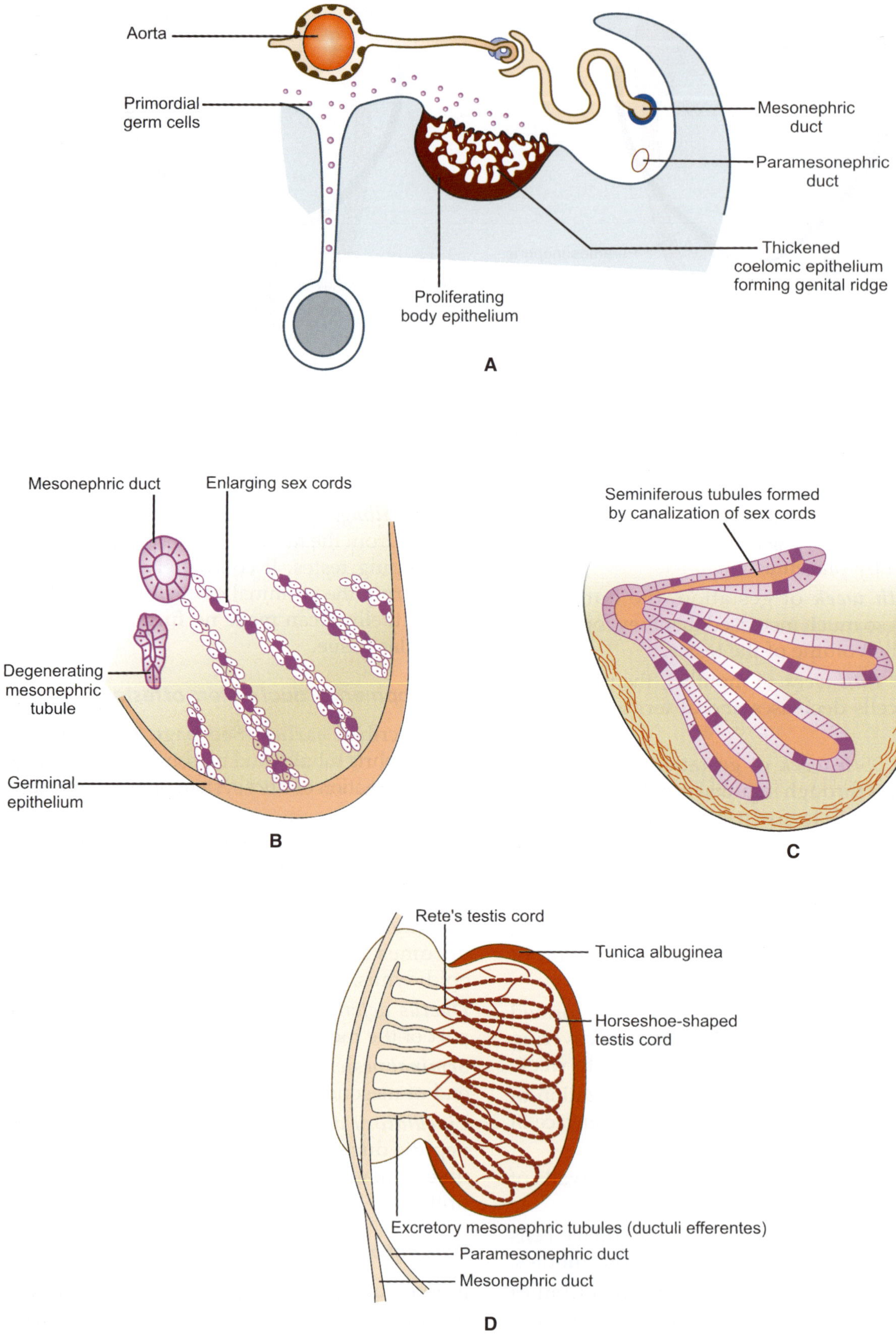

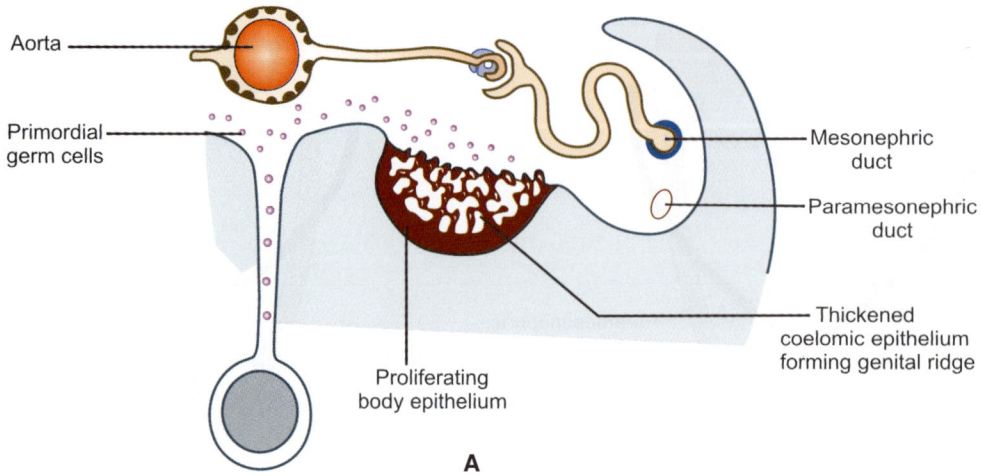

A

B

C

D

Fig. 12.22: Testicular differentiation: A, medulla of indifferent gonad showing proliferation of surface epithelium; B, formation of sex cords; C, formation of seminiferous tubules; D, formation of rete's-testis and tunica albuginea.

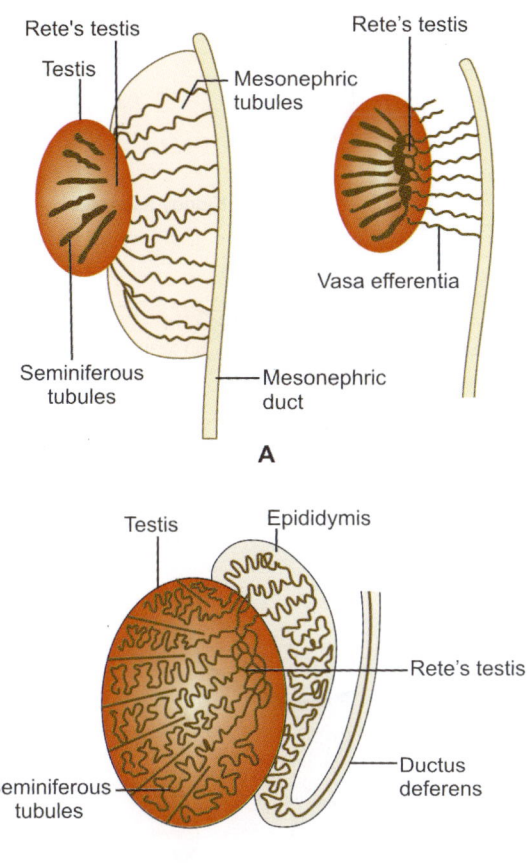

Fig. 12.23: Development of duct system of the testis: A, Vasa efferentia formed from the mesonephric tubules established connection with the rete's testis; B, Formation of epididymis, ductus deferens, seminal vesicle and ejaculatory duct from the mesonephric duct.

- *Urogenital mesentery* attaches each testis along with the mesonephros to the posterior abdominal wall by the end of 2nd month.
- *Mesorchium:* After the degeneration of mesonephros the urogenital mesentery becomes the mesorchium (mesentery of testis).
- *Caudal genital ligament* is the inguinal fold of peritoneum which extends from the caudal end of testis to the genital (secrotal) swelling.
- *Guberneaculum testis* refers to the band of mesenchymal condensation formed in the inguinal peritoneal fold. It initially extends from the caudal end of the testis to the inguinal region. After the test it starts descending, the extraabdominal portion of the guberneculum is formed which grows from the inguinal region towards the scrotal swelling. It plays important role in the descent of testis.

Iliac fossa is the region where the testes reach during 3rd month after they begin to descend. Here, the testes lie at the site of the deep inguinal ring upto the

7th month of intrauterine life. While the testis descends from the lumbar region to the iliac fossa, the metanephric (permanent) kidney ascends from the pelvis to the lumbar region. Eventually the vas deferens crosses ventral to the ureter close to superolateral angle of the base of urinary bladder, (Fig. 12.24B), since the ureteric bud shifts on the dorsolateral side of mesonephric duct.

Inguinal canal is formed by a fold of peritoneum which evaginates on each side of the midline into the ventral abdominal wall. This evagination further follow the course of gubernaculum testis into the scrotal swelling, where it is known as *processus vaginalis.* Inguinal canal is traversed by each testis during 7th month. At the time the testis passes through the inguinal canal, the extraabdominal portion of gubernaculum contracts the scrotal floor (Fig. 12.24C).

Scrotum is the final destination, where the testes reach at or shortly after birth (Fig. 12.24D) while traversing the inguinal canal to the scrotum, each testis is covered by the *processus vaginalis* and others layers from the abdominal wall which form the various coverings of testis as below (Fig. 12.25):

- *Tunica vaginalis* is a reflected fold of peritoneum from processus vaginalis the innermost covering in which the testis invaginates. The inner layer of tunica vaginalis which covers the testis is called *visceral layer* and the outer layer is called the *parietal layer.* The narrow canal connecting the lumen of tunica vaginalis with the peritoneal cavity is obliterated at birth or shortly thereafter.
- *Internal spermatic fascia* is the downward continuation of the transversalis fascia of anterior abdominal wall.
- *Cremasteric fascia and muscles* are derived from the internal abdominal oblique muscle.
- *External spermatic fascia* is the continuation of external abdominal oblique muscle into the scrotum.

Factors responsible for descent of testes

Though not exactly known, following factors are thought to play role in the descent of testes :

- *Enlargement of testes and atrophy of mesonephroi* allow downward movement of testes along the posterior abdominal wall.
- *Gubernaculum testis* as mentioned above, plays an important role in the descent of testes. Its intraabdominal portion guides the descent from the lumbar region to the inguinal ring. When the testis passes through the inguinal canal, the guber-

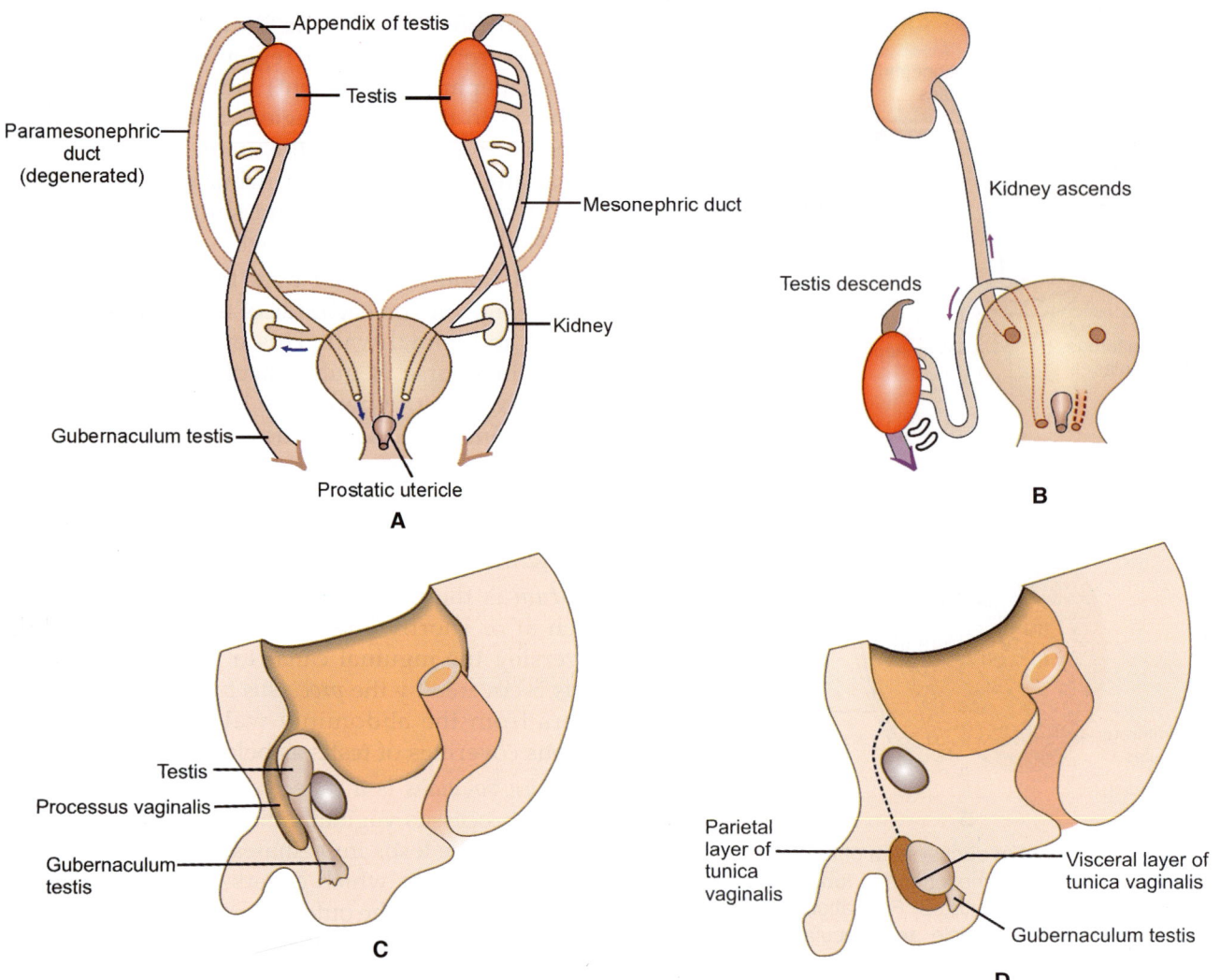

Fig. 12.24: Descent of testes: A, lumbar region; B, Iliac fossa; C, Inguinal canal; and D, scrotum.

naculum helps to dilate the canal. Extraabdominal portion of the gubernaculum guides the testis from the inguinal canal into the scrotum.

- *Atrophy of paramesonephric duct* induced by the *MIS*, enables the testes to move transabdominally to the deep inguinal rings.
- *Enlargement of processus vaginalis* guides the testis through inguinal canal into the scrotum
- *Increased intra-abdominal pressure* due to organ growth helps in passage of testis through the inguinal canal.
- *Differential growth of the abdominal wall* also plays some role in the descent of testes.
- *Contraction of arched fibres of internal oblique muscle* help in passage of testis through the inguinal canal.
- *Role of testicular hormones:* Testicular androgens are important driving force for descent. It is presumed that androgens act on the cell bodies of genito femoral nerve to release a peptide neurotrans-

mitter, which causes rhythmic contractions of cremasteric muscle. The contractions of cremasteric muscle pull the gubernaculum testis which helps in descent of testes.

Development of male glands

Prostate

Glandular part of prostate gland develops from multiple *endodermal buds* which arise from the prostatic urethra, i.e. from the caudal part of the vesico-urethral canal and from the pelvic part of the definitive urogenital sinus.

Fibromuscular part of the prostate develops from the surrounding mesenchyme.

Bulbo-urethral glands

Glandular tissue of these glands develop from the buds arising from the caudal part of the urogenital sinus.

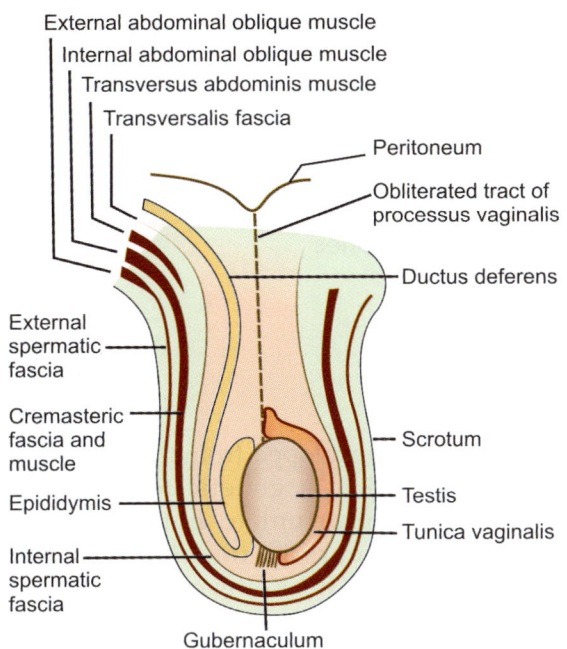

Fig. 12.25: Coverings of testis and the sources of their origin.

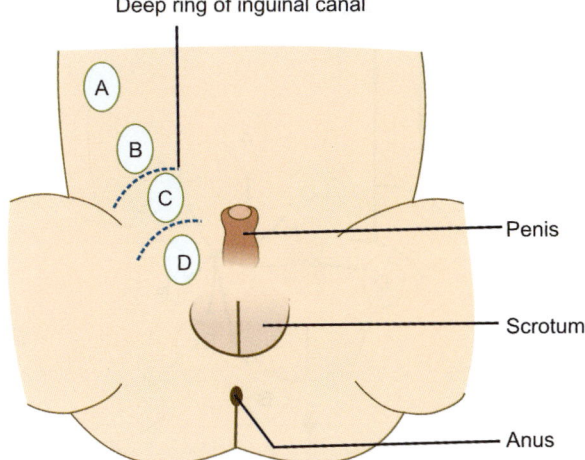

Fig. 12.26: Common sites of undescended testes (cryptorchidism): A, lumbar region; B, Iliac fossa; C, Inguinal canal; and D, upper part of scrotum.

Fibromuscular part develops from the surrounding mesenchyme.

Note. The bulbo-urethral glands of males correspond with the *Bartholin's* glands (greater vestibular glands) of females.

Anomalies of testes and male ductal system

Anomalies of testes

1. *Duplicated testes,* i.e. double testes may be present on one side or both sides.
2. *Synorchidism,* i.e. the two testes may be fused together.
3. *Cryptorchidism or undescended testis* occurs in about 3 to 4% of full term males and upto 30% of premature males.
   - May be bilateral (anorchidism) or unilateral (mono-orchidism).
   - May be completely undescended testis or partially descended testis.
   - Undescended testis may be located in the lumbar region, iliac fossa, in the inguinal canal or in the upper part of scrotum (Fig. 12.26).
   - Cause in most cases of cryptorchidism is unknown, but a deficiency of androgen production by fetal testis is an important factor.
   - Spermatogenesis often fails to occur in undescended testis.
   - Cryptorchidism is associated with an increased risk of developing testicular cancer.
   - Orchidopexy, i.e. surgical mobilisation of testis should be done as early as possible after birth.
4. *Ectopic testis.* After traversing the inguinal canal, the testis does not reach the scrotum and deviates from its usual path of descent. It occurs when a part of gubernaculum passes to an abnormal location and the testis follows it. Ectopic testis may occupy any of the following locations (Fig. 12.27):
   - *Interstitial ectopia,* i.e. external to aponeurosis of external oblique muscle (Fig. 12.27A).
   - *Perineal ectopia,* i.e. within the superficial perineal pouch (Fig. 12.27B).
   - *Prepenile ectopia,* i.e. dorsal to the penis in front of symphysis pubis (Fig. 12.27C).
   - *Crossed ectopia,* i.e. on the opposite side (Fig. 12.27D).
   - In the proximal part of the *medial thigh,* i.e. at the saphenous opening (Fig. 12.27E).
   - In the femoral canal (Fig. 12.27F).
   - Rarely, in the anterior superior iliac spine.
5. *Hydrocoele of testis,* i.e. collection of fluid in the processus vaginalis, may occur occasionally when the abdominal end of the processus vaginalis remains open (Fig. 12.28).
6. *Congenital inguinal hernia* may occur when the communication between the tunica vaginalis and the peritoneal cavity fails to close. A loop of intestine may herniate through it into the scrotum (Fig. 12.29).

Anomalies of duct system of testis

Failure of seminiferous tubules in establishing connection with the vas efferentia.

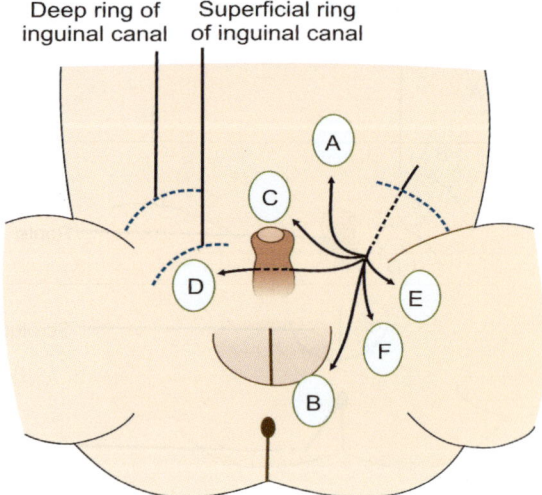

Fig. 12.27: Usual location of ectopic testis; A, interstitial ectopia; B, perineal ectopia; C, pre-penile ectopia; D, crossed ectopia; E, at saphenous ring; and F, in the femoral canal.

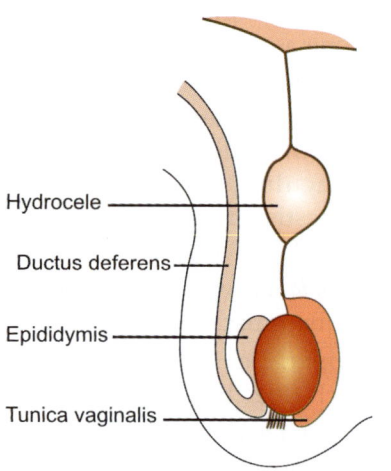

Fig. 12.28: Hydrocele of testis.

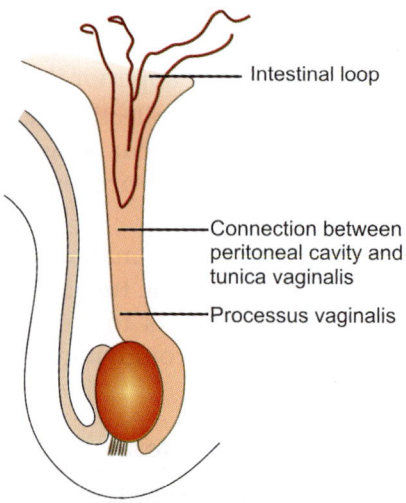

Fig. 12.29: Congenital inguinal hernia.

Ductus deferens may show following anomalies:

- *Absence,* which may be partial or complete, and unilateral or bilateral.
- *Failure to establish connection* with the epididymis.

DEVELOPMENT OF OVARIES AND FEMALE DUCT SYSTEM

Development of ovaries

Indifferent stage

See page 185.

Definitive ovary

Definitive ovary is developed from the cortex of each indifferent gonad in a genetic female (44+XX) embryos. It is important to note that ovarian differentiation occurs in the absence of testis determining factor (TDF). Key events are: (Fig. 12.30):

- *Primordial female germ cells* which have migrated from the endodermal wall of the hindgut are present beneath the surface epithelium in the indifferent gonad.
- *Medullary sex cords* containing germ cells project from the surface epithelium towards the medulla and form cell clusters known as rete ovaries (Fig. 12.30A). Later they disappear and are replaced by a vascular stroma that forms *ovarian medulla.* Thus rete ovaries degenerates and fail to communicate with mesonephric tubules (e.g. rete's testis).
- *Cortical sex cords* (2nd generation of cords) are formed from the surface epithelium in 7th week only in a genetic female embryo. These project only upto cortex of the developing gonad (Fig. 12.30B).
- ***Primordial follicle.*** Soon the cortical sex cords become broken into small masses by the invading mesenchyme. The cells of each mass surround one primordial germ cell (oogonium) to form a primordial follicle. Later the oogonium undergoes meiotic division to form oocyte, which is the end point of ovarian differentiation (Fig. 12.30C).
- *Interstitial gland cells* later differentiate from the mesenchyme of gonad.
- *Tunica albuginea* is not a prominent feature in the female gonad; the surface epithelium may contribute to the ovary even in postnatal life, hence it is named the germinal epithelium.
- *At birth* (Fig. 12.30D), each ovary contains about 2 million primary follicles.

Descent of ovary

Lumbar region of the posterior abdominal wall is the area where the ovaries develop as retroperitoneal structures (Fig. 12.31A and B).

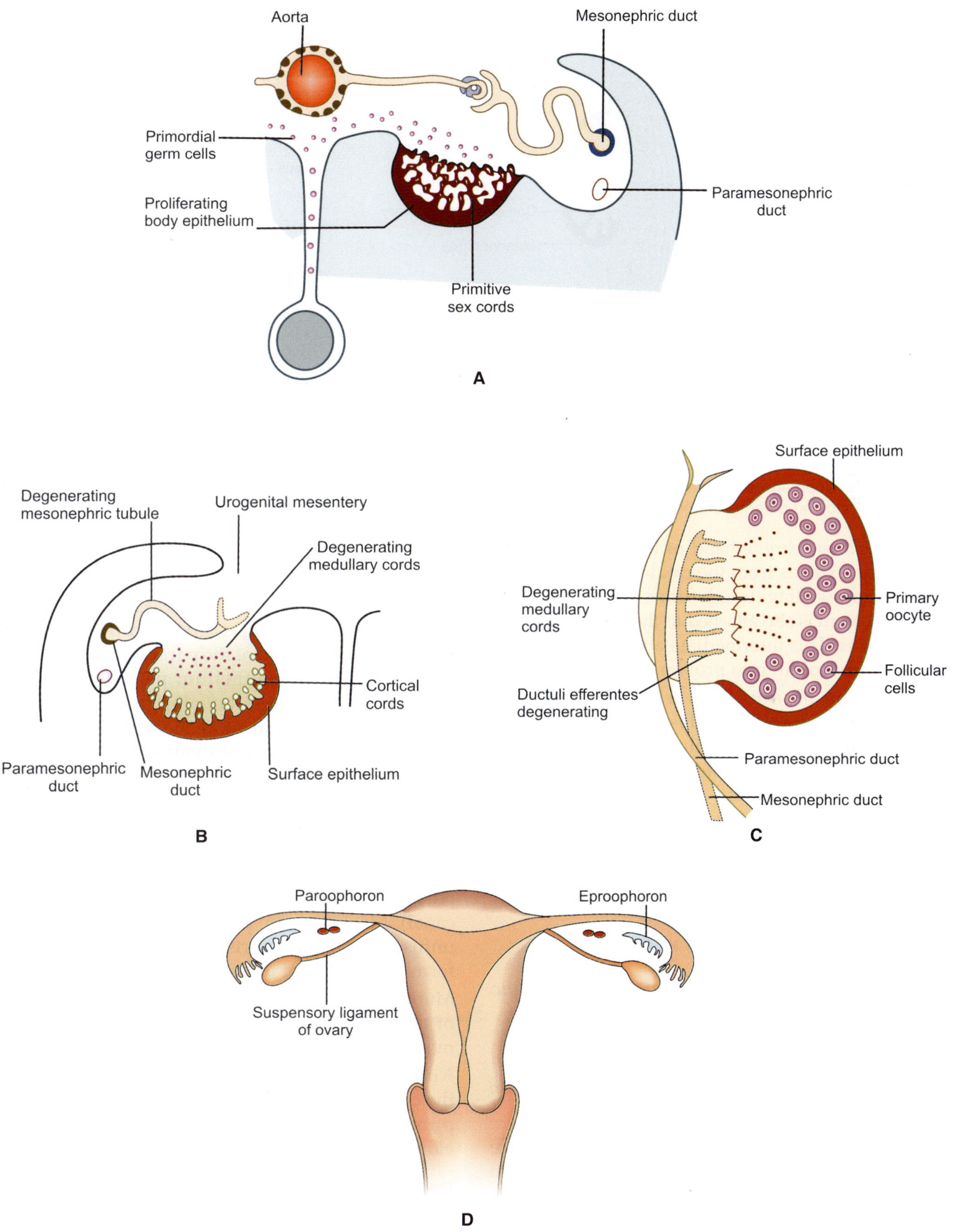

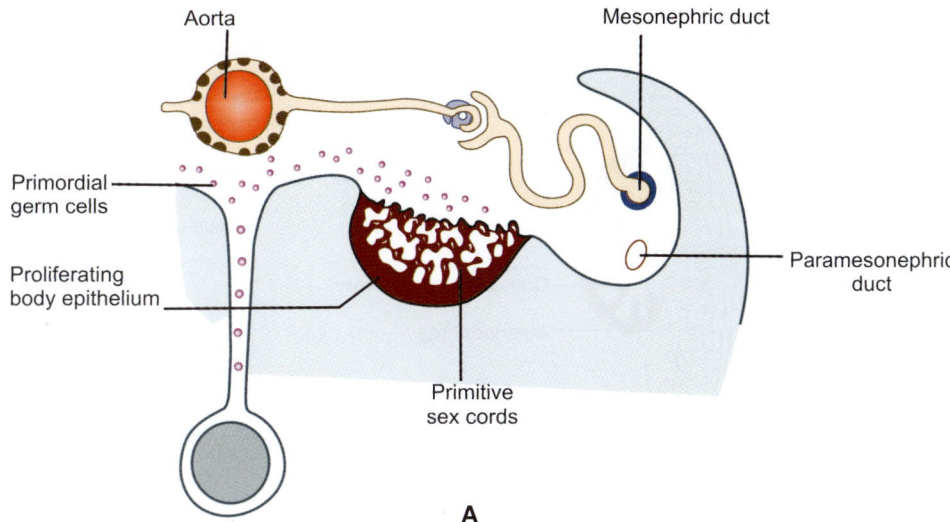

Aorta

Mesonephric duct

Primordial germ cells

Proliferating body epithelium

Paramesonephric duct

Primitive sex cords

A

Degenerating mesonephric tubule

Urogenital mesentery

Degenerating medullary cords

Cortical cords

Paramesonephric duct

Mesonephric duct

Surface epithelium

B

Surface epithelium

Degenerating medullary cords

Primary oocyte

Ductuli efferentes degenerating

Follicular cells

Paramesonephric duct

Mesonephric duct

C

Paroophoron

Eproophoron

Suspensory ligament of ovary

D

Fig. 12.30: Ovarian differentiation: A, indifferent gonads; B, transverse section of the developing ovary at 7th week showing degeneration of the primitive (medullary) sex cords and formation of the cortical cords; C, developing ovary at 5 months showing formation of oocytes and primordial follicles; D, ovary at birth.

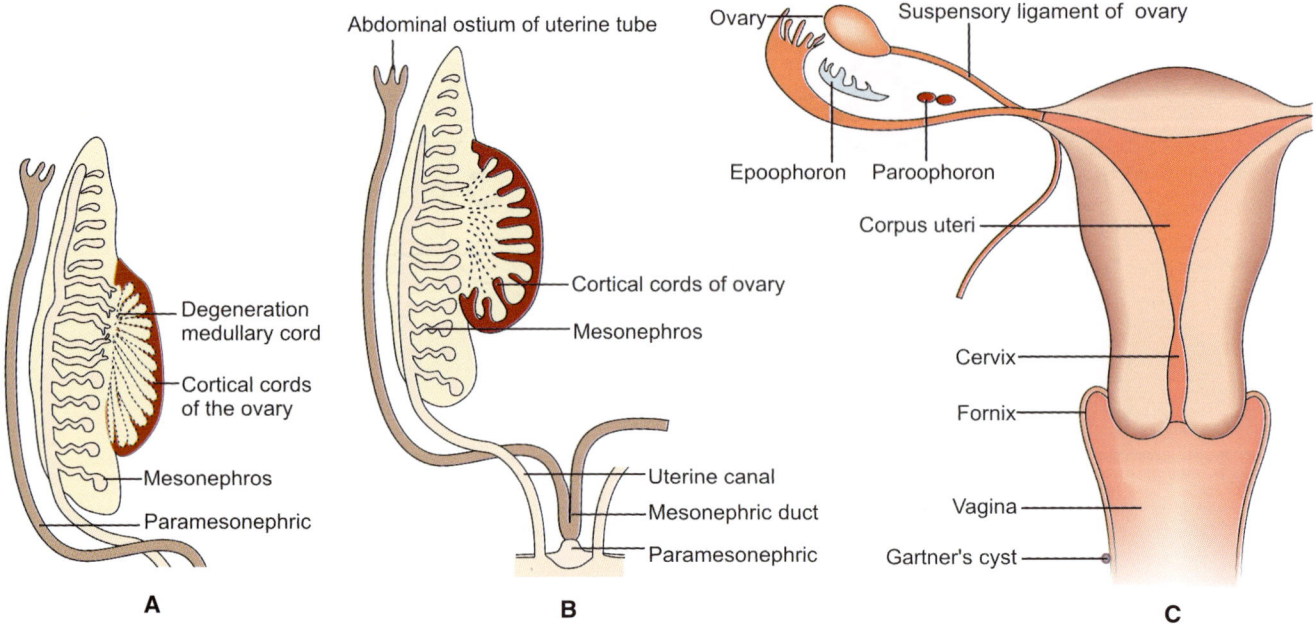

Fig. 12.31: Development of female internal genitalia: A, schematic frontal view to show the relationship of developing ovary with mesonephric and paramesonephric ducts; B and C, profile of developing uterine tubes before and after descent of ovaries.

- *Gubernaculum ovary*, a band of mesenchymal condensation extends from the caudal end of ovary to the genital swelling (which forms labia major). The gubernaculum is also attached to the angle of developing uterus. This intermediate attachment divides the gubernaculum into proximal and distal parts.

Area just below the rim of true pelvis forms the final destination of ovary after descent (Fig. 12.31C). Attachment of the gubernaculum to the developing uterus is responsible for the descent of ovary upto true pelvis. After descent:

- *Ligament of ovary* is formed by the proximal part of gubernaculum, and
- *Round ligament of uterus* is formed by the distal part of gubernaculum.

Development of female ductal system (internal genitalia)
Formation of paramesonephric and mesonephric ducts.

Revise from page 175 and 185.

Derivatives of paramesonephric (Müllarian) ducts in female

In the genetic female fetus (44 +XX), in the absence of Müllarian inhibiting substance (MIS), the Müllarian ducts (paramesonephric or female ducts) proliferate and give rise to:

- Uterine tubes,
- Uterus, and
- Vagina (upper two third).

Development of uterine tubes

Uterine tubes develop from the cephalic vertical and most of horizontal parts (i.e. infused parts) of the para mesonephric ducts (Fig. 12.31A and B). The original points of invagination of the parameso-nephric ducts into the coelomic epithelium persist as the *pelvic ostium* of uterine tubes opening into the peritoneal cavity. The fimbria around the ostium are formed later. With the descent of ovaries, the uterine tubes fall in the pelvic cavity and undergo for the most part a horizontal course (Fig. 12.31C).

Development of uterus

Epithelium of entire uterus is derived from the cranial part of fused paramesonephric ducts (utero-vaginal canal). Most cephalic point of fusion and adjoining unfused horizontal parts of paramesonephric ducts form the fundus of uterus (Fig. 12.31A and B).

Myometrium, i.e. musculature of uterus and stroma of endometrium are derived from the surrounding mesenchyme.

Note. In the fetus and earlier years of postnatal life the cervical part is larger than the body of uterus. At puberty, the body of the uterus becomes more elongated and larger than cervix.

Development of vagina

Vagina develop from two sources (Fig. 12.32):

- *Caudal part of utero-vaginal canal* forms upper two-thirds of vagina including the *vaginal fornices* (wing like expansion of vagina around the uterus.

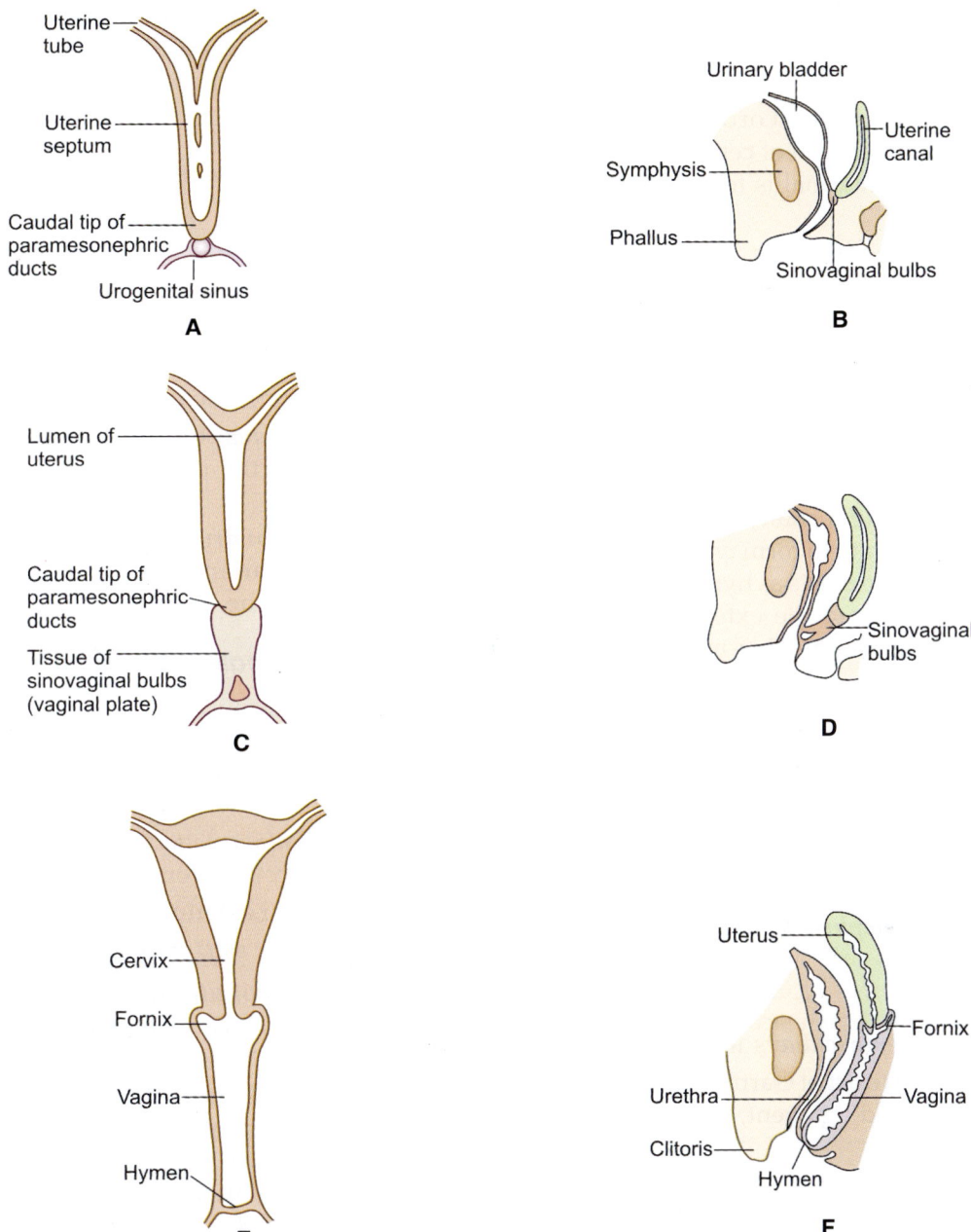

Fig. 12.32: Development of vagina: A and B, formation of sinovaginal bulbs from proliferation of endodermal lining of urogenital sinus as seen in front view and sagittal section respectively; C and D, formation of vaginal plate by fusion of sinovaginal bulbs and formation of vaginal cord by proliferation of mesodermal cells from the blind caudal end of utero-vaginal canal as seen in front view and sagittal section, E and F, front and sagittal view of formation of vaginal canal, vaginal fornices and hymen.

- *Sinovaginal bulb* forms lower one-third of the vagina.

Main steps in the development of vagina are as follows:

- *Formation of sinovaginal bulb.* The sinovaginal bulbs arise as two swellings by proliferation of endodermal cells of phallic part of urogenital sinus in the region where the blind lower end of the uterovaginal canal projects into the urogenital sinus (Fig. 12.32A and B).

- *Formation of vaginal plate.* The sinovaginal bulbs soon fuse to form a solid *vaginal plate*, which later assumes cylindrical outline as the cells proliferate (Fig. 12.32C and D). Proliferation continue at the cranial end of the vaginal plate, increasing the distance between the urogenital sinus and caudal end of the utero-vaginal canal.

- *Formation of vaginal cord.* Simultaneous with the formation of vaginal plate, the mesodermal cells from the blind caudal end of utero-vaginal canal proliferate and convert it into a solid bar of tissue called *vaginal cord* (Fig. 12.32C and D).

- *Formation of vaginal canal.* The solid vaginal plate fuses with solid vaginal cord which are later canalized by degeneration of central cellular mass and thus the vaginal canal is formed (Fig. 12.32E and F).

- *Formation of vaginal fornices.* Upper end of the vaginal canal advances around the cervix to form *vaginal fornices* (Fig. 12.32E and F).

- *The hymen.* The lower end of the vaginal canal remains separated from the urogenital sinus by the hymen a bilaminar membrane consisting of inner layer of vaginal cells and outer layer of epithelial lining of urogenital sinus (Fig. 12.32E and F). During perinatal life, usually the central cells of the hymen degenerate to form *orifice of hymen* and the peripheral part persists as hymenal membrane. The vagina opens into the exterior through the *vestibule* (a cleft between labia minora) (see page 200).

Derivatives of mesonephric (Wolffian) ducts in female.

In the genetic female fetus (44 +XX), due to absence of testosterone the mesonephric (wolffian) ducts and the mesonephric tubules mostly degenerate except for the following (Fig. 12.33):

Derivatives of mesonephric tubules include:
- Epoophoron, and
- Paroophoron.

Derivates of mesonephric ducts include:
- *Duct of epoophoron* (duct of Gartner), a vestigial part present in the broad ligament, and

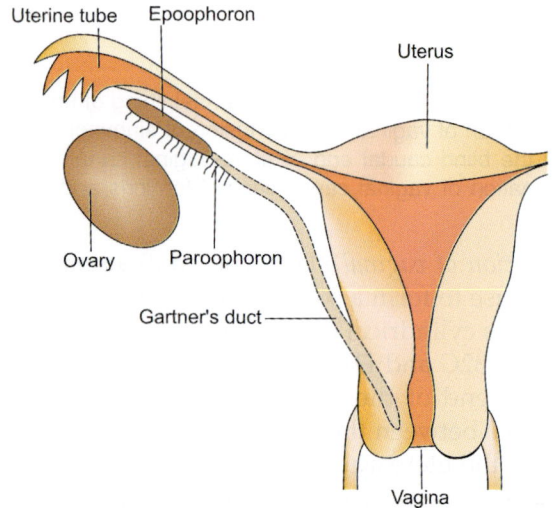

Fig. 12.33: Derivatives of mesonephric tubules and mesonephric (Wolffian) duct in female.

- *Ureteric buds,* which arise from the caudal part of mesonephric ducts and take part in the formation of collecting system of kidney as described on page 175.

Anomalies of ovaries and female ductal system (internal genitalia)

Anomalies of ovaries

1. **Absence of ovary** on one side or both may occur rarely.
2. **Duplicated ovary,** i.e. double ovary may be present on one or both sides.
3. **Ectopic ovaries,** e.g. one or both ovaries may descend into the inguinal canal or even into the labia majora.
4. **Teratoma of ovary,** i.e. a tumour like condition in which the ovarian cells differentiate into various tissues like bone, cartilage, hair, etc.

Anomalies of female duct system (internal genitalia)

I. **Anomalies of uterine tubes** include:
   1. *Absence of uterine tubes* segmental or complete may occur on one side or both sides.
   2. *Duplication of uterine tubes* partial or complete may occur on one or both sides.
   3. *Atresia,* i.e. failure of the tube to canalize
   4. *Accessory ostia* may be present in the tubes

II. **Anomalies of uterus** includes:
   1. *Absence of uterus* may occur rarely.
   2. *Duplication of uterus,* may be complete or partial. Duplication results from lack of fusion of paramesonephric ducts which may be partial or complete. Some forms of duplicate uterus are as below:
      - *Uterus didelphys,* an extremely rare anomaly results from complete failure of fusion of paramesonephric ducts. It is characterized by double uterus, double cervix and double vaginal canal (Fig. 12.34A). In marsupials, *didelphys* is of normal occurrence.
      - *Uterus bicornis,* a relatively common anomaly, is characterised by presence of double uterus and double cervix opening in single vagina (Fig. 12.34B). This condition is normal in many mammals below the primates.
      - *Uterus arcuatus* is a milder form of uterus duplication in which there is slight indentation in the middle (Fig. 12.34C).

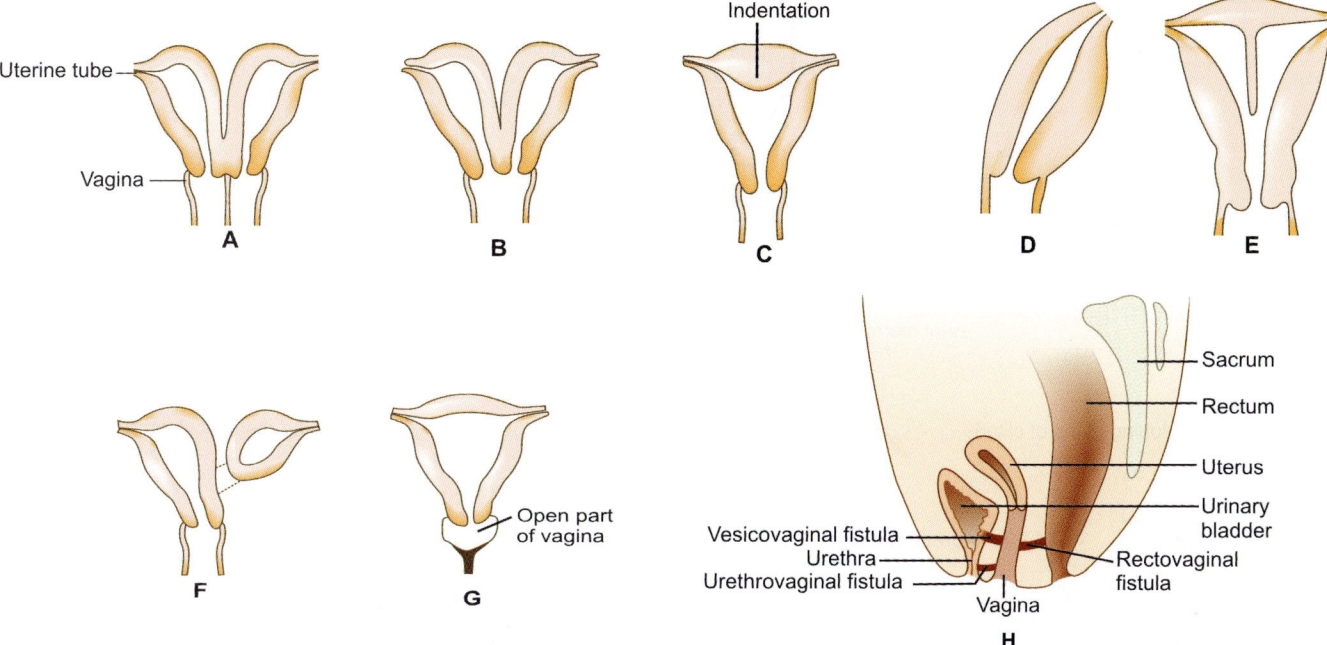

Fig. 12.34: Some anomalies of uterus and vagina: A, uterus didelphys, B, uterus bicornis; C, uterus arcuatus; D, unicornuate uterus; E, septate uterus; F, uterus bicornil unicollis; G, atresia of vagina; H, vaginal fistulae (vesicovaginal, urethrovaginal and rectovaginal).

3. **Unicornuate uterus,** i.e. one half of the uterus is absent (Fig. 12.34D). This occurs due to unilateral suppression of paramesonephric duct.

4. **Septate uterus:** Externally the uterus looks normal but its lumen is completely divided by a septum into two parts (Fig. 12.34E). In *subseptate uterus* the division is incomplete.

5. **Atresia of uterus** may be complete or incomplete. Example is:
   - *Uterus bicornis unicollis* with one rudimentary horn (Fig. 12.34F).

III. **Anomalies of vagina** include:
   1. *Duplication of vagina:* This anomaly is usually associated with duplication of uterus (didelphys, see above, Fig. 12.34A). Double vagina is formed when the sinovaginal bulbs fail to fuse.
   2. *Vaginal atresia* occurs when the sinovaginal bulbs fail to develop. In this condition a small vaginal pouch originating from the paramesonephric ducts usually surrounds the opening of cervix (Fig. 12.34G).
   3. *Septate vagina* occurs due to persistence of the median partition in the caudal part of uterovaginal canal.
   4. *Imperforate hymen* occur due to failure of disintegration of the central cells of Müllerian eminence. After puperty, the imperforate hymen leads to crypto-menorrhoea.

5. *Vaginal fistulae* include (Fig. 12.34H):
   - *Vesicovaginal fistula,* i.e. abnormal communication of vagina with urinary bladder. It occurs due to rupture of Müllerian eminence in the vesicourethral part of cloaca, instead of the urogenital sinus.
   - *Rectovaginal fistula,* i.e. abnormal communication of vagina with rectum. It occurs when the Müllerian eminence projects into the rectal segment of the cloaca due to incomplete development of the urorectal septum.

DEVELOPMENT OF EXTERNAL GENITALIA

INDIFFERENT EXTERNAL GENITALIA

Common anlagen from which both male and female external genitalia develop include (Fig. 12.35):
- *Phallus part of urogenital sinus,* which has been described earlier (page 181).
- *Urogenital membrane,* refers to the ventral part of the cloacal membrane which bounds the phallus (caudal) part of definitive urogenital sinus (see page 181, Fig. 12.13).
- *Cloacal folds:* In the 3rd week the mesenchyme cells originating in the region of primitive streak migrate around the cloacal membrane to form a pair of slightly elevated folds, the cloacal folds (Fig.

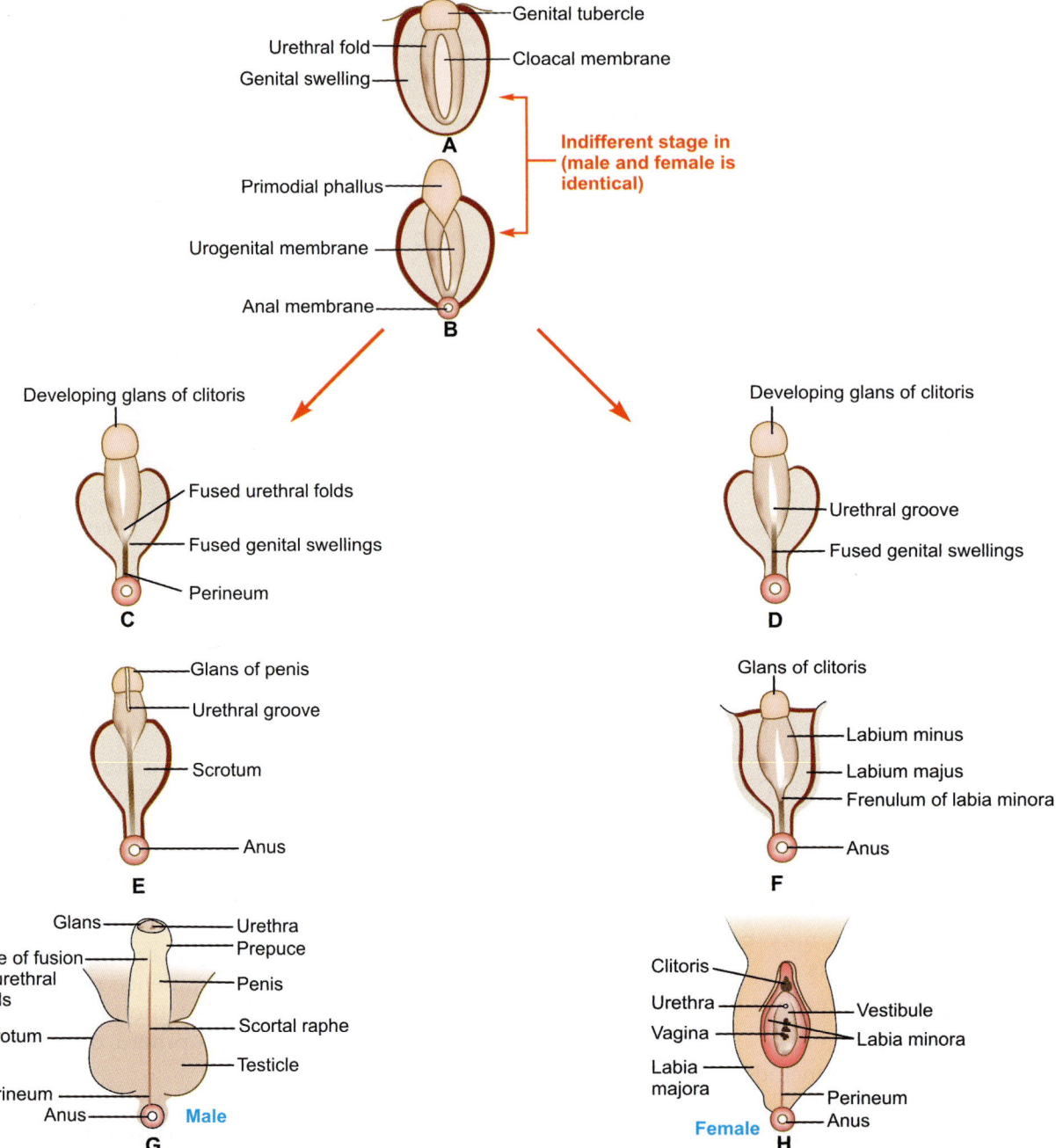

Fig. 12.35: Development of male and female external genitalia: A and B, indifferent stage of external genitalia. Common analgen include phallic part of urogenital sinus bounded by urogenital membrane, cloacal folds, genital tubercle and genital swellings; C, E, G, stages in development of male external genitalia; D,F,H, stages in development of female external genitalia.

12.35A). In the 6th week, the cloacal folds are divided into two parts:

– *Urethral folds*, the anterior parts, and
– *Anal folds*, the posterior parts (Fig. 12.35B).

• *Genital tubercle*, a midline structure, situated between the urogenital membrane and the lower part of the anterior abdominal wall is formed by union of the cloacal folds cranial to the cloacal membrane.

• *Genital swellings* (a right and a left) appear on each side of urethral folds (Fig. 12.35A).

Note: Till the end of 6th week the external genitalia are bipotential, i.e. they can develop along either male or female lines.

Derivation of external genitalia from the common anlagen in male and female are shown in Table 12.1.

Table 12.1: The male and female external genitalia derived from the common anlagen

Anlagen part	Male derivative	Female derivative
Urogenital sinus	Prostate and prostatic urethra	Urethra
Urethral fold	Penile urethra and shaft of penis	Labia minora
Genital swelling	Scrotum	Labia majora
Genital tubercle	Glans penis	Clitoris

DEVELOPMENT OF MALE EXTERNAL GENITALIA

In the genetic male fetus having functional testes secreting testosterone and dihydrotestosterone (DHT), the external genitalia acquire male characteristics by the 5th month of gestation. The main steps of development of male external genitalia are described here briefly (Fig. 12.35 C, E and G):

Development of penis and penile urethra

Penis is developed from the genital tubercle. The genital tubercle enlarges, becomes cylindrical and is called *phallus*. The rapid elongation of the phallus forms the penis. Appearance of coronary sulcus distinguishes the glans part of the penis. The *corpora cavernosa* and *corpus spongiosum* of the penis develop from the mesenchyme in the phallus. *Prepuce* is later formed by reduplication of the ectoderm covering the glans penis (Fig. 12.36).

Penile urethra develops from two sources:

Most of penile urethra except the terminal part is developed from the phallic part of definitive urogenital sinus (*endodermal*). Steps involved are:

- When the phallus elongates rapidly to form penis, it also drags the *urethral folds* along with. In this way the *primary urethral groove* bounded by urethral folds extend onto the undersurface of developing penis but does not reach its most distal part (i.e. glans).

- The urogenital membrane bounding the phallic part of urogenital sinus breaks down, opening the sinus into the caudal part of *primitive urethral* groove.

- The endodermal cells of the phallic part of urogenital sinus proliferate and grow in the urethral groove as solid *urethral plate*. Later the cells of the urethral plate degenerate to form the *secondary urethral groove* lined by endodermal cells.

- The urethral folds then close converting secondary urethral groove into penile urethra. At this juncture the surface ectoderm fuses in the median plane of the penis, forming the *penile raphe* and enclosing the spongy urethra within the penis.

- *The terminal part of urethra,* that lies in the glans of the penis is derived from a solid cord of ectodermal cells that grows from the tip of the glans and joins rest of the penile urethra during fourth month. This cord is later canalized and form the external urethral meatus at the tip of glans (Fig. 12.35G).

Development of scrotum

Scrotum of scrotal sac, into which the testes later descend are derived from the *genital swellings*. The genital swellings arise in the inguinal region and with further development they move caudally and unite with each other to form the scrotum but the two halves of the scrotal sac are separated by the scrotal septum (Fig. 12.35G). Externally the line of fusion of two scrotal swellings is clearly visible as *scrotal raphe*.

Anomalies of male external genitalia

Anomalies of penis

Anomalies of penis include:

1. *Agenesis of penis,* either completely or partially may be noted. In partial absence, either the corpora cavernosa or the prepuce may be missing. Complete agenesis of penis and urethra is associated with *anourethral fistula*.

2. *Micropenis,* i.e. very small penis occurs due to fetal testicular failure and is commonly associated with hypopituitarism.

3. *Duplicated* or *bifid penis* may be noted rarely when two genital tubercles develop. The condition is usually associated with *exostrophy* of the bladder with other urinary tract abnormalities and imperforate anus.

4. *Posteriorly located penis:* Rarely penis may be located posterior to scrotum.

5. *Phimosis* refers to marked narrowing of opening of prepuce in which retraction of prepuce is not possible. It is seen quite oftenly.

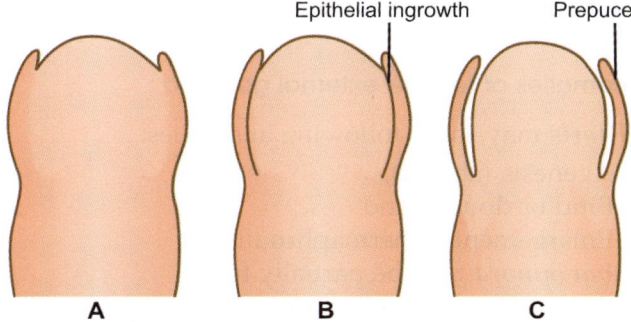

Fig. 12.36: Formation of prepuce of penis.

Anomalies of male urethra

Some anomalies of urethra have been described earlier (see page 184) and a few are described below:

1. **Hypospadias** refers to a condition in which the urethra opens on the undersurface of penis or in the perineum instead of the tip of glans penis. It is the most common anomaly of penis and urethra. It may be of following types (Fig. 12.37A):

   • *Balanic hypospadias* occurs due to failure of development of ectodermal urethra in the region of glans penis. In this condition the urethra opens on the under surface of glans penis.

   • *Penile hypospadias* occurs due to failure of fusion of anterior part of the genital folds. In this condition the urethra presents as a longitudinal groove on the undersurface of the body of penis.

   • *Penoscrotal hypospadias:* In it the urethral opening is at the junction of penis and scrotum.

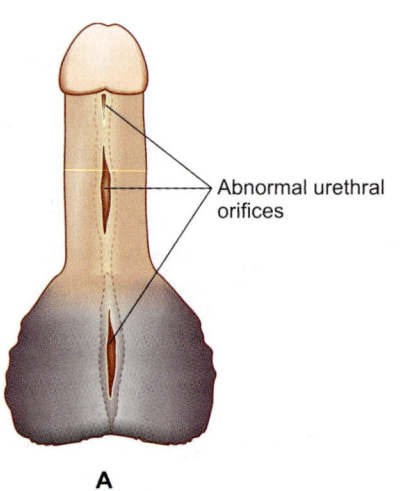

A

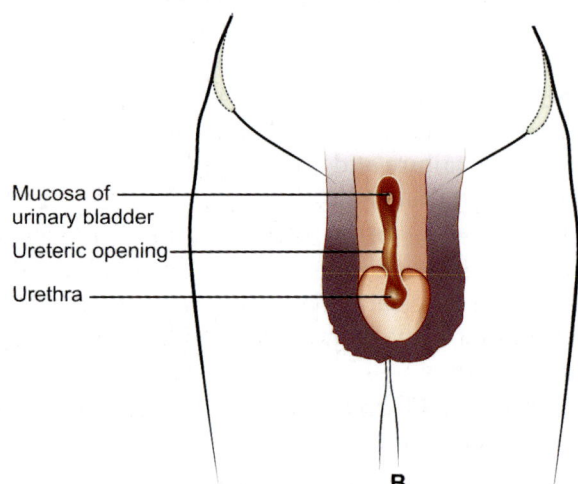

Mucosa of urinary bladder

Ureteric opening

Urethra

B

Fig. 12.37: Anomalies of male external genitalia: A, hypospadias and B, epispadias.

• *Complete perineal hypospadias* occurs due to failure of fusion of scrotal folds. The urethral opening is located between the unfused halves of scrotum. It is usually associated with malformed penis and undescended testis and therefore some times diagnosed as male pseudohermaphroditism.

2. **Epispadias** refers to a condition in which the urethra opens on the dorsal aspect of penis (Fig. 12.37B). It may occur as an isolated anomaly or in association with *ectopia vesicae* (see page 183).

3. **Congenital stenosis of urethra** may occur due to failure of canalization of some part of the urethral plate.

DEVELOPMENT OF FEMALE EXTERNAL GENITALIA

In the genetic female fetus (44+XX), i.e. in the absence of testicular hormones (DHT testosterone and MIS) the differentiation of common analgen into external genitalia occurs along the female line as below (Fig. 12.35D, F and H):

1. **Clitoris** is developed from the *genital tubercle* which elongates only slightly and become cylindrical. In early stages of development the clitoris is relatively large than the penis in male embryo.

2. **Vestibule and labia minora.** After the break down of urogenital membrane, a continuity is established between the urogenital sinus (which form the vestibule) and the exterior. The *primitive urethral folds* do not fuse (as in the male) and form the *labia minora;* except posteriorly where they join to form the *frenulum of labia minora*. It is important to note that minora are lined on outside by ectoderm and inside by endoderm. Thus the cleft between the labia minora, the vestibule receives the openings of urethra and vagina.

3. **Labia majora** are developed from the enlargement of genital swellings which do not fuse (homologous to the scrotum in male). The genital swellings (labioscrotal folds) fuse posteriorly to form the *posterior labial commissure* and anteriorly to form the *anterior labial commissure* and *mons pubis*.

Anomalies of female external genitalia

Clitoris may show following anomalies:

• Agenesis (absent),
• Bifid or double, and
• Enlargement in hermaphroditism

Labia minora may be partially fused.

Urethra may open on the anterior wall of the vagina. In the female this is equivalent of male hypospadias.

Development of Respiratory System

GENERAL CONSIDERATIONS
- Respiratory primordia
- Formation of respiratory diverticulum and outlines of development of respiratory organs
- Control of respiratory development

DERIVATION OF RESPIRATORY ORGANS

Larynx
- Primordia
- Derivation of laryngeal structure

Trachea and bronchi
- Trachea

- Main (primary) bronchus
- Lobar (secondary) bronchi,

Lungs
- Development of bronchial tree and lung parenchyma
- Development of pleura
- Maturation of lungs

ANOMALIES OF RESPIRATORY SYSTEM
- Anomalies of larynx
- Anomalies of trachea
- Anomalies of lungs and bronchi

GENERAL CONSIDERATIONS

The respiratory system can be divided into upper and lower respiratory organs.

- *Upper respiratory organs* include nose, nasal cavities and nasopharynx. Their development is described in chapter 10.
- *Lower respiratory organs* include larynx, trachea, bronchi and lungs. Their development is described in this chapter.

Respiratory primordia

Primordia from which lower respiratory organs develop include:

Respiratory diverticulum (lung bud), an endodermal structure which arises from the foregut and forms the epithelial lining of the respiratory organs,

Splanchnic mesoderm surrounding the part of foregut (from which respiratory diverticulum arises) forms the cartilagenous, muscular and connective tissue components of the trachea, bronchi and lungs.

Fourth and sixth pharyngeal arches contribute cartilages and muscles of the larynx.

Formation of respiratory diverticulum and outlines of development of respiratory organs

Formation of respiratory diverticulum

- *Respiratory diverticulum* (lung bud) appears during 4th week as laryngotracheal groove, (a median evagination), in the caudal end of the ventral wall of the pharyngeal part of the foregut located caudal to the hypopharyngeal eminence (Fig. 13.1). Thus, initially the lung bud is a open communication with the foregut (Fig. 13.2A).

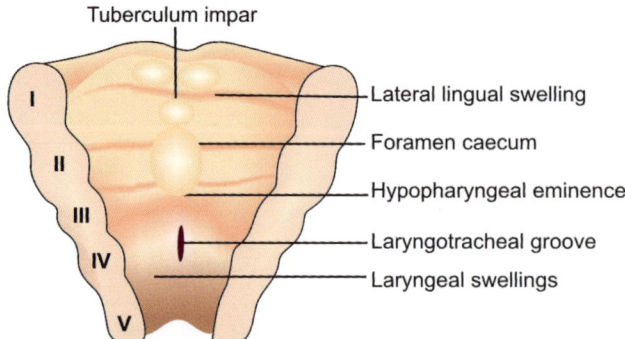

Fig. 13.1: Floor of the primordial pharynx depicting location of the laryngotracheal groove caudal to the hypopharyngeal eminence.

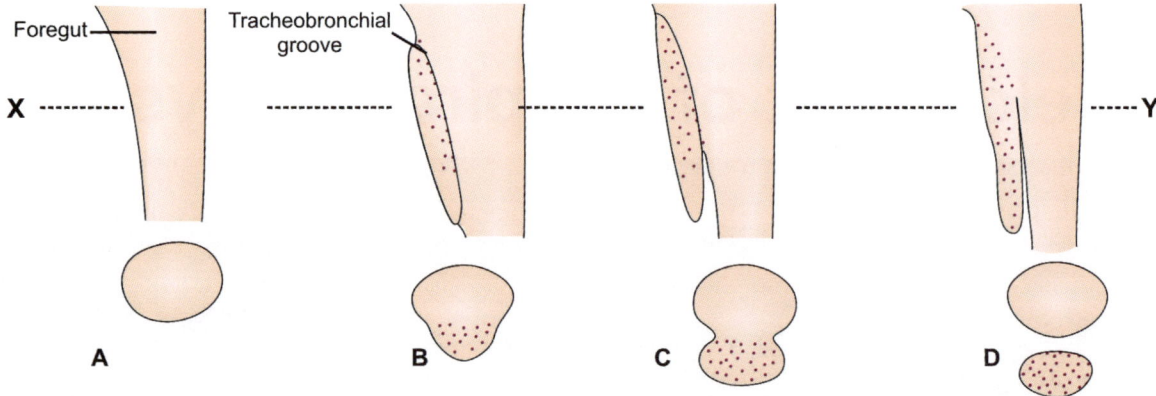

Fig. 13.2: Schematic sagittal (upper drawing) and transverse section (lower drawing) to show successive stages of development of respiratory diverticulum from pharyngeal part of foregut: A, stage of laryngotracheal groove — an open communication with foregut; B, formation of tracheooesophageal folds; C, tracheooesophageal septum dividing foregut into ventral and dorsal parts; and D, separation of laryngotracheal tube (ventral part) from the primordium of oesophagus (dorsal part).

- *Tracheoesophageal* folds appear soon and make a demarcation between the respiratory diverticulum and the foregut (Fig. 13.2B).
- *Tracheoesophageal septum* is then formed by fusion of the tracheoesophageal ridge (Fig. 13.2C). The septum, thus divides the pharyngeal part of foregut into two parts (Fig. 13.2D).
- *Ventral part, the laryngotracheal tube* which forms the respiratory organs, and
- *Dorsal part, the primordium of oropharynx and oesophagus.*

Outlines of development of respiratory organs

The upper end, which opens into the *primordial laryngeal inlet* is formed by the opening of cephalic end of laryngotracheal tube into the pharynx.

- *Larynx* is developed from the cephalic part of the laryngotracheal tube.
- *Trachea* is formed by the part of the tube which succeeds the larynx.
- *Bronchial tree and lungs* develop from the right and left *primary bronchial buds* which arise from the caudal end of the laryngotracheal tube.

Molecular control of respiratory development

- *Transcription factor TBX$_4$,* expressed in the endoderm of gut tube at the site of respiratory diverticulum induces formation of lung bud and is also responsible for continued growth and differentiation of lungs.
- *Fibroblast growth factor (FGF)-10* and other signals from splanchnic mesenchyme probably induce the outgrowth of tracheal bud.
- *Sonic hedgehog (SHH-GLi)* and other signaling pathway are involved in the epithelial mesenchyme interaction which governs the branching of tracheal bud and its proliferation.

DERIVATION OF RESPIRATORY ORGANS

LARYNX

Primordia from which larynx develops are:
- Cephalic most part of laryngotracheal tube, and
- Fourth and sixth pharyngeal arches.

Derivations of laryngeal structures is as below:

- *Epithelial lining* of the larynx develops from the endoderm of cephalic part of laryngotracheal tube.
- *Cartilages of larynx* develop from the cartilages in the 4th and 6th pharyngeal arches.
- *Muscles of larynx* develop from the mesenchyme of 4th and 6th pharyngeal arches and are thus supplied by laryngeal branches of vagus nerve.
- *Inlet of larynx* is formed by the communication between the cephalic end of laryngotracheal tube and the pharynx; which is initially slit like (Fig. 13.3A). As a result of rapid proliferation of mesenchyme of 4th and 6th pharyngeal arches, the slit shaped laryngeal inlet (*primordial glottis*) is converted into a T-shaped opening (Fig. 13.3B). Subsequently, when mesenchyme of the two arches transforms into the thyroid, cricoid, and arytenoid cartilages, the characteristic adult shape of the laryngeal inlet (glottis) can be recognized (Fig. 13.3C).
- *Formation of vocal folds (cords) and vestibular folds.* At about the time that cartilages are formed, the laryngeal epithelium proliferates rapidly resulting in temporary occlusion of the laryngeal lumen. Subsequently, recanalization occurs and during this process, a pair of lateral recesses, the *laryngeal ventricles* are formed. The mucous folds bounding the laryngeal ventricles develop into vocal folds and vestibular folds.
- *Epiglottis* develops from the caudal part of the hypopharyngeal eminence.

TRACHEA AND BRONCHI

Trachea, bronchi and lungs develop from the laryngotracheal tube distal to the larynx:

- *Endoderm* forming laryngotracheal tube differentiates into epithelial lining of trachea, bronchi and lung.
- *Splanchnic mesenchyme* surrounding the laryngotracheal tube form the cartilages, connective tissue and muscles of trachea and bronchi.

Major events in the development of trachea and bronchi

Trachea. The caudal end of the laryngotracheal tube divides into two primary bronchial buds (Fig. 13.4A). Trachea develops from the part of laryngotracheal tube that lies between the point of its bifurcation and the larynx.

Main bronchi. The two primary bronchial buds enlarge to form the right and left main bronchus during 5th week.

Secondary bronchi develop from each main bronchus (Fig. 13.4B):

- *Right main bronchus* divides into three secondary (lobar) bronchi around which three lobes of the right lung develop.
- *Left main bronchus* divides into two secondary (lobar) bronchi around which two lobes of the left lung develop.

LUNGS

Development of bronchial tree and lung parenchyma

Tertiary (segmental) bronchi are formed by repeated division of secondary bronchi in a dichomatous fashion. A total of ten segmental bronchi are formed in right and eight in left lung (Fig. 13.4C).

Bronchopulmonary segments form the substance of the lung. Each segmental bronchi with its surrounding mass of mesenchyme forms the primordium of a bronchopulmonary segment. By the end of 6th month, approximately 17 generations of subdivisions of bronchial tree have formed and respiratory bronchioles have developed. Additional 6

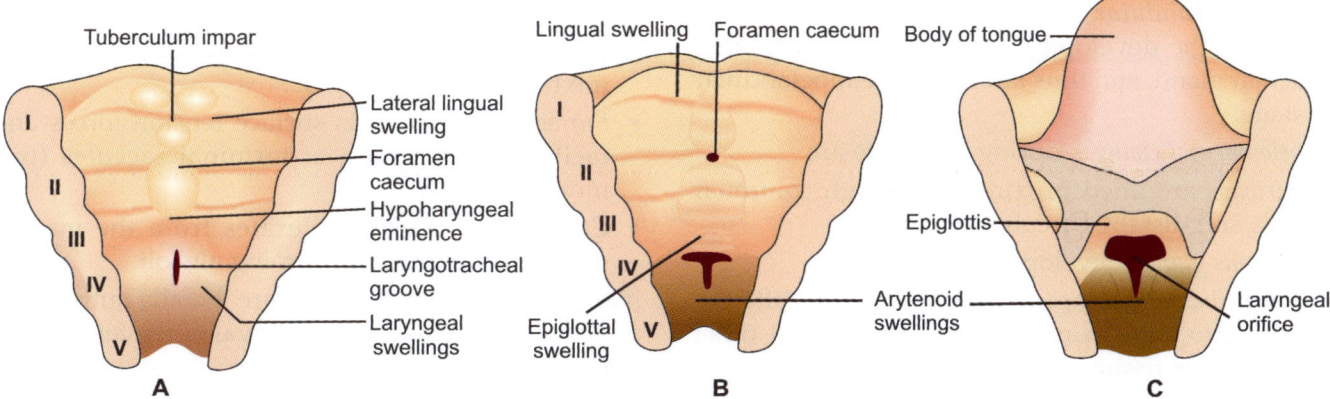

Fig. 13.3: Laryngeal inlet as seen in successive stages of development of larynx; A, slit shaped (4 weeks); B, t-shaped (6 weeks) and C, adult shape (12 weeks).

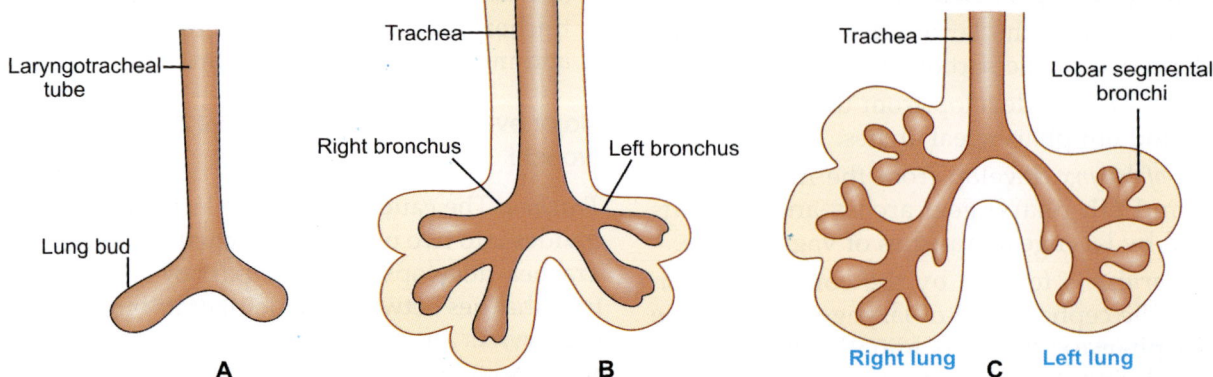

Fig. 13.4: Development of trachea and bronchi: A, primary bronchial buds arising from the lower end of laryngotracheal tube; B, lobar bronchi, three from the right main bronchus and two from the left main bronchus; C, segmental bronchi (ten in right and eight in left lung) established.

generations of subdivisions are formed after birth, completing the bronchial tree.

Alveoli are formed by expansion of the terminal parts of bronchial tree.

Development of pleura

The developing lungs acquire a layer of *visceral pleura* from the splanchnic mesoderm. As the pleura lines the surface of each lobe separately, the lobes come to be separated by *tissues*.

For details of development of visceral and parietal pleura and pleural cavity, see page 97.

Maturation of lungs

Maturation of lungs, which includes ramification of the bronchial tree, begins at 6th week of gestation and is completed at the age of about 8 years and can be divided into four stages:

- Pseudoglandular stage (6 to 16 weeks),
- Canalicular stage (16 to 26 weeks),
- Terminal saccular stage, (26 weeks to birth), and
- Alveolar stage (32 weeks to 8 years).

1. **Pseudoglandular stage:** During this stage (6 to 16 weeks) the developing lungs resemble a tubulo-acinar gland, and thus known as pseudoglandular stage.

Developmental changes during this stage are:

- *Airways* are lined proximally by high columnar cells and distally by cuboidal cells.
- *Mucous glands* develop by 12th week.
- *Mesenchymal cells* around the epithelium differentiate into smooth muscles, cartilages, and other connective tissue cells.

Note: By the end of this stage all major elements of the lung have formed except those involved with gas exchange. Therefore, fetuses born during this stage can not survive, as respiration is not possible.

2. **Canalicular stage** extends from 16th to 26 weeks.

Developmental changes of this stage are:

- *Lumina* of bronchi and terminal bronchioles becomes larger.
- *Respiratory bronchioles* and alveolar ducts develop.
- *Vascularity* of the lung tissue increases markedly.

Note: Respiration is possible at the end of this stage. However, most of the fetuses born at the end of this stage die because the respiratory and other systems are still relatively immature.

3. **Terminal saccular stage** (26 weeks to birth)

Developmental changes of this stage are:

- *Terminal saccules* (primordial alveoli) are developed from the alveolar ducts.
- *Epithelial lining* of the terminal saccules, which is initially cuboidal changes to squamous epithelial cells of endodermal origin *type-I alveolar cells* or pneumocytes across which gas exchange occurs. Scattered among these cells are rounded secretory epithelial cells - *type-II alveolar cells* or pneumocytes which secrete *pulmonary surfactant*, a complex mixture of phospholipids.
- *Surfactant* counteracts surface tension forces and facilitates expansion of terminal saccules (primordial alveoli).
- *Capillary network* proliferates from the mesenchyme around the developing alveoli.

Note: By 26 weeks the lungs are usually sufficiently well developed to permit survival of the fetus if it is born prematurely.

4. **Alveolar stage** of lung development extends from 32 weeks of gestation to 8 years of age.

Developmental changes during this stage are:

- *Upto 32 weeks the alveolar capillary membrane* (pulmonary diffusion barrier or respiratory membrane) becomes sufficiently thin to allow gas exchange.
- *Before birth* breathing movements begin and due to aspiration the lungs are filled with fluid having little protein, some mucus and the surfactant produced by type II alveolar epithelial cells.
- *During first three days after birth,* all the alveoli are inflated with air and the fluid is reabsorbed by the blood and lymph capillaries.
- *Upto eight years after birth* lungs keep on growing primarily due to an increase in the number of respiratory bronchioles and alveoli and not to an increase in the size of the alveoli. About 17 to 18 generations of bronchi are formed upto birth, and about 7–8 more generations are formed from birth to eight years of age. In newborn the number of alveoli in both lungs is about 20 million which increases to about 300 million at the age of 8 to 10 years.

ANOMALIES OF RESPIRATORY SYSTEM

ANOMALIES OF LARYNX

1. *Laryngeal atresia* results from failure of recanalization of the larynx. The clinical presentation is termed as *congenital high airway obstruction syndrome* (CHAOS).
2. *Laryngeal web* is characterized by formation of a membranous web at the level of the vocal folds which partially obstructs the airway. It results from partial recanalization of the larynx.

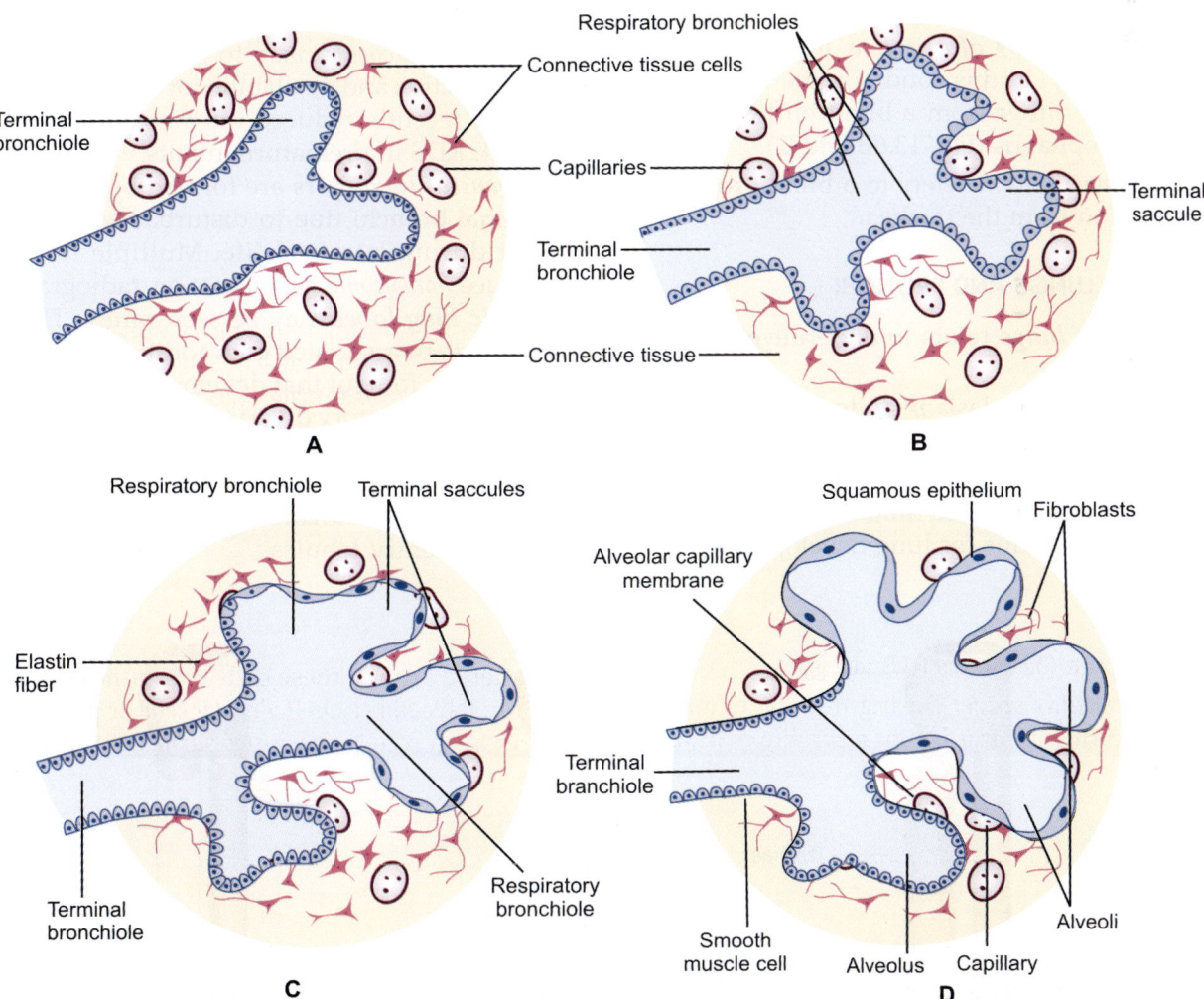

Fig. 13.5: Histological characteristics of terminal bronchioles and respiratory bronchioles during maturation of lung; A, pseudoglandular stage; B, canalicular stage. Note cuboidal cells lining the respiratory bronchiole; C, terminal saccular stage. Note change of cuboidal epithelium to squamous epithelium and proliferation of capillaries around the developing alveoli; D, alveolar stage. Note formation of alveolocapillary membrane.

3. *Laryngocoele* is characterized by an abnormally large laryngeal saccule which may form a swelling in the neck.

4. *Laryngoptosis* refers to the condition in which larynx lies low down in the neck.

5. *Duplication* of entire larynx or part of it (e.g. vocal cords) may occur rarely.

ANOMALIES OF TRACHEA

1. *Tracheo-esophageal fistula (TEF)* the most common anomaly of lower respiratory tract occurs once in 3000–4500 live births (Fig. 13.6). For details see page 154.

2. *Tracheal stenosis and atresia,* i.e. narrowing and obstruction of trachea occurs due to unequal partitioning of foregut into trachea and oeso-phagus. These anomalies are rare and are usually seen in association with tracheo-esophageal fistula (Fig. 13.6).

3. *Absence (agenesis) of trachea* may be noted extremely rarely. In this condition the bronchi to the lung arise either from a blind bifurcation or from the oesophagus (Fig. 13.6B and C).

4. *Tracheal diverticulum* refers to a blind bronchus like projection from the trachea.

ANOMALIES OF LUNGS AND BRONCHI

1. *Hypoplasia of lungs* refers to underdevelopment of lung tissue.

   Causes of lung hypoplasia include:
   • *Oligohydramnios:* One of the important cause of hypoplasia of lungs is severe and chronic oligohydramnios (since fluid in the lungs is an important stimulus for lung development).

• *Congenital diaphragmatic hernia* (CDH) may be associated with lung hypoplasia. In CDH lung is not able to develop properly because it is compressed by the abnormally placed abdominal viscera.

2. *Agenesis of lungs* may be unilateral or bilateral. It results from failure of the bronchial buds to develop.

3. *Respiratory distress syndrome (RDS)* also known as hyaline membrane disease (HMD) affects about 2% of the live newborn infants.
   • *Cause* of RDS is deficiency of surfactant, because of which the air-water (blood) surface membrane tension becomes high. As a result the lungs remain uninflated and the alveoli contain a fluid with a high protein content that resembles a glassy or hyaline membrane and hence the name HMD.
   • *Premature infants* have high mortality because of surfactant deficiency.
   • *Role of glucocorticoids* to stimulate surfactant production and availability of *artificial surfactant* have recently reduced the mortality associated with RDS in premature infants.

4. *Congenital lung cysts* are formed by dilatation of terminal bronchi due to disturbance in development during late fetal life. Multiple lung cysts produce *honeycomb appearance* on radiographs.

5. *Ectopic lung lobes* may be seen rarely. These are thought to be associated with additional respiratory buds of the foregut that develop independently of the main respiratory diverticulum. These may arise from trachea or oesophagus.

6. *Abnormal divisions of bronchial* tree may be seen. Some of the abnormal bronchi may result in supernumerary lobules.

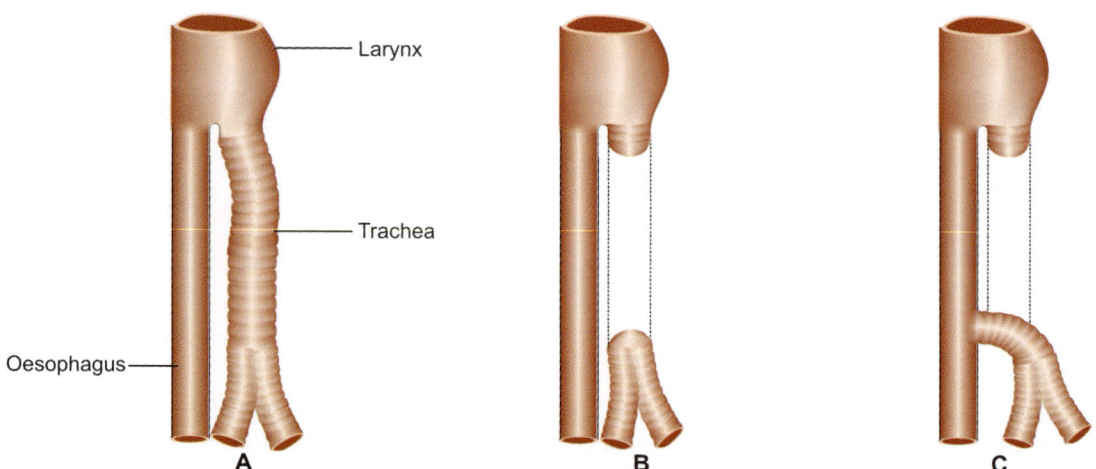

Fig. 13.6: Anomalies of trachea; A, normal, B, agenesis; and C, agenesis with tracheo-esophageal fistula.

14

Development of Cardiovascular System

CARDIOVASCULAR SYSTEM OF HUMAN EMBRYO
- Primordia of cardiovascular system
- Primordial heart and blood vessels

DEVELOPMENT OF THE HEART
- Formation of tubular heart
- Formation of cardiac loop and establishment of regional divisions of heart
- Formation of definitive chambers and conduction system of heart

DEVELOPMENT OF VASCULAR SYSTEM

Arterial system
- Aortic arches and their derivatives
- Derivatives of aortic sacs
- Development of major arteries
- Dorsal aortae and their branches

Venous system
- Derivatives and fate of vitelline veins
- Derivatives and fate of umbilical veins
- Derivatives and fate of cardinal subcardinal and supra cardinal veins

Fetal Circulation

ANOMALIES OF CARDIOVASCULAR SYSTEM
- Anomalies of heart
- Anomalies of arterial system
- Anomalies of veins

DEVELOPMENT OF LYMPHATIC SYSTEM
- Development of lymph sacs
- Development of lymph vessels
- Development of lymph nodes
- Maturation of other lymph organs

CARDIOVASCULAR SYSTEM OF HUMAN EMBRYO

PRIMORDIA OF CARDIOVASCULAR SYSTEM

Primordia of cardiovascular system from which the heart, blood vessels, and blood cells develop is the mesoderm. The cardiovascular system is derived mainly from:

- *Splanchnic mesoderm* related to that part of the intraembryonic coelome that forms the pericardial cavity forms the primordium of heart. This part of splanchnic mesoderm is termed the *cardiogenic area*.

- *Paraxial and lateral mesoderm* near the otic placodes also forms the primordium of cardiovascular system (CVS).

- *Neural crest cells* from the region between the otic vesicles and the caudal limits of the third pair of somites also take part in the development of CVS.

Time table for key events during development of CVS is as follows:

- *Third week* marks the beginning of development of the cardiovascular system. At the end of this week the cardiogenic area, heart tubes and pericardium are formed.

- *Fourth week* beginning marks the functioning of the primitive heart.

207

- *During 4th to 7th weeks* the heart divides into a typical four chambered structure by the formation of septa. Aortic arches are established during the 4th to 5th weeks. Veins are also established during this period. Lymphatic sacs form in the 5th week.

PRIMORDIAL HEART AND BLOOD VESSELS

Primordial heart and blood vessels appear in the middle of third week when the rapidly growing embryo is no longer able to meet its nutritional and oxygen requirements by diffusion alone. The primordial cardiovascular system differentiates from the *angioblast cells* which are derived from the mesoderm forming the primordia for the cardio-vascular system.

The primitive cardiovascular system during embryonic stage consists of primordial heart and vessels from which the definitive cardiovascular system develops (Fig. 14.1):

Primordial heart

Primordial heart, as mentioned above, develops from the splanchnic mesoderm forming the cardiogenic area. The primitive heart has an arterial and a venous end.

Veins associated with primordial heart

Veins of primitive cardiovascular system which drain into the primitive heart of a 4 week embryo include (Fig. 14.1):

Vitelline veins. These arise from the capillary plexus in the wall of yolk sac and after traversing the septum transversum drain into the venous end of the primitive heart. Later on these veins will form the hepatic veins and portal veins (See page 226).

Umbilical veins develop in the chorionic sac (primordial placenta), travel in the umbilical cord and after running on each side of the developing liver drain into the venous end of heart (sinus venosus). These veins bring well-oxygenated blood from the placenta into the sinus venosus.

- *Common cardinal veins* (right and left) return poorly oxygenated blood from the body of embryo to the heart. Each common cardinal vein is formed by the union of anterior and posterior cardinal veins which drain cranial and caudal parts of the embryo, respectively.

Arteries associated with primordial heart

Arteries associated with the primitive heart in a 4 week embryo are (Fig. 14.1):

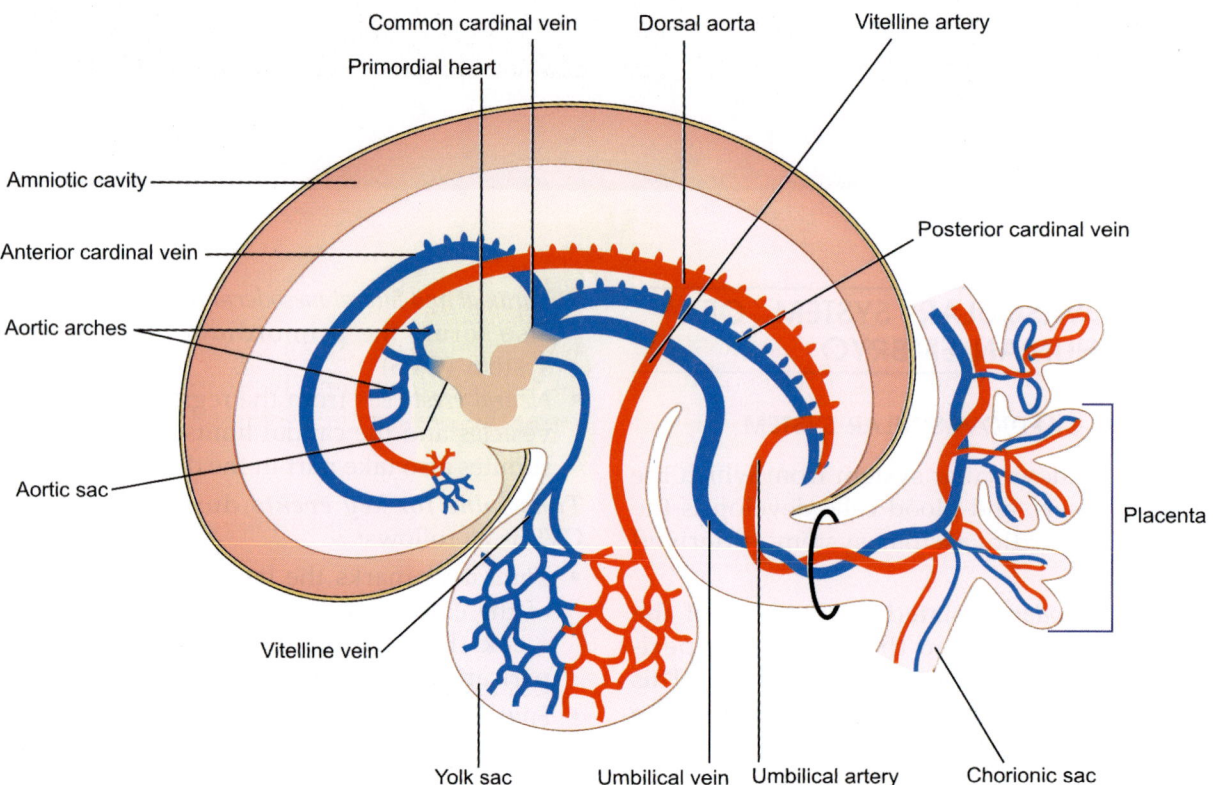

Fig. 14.1: Cardiovascular system of 4 weeks human embryo.

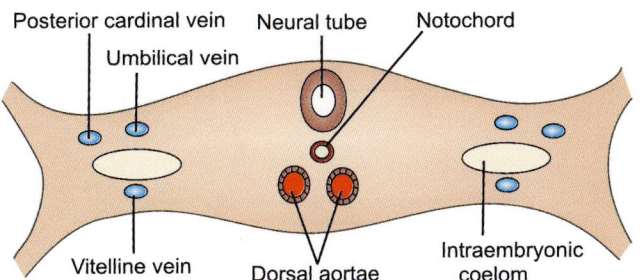

Fig. 14.2: Transverse section of the human embryo. Note location of dorsal aortae, umbilical vein, vitelline vein and anterior, posterior and common cardinal veins.

Dorsal aortae, are two longitudinal vessels which run through the entire length of the embryo one on each side of the notochord (Fig. 14.2) and along the dorsal wall of the yolk sac. Soon the paired dorsal aortae fuse to form a single dorsal aorta, just caudal to the pharyngeal arches.

Aortic arches (arteries of the pharyngeal arches which develop during 4th and 5th week) arise from the aortic sac on each side and terminate into the dorsal aortae (Fig. 14.1).

Vitelline artery arises from the ventral surface of dorsal aorta and supply the yolk sac, allantois, and chorion. These arteries pass to yolk sac and later the primordial gut, which is formed from the part of yolk sac incorporated into the body. The vitelline arteries form the:

• Celiac trunk to foregut,
• Superior mesenteric artery to midgut, and
• Inferior mesenteric artery to hindgut.

Umbilical arteries. The umbilical arteries arise from the caudal end of dorsal aorta and pass through connecting stalk (later the umbilical cord) and break up into the capillaries of the chorionic villi (embryonic part of placenta (Fig. 14.1). These arteries carry poorly oxygenated blood to the placenta. Later on, these form the internal iliac arteries and the vesical arteries (see page 226).

DEVELOPMENT OF THE HEART

FORMATION OF TUBULAR HEART

Development of primitive heart from the splanchnic mesoderm forming cardiogenic area is induced by anterior endoderm. Key events are as follows:

Angioblasts cords, a paired endothelial strands are formed in the cardiogenic area during third week.

Heart tubes, are then formed after canalization of these angioblastic cords (Fig. 14.3A).

Tubular heart is formed at the end of 3rd week. The cephalic and lateral foldings of the embryo bring the two heart tubes closer in the thoracic region, where they meet and fuse in a cranio-caudal direction to form a single tubular heart (Fig. 14.3B). The endothelial heart tube is separated from the developing pericardial sac by a thickened plate of mesodermal tissue known as *myo-epicardial mantle* which soon surrounds the endothelial tubular heart. The myocardium then thickens and secretes a thick layer of extracellular matrix rich in hyaluronic acid (cardiac jelly) that separates it from the endothelial tubular heart. The developing heart then bulges more and more into the pericardial cavity till it is invaginated and is lined by the visceral layer of pericardium, also known as epicardium. Thus the developing heart now consists of three layers (Fig. 14.4):

• *Endocardium,* the internal endothelial lining of the heart;
• *Myocardium,* forming the muscular wall of the heart, and
• *Epicardium* or visceral pericardium which is derived from the mesothelial cells. At this stage the tubular heart is suspended from the dorsal wall by a mesentery the *dorsal mesocardium* (Fig. 14.4).

Changes in position of the developing heart

Before folding of the embryo the developing heart and pericardial cavity lie anterior to the bucco-pharyngeal membrane and the primordial brain (Fig. 14.5A).

After folding of the embryo, as mentioned above the developing heart and pericardial cavity come to lie ventral to the foregut and caudal to the bucco-pharyngeal membrane and cranial to the septum transversum (Fig. 14.5B and C). As shown in Fig. 14.5C, the developing heart is separated ventrally from the pericardial cavity by the myoepicardial mantle.

Components of tubular heart

The developing tubular heart shows four dilatations, which cranio-caudally form the following parts (Fig. 14.3C):

• Bulbus cordis,
• Primitive ventricle,
• Primitive atrium, and
• Sinus venosus.

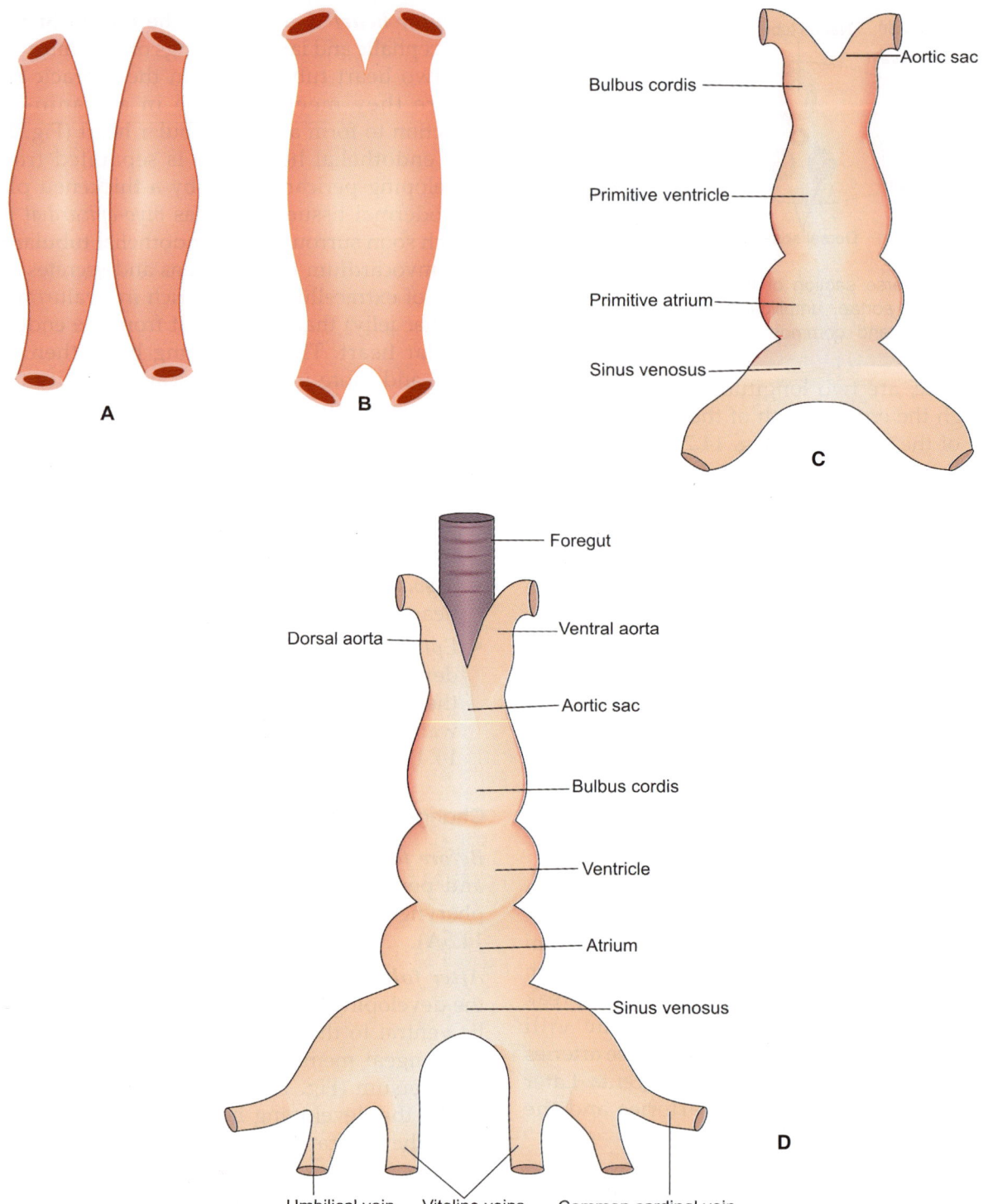

Fig. 14.3: Development and components of the tubular heart: A, right and left heart tubes; B, fused heart tubes; C, components of heart tube; D, attachment of aortic arches with aortic sac, limb and sac veins opening in the two horns of sinus venosus.

1. **Bulbus cordis** the cranial most part of the tubular heart, subsequently is subdivided into three parts (Fig. 14.3C):
   - *Proximal part,* which will later form the trabeculated part of the right ventricle,

   - *Mid portion, the conus cordis,* which will later form the outflow tracts of both ventricles, and
   - *Distal part,* the *truncus arteriosus,* which will later form the ascending aorta and pulmonary trunk. At this *juncture,* distally the trunctus arteriosus

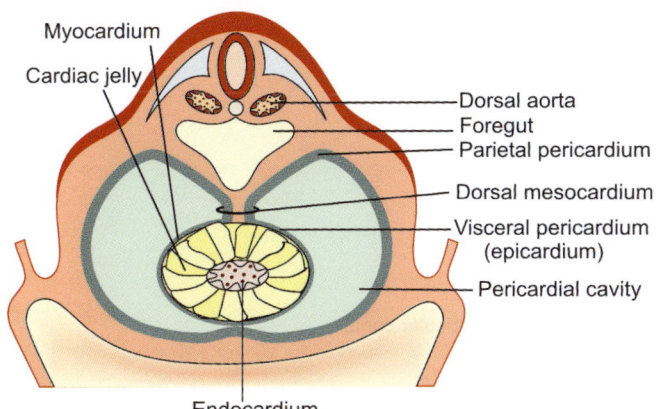

Fig. 14.4: Three layers of primitive heart and dorsal mesocardium.

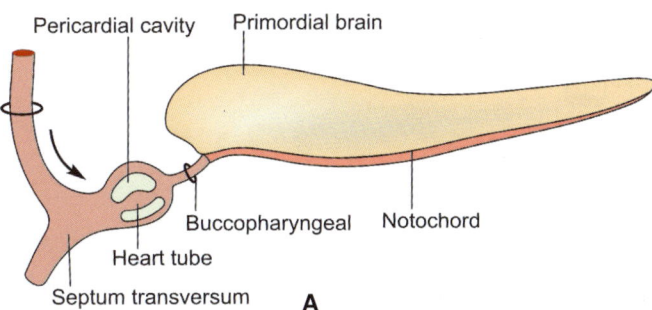

A

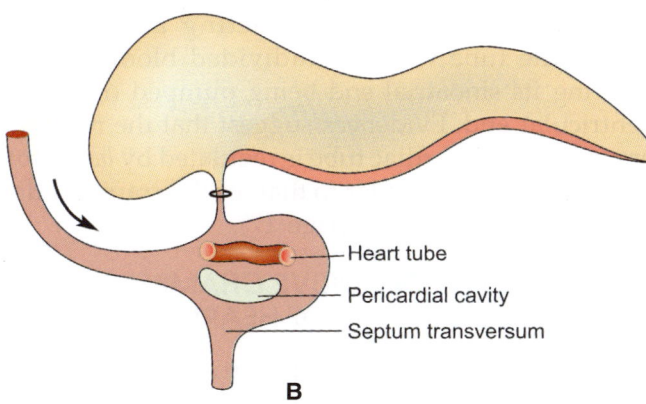

B

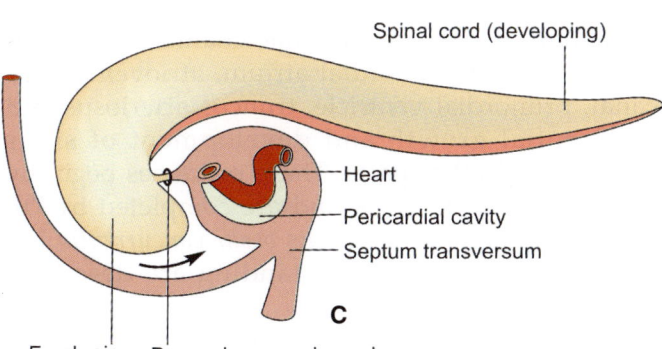

C

Fig. 14.5: Position of developing heart before (A) and after folding (B and C) of embryo.

is continuous with *aortic sac* which divides into right and left limbs (Fig. 14.3C). Each limb is connected with the corresponding dorsal aorta through six aortic arches (arteries of pharyngeal arches) (Fig. 14.3D).

2. ***Primitive ventricle*** along with the conus cordis will form the right and left ventricles. Junction of the primitive ventricle with the bulbus cordis, externally indicated by the *bulboventricular sulcus* remains narrow. It is called *primary interventricular foramen.*

3. ***Primitive atrium*** is connected with the primitive ventricle through *atrioventricular canal.* The primitive atrium will later form the right and left atria.

4. ***Sinus venosus,*** the caudal most part of the tubular heart is also called its venous end. At its lower end the sinus venosus presents right and left horns (Fig. 14.3C). Each horn receives blood from following three veins (Fig. 14.3D).

• *Vitelline vein* from the yolk sac,

• *Umbilical vein* from the placenta, and

• *Common cardinal vein* from the body wall.

Note: The arterial end of the developing heart is fixed by pharyngeal arches and the venous end by the septum transversum (Fig. 14.3D).

Fate of the various parts of the heart tube as described above is summarized in Fig. 14.6.

FORMATION OF CARDIAC LOOP AND ESTABLISHMENT OF REGIONAL DIVISIONS OF THE HEART

Formation of cardiac loop

The tubular heart elongates rapidly and increases in length so much faster than the chamber in which it lies that it first bends to the side and then twisted into a loop. As a result the tubular heart bulges ventrally and some what caudally in a V-shaped manner. The bend occurs in the mid portion that is between bulbus cordis and primitive ventricle, hence also called *bulboventricular loop.* As a result of cardiac looping following positional changes occur (Fig. 14.7):

• Bulbus cordis is displaced caudally, ventrally and to the right,

• Primitive ventricle is displaced to the left

• Primitive atrium and sinus venosus are shifted postero-superiorly and come to lie dorsal to the bulbus cordis and ventricle. The continuous growth of the cardiac loop produces degeneration of the central part of dorsal mesocardium,

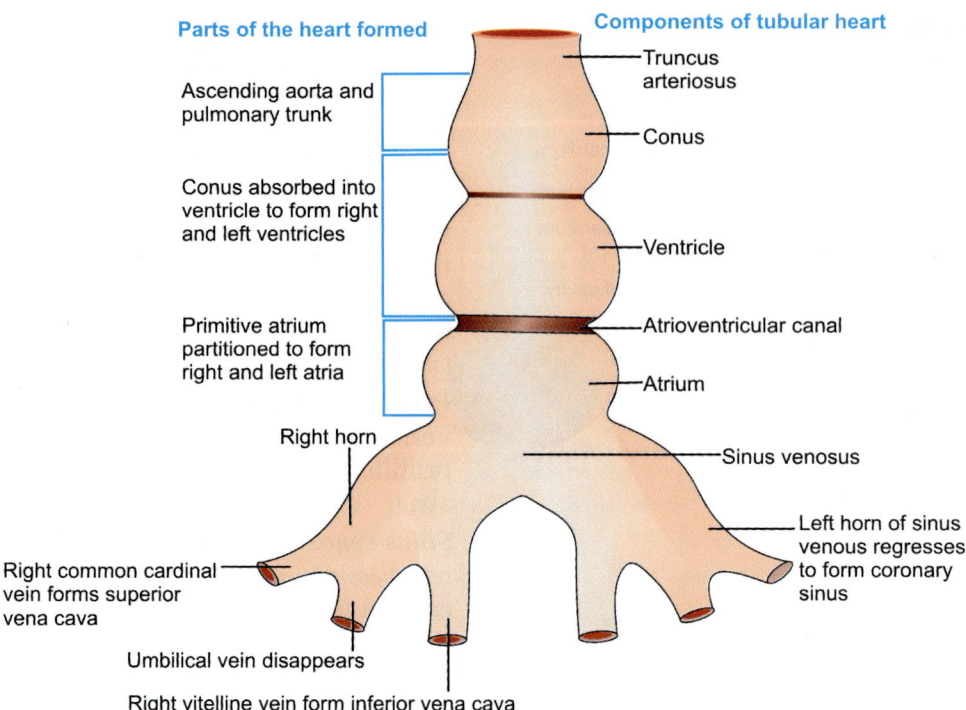

Parts of the heart formed — Components of tubular heart

Ascending aorta and pulmonary trunk

Conus absorbed into ventricle to form right and left ventricles

Primitive atrium partitioned to form right and left atria

Right horn

Right common cardinal vein forms superior vena cava

Umbilical vein disappears

Right vitelline vein form inferior vena cava

Truncus arteriosus

Conus

Ventricle

Atrioventricular canal

Atrium

Sinus venosus

Left horn of sinus venous regresses to form coronary sinus

Fig. 14.6: Fate of various components of heart tube.

forming a communication, the *transversus pericardial sinus* between the right and left sides of the pericardial cavity (Fig. 14.8).

Note: The process of cardiac looping is completed by the end of 4th week.

Establishment of regional divisions of the heart

As a result of cardiac loop formation and local expansion of some parts of the heart tube, the primary regional divisions of the heart become clearly differentiated as below (Fig. 14.7):

- *Atrial region* is established by transverse dilatation of the tubular heart which bulges out on either side of midline. Its bilobed configuration is emphasized by the manner in which the truncus arteriosus compresses it mid ventrally.

- *Ventricle* is formed by the bend in the midportion of original cardiac tube. As a result of cardiac loop formation the ventricle originally situated cephalic to atrium is brought into its characteristic adult position caudal to the atrium (Fig. 14.7). A distinct median furrow, an external indication of the impending division of heart into right and left sides, appears at the apex of ventricular loop.

- *Truncus arteriosus*, the most cephalic part of cardiac tube, connecting the ventricle with the ventral aortic roots undergoes least change in appearance.

Regulation of regional organization of cardiac tube

Thus by the end of 4 weeks the principal regional divisions of the heart are recognizable. Functionally, however, the heart is still acting as a simple contractile tube with an undivided blood stream entering its sinoatrial end being pumped out of its ventricular end. Evidences suggest that the regional organization of cardiac tube is regulated by *homeobox genes* in a manner similar to that for the craniocaudal axis of the embryo (see page 17).

FORMATION OF DEFINITIVE CHAMBERS AND CONDUCTION SYSTEM OF HEART

The single heart tube is partitioned into four chambers, with systemic outflow on the left and pulmonary outflow on the right. The process of formation of definitive cardiac chambers involves partitioning of primordial atrium, atrioventricular canal, primordial ventricle, truncus arteriosus and differential growth and development of sinus venosus and other parts. These processes begin by the middle of 4th week and are completed by 7th week. Although *all the events occur concurrently* but for the purpose of understanding are described separately.

FORMATION OF ATRIA

Formation of atria involves following processes:

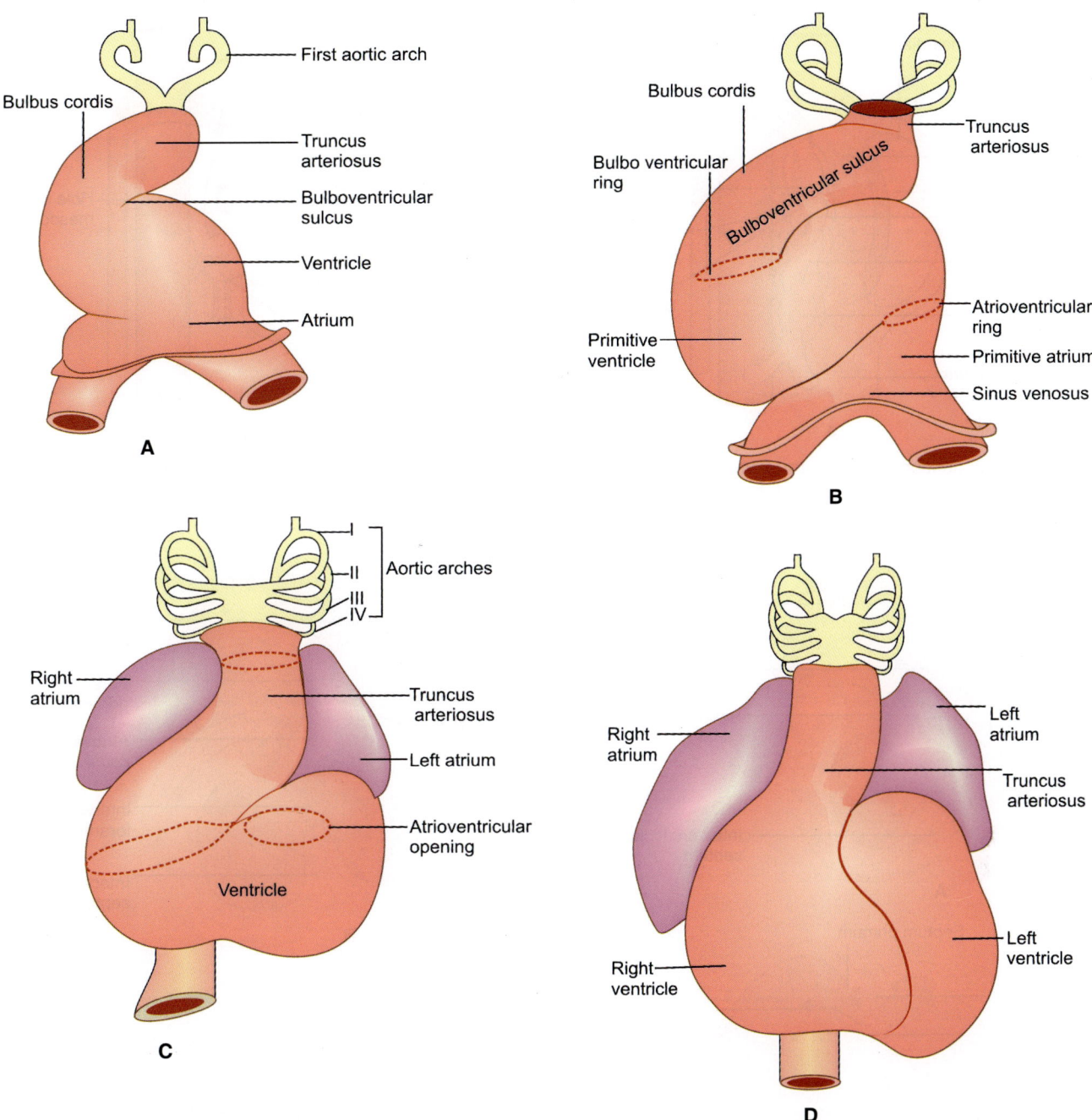

Fig. 14.7: Stages in the formation of cardiac loop and establishment of regional divisions to take adult external form.

- Septation of atrioventricular canal,
- Septation of primordial atrium,
- Incorporation of sinus venosus into right atrium, and other changes in it.
- Incorporation of pulmonary veins into left atrium.
- Formation of atrioventricular valves.

Septation of atrioventricular canal

Atrioventricular (AV) canal is divided into right and left canals by fusion of *endocardial cushions* which arise from its dorsal and ventral walls by the end of 4th

week. The fused cushions form the so called *septum intermedium* (Figs 14.9 and 14.10).

Septation of primordial atrium

Begins at the end of 4th week. The primordial atrium is divided into right and left atria by the formation, subsequent modification of two septa, the septum primum and septum secundum (Figs 14.9 and 14.11).

Septum primum arises from the roof of the common atrium (Fig. 14.11A) and grows caudally towards the septum intermedium formed by fusion of the

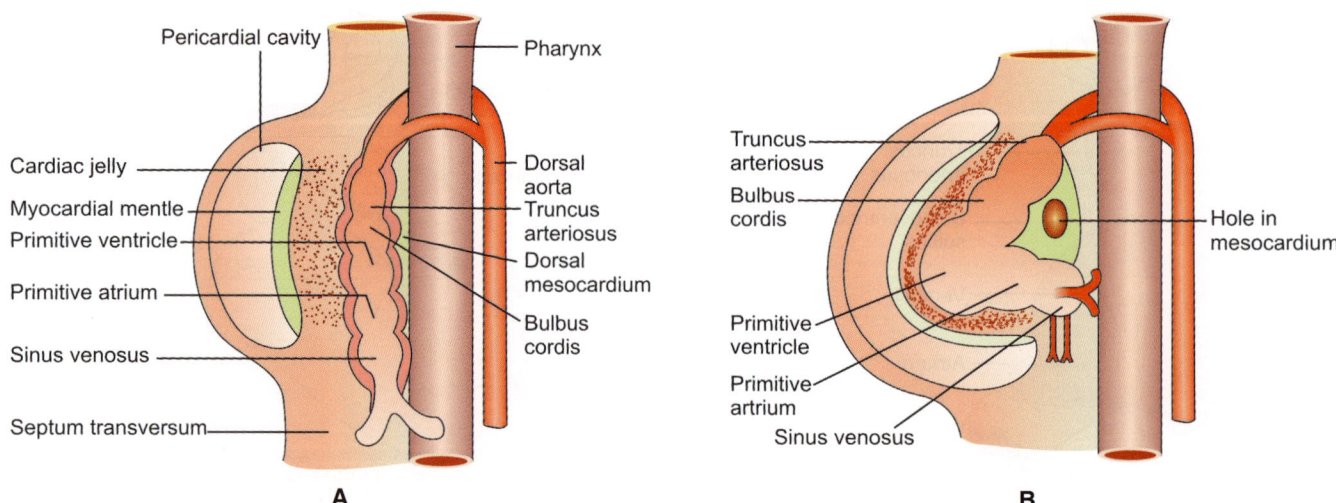

Fig. 14.8: Cut section of left lateral view depicting dorsal mesocardium of a tubular heart (A) and formation of sinus transversus during the formation of bulboventricular loop (B).

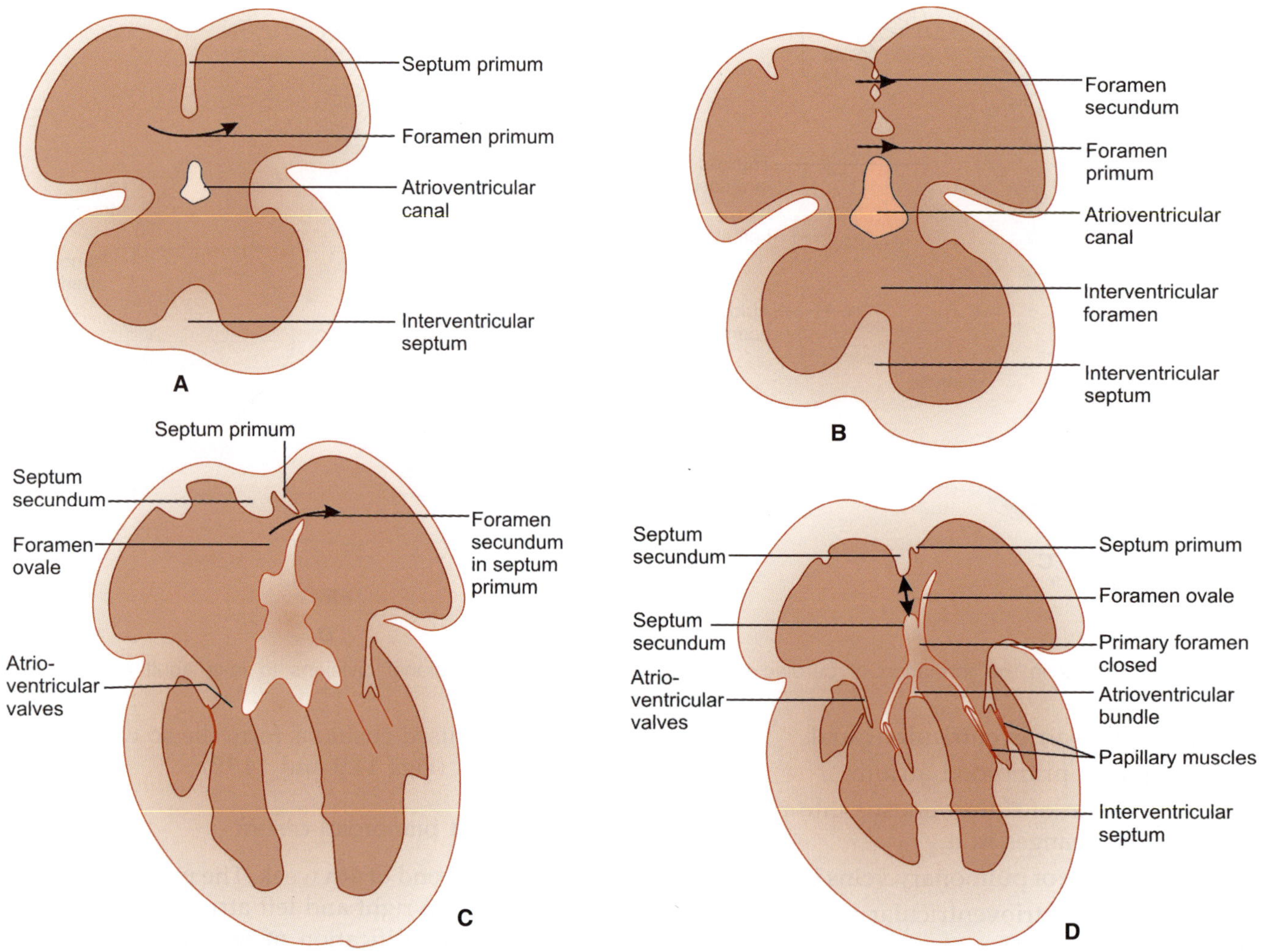

Fig. 14.9: Formation of definitive cardiac chambers and major vascular trunks; (note the various events occuring concurrently): A, appearance of septum primum, foramen primum, septum intermedium, and interventricular septum; B, appearance of septum secundum and foramen secundum, closure of foramen primum; C, further downgrowth of septum secundum resulting in formation of foramen ovale; D, completion of inter atrial septa formation and interventricular septum (muscular part as well as membraneous part) formation.

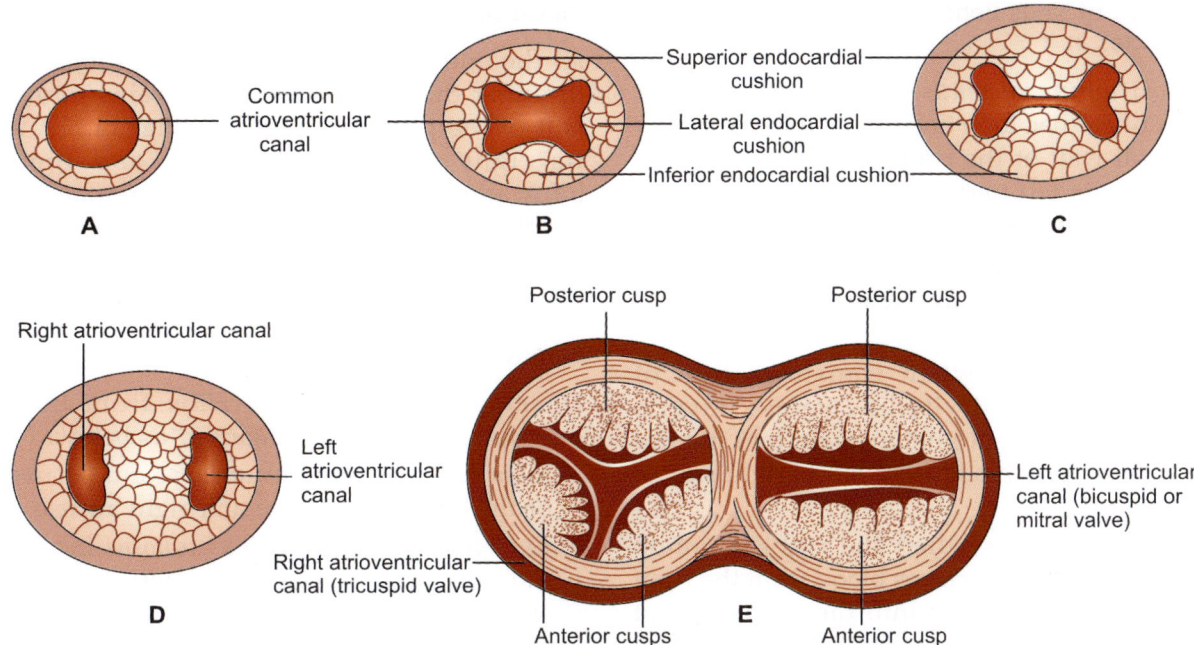

Fig. 14.10: Septation of arterioventricular canal (A to D) and formation of tricuspid and mitral valves (E).

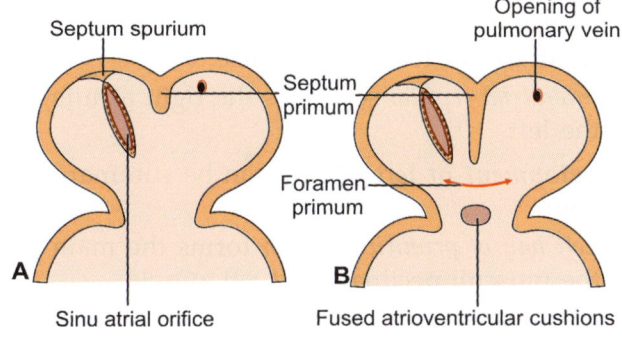

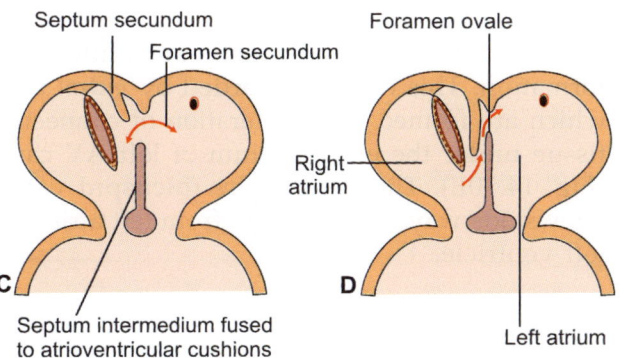

Fig. 14.11: Stages of formation of interatrial septum: A, formation of septum primum; B, formation of septum intermedium and foramen primum; C, appearance of septum secundum, formation of foramen secundum and closure of foramen primum; D, further downgrowth of septum secundum and formation of foramen ovale.

endocardial cushions. It is a thin crescent shaped membrane.

• *Foramen primum* is formed between the free borders of growing septum primum and the fused A-V cushions, which serves as a shunt allowing oxygenated blood to pass from the right to the left atrium (Fig. 14.11B). Shortly afterwards the septum primum fuses with septum intermedium (fused AV cushions), obliterating foramen primum.

• *Foramen secundum,* however, is formed by the degeneration of cranial part of septum primum, before the complete closure of foramen primum and ensures a continuous flow of oxygenated blood from the right to left atrium (Fig. 14.11C).

Septum secundum, a thick muscular septum grows caudally to the right of septum primum and overlaps the foramen secundum. The oxygenated blood now passes between septum secundum and septum primum through the foramen secundum. This whole passage between the two septa is called *foramen ovale* (Fig. 14.11D). Since the septum primum is a thin membrane, it allows passage of blood from right to left and not from the left to right. Thus, the foramen ovale is a valvular aperture, which is patent throughout fetal life. *After birth,* the left atrium starts receiving oxygenated blood from the lungs, and the foramen ovale closes by fusion of septum primum with the septum secundum.

Incorporation of sinus venosus into right atrium and other changes in it

Dorsal positioning of sinus venosus occurs after formation of cardiac loop and opens into the center of the dorsal wall of the primordium atrium (Fig. 14.12A) with its left and right horns being about the same size (Fig. 14.12A).

Transpositioning of sinus venosus to the right occurs during 5th week due to following two *left-to-right extra cardiac shunts* of blood:

- *First shunt* occurs when transformation of umbilical veins and vitelline veins converts proximal part of right vitelline vein into inferior vena cava shifting blood from left to right side of sinus venosus.

- *Second shunt occurs* when the right common cardinal vein which receives blood from the right side of body and drains into the right horn of sinus venosus, also starts receiving blood from the left side of the body due to establishment of an oblique communication between the right and left anterior cardinal veins cephalic to heart (Fig. 14.12C). Subsequently the part of left anterior cardinal vein caudal to the oblique communication obliterates. Later the right common cardinal vein and caudal part of right anterior cardinal vein form the *superior vena cava.*

Changes in the sinus venosus occurring as a result of the above two left-to-right shunts can be summeri-zed as below:

- *Right horn enlarges,* as it receives all the blood from the head and neck through superior vena cava and from the placenta and caudal region of the body through inferior vena cava.

- *Sinoatrial orifice* as a result of enlargement of right horn, moves to the right and opens in the part of primordial atrium that will become the adult right atrium. Sinoatrial orifice, which initially was wide, becomes a narrow slit. This orifice is guarded by right and left venous valves, cranially these two valves fuse to form the *septum spurium* (Fig. 14.12B).

- *Incorporation of right enlarged horn* of the sinus venosus then occurs into the right atrium forming its posterior smooth part, the *sinus venarum* (Fig. 14.12E), which is separated from the rest of rough right atrium by *crista terminalis,* a remnant of right venous valve.

- *Left horn and body of sinus venosus* become a narrow tube and form the coronary venous sinus (Fig. 14.12E).

Incorporation of pulmonary veins into left atrium

At the end of 4th week, a single pulmonary vein draining the early lung buds, drains into the left half of the primordial atrium (Fig. 14.13A and B). Its right and left tributaries and their first bifurcations, are successively incorporated into the left atrium, forming its smooth part the *sinus venarum* (Fig. 14.13C to F). Thus, at 8 weeks four pulmonary veins open into the left atrium (Fig. 14.13E and F).

Summary of development of atria

Development of right atrium from the above description, can be summarised as below:

- *Right half of the primitive atrium* form the main part of the muscle pectinate and right auricle.

- *Enlarged right horn of sinus venosus* incorporated into the atrium forms the posterior smooth part-sinus venarum. Superior vena cava and inferior vena cava open in this part.

- *Right atrioventricular canal* is also absorbed to some extent into the right atrium. The right AV canal is guarded by the *tricuspid valves* which are formed by proliferation of connective tissue under the endocardium of right AV canal (Fig. 14.10E). The tricuspid valve allows one way flow of blood from right atrium to right ventricle.

- *Interatrial septum* separates the right atrium from the left.

Development of left atrium can be summarised as below:

- *Left half of primitive atrium* forms the main part-the musculi pectinate and left auricle.

- *Absorbed part of pulmonary veins* form the smooth part (sinus venarum). Four pulmonary veins bringing oxygenated blood from the lungs drain into this part.

- *Left atrioventricular canal* also contribute in its formation. This canal is guarded by *mitral valve* which are formed by proliferation of connective tissue under the endocardium of left AV canal (Fig. 14.10E). The *mitral valve* (bicuspid valve) allows one way flow of blood from left atrium to left ventricle.

FORMATION OF VENTRICLES

Formation of ventricles is accomplished by following processes which depend on the blood stream flowing through the bulboventricular loop (Fig. 14.9 and 14.14).

- Developmental changes in bulbus cordis, and
- Formation and septation of bulboventricular chamber.

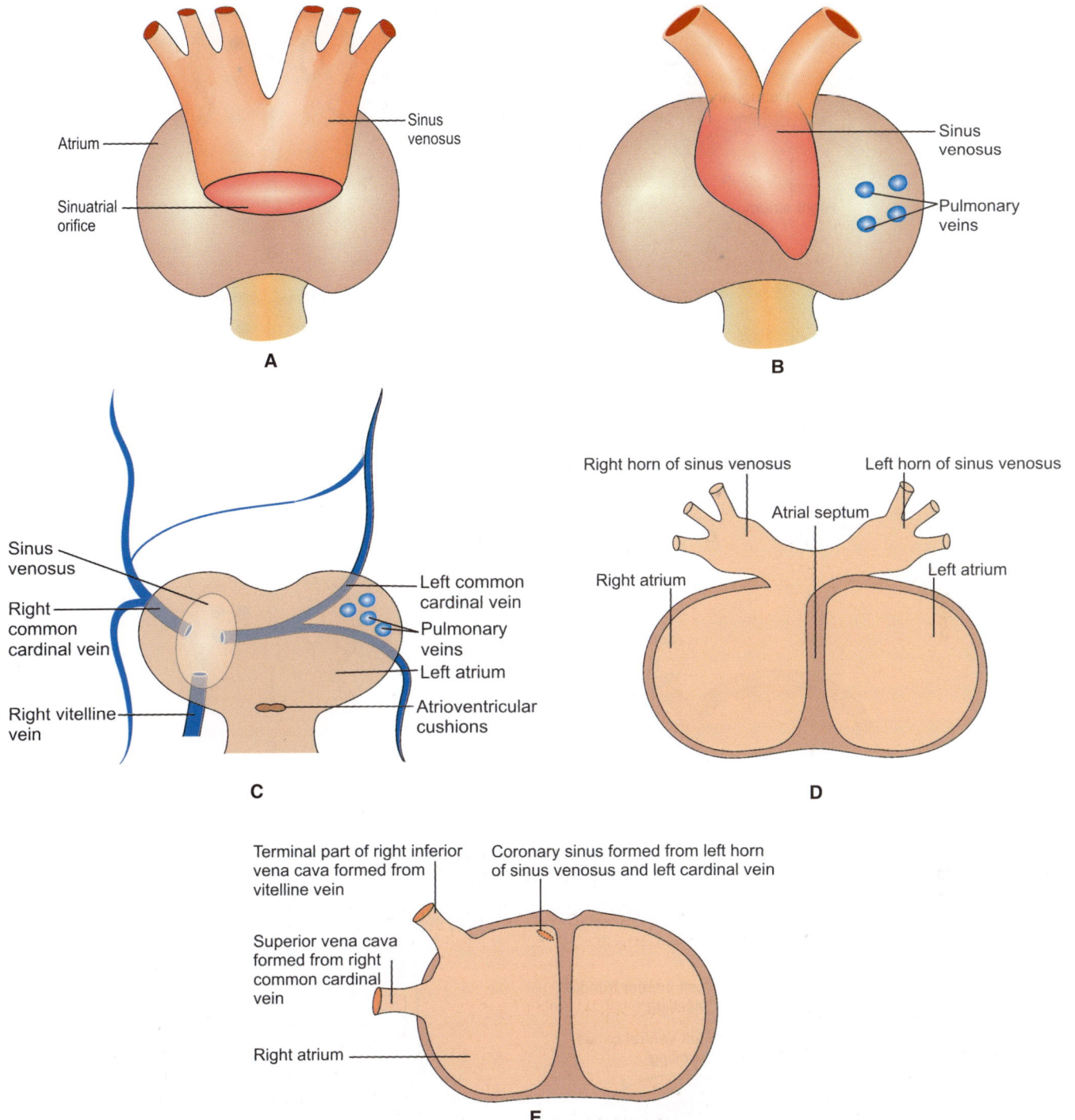

Fig. 14.12: Changes in sinus venosus leading to its incorporation into the right atrium; A, sinus venosus positioned dorsal to the primitive atrium and opening in it by a single central transverse orifice; B, shifting of sinuatrial orifice towards right and with vertical orientation; C, depicting formation of right to left shunt between the anterior cardinal veins; D, enlargement of right horn and shrinking of left horn; E, incorporation of right horn of sinus into the right atrium. Note, superior vena cava is formed by right common cardinal vein, terminal part of inferior vena cava is formed by part of right vilelline vein, coronary sinus is formed by body and left horn of sinus venosus.

Developmental changes in bulbus cordis

Bulbus cordis, the most cephalic part of heart tube is craniocaudally divisible in three parts (Fig. 14.6).

- Truncus arteriosus,
- Conus cordis, and
- Proximal part of bulbar cordis.

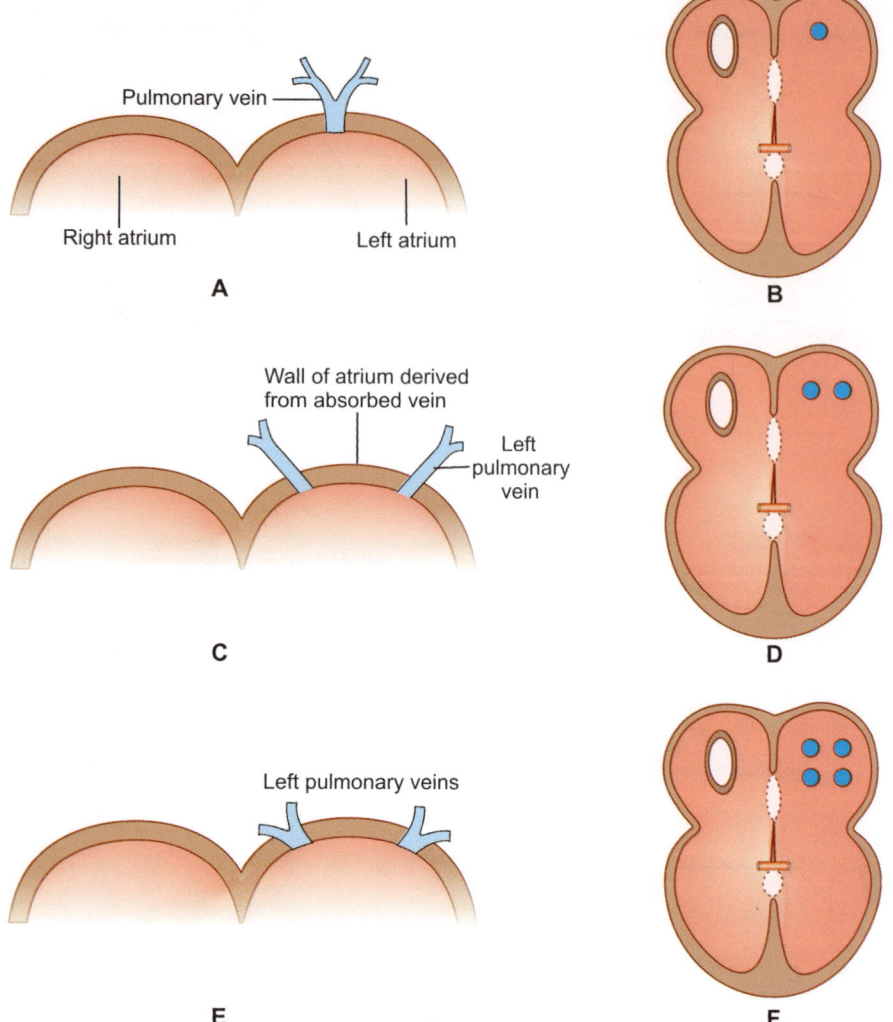

Fig. 14.13: Incorporation of pulmonary veins into left atrium as seen in tranverse section and vertical sections, respectively: A and B, single vein; C and D, two veins; and E and F, four veins.

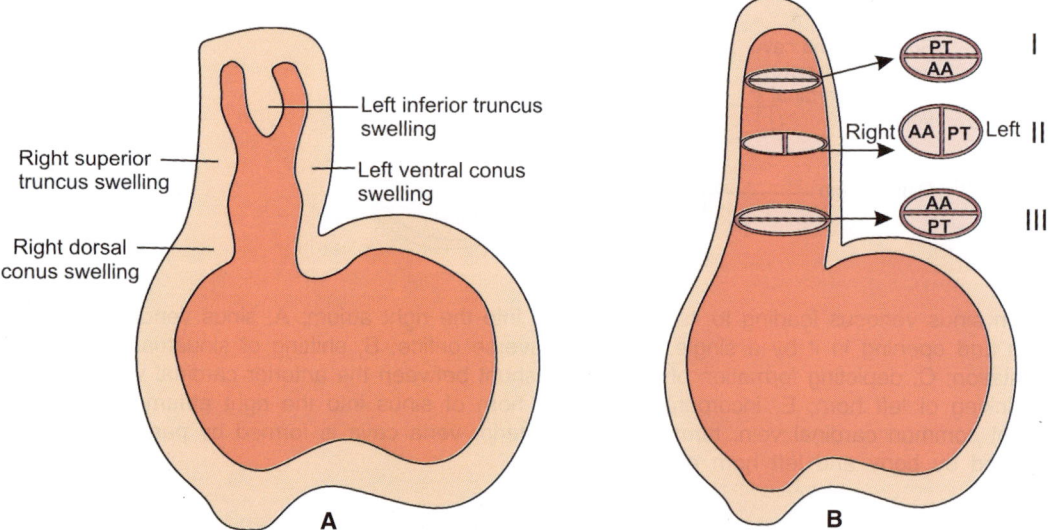

Fig. 14.14: Septation of truncus arteriosus: A, appearance of truncal swellings (ridges); B, formation of spiral aorticopulmonary septum which is oriented coronally in the proximal part, with pulmonary trunk (PT) ventral and ascending aorta (AA) dorsal (I). In the central part the septum is in anteroposterior position with PT left and AA right (II), distally again the septum is coronally oriented with PT dorsal and AA ventral (III).

Septation of truncus arteriosus

Truncal ridges (two swellings) appear in the walls of truncus arteriosus during 5th week. These ridges are formed by the *neural crest cells* which have migrated from the edges of the neural folds in the hind brain region through the pharyngeal arches. These ridges are (Fig. 14.14A):

- *Right superior truncus swelling,* appearing in the right superior wall, and
- *Left inferior truncus swelling* appearing in the left inferior wall.

Spiral aorticopulmonary septum is formed by the fusion of these truncus swellings after they grow towards each other in a spiral fashion. The spiral septum divides the truncus arteriosus into ascending aorta, and pulmonary trunk (Fig. 14.14B).

- *Proximally* the spiral septum becomes continuous with the distal bulbar septum and is coronally oriented, pulmonary trunk being ventral and aorta dorsal (Fig. 14.14B-I)
- *Centrally,* the septum is anteroposterior position with pulmonary trunk on the left side and aorta on the right side (Fig. 14.14B-II).
- *Distally,* the septum is again coronally oriented, but the aorta here is ventral and pulmonary trunk dorsal (14.14B-III).

Cephalic end of the spiral septum fuses with the dorsal wall of the aortic sac between the 5th and 6th pair of aortic arches. As a result:

- Upper five pairs of aortic arches are connecting to ascending aorta and left ventricle (i.e. systemic circulation), sixth pair of aortic arches is connected

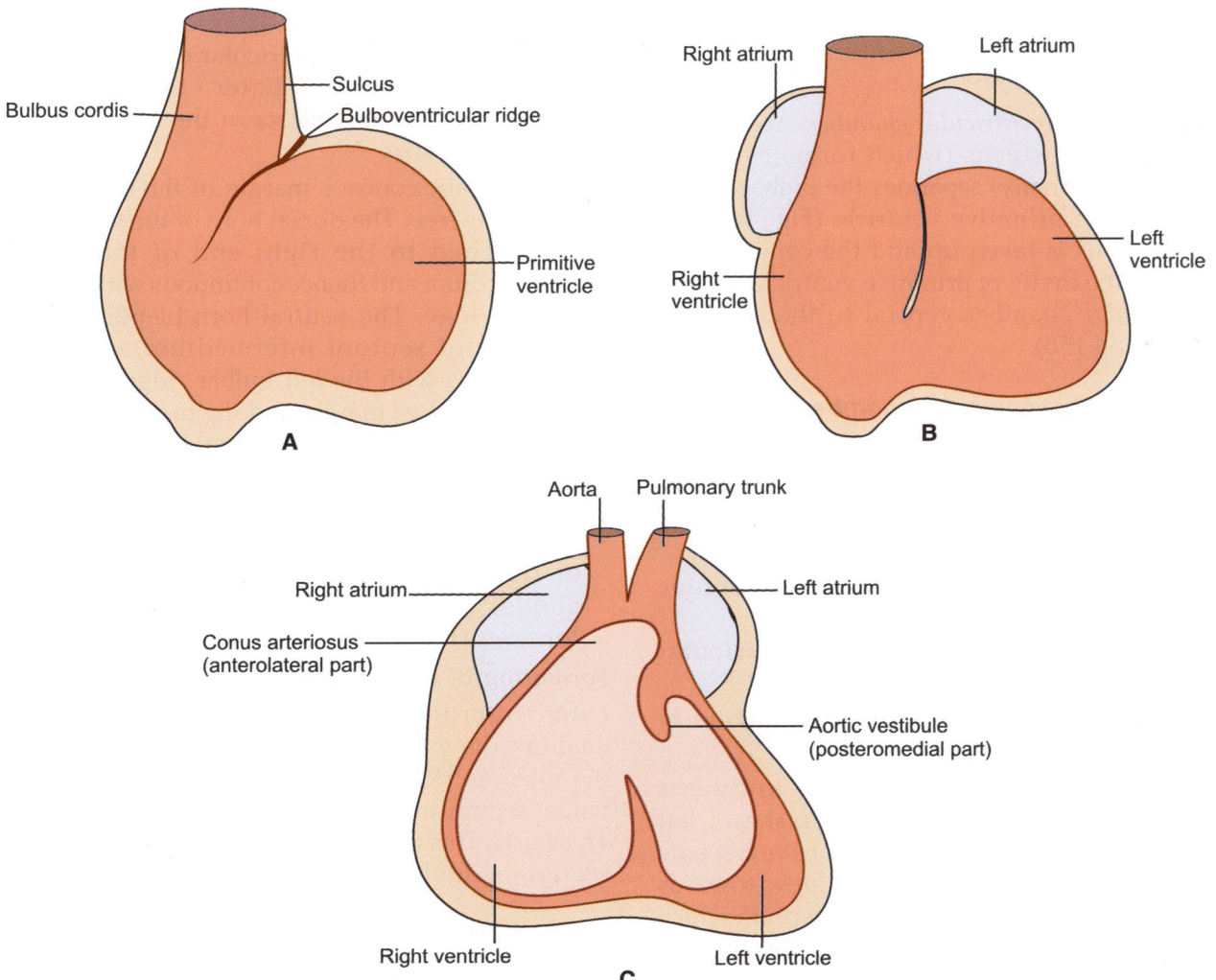

Fig. 14.15: Formation of bulboventricular chamber and proximal bulbar septum: A, bulbar cordis opening in primitive ventricle, note bulboventricular ridge and sulcus; B, disappearance of bulboventricular ridge and sulcus leading to formation of bulboventricular chamber; C, formation of proximal bulbar septum dividing conus cordis part into conus arteriosus (anteriolateral part) and aortic vestibule (posteromedial part).

to pulmonary trunk and right ventricle (pulmonary circulation).

Formation of aortic and pulmonary valves

At the lower end of the truncus arteriosus at its junction with the conus cordis four cushions (swellings) — right and left bulbar ridges and dorsal and ventral are formed. With separation of aortic and pulmonary openings the fused right and left bulbar cushions are subdivided into two parts, one part going to each orifice (Fig. 14.14C). In this way each orifice has three cushions from which the three cusps of the corresponding valve develop (Fig. 14.14D).

- *Aortic valve* has one anterior and two posterior cusps, while
- *Pulmonary valve* has two anterior and one posterior cusp.

Formation and septation of bulboventricular chamber

Formation of bulboventricular chamber: At 4 weeks, externally a deep sulcus (which forms *bulboventricular* ridge internally) separates the bulbar cordis proper from the primitive ventricle (Fig. 14.15A). Soon this sulcus is taken up and the conus cordis merges with the cavity of primitive ventricle to form *bulboventricular* chamber ventral to the common atrium (Fig. 14.15B).

Septation of bulboventricular chamber

Septation of bulboventricular chamber formed above involves three processes:
- Septation of conus cordis part by formation of proximal bulbar septum,
- Formation of muscular interventricular septum, and
- Formation of membranous interventricular septum.

Septation of conus cordis part by formation of proximal bulbar septum

Conus (bulbar) ridges cushions (similar to truncus swellings) appear along the right dorsal and left ventral walls of conus cordis which have become continuous with the ventricle. These grow towards each other and fuse to form the bulbar septum which divides the conus cordis into two parts (Fig. 14.15C).

- *Anterolateral portion of conus cordis* forms the *conus arteriosus* the outflowing smooth part of the right ventricle which cranially becomes continuous with pulmonary trunk with semilunar valves intervening.

- *Posterior medial portion* of conus cordis forms the *aortic vestibule* the outflowing smooth part of left ventricle which cranially becomes continuous with ascending aorta with semilunar valves intervening.

Formation of muscular ventricular septum (Figs 14.9 and 14.16)

- Division of primitive ventricle into right and left chambers by the appearance of *primordial ventricular septum* at the apex of ventricular bend becomes recognizable about the same time that the interatrial septum primum appears and the atrio-ventricular canal is divided into right and left canals by the formation of *intermediate septum* (fused atrio-ventricular cushions). Infect the medial walls of the enlarging ventricles approach each other and gradually merge to form the muscular interventricular (IV) septum.

- Initially, most of the increase in height of the IV septum results from the downward enlargement of the right and left ventricular cavities on either side of the septum. Later, there is active proliferation of myoblasts in the septum which increase its size.

- The cephalic concave margin of the muscular IV septum is free. The dorsal horn of the free margin is attached to the right end of the septum intermedium and thence continuous with the right bulbar ridge. The ventral horn blends with the left end of septum intermedium and thence continuous with the left bulbar ridge. The space between its free margin and the fused endocardial cushions (septum intermedium) is called *interventricular foramen,* which permits communication between the two ventricles (Fig. 14.16A and B).

- The proximal bulbar septum formed by the fusion of right and left bulbar ridges (as described above) partially closes the interventricular foramen (Fig. 14.16C and D).

Formation of membranous interventricular septum

Later, from the right edge of the septum intermedium the endocardial cells proliferate and close the interventricular foramen between the proximal bulbar septum and muscular interventricular septum. This part forms the *membranous part* of the ventricular septum of adult heart (Fig. 14.16C and D).

FORMATION OF CONDUCTION SYSTEM OF HEART

Sinoatrial (SA) node is formed from the pacemaker which occupies following positions:
- Caudal part of left cardiac tube initially.
- Sinus venosus part of tubular heart after fusion of the two heart tubes, and

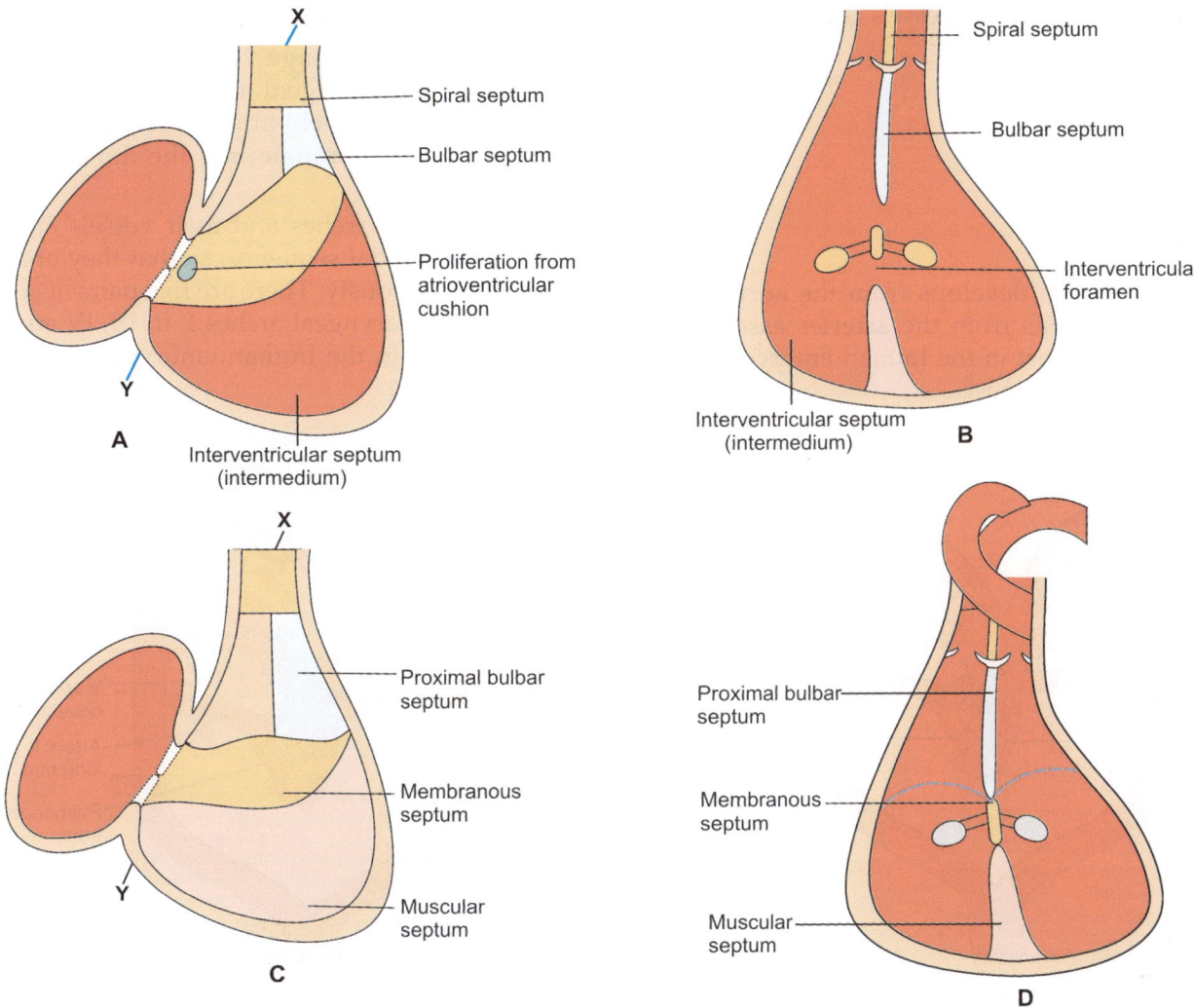

Fig. 14.16: Formation of interventricular septum (bulbar, membranous and muscular parts); A and B, early stage, note presence of interventricular foramen; C and D, late stage; *Note:* B and D are sections along axis XY of A and C.

• Right atrium, near the opening of superior vena cava, after incorporation of sinus venosus into the right atrium.

Atrioventricular (AV) node and bundle of His are formed from two sources:

• Left wall of sinus venosus, and
• Atrioventricular canal.

After incorporation of sinus venosus into the right atrium, the final position taken of by these cells is at the base of the interatrial septum.

MOLECULAR REGULATION OF CARDIAC DEVELOPMENT

Genes involved in cardiac development are :

• *NKX-2* is the master gene regulating development of heart.
• *HAND-1 and HAND-2* are other genes involved in cardiac development.

Signaling molecules involved are:

• *BMPs 2 and 4* secreted by the endoderm and lateral plate mesoderm which induce the heart forming region of splanchnic mesoderm.
• *Crescent and cerebrus* produced by endoderm cells inhibit WNT proteins 3a and 8 secreted by neural tube (which inhibit heart development).

DEVELOPMENT OF VASCULAR SYSTEM

Vessels are formed by two mechanisms:

1. *Vasculogenesis* refers to a process in which blood vessels differentiate from the angioblasts. Most of the major vessels including the dorsal aortae, and cardinal veins are formed by vasculogenesis.

2. *Angiogenesis* refers to the process in which vessels sprout from the pre-existing blood vessels. Most of the vessels (except those formed by vasculogenesis in embryo), are formed by this:

Derivation of important vessels is described here briefly in following sections:

- Arterial system,
- Venous system, and
- Lymphatic system

ARTERIAL SYSTEM

The arterial system develops from the aortic sacs and by angiogenesis from the arteries associated with primordial heart in the human embryo which develop by vasculogenesis.

AORTIC ARCHES AND THEIR DERIVATIVES

As described earlier (page 209), the aortic arches (arteries of the pharyngeal arches which develop during 4th and 5th week) arise from the aortic sac on each side and terminate into the dorsal aortae (Fig. 14.17A).

The pharyngeal arches and their vessels appear in a cranial to caudal sequence, so that they are not present simultaneously. There are five pairs of aortic arches for the pharyngeal arches I, II, III, IV and VI (V being absent in the human embryo), which are present as below:

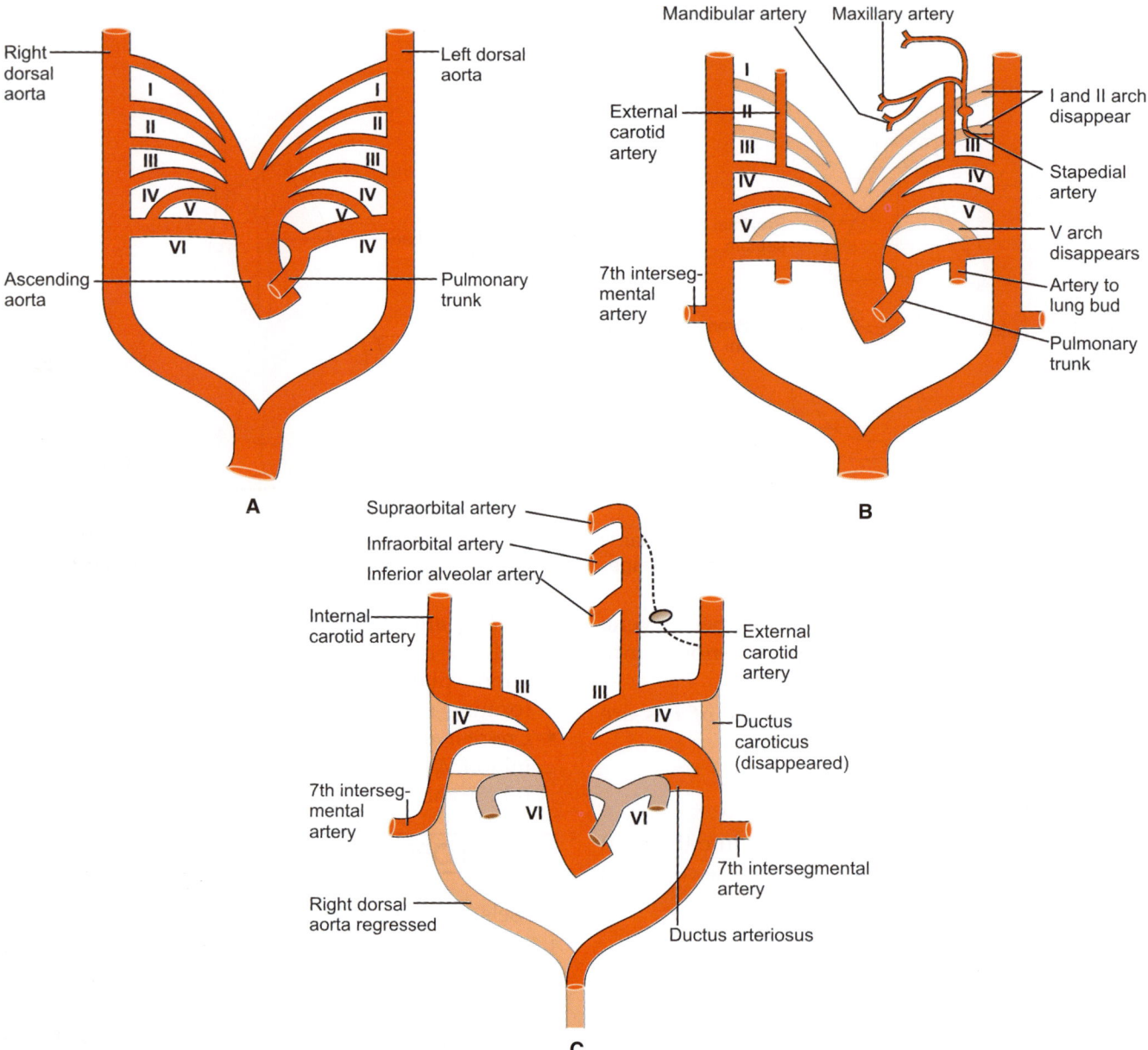

Fig. 14.17: Aortic arches, ascending aorta, aortic sac pulmonary trunk from dorsal aortae above the fusion and their derivatives: A, schematic connections of the above structures; B, disappearance of I, II, V aortic arches and appearance of external carotid arteries as sprouts from III aortic arch; C, disappearance of ductus caroticus on both sides, part of right dorsal aorta, and part of right VI aortic arch leading to formation of major vessels.

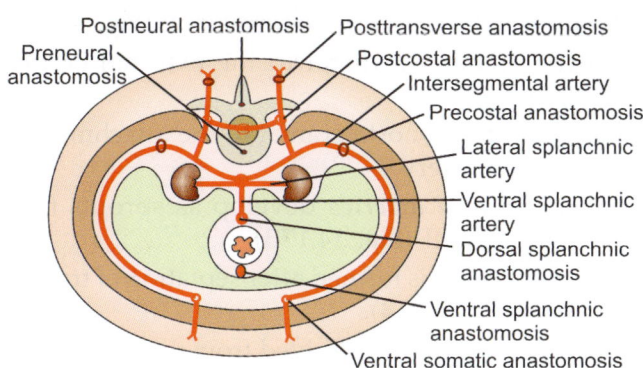

Fig. 14.18: Schematic transverse section of abdomen depicting general plan for the branches of the dorsal aorta.

- *At 4 weeks,* arch arteries I, II and III are present.
- *During 5th and 6th weeks* the arch arteries IV and VI appear, and I and II atrophy (Fig. 14.17B).
- *During 7th and 8th weeks,* III, IV and VI are modified into the definitive great arteries (Fig. 14.17C).

Fate of aortic arches

Aortic arch I. Mainly disappears, the small remaining part forms:

- Inferior alveolar artery, branch of maxillary artery.

Aortic arch II. Mainly disappears, remaining part forms:

- Hyoid artery, and
- Stapedial artery

Aortic arch III. Persists and forms:

- Common carotid artery, and
- First part of internal carotid artery. Rest of internal carotid artery is formed by cranial portion of dorsal aorta (Fig. 14.17C).
- External carotid artery develops as a sprout of aortic arch III (Fig. 14.17B and C).

Aortic arch IV. The right and left side develop differently.

Left aortic arch IV forms:

- Part of arch of aorta, between the left common carotid and left subclavian arteries.

Right aortic arch IV forms:

- Most proximal part of right subclavian artery, (dorsal part is formed by a portion of right dorsal aorta and 7th intersegmental artery). The left subclavian artery is formed by left 7th intersegmental artery.

Aortic arch V, does not develop in human embryo.

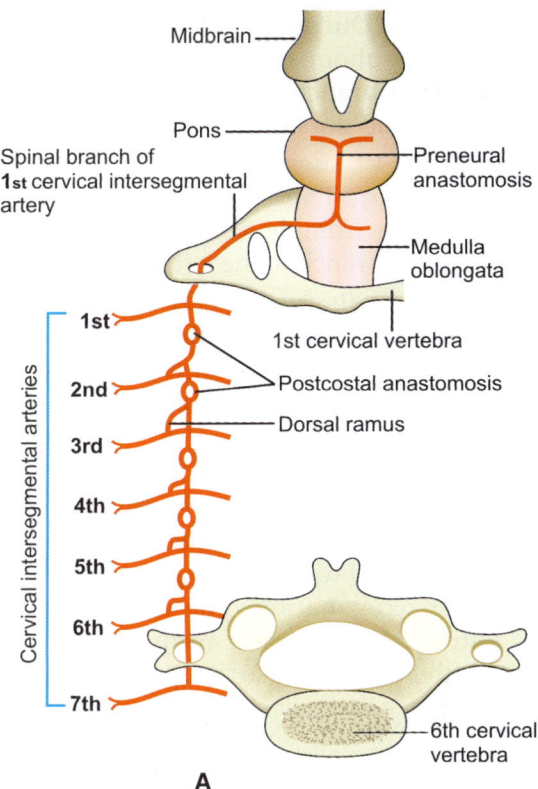

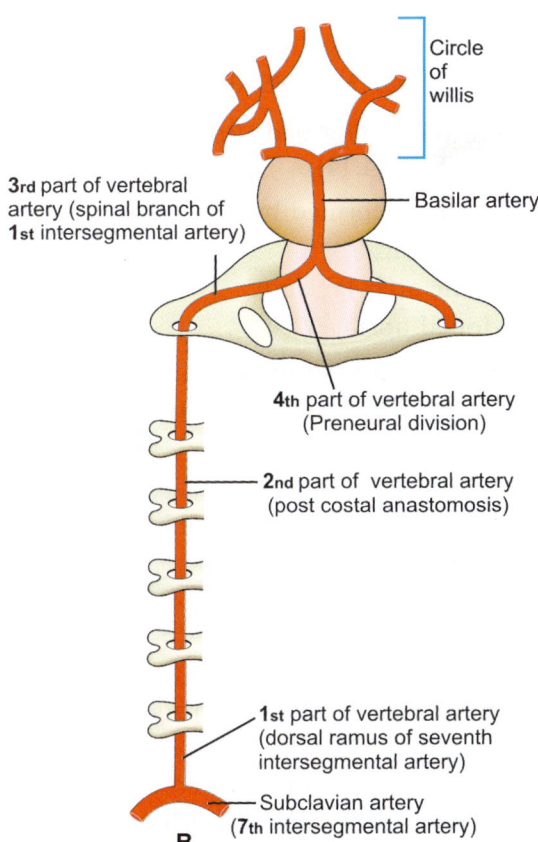

Fig. 14.19: Stages of development of vertebral artery; early (A) and late (B).

Aortic arch VI. During septation of the truncus arteriosus, the pulmonary flow ends in aortic arch VI. They give a branch to the corresponding lung buds and join the dorsal aortae (Fig. 14.17B).

Right aortic arch VI loses connection with the dorsal aorta (6th week). The right pulmonary artery, therefore, derives from the ventral part of right arch artery VI and its branch to the left lung (Fig. 14.17C).

Left aortic arch VI, its ventral part and its branch to the lung bud form the left pulmonary artery, but the connection with the dorsal aorta is not lost. It persists as the *ductus arteriosus* during the fetal period (Fig. 14.17C).

The *ductus arteriosus,* an important fetal adaptation to intrauterine life, enables venous blood to be diverted from the functionless lungs into the descending aorta. From there it goes directly to the placenta for oxygenation. The ductus arteriosus closes within 12 hours after birth, and undergoes fibrosis in the first 6 weeks postpartum, to become the *ligamentum arteriosum.*

DEFINITIVE DERIVATIVES OF AORTIC SACS

Right aortic sac becomes the brachiocephalic artery.

Left aortic sac forms part of arch of aorta.

DEVELOPMENT OF MAJOR ARTERIES

Ascending aorta is formed after septation of truncus arteriosus (Fig. 14.14).

Arch of aorta is formed by (Fig. 14.17C):
- Left aortic sac,
- Left aortic arch IV, and
- Left dorsal aorta.

Descending aorta is formed by (Fig. 14.17C):
- Left dorsal aorta below the attachment of aortic arch IV, and
- Fused dorsal aortae

Brachiocephalic artery is formed by the right aortic sac (Fig. 14.17C).

Subclavian artery is derived differently on right and left sides.

- *Right subclavian artery:* Proximal part from the right aortic arch IV and remaining part from 7th intersegmental artery.
- *Left subclavian artery* is derived entirely from the 7th cervical intersegmental artery (Fig. 14.17C):

Common carotid arteries are formed by aortic arches III, proximal to the external carotid bud (Fig. 14.17C).

Internal carotid arteries are formed by (Fig. 14.17C)
- Aortic arches III, distal to the external carotid bud, and
- Original dorsal aorta cranial to the attachment of third arch artery.

External carotid arteries develop as sprouts from the aortic arch III (Fig. 14.17B).

Pulmonary trunk is formed after septation of truncus arteriosus (Fig. 14.14).

Pulmonary arteries are derived from the ventral part of aortic arch VI and its branch to the lung bud (Fig. 14.17C).

DORSAL AORTAE AND THEIR BRANCHES

As described earlier (page 209), the dorsal aorta is a paired vessel in the early human embryo and persists bilaterally in the head and neck as internal carotid arteries. In the 5th week, the two aortae fuse caudal to T_4, forming a single aorta in the developing thoracic and abdominal regions. Opposite the sacral segments, the fused aortae persists in rudimentry form as median sacral artery.

Branches of dorsal aortae and their fate

Each dorsal aorta, even before the stage of fusion gives numerous branches which arise at right angles to the long axis, and in fused dorsal aorta they appear as right and left branches, which can be arranged in three groups (Fig. 14.18):
- Intersegmental arteries,
- Lateral splanchnic branches, and
- Ventral splanchnic branches.

Fate of intersegmental arteries

About 30 or so somatic intersegmental arteries arising from the dorsal aorta supply the blood to developing somites and their derivatives. Most of the original connections of the intersegmental arteries to the dorsal aorta disappear, and they form the following definitive arteries :
- *In the neck,* thin postcostal anastomosis (C_1 to C_8) form the vertebral artery along with dorsal division of 7th cervical intersegmental artery (Fig. 14.19).
- *In the thorax,* they persist as *intercostal arteries.* Anastomosis between their ventral divisions along with the ventral division of 7th cervical intersegmental artery (which forms mainstem) form the internal thoracic artery (Fig. 14.20).
- *In the abdomen,* they form *lumbar arteries,* but the 5th pair of lumbar intersegmental arteries remain as the *common iliac arteries* (Fig. 14.21).

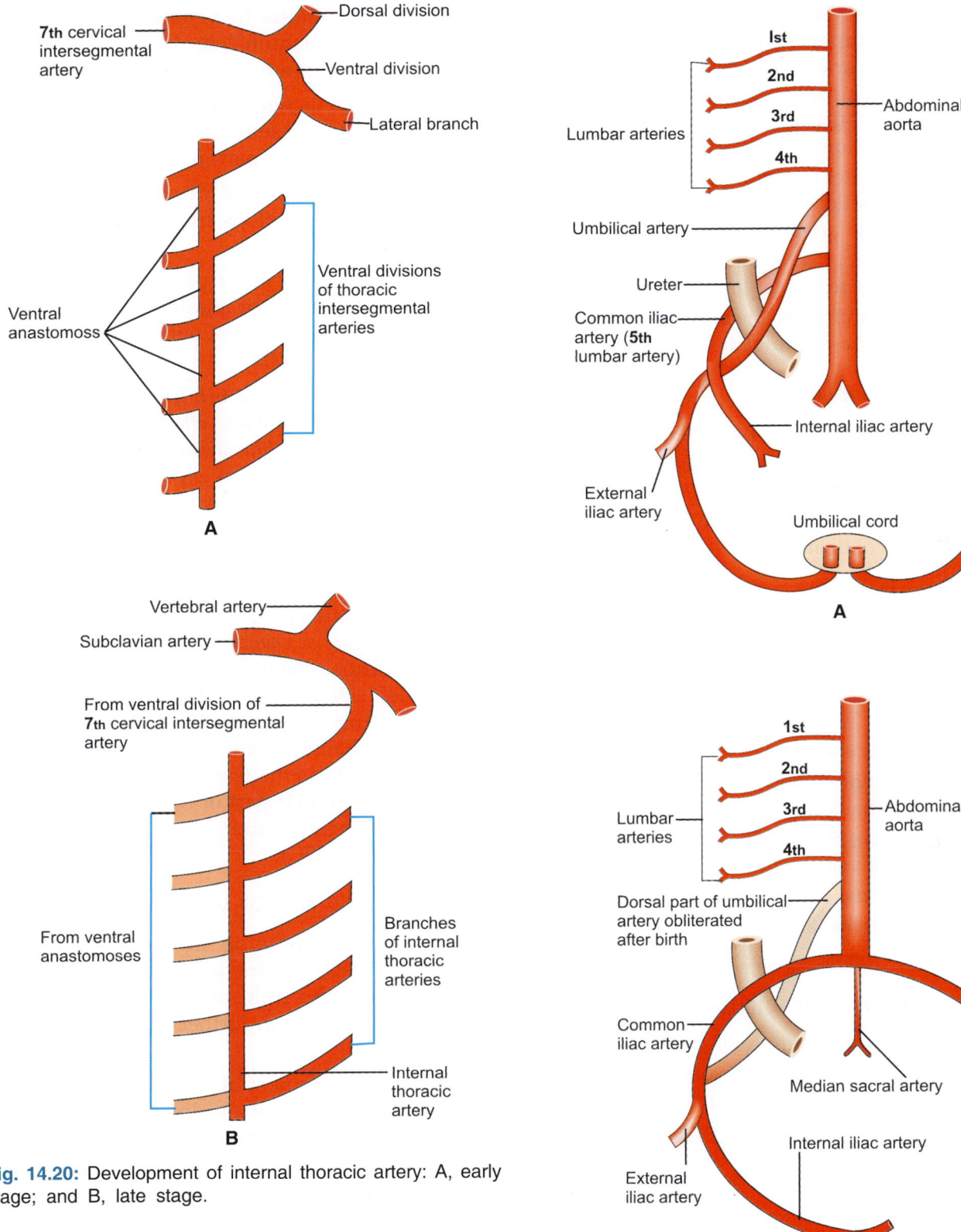

Fig. 14.20: Development of internal thoracic artery: A, early stage; and B, late stage.

- *In the sacral region,* they form the lateral sacral arteries (Fig. 14.21):

Fate of vitelline arteries

As described earlier (page 209) the vitelline arteries are unpaired ventral branches of the dorsal aorta that supply yolk sac, allantois and chorion and later

Fig. 14.21: Fate of intersegmental arteries in lumbar and sacral regions, and development of iliac and umbilical arteries.

to the primitive gut. Three vitelline arteries persist as; celiac trunk, superior mesenteric artery and inferior mesenteric artery. The origin of these three trunks migrate caudally from their primitive positions, due to successive growth of the new caudal stems, as below:

- *Celiac trunk* migrates from the 7th cervical segment to the adult position opposite the 12th thoracic segment. It is the artery of foregut.
- *Superior mesenteric artery* to midgut, shifts from 3rd thoracic segment to the Ist lumbar segment, and
- *Inferior mesenteric artery* to the hindgut, shifts from 5th thoracic to the 3rd lumbar segment.

Fate of umbilical arteries

Fate of umbilical arteries (see page 209), is as below:
- *Proximal parts* persist as internal iliac arteries and superior vesical arteries (Fig. 14.21).
- *Dorsal parts* obliterate after birth and become the medial umbilical ligaments.

VENOUS SYSTEM

Veins of primitive cardiovascular system which drain into the primitive heart of a 4 week embryo include following three pairs (Fig. 14.1):
- Vitelline veins,
- Umbilical veins, and
- Common cardinal veins formed by anterior and posterior cardinal veins.

However, during 5th to 7th weeks, a number of additional pairs of veins are formed, which include:
- Subcardinal veins,
- Sacrocardinal veins, and
- Supracardinal veins.

DERIVATIVES AND FATE OF VITELLINE VEINS

The right and left vitelline veins arise from the capillary plexus in the wall of yolk sac and after traversing the septum transversum drain into the right and left horns of sinus venosus, respectively (Fig. 14.22A). The appearance of hepatic buds in the septum transversum subdivides the vitelline veins into three parts:
- Infrahepatic part,
- Intrahepatic part, and
- Suprahepatic part

Infrahepatic part of right and left vitelline veins develop three sets of transverse anastomosis between each other around the duodenum, upper

and lower anastomoses lie ventral and middle one dorsal to the duodenum (Fig. 14.22B). Derivatives of infrahepatic part are as below (Fig. 14.22B):

- *Portal vein* and its right and left branches develops from the transverse anastomotic channels and parts of those veins taking part into these anastomoses.
- *Superior mesenteric vein* draining the primary intestinal loop develops from the anterior limb of lower anastomosis.
- *Distal portions* and other parts of right and left vitelline veins and their anastomotic channels not forming portal vein and superior mesenteric vein disappear (Fig. 14.22C).

Intrahepatic parts of the vitelline veins just after entering the liver divide into *afferent branches* (which persist as *intrahepatic branches of portal vein*) which break up into a network of capillary plexuses and join secondarily with the *hepatic sinusoids* which develop in situ between the rows of liver cells. The efferent vessels arising from the capillary plexus form the *tributaries of the hepatic vein* (Fig. 14.22B).

Suprahepatic part of vitelline veins form the right and *left hepatocardiac channels* (Fig. 14.22B). Soon, the left hepatocardiac channel disappears and the blood from the left side of liver is rechanneled toward the right resulting in an enlargement of the right *hepatocardiac* channel (common hepatic vein) which persists in adults as the *terminal part of inferior vena cava* opening into that part of right atrium which is formed after incorporation of right horn of sinus venosus (Fig. 14.22C).

DERIVATIVES AND FATE OF UMBILICAL VEINS

Umbilical veins develop in the chorionic sac (primordial placenta), travel in the umbilical cord and drain into the right and left horns of sinus venosus (Fig. 14.1). Their further fate and derivatives are as below:

- With the development of liver the umbilical vein pass on each side of the liver, but also make connection with the hepatic sinusoids (Fig. 14.22B).
- Soon, whole of the right umbilical vein and proximal part of the left umbilical vein disappear. Thus, the left vein is the only one to carry oxygenated blood from the placenta to liver.
- *Ductus venosus*, a direct passage between the left umbilical vein and right hepatocardiac channel is later developed, which bypasses the sinusoidal plexus of liver and thus facilitates the passage of

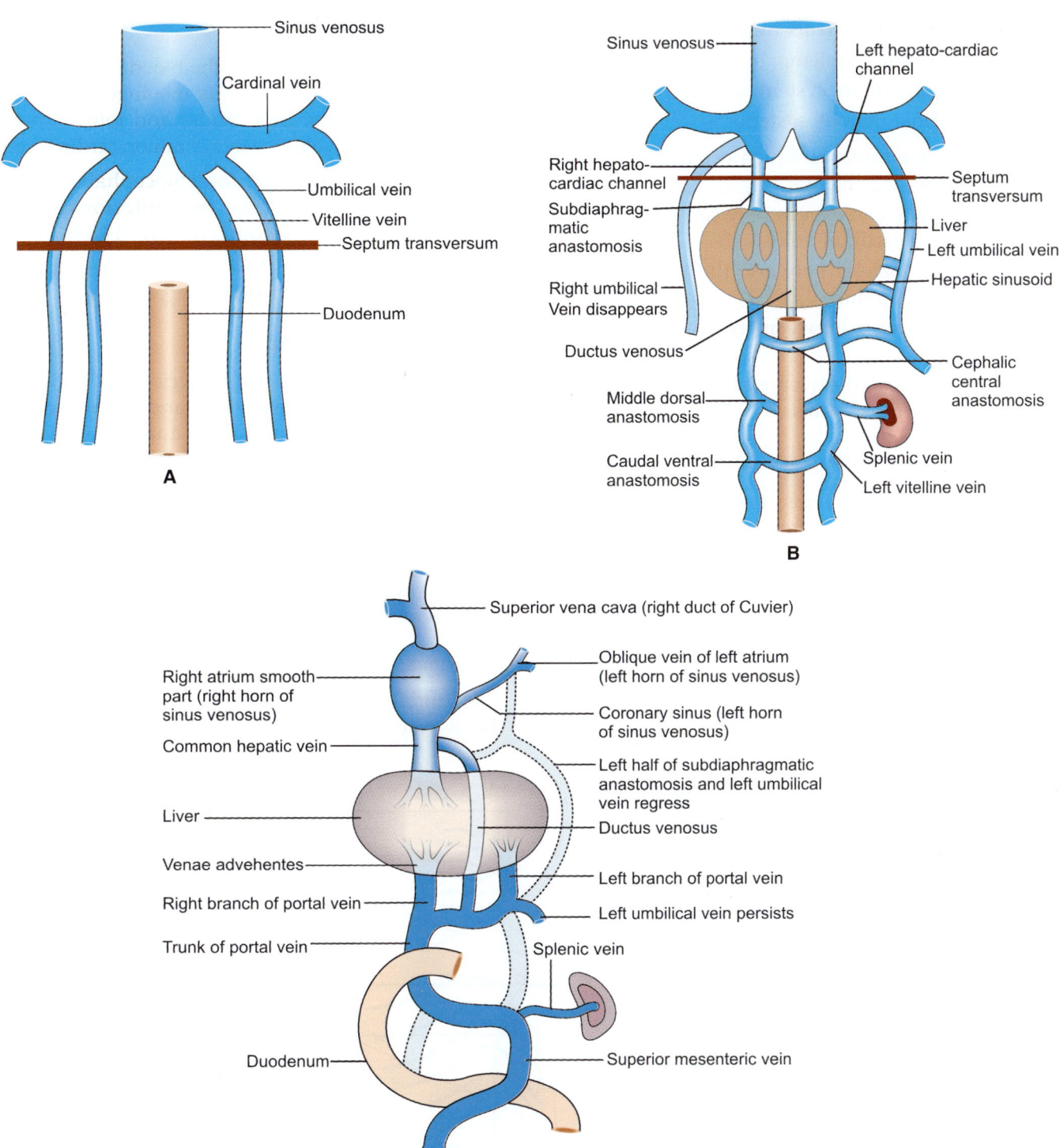

Fig. 14.22: Development and derivatives of vitelline and umbilical veins: A, vitelline and umbilical veins opening in the horns of sinus venosus along with the common cardinal veins; B, anastomosis of vitelline veins and formation of hepatic sinusoids; C, development of portal vein, ductus venosus, and hepatic veins.

blood from the increasing placental circulation (Fig. 14.22C).

- After birth, the left umbilical vein and ductus venosus are obliterated and form the *ligamentum teres hepatis* and *ligamentum venosum*, respectively.

DERIVATIVES AND FATES OF CARDINAL, SUBCARDINAL, SACROCARDINAL AND SUPRACARDINAL SYSTEMS OF VEINS

Adults venous pattern is developed from the three embryonic venous systems and four major transverse anastomoses between them.

Embryonic venous systems include:
- Cardinal venous system,
- Subcardinal venous system, and
- Supracardinal venous system

Transverse anastomoses which occur between the above venous systems are:
- *Brachiocephalic anastomosis* between the right and left anterior cardinal veins,
- *Azygos anastomosis* between the right and left supracardinal veins,
- *Renal anastomosis* between the two subcardinal veins, and
- *Iliac anastomosis* between caudal ends of two posterior cardinal veins.

Cardinal venous system

Initially the cardinal veins form the main venous drainage system of the embryo. It consists of (Fig. 14.23):

Common cardinal veins

Common cardinal veins are formed by the union of anterior and posterior cardinal veins. The right and left common cardinal veins drain into the right and left horns of sinus venosus, respectively.

Anterior cardinal veins

Anterior cardinal veins drain the blood from cephalic parts (developing brain and its meninges, head and neck and the upper limb buds) and join with the posterior cardinal veins to form common cardinal vein.

Oblique cross connection (brachiocephalic anastomosis) occurs between the two anterior cardinal veins during later development (Fig. 14.24).

Intersegmental veins (1 to 7 cervical) are tributaries of the anterior cardinal veins (Fig. 14.23).

Posterior cardinal veins

At their cephalic ends the posterior cardinal veins end in common cardinal veins and at their caudal ends they make a transverse anastomosis (*iliac anastomosis*) with each other, twelve thoracic and five lumbar *intersegmental veins* form their tributaries. Posterior cardinal vein initially drains rest of the embryo (Fig. 14.23). However, after development of subcardinal and supracardinal veins (between 5th to 7th week) they cease to drain the urogenital ridge and largely degenerate (Fig. 14.25).

Derivatives of cardinal venous system

The caudal part of left anterior cardinal vein and the whole left common cardinal vein undergo

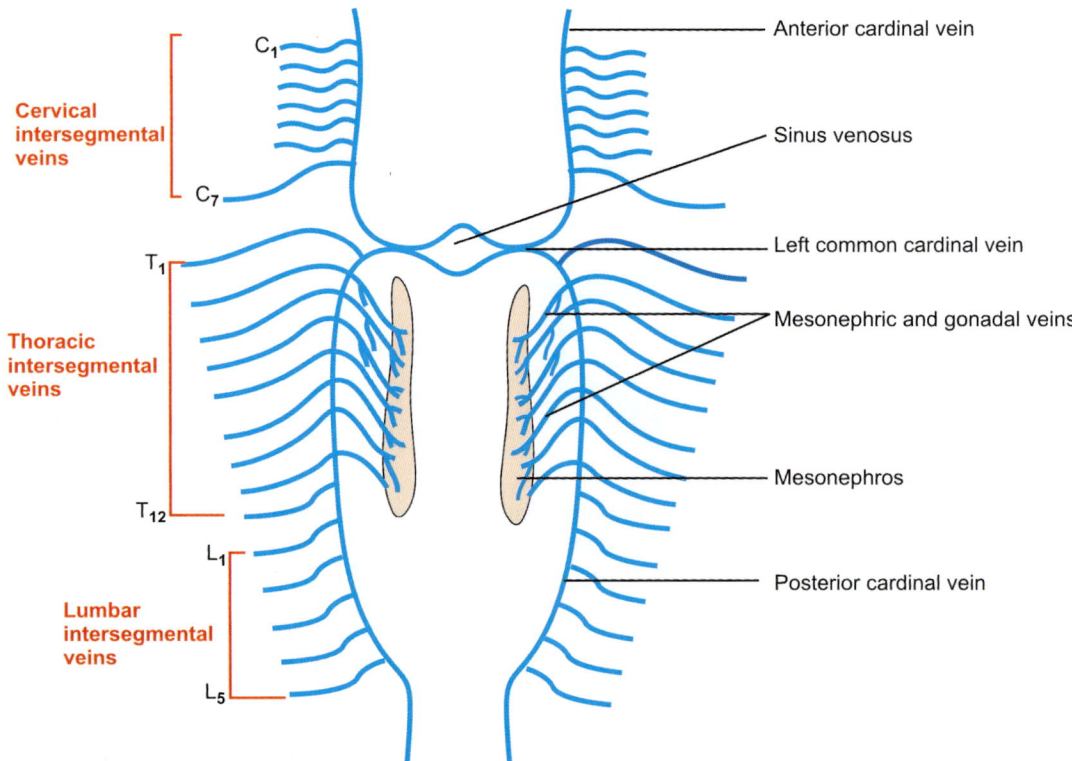

Fig. 14.23: The cardinal venous system draining the body wall and urogenital ridges at 4 weeks.

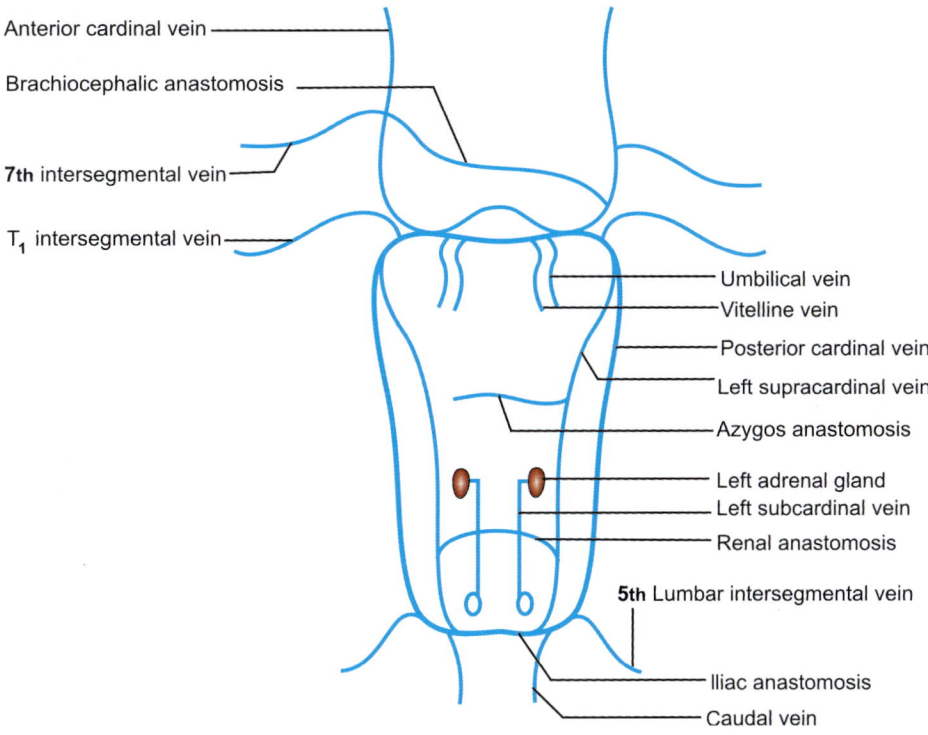

Fig. 14.24: The cardinal, subcardinal, and supracardinal systems and their transverse anastomosis.

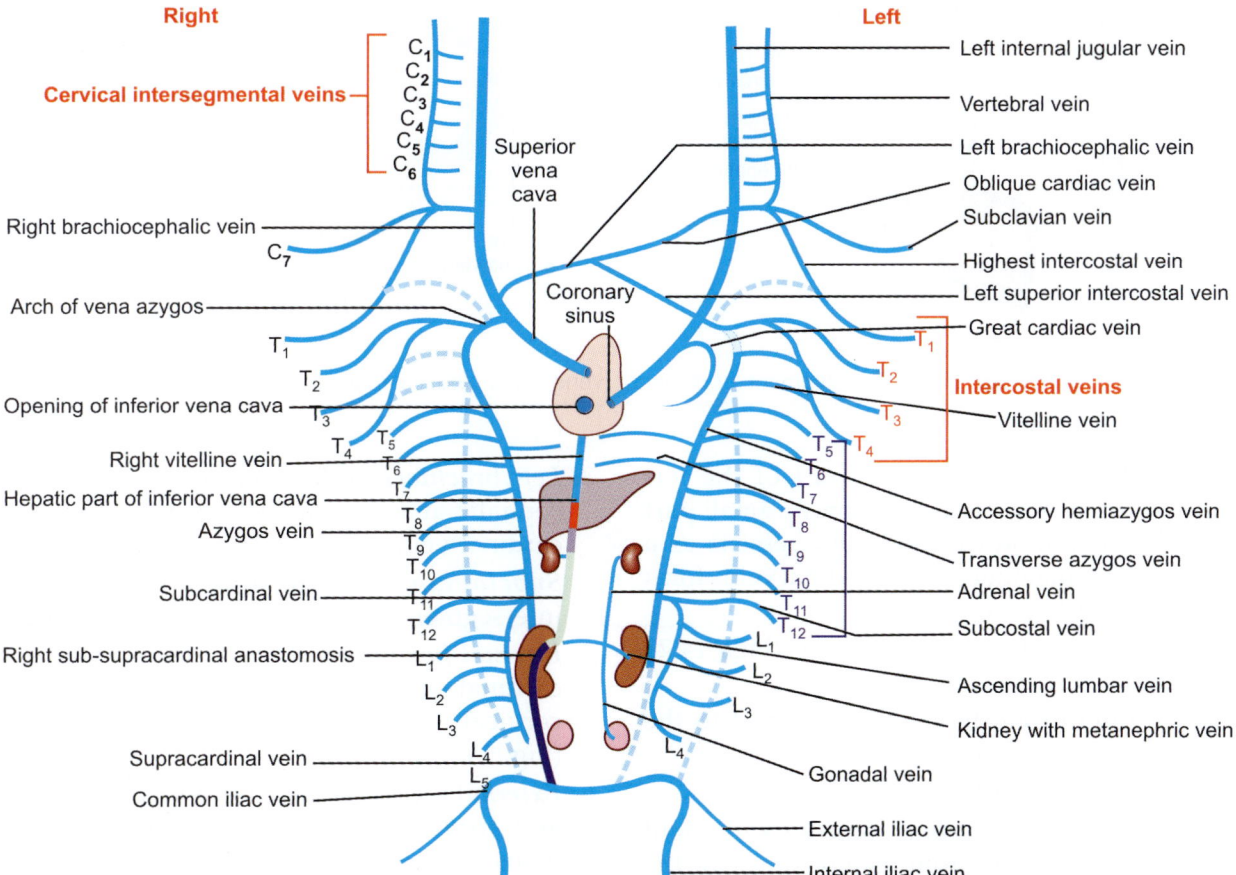

Fig. 14.25: Development of adult veins from cardinal, (blue color) subcardinal (green color) and supracardinal (voilet) system. Atrophied veins are shown in broken lines. New formed vessels are shown in light blue color and right vitelline derivatives in light green.

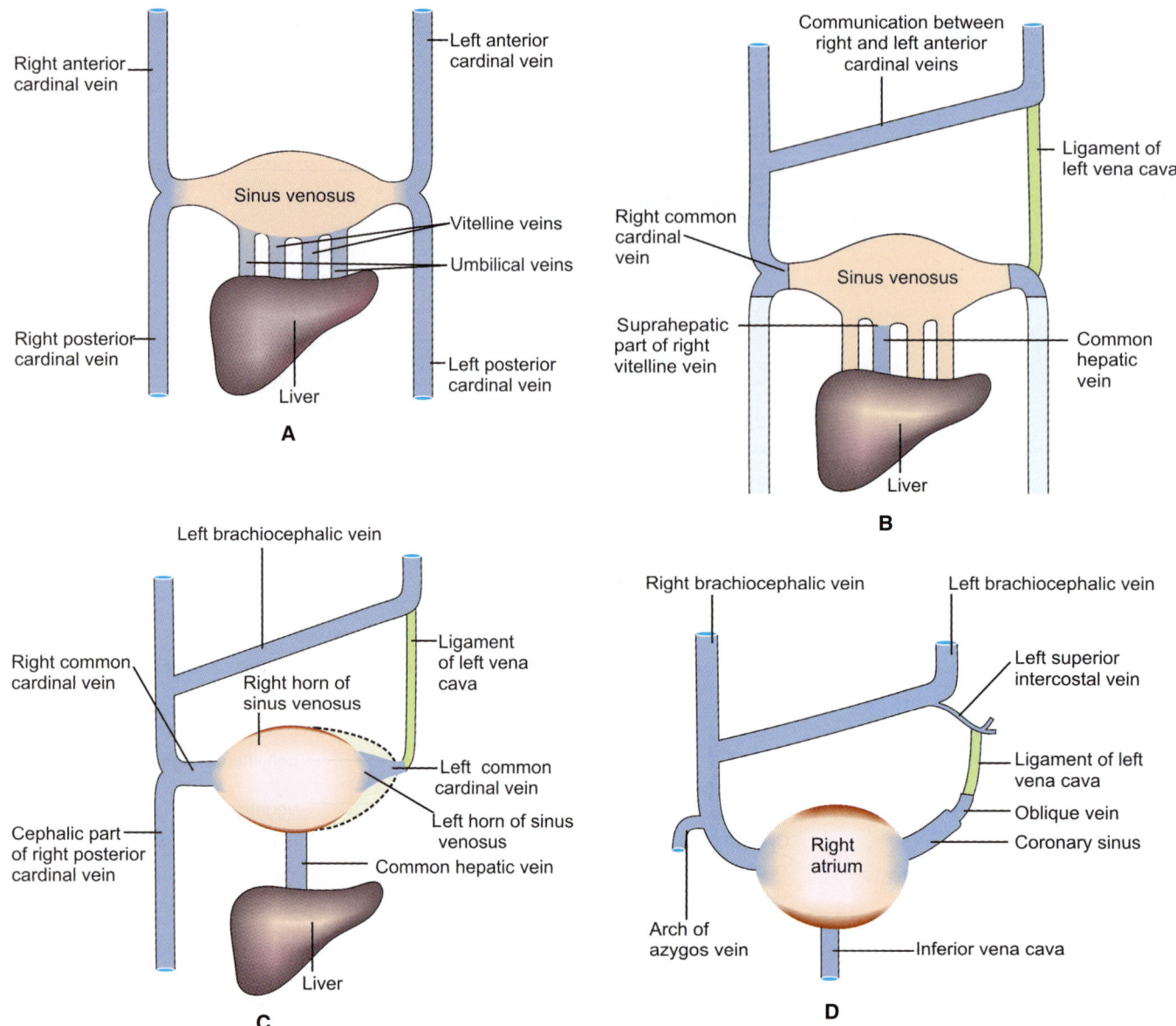

Fig. 14.26: Development of superior vena cava and its main tributaries.

marked regression. The greater part of the left posterior cardinal vein disappears, only a small part adjoining the common cardinal vein persists as a small vein. The remaining part of cardinal veins form the following derivatives.

1. **Superior vena cava** is derived from (Figs 14.25 and 14.26):
   • Right anterior cardinal vein proximal to the brachiocephalic anastomosis, and
   • Right common cardinal vein.

2. **Right brachiocephalic vein** is formed by the right anterior cardinal vein, from its junction with the right 7th cervical intersegmental vein down to the brachiocephalic anastomosis (Figs 14.25 and 14.26).

3. **Left brachiocephalic vein** is formed by brachiocephalic anastomosis between the two anterior cardinal veins (Figs 14.25 and 14.26).

4. **Subclavian veins** are formed by 7th cervical intersegmental veins of right and left side.

5. **Internal jugular veins** are formed by the anterior cardinal veins cranial to their junction with 7th cervical intersegmental (adult subclavian) vein (Fig. 14.25).

6. **External jugular veins** arise as secondary channels and are not derived from the anterior cardinal veins.

7. **Left superior intercostal vein** is formed by regressed part of left anterior cardinal vein caudal to the transverse anastomosis and the most

cranial part of left posterior cardinal vein. It drains into left brachiocephalic vein and received 2nd and 3rd intercostal veins as tributaries (Fig. 14.25).

8. *Vertebral vein* on each side is formed by a longitudinal anastomosis which develops between the C_1 to C_7 and intercostal veins (Fig. 14.25).

9. *Spiral veins* in the cervical region represent the persisting intersegmental veins as tributaries of vertebral vein (Fig. 14.25).

Subcardinal veins

The subcardinal veins are formed in relation to the urogenital ridges which mainly drain the developing kidney. Cranially and caudally they communicate with the posterior cardinal veins.

- *Renal anastomosis* (inter-subcardinal anastomosis) refers to a transverse anastomosis that develops between the two subcardinal veins.

- Cranial part of the right subcardinal vein also establishes an anastomosis with right hepto-cardiac channel (see page 228).

Supracardinal veins

The supracardinal veins are longitudinal veins which communicate cranially and caudally with the posterior cardinal veins. They also communicate with the subcardinal veins through transverse anastomosis in the renal region. They drain the body wall by way of intercostal veins and thus take over the function of posterior cardinal veins which obliterate mostly.

Derivatives of posterior cardinal veins, subcardinal veins and supracardinal veins

Many parts of these longitudinal venous channels disappear (Fig. 14.25). Derivatives of the remaining parts are:

1. *Inferior vena cava (IVC)* is derived from the following in craniocaudal sequence (Figs 14.25 and 14.27):
   - *Hepatic segment* of IVC is derived from:
     - Right hepatocardiac channel (that develops from suprahepatic part of right vitelline vein) and
     - Anastomotic channel between the sub-cardinal vein and hepatocardiac channel.
   - *Renal segment* of IVC is formed by upper part of the right subcardinal vein. This part receives both renal and right suprarenal veins.

- *Post-renal segment* of IVC is formed cranio-caudally by:
  - Anastomosis between right supracardinal and subcardinal veins,.
  - Lower part of right supracardinal vein, and
  - Lowest part of right posterior cardinal vein.

2. *Right renal vein* is a mesonephric vein that originally drains into that part of subcardinal veins which forms the renal segment of the IVC (Fig. 14.27).

3. *Left renal vein* develops from three sources:
   - *Mesonephric vein* that originally drains into left subcardinal vein,
   - *A small part of left subcardinal vein* where the mesonephric vein originally opens, and
   - *Pre-aortic intersubcardinal anastomosis.*

4. *Left gonadal veins* develop from the distal part of subcardinal veins below the inter-subcardinal anastomosis. Note in Fig. 14.25 the left gonadal vein drains into left renal vein and right drains into inferior vena cava because of their developmental origin.

5. *Suprarenal veins* develop from the part of subcardinal veins above the inter-subcardinal anastomosis. Note in Fig. 14.25 the right vein opens in IVC and left in left renal veins because of their developmental origin.

6. *Right common iliac vein* is derived from the most caudal part of right posterior cardinal vein.

7. *Left common iliac vein* develops from the transverse anastomosis between the lower ends of two posterior cardinal veins. It joins the right common iliac vein to terminate in IVC.

Azygos system of veins

Veins forming azygos system of veins develop as below (Fig. 14.25):

1. *Azygos vein.* With the obliteration of the posterior cardinal veins, the supracardinal veins take over their function and drain the body wall. The 4th to 11th right intercostal veins empty into the right supracardinal vein which together with cranial part of right posterior cardinal vein (arch of azygos) forms the azygos vein.

2. *Hemiazygos* vein develops from the left supra-cardinal veins which receives 4th to 7th left intercostal veins as tributaries. It drains into azygos veins through transverse azygos vein.

3. *Transverse azygos* vein develops from the transverse anastomosis between the supra-cardinal veins (Fig. 14.25).

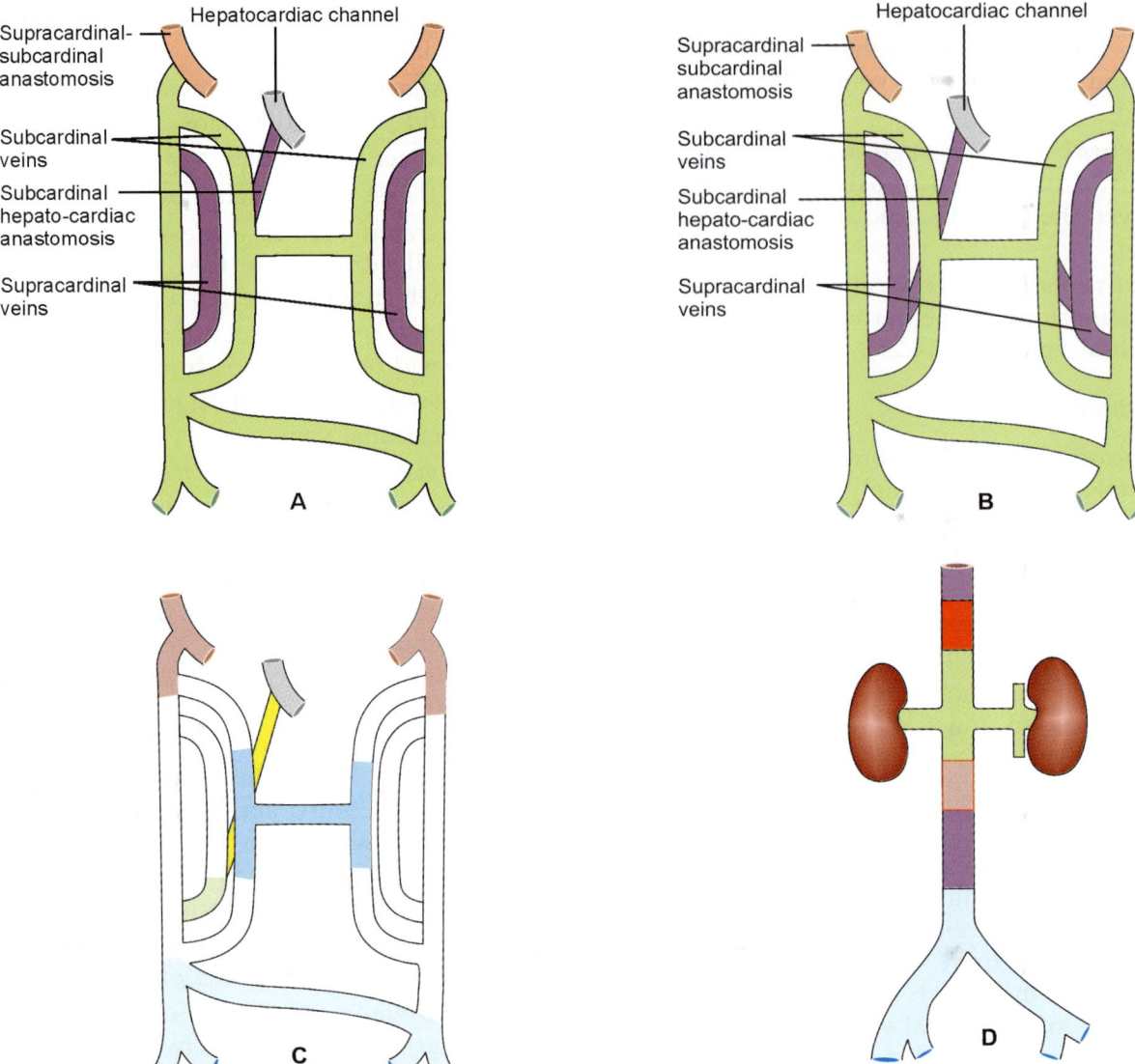

Fig. 14.27: Colour coded diagram to show development of various segments of inferior vena cava from different veins. For understanding correlate this figure with Fig. 14.25.

FETAL CIRCULATION

Pattern of fetal circulation

Pattern of fetal circulation shown in Fig. 14.28 and represented diagrammatically in Fig. 14.29 is:

Umbilical vein brings oxygenated blood from the placenta, which acts as lungs for the fetus. This blood is 80% saturated with O_2 (compared with 98% saturation in the arterial circulation in adults). The umbilical vein, before supplying the blood to liver, bypasses some of the blood to the inferior vena cava through *ductus venosus* (Fig. 14.28).

Inferior vena cava thus receives some blood (80% saturated with O_2) from the umbilical vein through ductus venosus, and other blood from the hepatic veins and systemic veins draining from the trunk

and inferior extremities (26% saturated with O_2).The mixed blood from inferior vena cava (with approximate 67% saturation) then enters the right atrium.

Right atrium receives blood from the inferior vena cava (saturation 67%) as well as superior vena cava (saturation 26%). The fate of blood entering the right atrium is very different from that in adult:

• From the right atrium, majority of the blood coming from the inferior vena cava (saturation 67%) passes to the left atrium directly through the foramen ovale (an opening in the interatrial septum), and joins the blood coming from the pulmonary vein (saturation 42%). The mixed blood from left atrium (saturation 62%) passes on to the left ventricle.

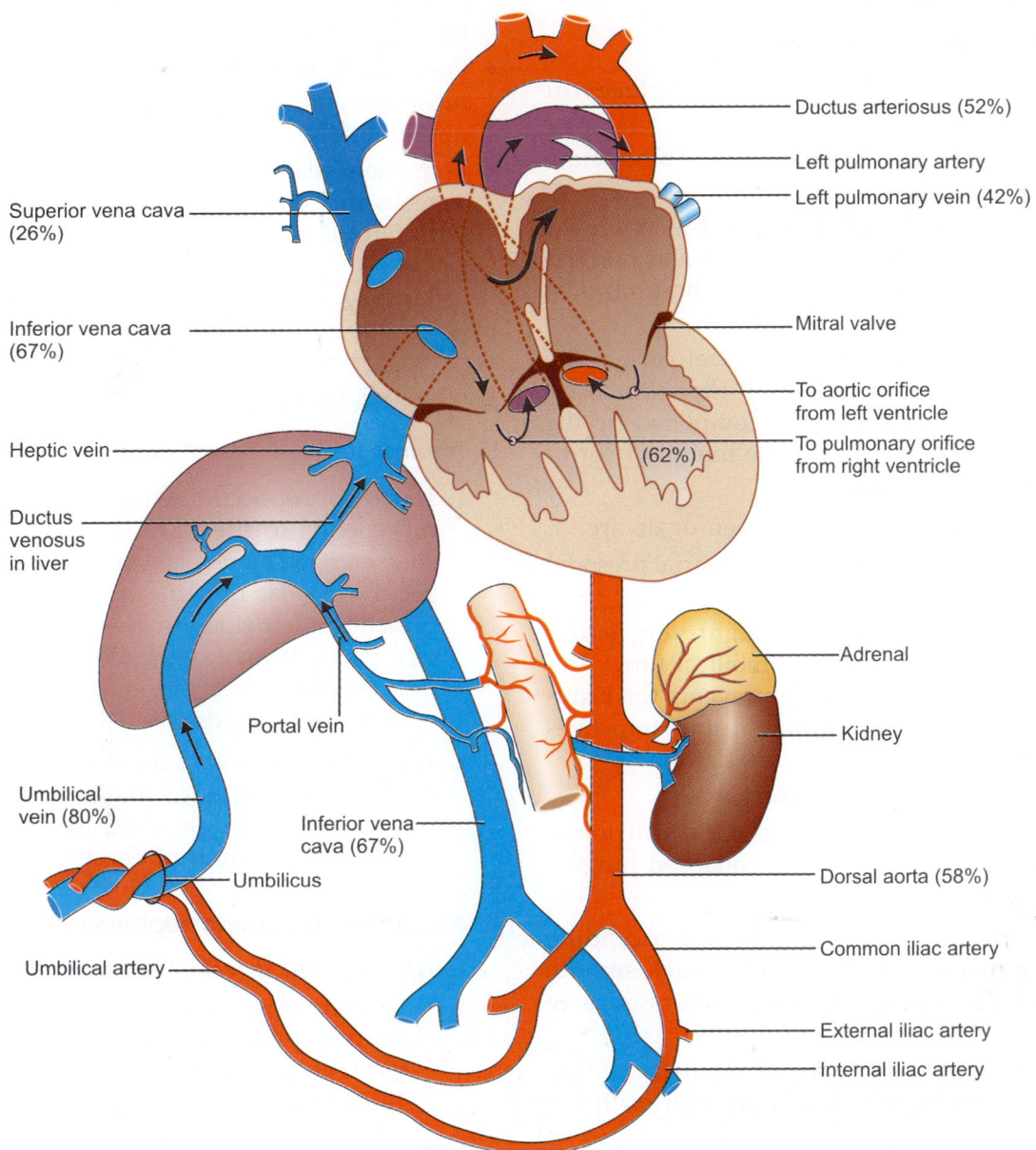

Fig. 14.28: Pattern of fetal circulation with pO₂ in different components.

- From the right atrium, most of the blood coming from superior vena cava (26% saturation) and small amount of that coming from the inferior vena cava (saturation 67%), passes into the right ventricle. This mixed blood from the right ventricle (saturation 52%) is pumped into the pulmonary artery. But, since the fetal lungs are collapsed, their vascular resistance is very high. Hence only a small fraction of blood passes through the lungs to reach the left atrium via the pulmonary veins. Bulk of the pulmonary artery blood enters the descending aorta directly by a vascular connection called the *ductus arteriosus*.

Left ventricle pumps the blood (with saturation 62%) into the ascending aorta, from where most of the blood goes into the vessels of the head and neck and forelimbs and only a small amount of blood goes to the descending aorta.

Descending aorta, thus receives blood mainly from the pulmonary artery through ductus arteriosus (with saturation 52%) and only a small amount from the left ventricle (with saturation 62%). The descending aorta then supplies the blood (with saturation 58%) to the whole of body (minus head and neck and forelimbs) and also to the placenta via umbilical arteries for oxygenation.

NEONATAL CIRCULATION

Changes in circulation after birth

1. *Arrest of umbilical blood flow and placental transfusion*

Factors responsible for arrest of umbilical blood flow and placental transfusion are:

- Vasoconstriction of umbilical vessels—Immediately after birth, there occurs sudden and marked reduction in blood flow through the umbilical vessels.
- Tieing and cutting of the umbilical cord—The process which is initiated by the nature by producing vasoconstriction is completed by the doctor by tieing and cutting the umbilical cord.

2. *Closure of foramen ovale*

Factors leading to closure to foramen ovale are:

- Reduction in inferior vena cava-left atrial pressure gradient.
- Decrease in right atrial and right ventricular pressure following arrest of umbilical flow. Closure of the foramen ovale prevents the right-to-left flow of venous blood and thus improves the oxygenation of systemic arterial blood.

3. *Changes in pulmonary circulation*

Rapid fall in pulmonary artery pressure which occurs following inflation of previously collapsed lungs.

4. *Closure of ductus arteriosus*

The ductus arteriosus is almost as large as ascending aorta of the mature fetus and has a thick smooth muscle wall. The closure of ductus occurs in three steps:

- Vasoconstriction of ductus arteriosus occurs rapidly during the first few hours after birth but final functional closure takes place gradually over the next 1–3 days.
- Functional closure of the ductus with complete muscular contraction occurs gradually over the next 1–8 days.
- Permanent sealing of the ductus lumen occurs 2–3 weeks after birth by replacement of musculature with fibrous tissue.

ANOMALIES OF CARDIOVASCULAR SYSTEM

ANOMALIES OF HEART

I. Anomalous positions of heart

1. *Dextrocardia* occurs when the primitive heart tube bends to the right, instead of left. It is characterized by reversal of heart chambers and great vessels, i.e. the structures normally present on left side are seen on right side and vice versa. It may occur alone or as a part of *situs inversus* viscerum in which all the body organs are transpose.

2. *Ectopia cordis* occurs due to faulty apposition of the lateral folds of the body leading to a sternal cleft through which heart is exposed and lies on the front of chest.

II. Anomalies of cardiac septation

1. *Atrial septal defect (ASD)* may occur due to:
   - Persistent osteum primum occurs when septum primum fails to fuse with atrio-ventricular endocardial cushions (Fig. 14.30A).

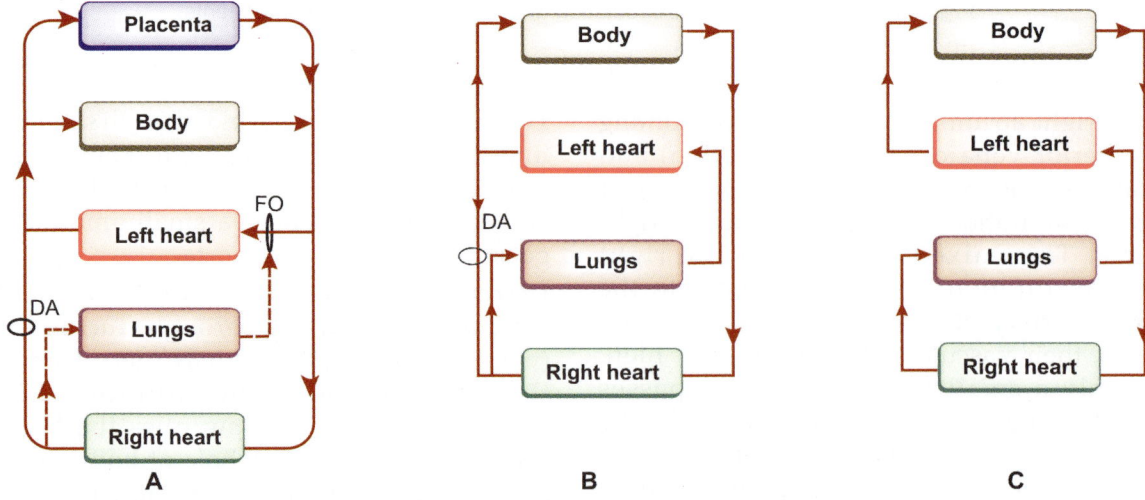

Fig. 14.29: Circulatory pattern in: A, fetus just before birth; B, newborn; C, adult.

- *Persistent osteum secundum* occurs when septum secundum fails to develop (Fig. 14.30B).
- *Patent foramen ovale* is comparatively more common cause of ASD. It may occur in two forms:
  - *Probe patency of foramen ovale:* In this condition the foramen is closed functionally after birth but remains patent anatomically which can be ascertained by passage of a probe. It is a symptomless condition.
  - *Functional and anatomical patency* (Fig. 14.30C) is usually associated with symptom *consequences.* A large ASD causes problem due to shunting of large volume of blood from left to right atrium, then to right ventricle and pulmonary arteries. Thus, initially right ventricle is overburdened, and later on pulmonary hypertension may develop.
2. *Ventricular septal defect (VSD)* occurs due to defective development of membranous part of interventricular septum leading to persistent interventricular foramen (Fig. 14.30D). The VSD may be small and isolated or a part of complex heart disease. It is the most common congenital cardiac defect occurring in 1:500 live births. It is an acyanotic heart defect with left to right (L → R) shunt.
3. *Truncal septal defect* include:
   - *Undivided truncus arteriosus* occurs due to failure of aortic-pulmonary septum to develop. The undivided truncus arises above the patent interventricular foramen and convey the blood from both ventricles.
   - *Transpositioning of ascending aorta and pulmonary trunk*—It occurs due to reverse attachment of the aorto-pulmonary septum. In it ascending aorta arises from the right

ventricle and the pulmonary trunk from the left ventricle. When associated with patent interventricular foramen the condition is known as *Tausig-Bing syndrome.*
4. *Intermediate septal defect,* i.e. defective fusion of atrioventricular endocardial cushions may result in:
   - Atrioventricular canal defect, or
   - Persistent atrioventricular canal.

In this condition atrial septum as well as ventricular septum are incomplete due to failure of intermediate septum. So all the four chambers communicate with each other.

III. Valvular defects

1. *Valvular stenosis of pulmonary orifice* occurs when the semilunar pulmonary cusps are fused forming a conical diaphragm perforated at the center when the orifice is closed (*tricuspid stenosis*). There occurs increased pressure in the right atrium, resulting in failure of closure of foramen ovale. In this condition *patent ductus arteriosus* persists to convey the blood to both lungs.
2. *Valvular stenosis of aortic orifice* occurs when the aortic cusps fuse and produce a pin-hole opening through which only a small amount of blood reaches the ascending aorta. Persistence of patent ductus arteriosus (PDA) is the only avenue through which the blood reaches the distal part of arch of aorta.

IV. Combined defects

1. *Tetralogy of Fallot.* It occurs due to defective development of embryonic heart and as the name indicates, consists of four components:
   - Ventricular septal defect (VSD),
   - Overriding of the aorta at the level of VSD

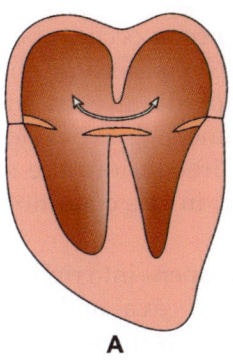 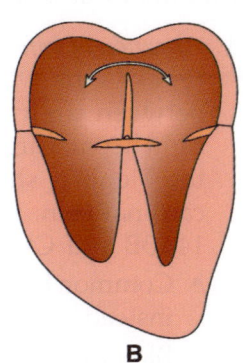 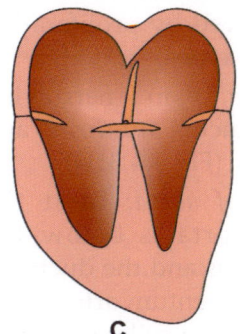 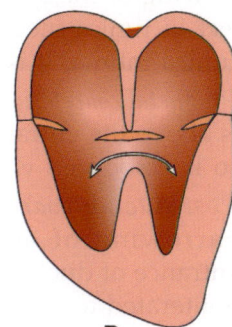

| A | B | C | D |

Fig. 14.30: Cardiac septal defects: A, septum primum defect; B, septum secundum defect; C, patent foramen ovale; D, interventricular septum defect.

- Pulmonary stenosis (subvalvular), and
- Right ventricular hypertrophy

Due to pulmonary stenosis and large VSD, the right ventricular pressure is elevated and leads to right-to-left shunt resulting in mixing of unoxygenated and oxygenated blood that is pushed into the overrided aorta. Thus there occurs tissue hypoxia, which produces cyanosis (bluish discolouration of skin) and clubbing of the fingers in infancy or after first year of life. Capacity for physical exercise is limited.

2. *Eisenmerger's complex* is a combination of pulmonary hypertension due to hypoplasia of pulmonary complex, dilatation of the pulmonary trunk, and hypertrophy of the right ventricle. When associated ASD, VSD and PDA the condition is termed Eisenmerger's syndrome.

ANOMALIES OF ARTERIAL SYSTEM

Developmental anomalies of aortic arches

1. *Double aortic arch* results when the right dorsal aorta also persists distal to the origin of the right intersegmental artery and its junction with the left dorsal aorta (Fig. 14.31A). The vascular rings so formed embraces the trachea and oesophagus and may cause difficulty in breathing and swallowing due to compression.

2. *Right aortic arch* results when the right dorsal aorta persists and the corresponding portion of the left dorsal aorta disappears (Fig. 14.31B).

3. *Interrupted aortic arch,* i.e absence of segment of arch results due to obliteration of the 4th aortic arch on the left side. In this condition the ascending aorta ends by supplying the left common carotid artery. The left subclavian artery arises from the distal segment which receives blood through the patent ductus arteriosus (PDA) (Fig. 14.31C).

4. *Coarctation of the aorta* refers to congenital narrowing of the arch of aorta. It occurs due to a defect in tunica media followed by proliferation of tunica intima. It is of two types:
   - *Preductal coarctation of aorta,* i.e. in it narrowing is above the entrance of ductus arteriosus and so is associated with PDA (Fig. 14.31D).
   - *Post-ductal coarctation of aorta:* In it the narrowing of arch of aorta is below the entrance of ductus arteriosus and the ductus is obliterated to form the ligamentum arteriosum (Fig. 14.31E). In this condition a collateral circulation is established between the branches of aorta, proximal and distal to the obstruction,

i.e. through the internal thoracic, epigastric and intercostal arteries.

Characteristic features of coarctation of aorta are:
- Higher arterial pressure in arms than in femoral arteries,
- Grooving of the lower borders of the ribs by enlarged intercostal arteries and
- Occasional visible pulsations on the back.

5. *Patent ductus arteriosus (PDA)* is one of the most frequently occurring abnormalities of the great vessels (8/10000 live births). It is more common in premature infants and in females than males. It may occur alone or in association with other anomalies. PDA establishes a left-to-right shunt.

6. *Abnormal origin of right subclavian artery—* Normally right subclavian artery is formed by right 4th aortic arch (Fig. 14.31F). However, sometimes the right 4th arch and proximal part of the right dorsal aorta obliterate and the right 7th intersegmental artery and the right dorsal aorta caudal to it are continued as right subclavian artery (Fig. 14.31G).

ANOMALIES OF VEINS

I. Anomalies of superior vena cava

1. *Left superior vena cava* is formed when the left anterior cardinal and common cardinal veins persist and the right ones obliterate. Left superior vena cava opens into right atrium through the coronary sinus (formed by left horn of sinus venosus) (Fig. 14.32B).

2. *Double superior vena cava* is characterized by persistence of left anterior cardinal vein and failure of the left brachiocephalic vein to form. The right superior vena cava opens directly into the right atrium while the left one opens through coronary sinus (Fig. 14.32C).

II. Anomalies of inferior vena cava

1. *Absence of inferior vena cava* occurs above the renal veins when the anastomotic channel between the right subcardinal vein and the right hepatocardiac channel fails to develop and the blood is shunted directly into the supra-cardinal vein. Therefore, in this condition (Fig. 14.33B and C):
   - Common hepatic vein opens into right atrium instead of inferior vena cava, and
   - Blood from caudal part of the body reaches the heart through azygos vein and superior vena cava.

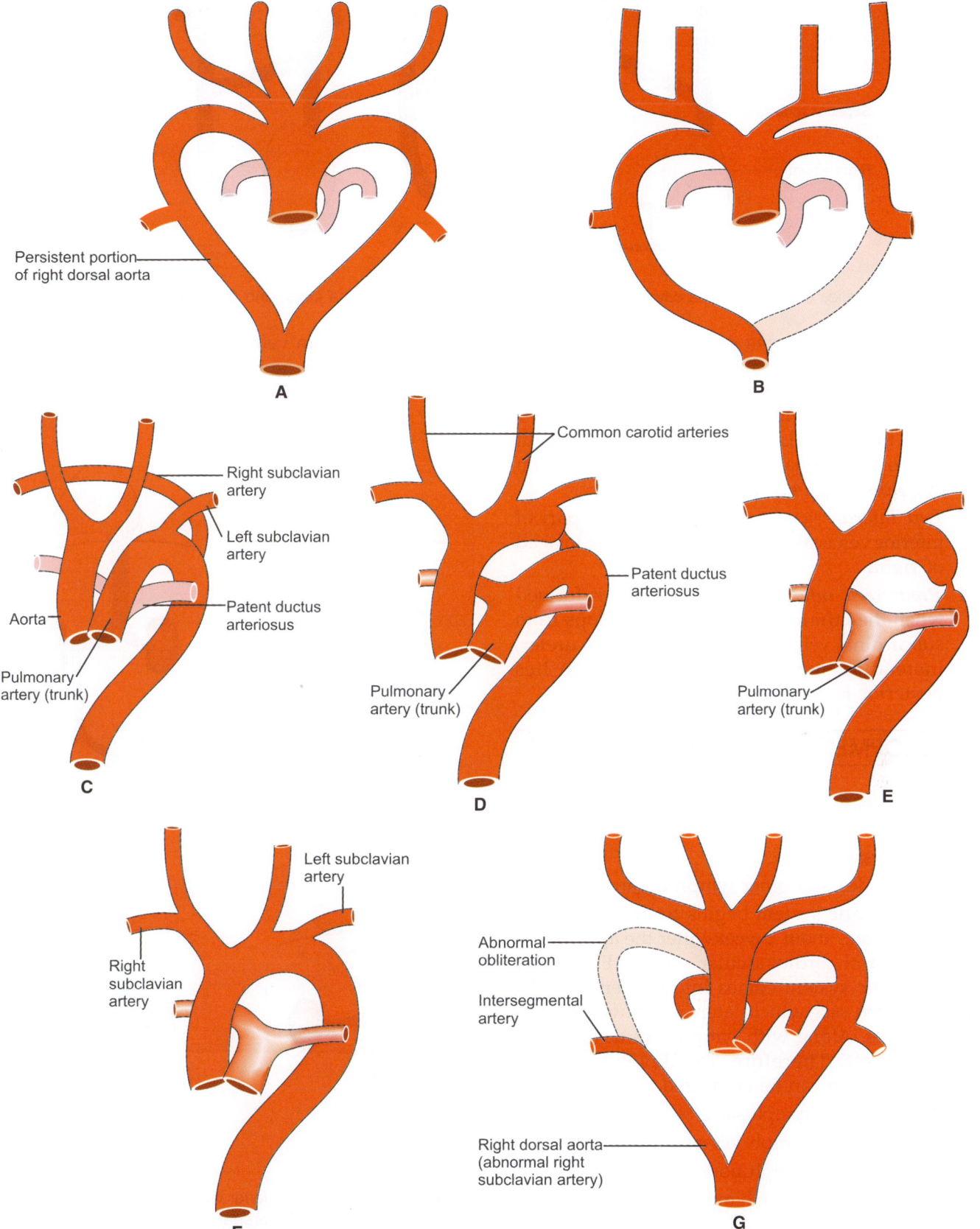

Fig. 14.31: Developmental anomalies associated with aortic arches: A, double aortic arch; B, right aortic arch; C, interrupted aortic arch; D, preductal coarctation of aorta; E, postductal coarctation of aorta; F, normal arch of aorta to compare with abnormal origin of right subclavian artery; G and abnormal origin of right subclavian artery.

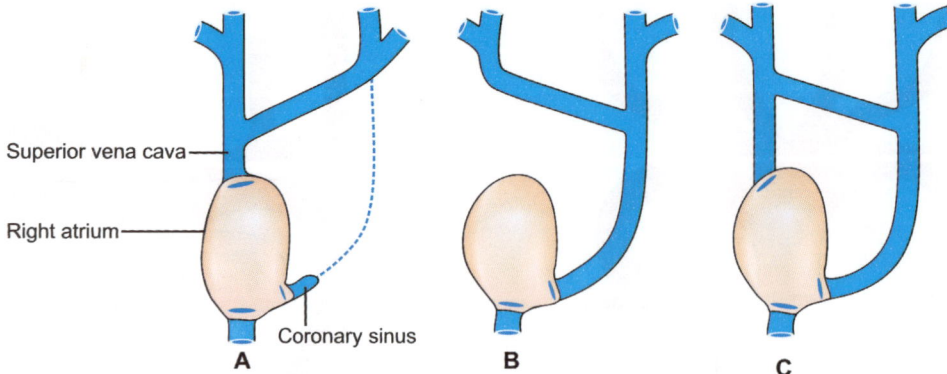

Fig. 14.32: Anomalies of superior vena cava: A, normal pattern B, Left superior vena cava; and C, Double superior vena cava.

2. ***Double inferior vena cava*** is usually formed below the level of renal veins. This occurs due to persistence of both the subcardinal and supracardinal veins below the level of kidneys. Both the channels may be present on the right side or additional channel may be present on left side (Fig. 14.33D).

3. ***Left inferior vena cava,*** i.e. infrarenal part of inferior vena cava is formed on left side instead of right.

4. ***Preureteric inferior vena cava*** (IVC) is formed when the infrarenal part of IVC develops from subcardinal vein (which lies anterior to ureter) instead of supracardinal vein (which lies posterior to the ureter).

DEVELOPMENT OF LYMPHATIC SYSTEM

The lymphatic system consists of:
- Lymph,
- Lymph vessels and
- Lymph nodes and other lymph organs

The lymphatic system begins to develop at the end of 6th week, about 2 weeks after the appearance of primordia of cardiovascular system. First of all the lymphatic system comes into existence in the form of *lymph sacs* which later get converted into lymph nodes. Along with lymph sacs develop the lymph vessels. Therefore, the development of lymphatic system can be organized as below:
- Development of lymph sacs,
- Development of lymph vessels,
- Development of lymph nodes, and
- Development of other lymph organs.

Development of lymph sacs

Lymph sacs, the endothelial lined sacs are thought to develop from the mesenchymal tissue rather than as outgrowths from veins. At the end of embryonic period six lymph sacs can be recognized (Fig. 14.34A):

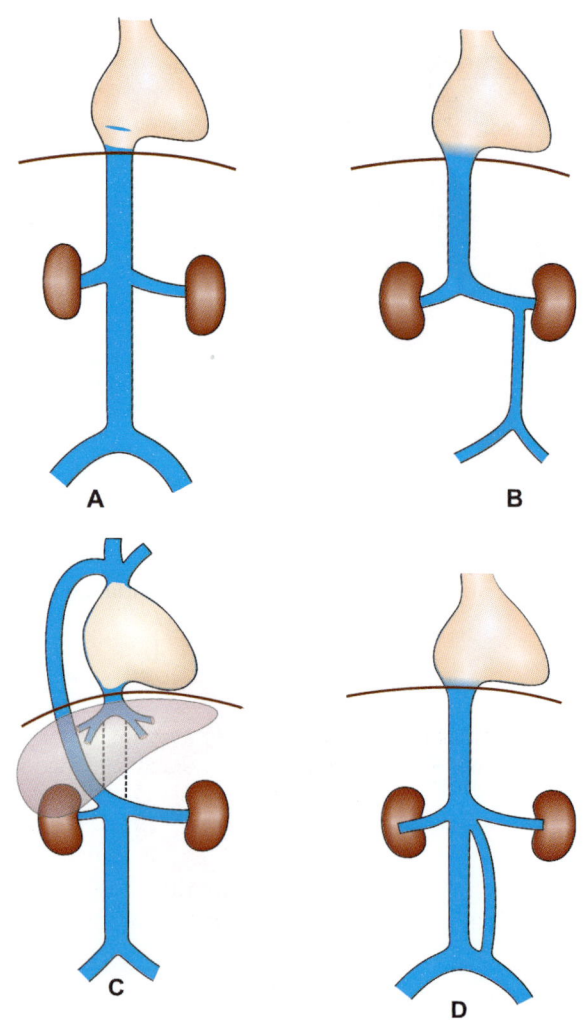

Fig. 14.33: Anomalies of inferior vena cava: A, normal pattern; B, absence of normal infrarenal segment, and replacement by another vessel on left-side; C, absence of normal hepatic segment. Blood from infra-renal segment of inferior vena cava is drained by enlarged vena azygos; and D, duplication of infra-renal segment.

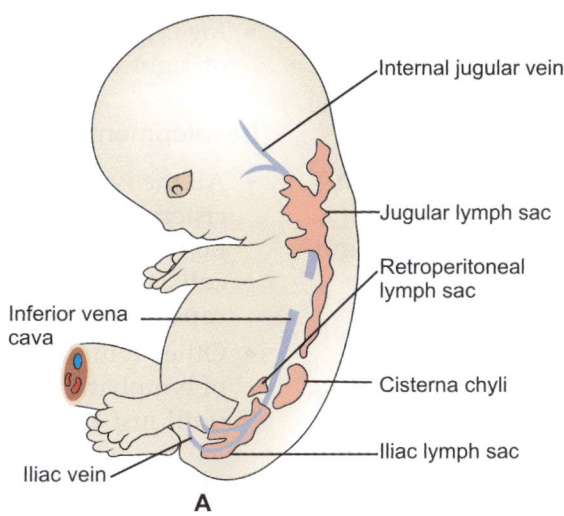

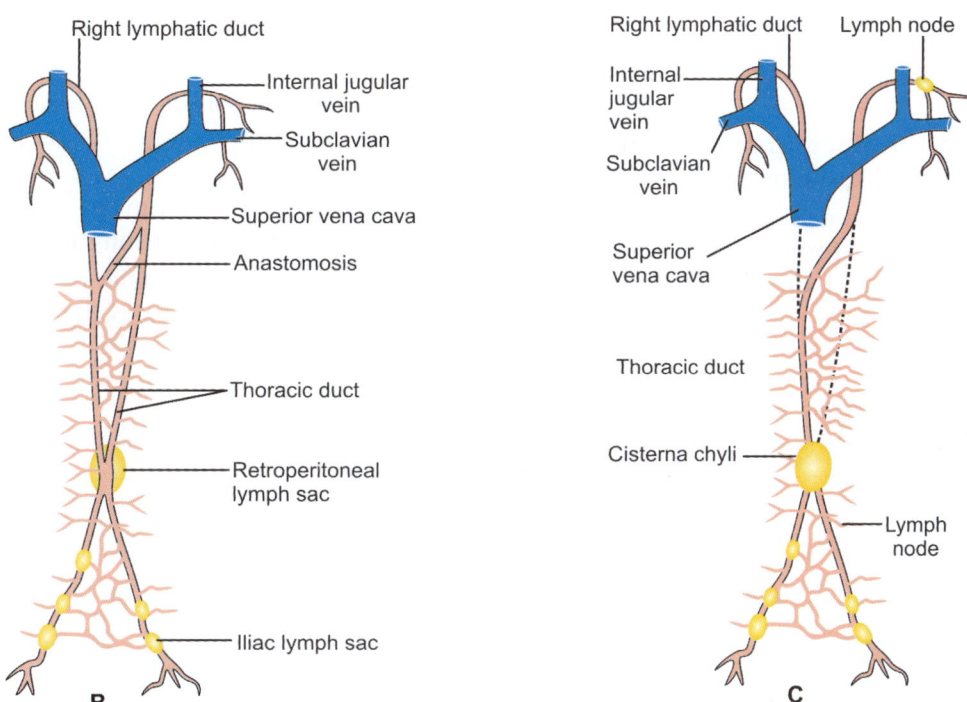

Fig. 14.34: Development of lymphatic system; A, location of primary lymph sacs; B, right and left lymphatic channels and their anastomoses, C, formation of thoracic duct and right lymphatic duct.

- *Jugular lymph sacs*, right and left, develop near the junction of the anterior cardinal veins (future internal jugular vein) and subclavian veins.
- *Iliac lymph sacs*, right and left, develop near the junction of the iliac veins with posterior cardinal veins.
- *Retroperitoneal lymph sac* (unpaired) develops in the root of the mesentery on the posterior abdominal wall.
- *Cisterna chyli* (unpaired) develops dorsal to the retroperitoneal lymph sac.

Development of lymph vessels

Lymph capillaries originate as closed endothelial buds from the angioblasts in the manner similar to that of blood vessels. The lymphatic capillaries develop in most tissues of the body except brain, cartilage, splenic pulp, bone marrow and avascular structures (cornea, crystalline lens, nail and hair).

Lymph vessels. The lymphatic capillaries join to form the lymph vessels. The lymphatic vessels are distributed throughout the body like veins.

The lymph vessels soon join and pass along the veins and join the lymph sacs as below:

- *Jugular lymph sacs* receives lymph vessels from the head, neck and upper limbs,
- *Iliac lymph sacs* from the lower trunk and lower limbs.
- *Retroperitoneal lymph sacs* from the primordial gut.
- *Cisterna chyli* from the primordial gut.

Lymphatic channels, the larger lymph vessels, are formed by the union of small and medium size lymph vessels and are named for the region with which they are associated. Initially two lymphatic channels are formed which connect the cysterna chyli to the corresponding jugular sacs. These are (Fig. 14.34B):

- Right lymphatic channel and
- Left lymphatic channel.

These lymphatic channels anastomose across the midline.

Collecting ducts, the thoracic duct and right lymphatic duct, are formed as below (Fig. 14.34C):

- *Thoracic duct* is formed from the caudal part of the right channel, the anastomosis between the right and left channels, and the cranial part of the left channel.

- *Right lymphatic duct* is formed by the cranial part of right channel.

Development of lymph nodes

- All the lymph sacs except the superior part of the cisterna chyli are converted into groups of lymph nodes by mesenchymal invasion. Mesenchymal cells form the connective tissue network and capsule of the lymph nodes.
- Other lymph nodes develop along the network of lymphatic vessels. Lymph nodes do not appear until just before birth or after birth.

Development of other lymph organs

Spleen develops from an aggregation of mesenchymal cells in the dorsal mesentery of the stomach.

Palatine tonsils are derived from second pair of pharyngeal arches (see page 134).

Pharyngeal tonsils (adenoids) are formed from the aggregation of lymphatic tissue in the wall of nasopharynx.

Lingual tonsil develops from an aggregation of lymph nodules in the root of tongue.

Mucosa associated lymph tissue (MALT) develop in the mucosa of respiratory and digestive systems.

15

Development of Nervous System

NEURULATION AND GENERAL OUTLINES OF DEVELOPMENT OF NERVOUS SYSTEM
- Formation of neural tube
- Neural crest and its derivatives
- Histogenesis of neural tube
- Derivatives of neural tube
- Molecular regulation of neurulation

DEVELOPMENT OF SPINAL CORD
- Histogenesis
- Changes in mantle layer: formation of anterior, lateral and posterior horns
- Changes in marginal layer: formation of white matter columns.
- Formation of dorsal root ganglia, nerve roots and spinal nerve trunks
- Positional changes in spinal cord

DEVELOPMENT OF BRAIN
General considerations
- Divisions and flexures of neural tube

- Development of external form of the brain
- Histogenesis of primary brain vesicles
- Development of ventricles of brain

Development of hindbrain
- Myelencephalon
  - Development of medulla oblongata
- Metencephalon
  - Pons
  - Cerebellum

Development of midbrain
- Mesencephalon : histogenesis

Development of forebrain
- Diencephalon
- Telencephalon

ANOMALIES OF SPINAL CORD AND BRAIN
- Anomalies of spinal cord
- Anomalies of brain

DEVELOPMENT OF AUTONOMIC NERVOUS SYSTEM
- Sympathetic nervous system
- Parasympathetic nervous system

NEURULATION AND GENERAL OUTLINES OF DEVELOPMENT OF NERVOUS SYSTEM

Neurulation refers to process of formation of neural plate and its infolding to form the neural tube.

FORMATION OF NEURAL TUBE

Induction of neural tube formation

Nervous system is developed from the ectoderm situated on the dorsal (amniotic) aspect of embryonic disc, in the midline. The ectoderm forming nervous system is called neuroectoderm. At the beginning of 3rd week the underlying notochord induces the process of neurulation.

Signaling molecules involved are transforming growth factor-β (TGF-β) family, which includes activin and fibroblast growth factors (FGFs).

Steps of neural tube formation

Steps involved in the formation of neural tube are:

Neural plate, a slipper-shaped area, is formed by thickening of neuroectoderm overlying the notochord, and therefore, extends from the prochordal plate to the primitive node (Fig. 15.1A and B). It is the first appearance of nervous system.

Neural groove, a longitudinal furrow, appears in the neural plate, which becomes progressively deeper and thus bound on each side by the neural folds. The tips of the neural folds have specialized neuro-ectodermal cells, known as the *neural crest cells* (Fig. 15.1C and D).

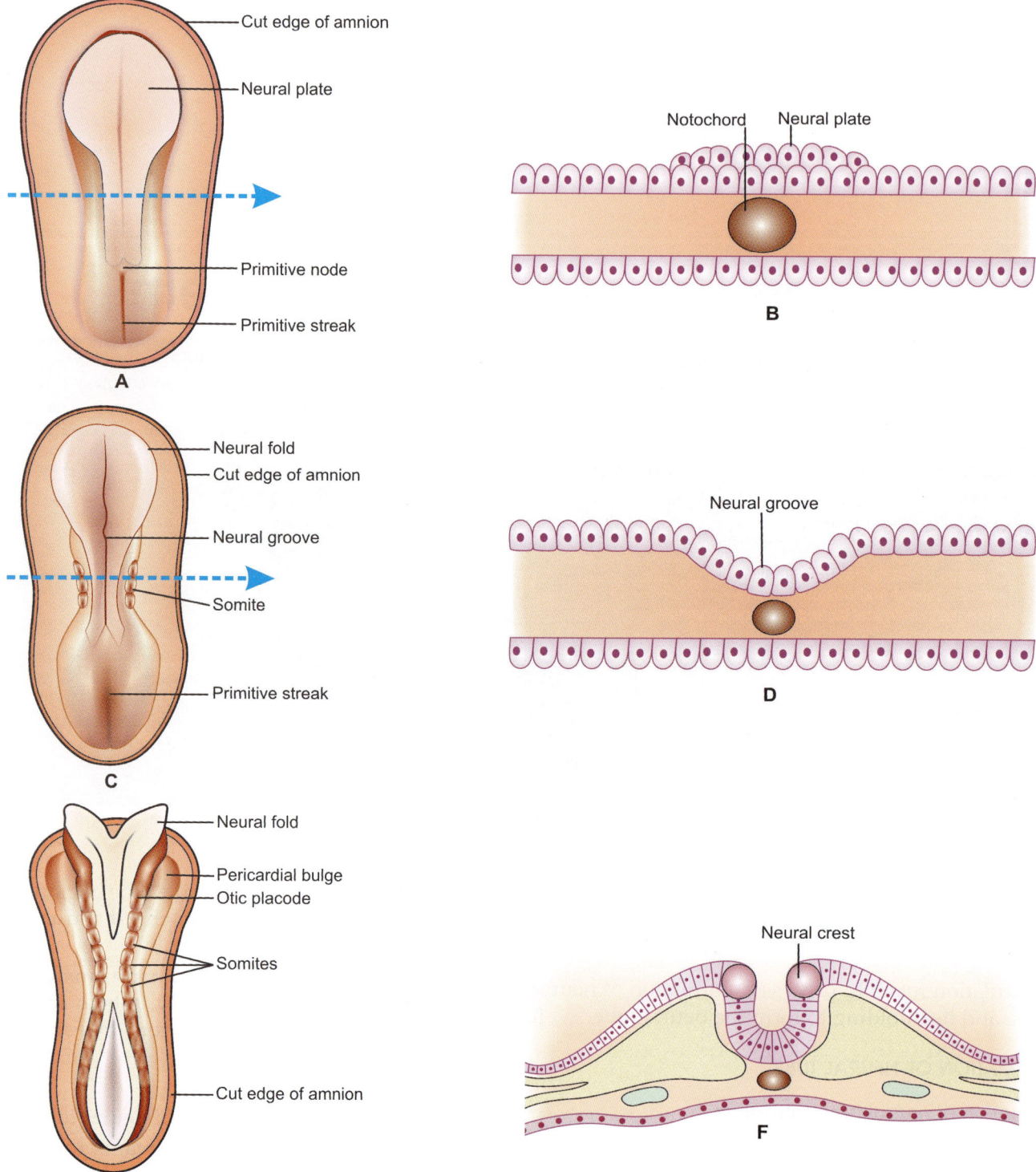

Fig. 15.1: Stages of formation of neural tube: A and B, formation of neural plate; C and D, formation of neural groove and folds; E and F, formation of neural tube; A, C and E are dorsal views of the embryo and B, D and F are transverse sections across axes XY.

Neural tube, the primordium from which central nervous system develops, is then formed by fusion of neural folds (Fig. 15.1E and D).

- The fusion begins in the middle part and slowly proceeds in cephalic and caudal direction, thus for sometime the tube is open cranially and caudally. The openings are called *cranial* and *caudal neuropores* through which the neural tube communicates with the amniotic cavity.
- *Cranial neuropore* closes at the 18 to 20 somite stage (25th day). Its position in the adult is represented by the lamina terminalis of the third ventricle.
- *Caudal neuropore* closes at 25 somite stage at the end of 4th week.

NEURAL CREST AND ITS DERIVATIVES

Neural crest. After fusion of the neural folds, the dorsal surface of the neural tube is detached from the surface ectoderm, and the neural crest cells proliferate to form a wedge shaped zone the *neural crest* which occupies the space between the surface ectoderm and the neural tube (Fig. 15.1F).

Primitive ganglia. Soon, this wedge shaped zone splits into two parts, which migrate dorsolaterally and arrange themselves as oval-shaped cell clusters known as primitive spinal ganglia. Each primitive ganglion differentiates into a dorsal and ventral mass of cells.

Derivatives of neural crest cells

Derivation of dorsal cell mass and ventral cell mass of primitive ganglia formed of neural crest cells are as below (Fig. 15.2):

Dorsal mass cells produce neuroblasts, spongioblasts and pluripotent cells, which inturn give rise to following structures.

- *Neuroblasts* give rise to dorsal root ganglia of all the spinal nerves, and sensory ganglia of V, VII, IX and X cranial nerves.
- *Spongioblasts* give rise to capsular cells and Schwann cells. The Schwann cells are responsible for formation of myelin and neurolemma sheaths around the peripheral nerves.
- *Pleuripotent cells* give rise to melanoblasts, odontoblasts, cartilage cells of branchial arches and *meninges*.

Ventral mass of neural crest undergoes wide range of migration and forms a syncytium of cells, which develop into sympathochromaffin organs that have small and large cells.

- *Small cells* (sympathoblasts) migrate laterally along the primitive dorsal aortae giving rise to sympathetic ganglion cells, which form the ganglionated trunk. They also form parasympathetic ganglion cells of ciliary, pterygopalatine, submandibular and otic ganglion.

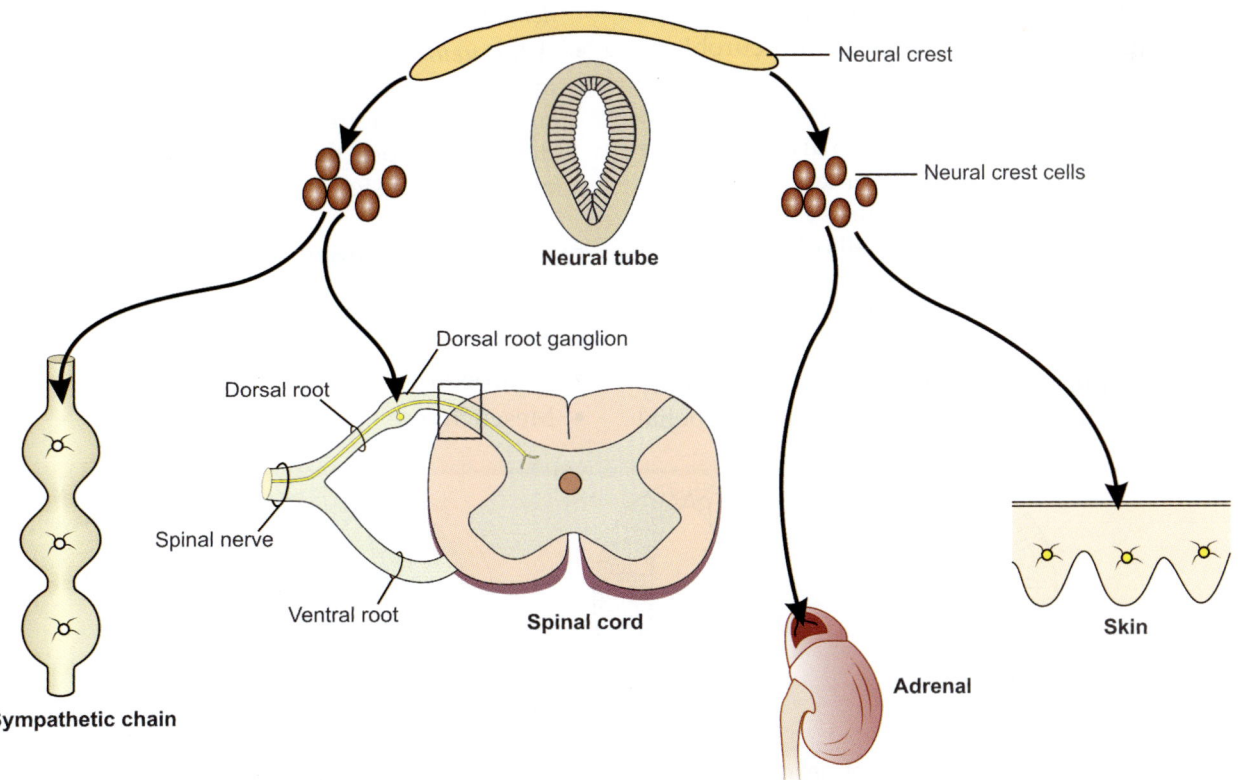

Fig. 15.2: Some derivatives of neural crest cells.

- *Large cells* contain brownish granules and form chromaffin cells or pheochromocytes, which secrete noradrenaline. Most of the cells enter the suprarenal ridge giving rise to chromaffin cells of adrenal medulla. They also form paraganglia, para-aortic body, argentaffin cells, and entro-chromaffin cells (APUD cells).

HISTOGENESIS OF NEURAL TUBE

The neurons and neuroglia are derived from the wall of neural tube. Histogenesis of neural tube can be discussed as:

- Formation of layers of neural tube wall, and
- Histological differentiation.

FORMATION OF LAYERS OF NEURAL TUBE WALL

1. *Neuroepithelial layer.* Initially the neural tube is lined by a single layer of cells, the neuroepithelial cells (Fig. 15.3A). These cells proliferate and form a thick pseudostratified epithelium known as neuroepithelial layer (Fig. 15.3B). This layer is also known as *matrix cell layer* or *germinal layer,* since these cells divide rapidly producing more and more cells including *neuroblasts* and neuroglia cells. When neural epithelial cells cease to produce neuroblasts and gliablasts, they differentiate into *ependymal* cells lining the lumen of tube and form the *ependymal* layer (Fig. 15.3C).

2. *Mantle layer.* This layer forms a zone around the neuroepithelial layer and consists of neuroblasts and neuroglial cells which have migrated from the neuroepithelial layer (Fig. 15.3C). The neuroblasts on reaching the mantle layer fail to divide and give rise to neurons. The mantle layer later forms grey matter of the central nervous system. In the cerebrum and cerebellum, the cells of mantle layer undergo mass migration and appear in the marginal layer giving rise to the cortical grey matter.

3. *Marginal layer.* This outer most layer initially contains cytoplasmic processes of neuroepithelial cells. Soon this zone is invaded by the nerve fibres emerging from the neuroblasts and processes of the neuroglial cells in the mantle layer (Fig. 15.3C). This layer contains no cells. The myelination of the nerve fibres, makes them appear white. Therefore, this layer is said to make *white matter* of the central nervous system.

Histological differentiation

Formation of neurons

Stages in the formation of a neuron are (Fig. 15.4):

- *Apolar neuroblasts.* Primitive nerve cells arise exclusively by division of neuroepithelial cells and migrate from neuroepithelial layer to the mantle layer. Once neuroblast is formed the ability of the cell of further division is lost. The newly formed neuroblasts have a central process extending into the lumen (*transient dendrites),* but when they migrate into the mantle layer, this process is lost and a round *apolar neuroblast* is formed (Fig. 15.4A).

- *Bipolar neuroblast* is formed from the apolar neuroblast by appearance of two processes on opposite side of the cell bodies (Fig. 15.4B).

- *Multipolar neuroblast* is formed when one of the processes of bipolar cell elongates to form *primitive axon* and the process at the other end shows a number of cytoplasmic arborization, the *primitive dendrites* (Fig. 15.4C).

- *Adult neuron* is then formed by further growth and appearance of *Nissel granules* in the cytoplasm. The further behaviour of axons and dendrites varies depending upon their fate in different components of nervous system.

Formation of glial cells

The glial cells of the nervous system are derived from two sources:

- Neuroepithelium, and
- Mesenchyme.

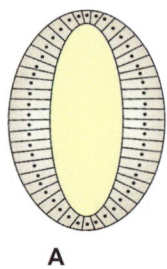 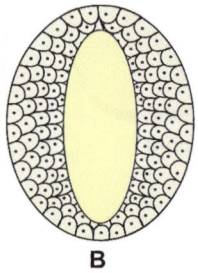 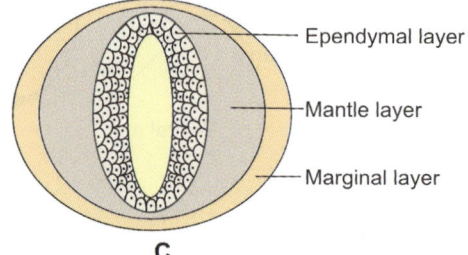

Ependymal layer

Mantle layer

Marginal layer

A	B	C

Fig. 15.3: Formation of layers of wall of neural tube: A, neural tube lined by single layer of neuroepithelial cells; B, neural tube lined by multilayered neuroepithelium; C, establishment of ependymal, mantle and marginal layers of neural tube.

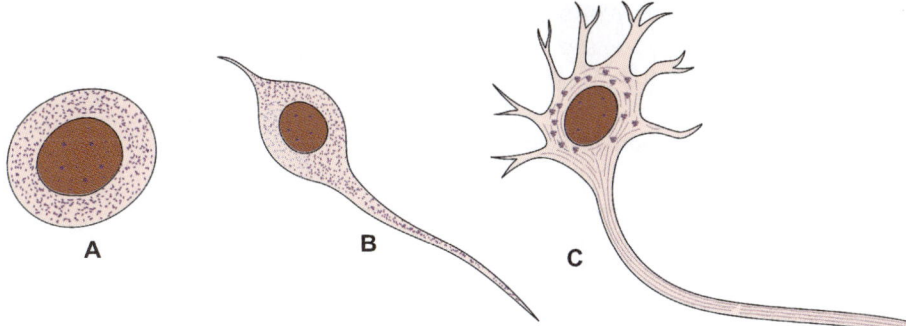

Fig. 15.4: Stages of development of a neuron: A, apolar neuroblast; B, bipolar neuroblast; and C, multipolar neuron.

Neuroepithelial derived glial cells

Neuroepithelial layer cells, after they cease producing neuroblasts (Fig. 15.5A) start producing primitive glial cells called the *gliablasts* (Fig. 15.5B), which migrate into mantle and marginal layers.

In mantle layer the gliablasts differentiate into (Fig. 15.5B):

- Protoplasmic astrocytes, and
- Fibrillar astrocytes

In marginal layer the gliablasts differentiate into (Fig. 15.5B)

- *Oligodendroglial cells,* which form myelin sheath around the ascending and descending axons.

Note. Oligodendrocytes form the myelin sheath in the central nervous system only. The myelin sheath of peripheral nerves are derived from Schwann cells (derived from neural crest cells).

Mesenchyme derived glial cells

Microglial cells, the third type of glial cells found in the CNS, are derived from mesenchyme (Fig. 15.5D). These cells are highly phagocytic and migrate into the CNS along with the blood vessels.

DERIVATIVES OF NEURAL TUBE

After studying the process of formation of neural tube and general outlines of development of layers of neural tube wall, neural crest cells, neurons, and glial cells; now it will be studied in the ensuing discussion, how these general developmental outlines apply to various derivatives of neural tube.

Derivatives of enlarged cephalic part of neural tube are various components of brain, i.e.:

- Forebrain,
- Midbrain, and
- Hindbrain, and

Derivative of tubular caudal part of neural tube is:

- Spinal cord.

MOLECULAR REGULATION OF NEURULATION

Induction of neural plate is regulated by inactivation of bone morphogenic protein 4 (BMP4).

Inactivation of BMP4 is caused by:

- *Noggin, chordin, and fallistatin* secreted by the node, notochord and prechordal mesoderm in the cranial region.
- *WNT 39 and FGF* in the hindbrain and spinal cord region.

DEVELOPMENT OF SPINAL CORD

The spinal cord develops from the caudal cylindrical part of neural tube.

Histogenesis

The histogenesis of the neural tube forming spinal cord occurs as described earlier and leads to formation of three zones of the wall (Fig. 15.6A):

- Ependymal layer,
- Mantle layer, and
- Marginal layer.

Change in mantle layer: formation of anterior, lateral and posterior horns

Roof plate and floor plate are formed respectively by the dorsal and ventral midline portions of the neural tube which remain thin (Fig. 15.6B). They do not contain neuroblasts and serve primarily as pathway of nerve fibres crossing from one side to the other.

Basal and alar plates. The neuroepithelial cells in the lateral wall proliferate add neuroblasts making it thick. A longitudinal sulcus known as *sulcus limitans* appears on the inner aspect of lateral wall, which converts the vertical oval central canal into diamond shape and divide the lateral wall into two functional areas (Fig. 15.6):

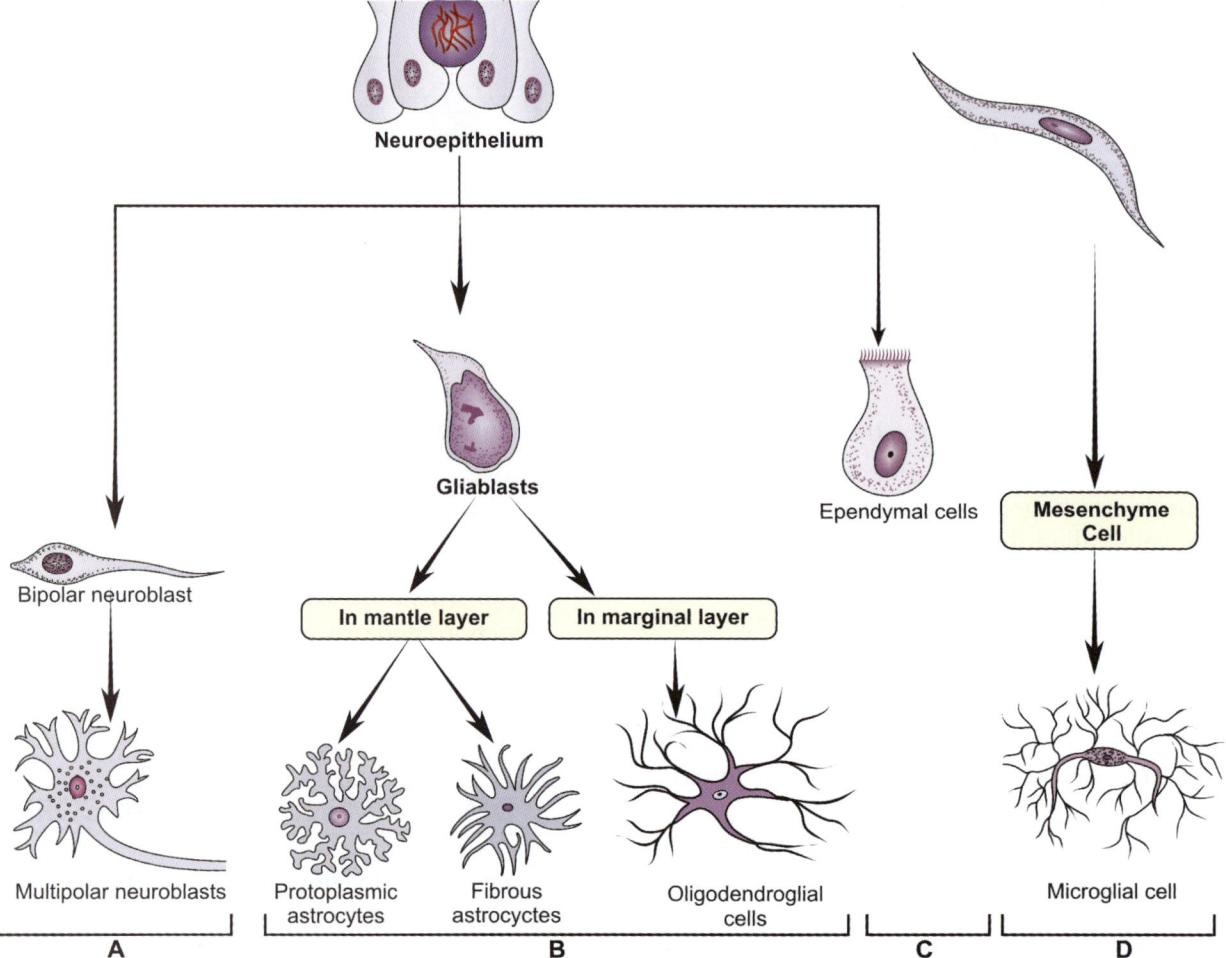

Fig. 15.5: Formation of glial cells. Note: Neuroepithelial cells first form neurons (A), then glial cells (B and C) and in the end get converted into ependymal cells. Microglia are derived from mesenchyme (D).

- *Basal plate* or the ventral lamina, is motor in function. Each basal plate bulges ventrolaterally and forms the anterior and lateral horns (Fig. 15.6C).

- *Alar plate* or *dorsal lamina* is sensory in function and forms the *posterior horn (grey column)*. The alar plates grow medially and fuse with each other to form the *posteromedian septum.* In this way, the dorsal part of central canal is obliterated and the diamond shaped canal is now reduced into a triangular form (Fig. 15.6C).

Note. Motor neurons of anterior and lateral horns differentiate earlier than the sensory neurons of posterior horn.

Changes in marginal zone: formation of white matter column

The marginal zone contains neurofibres emerging from the motor neurons (of anterior horn) and sensory neurons (of posterior horn) and those entering the spinal cord from the dorsal root ganglia which form various tracts. The marginal zone is converted into neurofibrous *white matter* as a result of myelination of nerve fibres of developing ascending and descending nerve tracts, including dorsal columns, spino-cerebellar and spino-thalamic tracts (sensory), and pyramidal and extra pyramidal tracts (motor). Tracts in the nervous system become myelinated at about the time they start to function. As the mantle layer take the shape of anterior and posterior grey columns, the white matter become subdivided with anterior, lateral, and posterior white columns (Fig. 15.6C).

Formation of dorsal root ganglia, nerve roots and spinal nerve trunks

Dorsal root ganglia, as described earlier, are formed by dorsolateral migration of neural crest cells. The bipolar cells of dorsal root ganglia are sensory and develop central and peripheral processes:

- *Axons,* the central processes, form the *dorsal root of spinal nerve* and penetrate the dorsal portion of

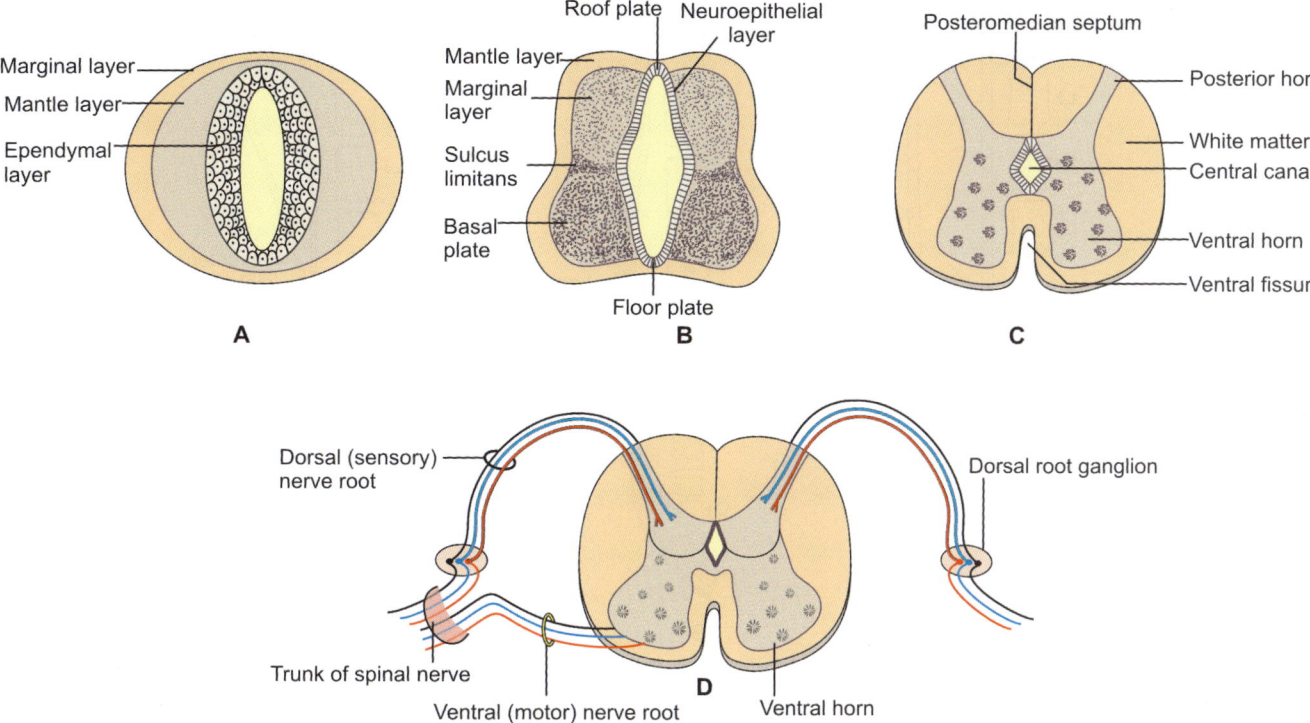

Fig. 15.6: Stages of development of spinal cord: A, neural tube with ependymal, mantle and marginal layers established; B, formation of alar plate, basal plate, roof plate and floor plate and convertion of central canal into diamond-shape by appearance of sulcus limitans; C, formation of anterior, lateral, and posterior horns of spinal cord; and D, formation of dorsal root ganglia, nerve roots and spinal nerve trunk.

spinal cord and either end in the dorsal horn or ascend through the marginal layer to one of the higher brain centres.

- *Dendrites,* the peripheral processes, form the sensory fibres of spinal nerves.

Nerve roots include (Fig. 15.6D):

- *Dorsal nerve root,* which consists of the central processes of neurons of dorsal root ganglia, as described above, and
- *Ventral nerve root* is formed by the axons of motor neurons of the anterior and lateral horns of spinal cord.

Spinal nerve trunk is then formed by (Fig. 15.6D):

- *Ventral nerve roots* which convey motor fibres to the somatic muscles and preganglionic motor fibres of the autonomic system to parasympathetic ganglion.
- *Sensory fibres* which are formed by peripheral processes of neurons of dorsal root ganglia and eventually terminate in the sensory receptors organs.

Positional changes in spinal cord

- *Upto 3rd month of development,* the spinal cord extends throughout the length of the developing

vertebral column and the spinal nerves pass outwards through the respective intervertebral column at right angles to the spinal cord (Fig. 15.7A).

- *At birth* spinal cord ends at the level of 3rd lumbar vertebra (Fig. 15.7B). This *recession of the spinal cord* occurs because of the fact that after 3rd month of gestation till birth, the vertebral column and dura increase in length more rapidly than that of the spinal cord.

- *In the adult,* i.e. at puberty the spinal cord reaches its final position opposite intervertebral disc between L1 and L2 vertebrae (Fig. 15.7C).

Effects of recession of spinal cord are:

- *Spinal nerves* run obliquely from their segment of origin in spinal cord to reach the corresponding inter vertebral foramina. This obliquity is least for cervical nerves and maximum for sacral and coccygeal nerves (Fig. 15.7B).
- As a result the bundle of nerves thus formed extends downward from the spinal cord to the periosteum of first coccygeal vertebra. It marks the tract of regression of the spinal cord (Fig. 15.7C).

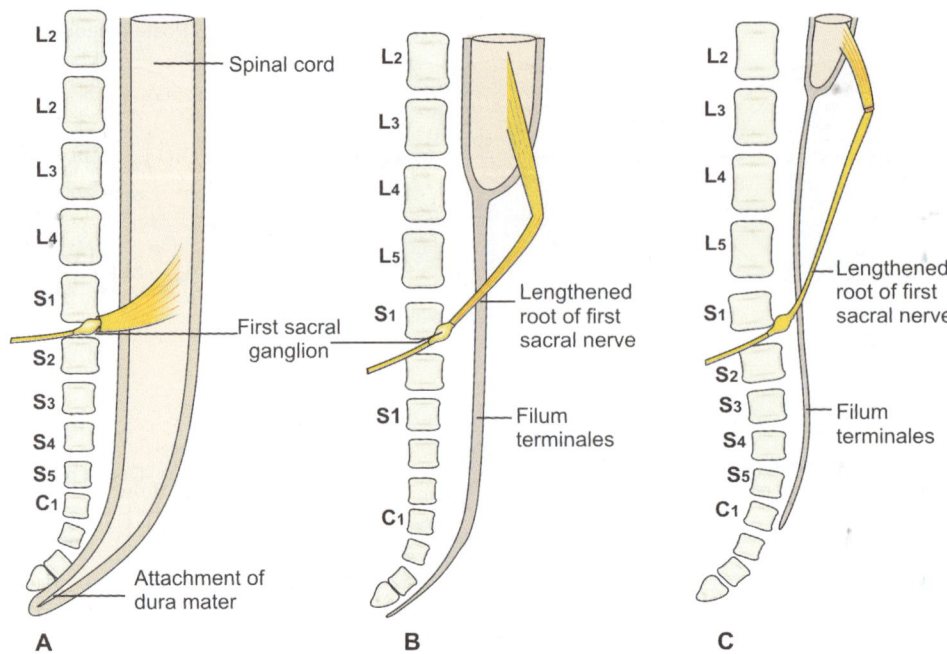

Fig. 15.7: Positional changes in spinal cord: A, at 3rd month the spinal cord extends throughout the length of the vertebral column; B, at birth spinal cord ends at L$_3$; and C, in adults the spinal cord extends upto between L$_1$ and L$_2$ vertebrae. Regression of spinal cord forms filum terminales, obliquity of spinal nerves and cauda equina.

DEVELOPMENT OF BRAIN

GENERAL CONSIDERATIONS

Divisions and flexures of neural tube

Due to differential growth, the neural tube is divisible into two parts (Fig. 15.8A):

- Enlarged cephalic part, which forms brain and
- Caudal tubular part which forms spinal cord.

Primary brain vesicles, the three dilatations, appear in the cephalic end of neural tube (Fig. 15.8B):

- *Prosencephalon* (forebrain vesicle) subdivides into (Fig. 15.8C):

  - Telencephalon and primitive cerebral hemisphere, and
  - Diencephalon which later forms thalamus and hypothalamus.

- *Mesencephalon* (midbrain vesicle),
  - Which later forms midbrain, and

- *Rhombencephalon* (hindbrain vesicle) which further subdivides into (Fig. 15.8C):

  - Metencephalon, which later forms the pons and cerebellum, and
  - Myelencephalon, which later forms medulla oblongata.

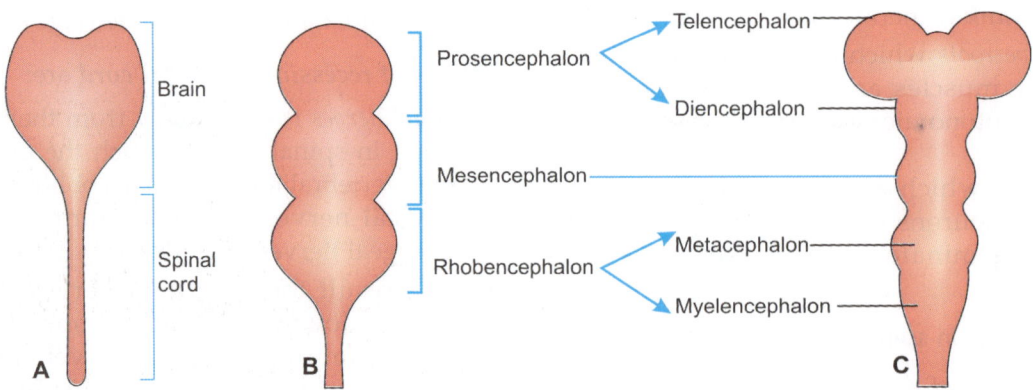

Fig. 15.8: Divisions of neural tube: A, enlarged cephalic part (primordium of brain) and caudal cylindrical part (primordium of spinal cord); B, primary brain vesicle; C, subdivisions of primary brain vesicle.

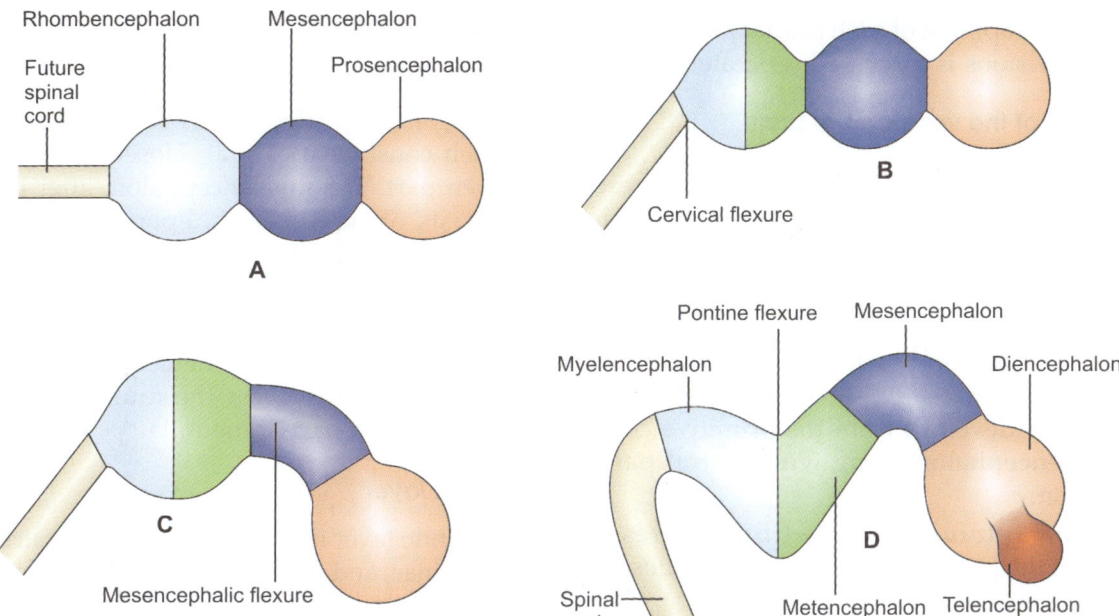

Fig. 15.9: Flexures of neural tube: A, neural tube before flexure; B, cervical flexure; C, mesencephalic flexure appeared and; D, pontine flexure formed.

Flexures of neural tube. The primary brain vesicles are at first arranged cranio-caudally (Fig. 15.9A). Their relative position is altered by the appearance of three flexures:

- *Cervical flexure* appears at the junction of hindbrain and spinal cord (Fig. 15.9B).
- *Mesencephalic or cephalic flexure* appears in the region of midbrain, (Fig. 15.9C) and
- *Pontine flexure* appears at the middle of rhomben-cephalon, dividing it into the metencephalon and myelencephalon (Fig. 15.9D).
- *Telencephalic flexure,* that occurs much later, between the telencephalon and diencephalon.

Development of external form of the brain

The various flexures of the brain, with further development result in adult orientation of the brain parts (Fig. 15.10).

Histogenesis of primary brain vesicles

Histogenesis of primary brain vesicles occurs on general lines as described earlier (page 245), and the wall of each primary vesicle is differentiated into three zones:

- Ependymal,
- Mantle, and
- Marginal.

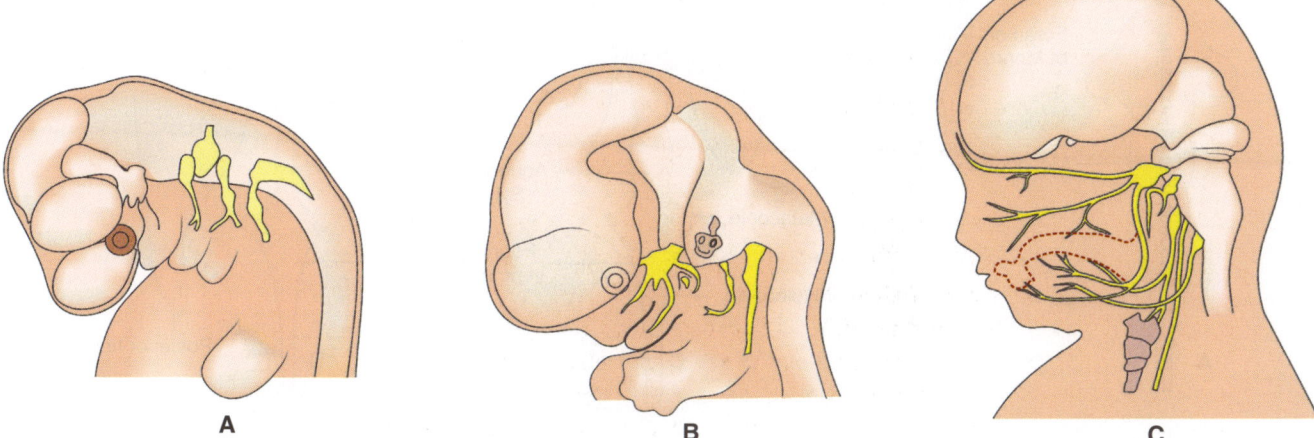

Fig. 15.10: Development of external form of brain. The adult orientation is achieved because of formation of various flexures and differential growth of some parts.

Further development of each primary brain vesicle and its subdivisions is discussed separately.

Development of the ventricles of brain

The primitive central cavity of neural tube is present in each primary and secondary brain vesicles and forms the various ventricles of the brain (Fig. 15.11):

Lateral ventricles are formed by the primitive central cavity of each telencephalic vesicle. The foramen of Monro is formed at the commencement of two cerebral hemispheres from the telencephalon.

Third ventricle develops from the primitive central cavity of diencephalon along with central part of telencephalon.

Aqueduct of Sylvius is formed by progressive narrowing of the primitive central cavity of mesencephalon.

Fourth ventricle develops from the primitive central cavity of rhombencephalon. The fourth ventricle, caudally is continuous with the central canal of spinal cord.

DEVELOPMENT OF HINDBRAIN

The hindbrain develops from the primary vesicle of rhombencephalon which consists of two secondary vesicles:

- Myelencephalon, and
- Metencephalon

Myelencephalon

Development of medulla oblongata

The myelencephalon gives rise to medulla oblongata which consists of caudal closed part and cephali-copen part. The myelencephalon, after histogenesis consists of three layers, ependymal, mantle and marginal (Fig. 15.12A):

Ependymal layer

Ependymal layer lines the central cavity, which is later stretched to form the fourth ventricle in the cephalic open part of medulla.

Mantle layer

- Mantle layer is arranged into *basal plates* or ventral laminae, and *alar plates* or dorsal laminae separated by sulcus limitans (Fig. 15.12B).
- Caudal closed part of the medulla contains central canal and resembles spinal cord developmentally and structurally. The cephalic open part of medulla forms caudal part of floor of fourth ventricle. In this area with the appearance of pontine flexure, the roof plate becomes greatly widened. As a result of this, the alar laminae come to lie dorsolateral to the basal laminae (Fig. 15.12B).
- Migration of some cells from alar laminae occurs into the marginal layer. These cells constitute the caudal part of the *bulbo-pontine extension* and develop into olivary nuclei (Fig. 15.12B and C).

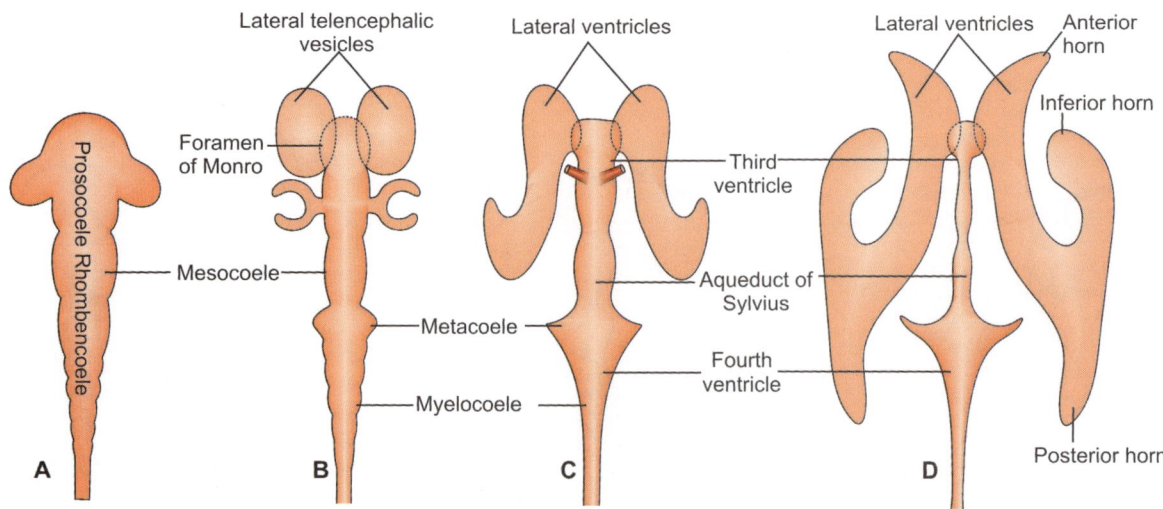

Fig. 15.11: Successive stages in the development of ventricles of brain: A, primitive three vesicles stage; B, early five vesicles stage; C, expansion of lateral telencephalic vesicles; and D, final arrangement.

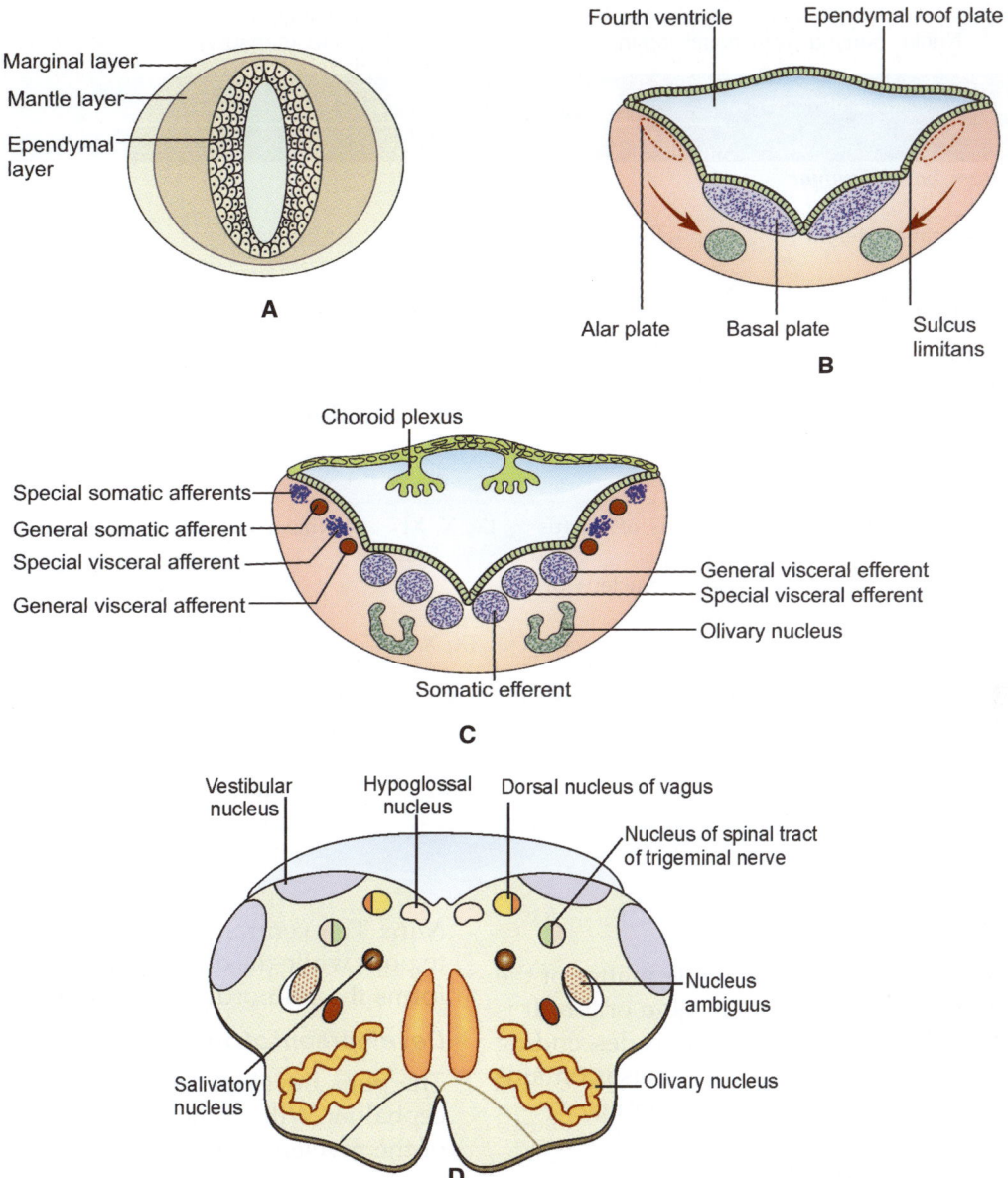

Fig. 15.12: Development of medulla oblongata (cross sections): A, primitive rhombencephalon; B and C, myelencephalon after pontine flexure. Note great widening of the roof plate; D, definitive position of various nuclei in upper medulla.

Basal plates or ventral laminae give rise to motor neurons which are arranged in three elongated but interrupted columns on each side. From medial to lateral, they are (Fig. 15.12C):

- General somatic efferent (GSE) column
- Special visceral efferent (SVE) column, and
- General visceral efferent (GVE) column

Nuclei and nerves associated with these columns are summarized in (Table 15.1)

Alar plates, or dorsal laminae give rise to sensory neurons that are arranged in four columns on each side. From medial to lateral they are (Fig. 15.12C).

- General visceral afferent (GVA) receiving impulses from the viscera,

- Special visceral afferent (SVA) receiving taste fibres,

- General somatic afferent (GSA) receiving impulses from the surface of head, and

- Special somatic afferent (SSA) receiving impulses from the ear.

Sensory nuclei and nerves associated with these columns are summarized in Table 15.1.

Migration of some nuclei ventrally from their primitive position in the floor of the fourth ventricle occurs. This process of migration is called neurobiotaxis. The definitive positions taken by various nuclei is shown in Fig. 15.12D.

Table 15.1: Nuclei derived from basal laminae (motor) and alar laminae (sensory) of medulla oblongata and pons

S.No. Functional component	Medulla oblongata		Pons	
	Nucleus	Cranial nerve	Nucleus	Cranial nerve
A. Derived from basal laminae				
1. General somatic efferent (GSE)	Hypoglossal	XII	Abducent	VI
2. Special visceral efferent (SVE)	Nucleus ambiguus	IX, X, XI	Motor nucleus of trigeminal nerve	V
			Motor nucleus of facial nerve	VII
3. General visceral efferent (GVE)	Dorsal nucleus of vagus	X	Superior salivary nucleus	
	Inferior salivary nucleus	IX	Lacrimatory nucleus	VII
B. Derived from alar laminae				
1. General visceral afferent (GVA)	Nucleus of tractus solitarius	IX, X, XI	Nucleus of tractus solitarius	VII
	Dorsal nucleus of vagus			
2. Special visceral afferent (SVA)	Nucleus of tractus solitarius	IX, X		
3. General somatic afferent (GSA)	Nucleus of spinal tract of trigeminal nerve	V	Main sensory nucleus and nucleus of spinal tract of trigeminal nerve	V
4. Special somatic afferent (SSA)	Vestibular	VIII	Vestibular cochlear	VIII

Marginal layer

Marginal layer, which forms the white matter of the medulla is predominantly extraneous in origin. It is made up of the fibres of ascending and descending tracts that pass through the medulla. It also contains olivary nuclei migrated from the alar laminae.

Roof plate of myelencephalon

Roof plate of the myelencephalon is greatly widened and consists of a single layer of ependymal cells covered by vascular mesenchyme, the *pia mater*, which combined constitute the *tela choroidea*. Tuft like invaginations, known as *choroid plexus*, is formed by active proliferation of vascular mesenchyme, which produce cerebrospinal fluid.

Development of metencephalon

The metencephalon like cephalic part of myelencephalon is characterized by (Fig. 15.13A):

- Greatly widened and thinned out roof plate,
- Alar laminae being placed dorsolateral to the basal laminae, i.e. (both basal and alar laminae lie in the floor of fourth ventricle).

In addition, the dorsolateral parts of the alar plates bend medially and form the *rhombic lips* (Fig. 15.13A).

Note: The ventral part of metencephalon gives rise to pons while the dorsal part containing rhombic lips forms the primordium of cerebellum.

Development of pons

The pons develops from the ventral part of metencephalon. With some contribution from alar plates of the myelencephalon.

Mantle Layer

Basal plates of metencephalon give rise to motor neurons which similar to medulla oblongata are arranged in three columns. From medial to lateral they are (Fig. 15.13A):

- General somatic efferent (GSE) column,
- Special visceral efferent (SVE) column, and
- General visceral efferent (GVE) column.

Nuclei and nerves associated with these motor columns are depicted in Table 15.1.

Alar plates give rise to sensory neurons that are arranged in four columns on each side. From medial to lateral they are (Fig. 15.13A):

- General visceral afferent (GVA),
- Special visceral afferent (SVA),
- General somatic afferent (GSA), and
- Special somatic afferent (SSA)

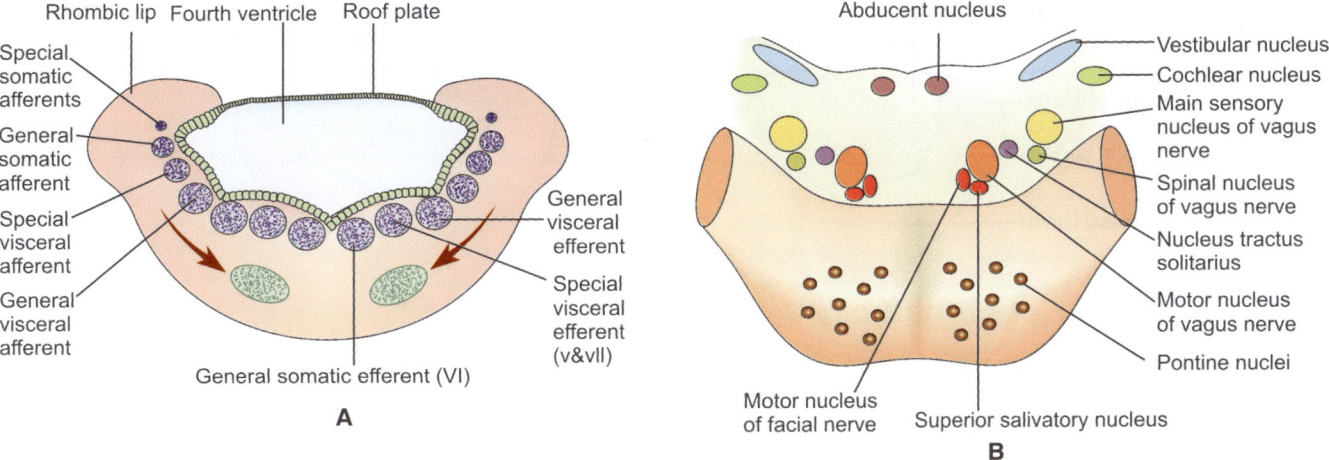

Fig. 15.13: Development of pons: A, cross section of metencephalon depicting differentiation of various motor and sensory nuclear columns in the basal and alar plates respectively and pontine nuclei in marginal layer (migrated as bulbo-pontine extension from the alar plate of myelencephalon. Note the position of rhombic lip (primordium of cerebellum); and B, Bilateral definitive position of nuclei in the pons.

Sensory nuclei and cranial nerves associated with these columns are depicted in Table 15.1.

Note. The nuclei derived from the basal plates and alar plates lie in the dorsal part or tegmental part of pons (Fig. 15.13B).

Marginal Layer

Marginal layer constitutes the ventral part of pons. It contains pontine nuclei and various nerve fibres (Fig. 15.13B):

Pontine nuclei are derived from the cranial bulbo-pontine extension which in turn develops from the sensory neurons migrated from the alar plates of myelencephalon.

Nerve fibres are in plenty in this part of pons. These include:

- *Axons of pontine nuclei* grow transversely and form the *middle cerebellar peduncle.*
- *Nerve fibres from cerebral cortex* to spinal cord (cotico-spinal), to medulla (cortico-bulbar) and to pontine nuclei (cortio-pontine), all pass through pons. Since the pons make a bridge for nerve fibres connecting cerebral cortex and cerebellar cortex with the spinal cord, hence its name (pons = bridge).

Development of cerebellum

Cerebellum develops from the posterior part of metencephalon.

Stages in the development of cerebellum

- *Rhombic lips* derived from the dorsolateral part of alar plates of metencephalon form the primordium of cerebellum (Fig. 15.13A). These lips are widely separated at the caudal part of metencephalon but meet in the midline close to the isthmus rhombencephali. The cells of rhombic lips proliferate forming cerebellar rudiments, which grow medially in the roof plate to meet in the midline (Fig. 15.14A to C).

- *Cerebellar plate* with dumb-bell shaped outline is then formed due to compression of rhombic lips cephalocaudally. This occurs as a result of further deepening of pontine flexure. This plate comprises of median vermis and bilateral rudiments of cerebellar hemispheres (Fig. 15.14D).

- *Flocculonodular lobe* is then formed by appearance of posterolateral fissure which separates the nodule from the vermis, and flocculus from the cerebellar hemisphere (Fig. 15.14E). Flocculo-nodular lobe is a component of *archicerebellum* and establishes connection with vestibular nuclei to regulate equilibrium and posture.

Anterior lobe, uvula and pyramid are then formed by further growth and appearance of fissura prima, fissura seconda and postpyramidal fissure (Fig. 15.14F). It is important to note that with the growth of cerebellum in dorsal caudal direction the flocculo-nodular lobe appears on the anterior part of inferior surface (Fig. 15.14F).

The anterior lobe plus the uvula and pyramid form the *paleo-cerebellum* which receives connections from the spinal cord and regulate tone and posture.

- *Neocerebellum* is constituted by the remaining part of cerebellum which connects with the cerebral cortex and helps in co-ordination of voluntary movements to perform skillful acts with precision.

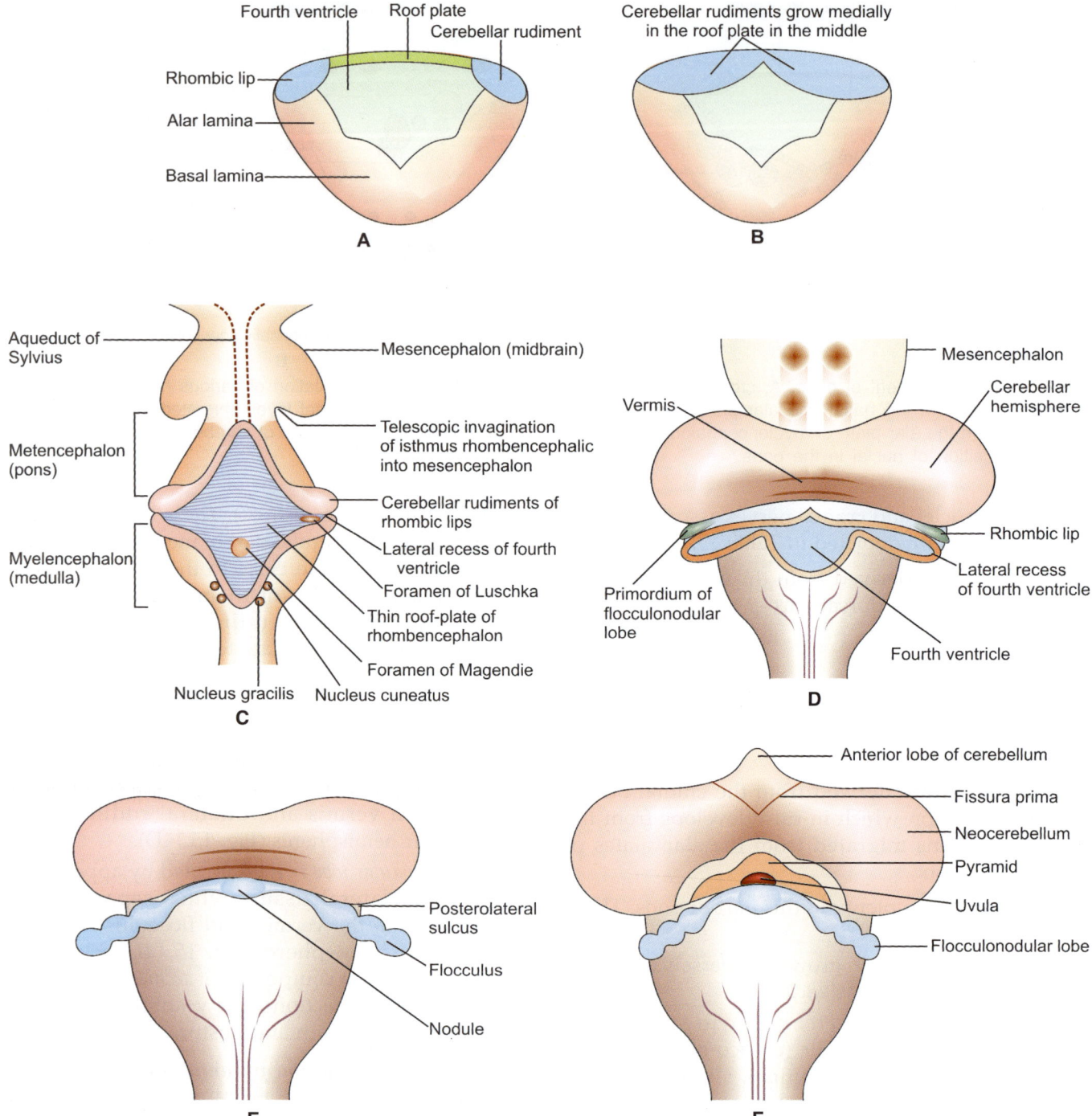

Fig. 15.14: Development of cerebellum: A, Cerebellar rudiments appear from alar laminae of metencephalon, B and C cerebellar rudiments meet with midline as seen in cross section and dorsal view, respectively; D, Formation of dumbel shaped cerebellar plate; E, Formation of flocculonodular lobe; F, Formation of anterior lobe, pyramid and uvula.

Histogenesis of developing cerebellum

Cerebellar plate, initially consists of ependymal, mantle and marginal layer (Fig. 15.15A).

Mantle layer. Neuroblasts of mantle layer form cerebellar cortex and deep cerebellar nuclei.

- *Formation of cerebellar cortex:* Some neuroblasts from the mantle layer migrate to the surface through the marginal zone and form the *external granular layer* of cerebellar cortex (Fig. 15.5B and C). Cells of this layer retain their ability to divide and form a proliferative zone on the surface of the cerebellum and release inward purkinje cells, granule cells, golgi cells, basket cells, and stellate cells (Fig. 15.5D). The cerebellar cortex reaches its definitive size after birth.

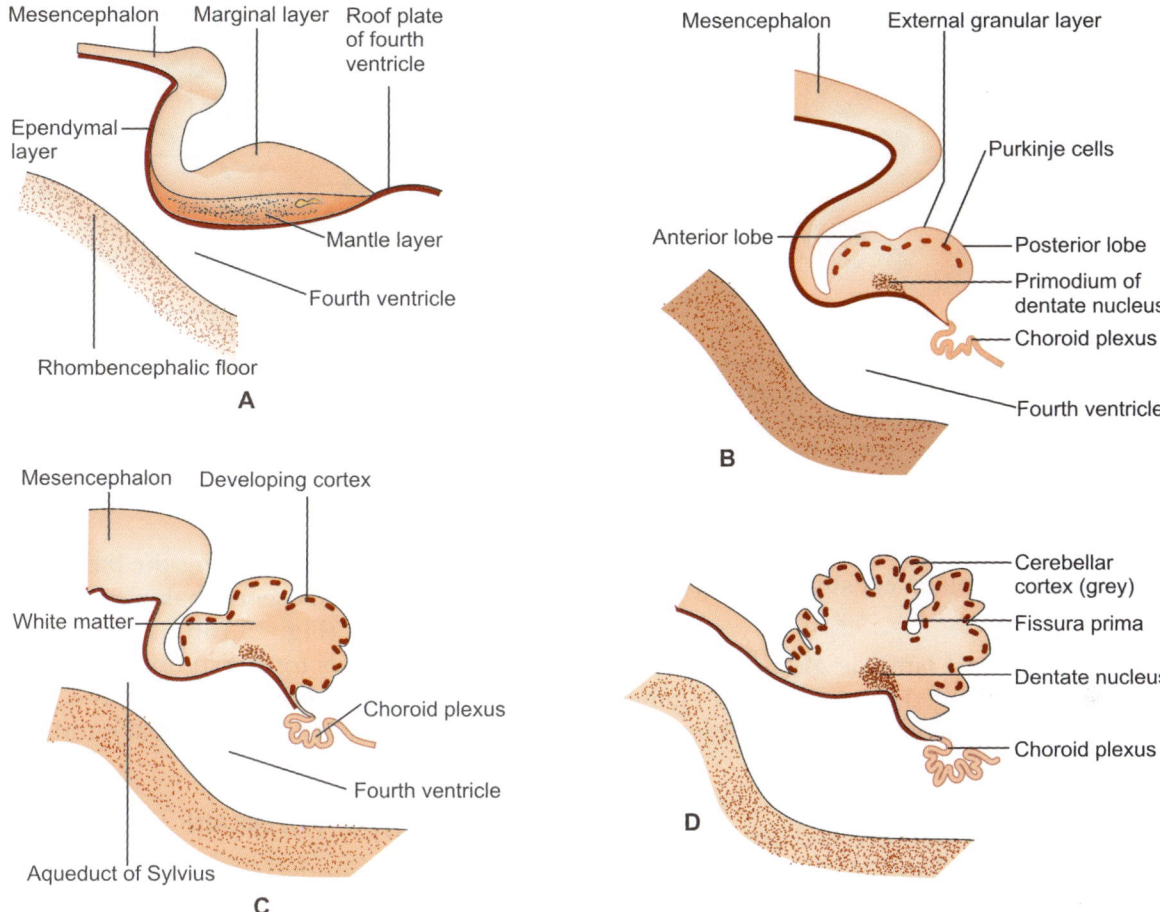

Fig. 15.15: Sagittal section showing the histogenesis of developing cerebellum from metencephalon: A, cerebellar plate consisting of ependymal, mantle and marginal layers; B, formation of cerebellar cortex by the neuroblasts migrating from the mantle layer to the surface; C and D; formation of deep nuclei.

- *Deep cerebellar nuclei* are formed by rest of the neuroblasts of mantle layer. These include dentate, emboliformis, globosus and fastigial. The deep cerebellar nuclei reach their final position before birth (Fig. 15.5D).

Marginal layer. Underneath the cerebellar cortex the marginal layer is formed by the axons. The axons also form the cerebellar peduncles:

- *Superior cerebellar peduncle* is formed mainly by the axons growing out of the dentate nucleus,
- *Middle cerebellar peduncle* is formed by the axons growing in the cerebellum from the cells of pontine nuclei, and
- *Inferior cerebellar peduncle* is formed by the axons that grow into the cerebellum from the spinal cord and medulla.

DEVELOPMENT OF MIDBRAIN

The midbrain develops from the *mesencephalon* and isthmus rhombencephali which during development gets incorporated with the caudal part of developing midbrain.

Mesencephalon: Histogenesis and salient features of development

Histogenesis of the part of neural tube forming midbrain (mesencephalon) occurs as described earlier (page 248) and leads to formation of three zones of the wall (Fig. 15.16A):

- Ependymal layer,
- Mantle layer, and
- Marginal layer.

Ependymal layer

Ependymal layer lines the central cavity of mesencephalon which is progressively narrowed by the growth of the walls, and forms the *aqueduct of Sylvius*.

Mantle layer

Lateral walls of mantle layer are arranged into *basal plates* or ventral laminae, and *alar plates* or dorsal laminae separated by sulcus limitans. *Roof plates* and *floor plates* are formed, respectively by the dorsal and

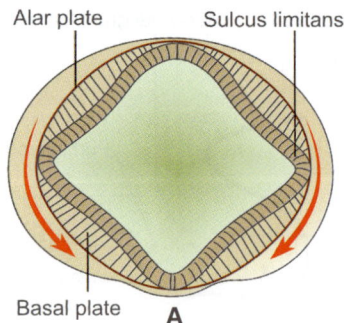

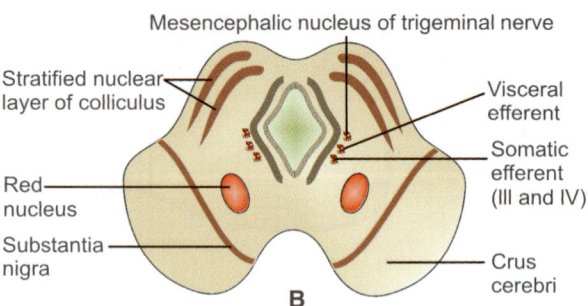

Fig. 15.16: Development of midbrain: A, primitive mesencephalon showing ependymal layer, mantle layer (arranged as basal plates and alar plates) and marginal layer. Arrows indicate the path followed by the migrating neuroblasts from alar plates which form the red nucleus and substantia nigra; B, definitive position of masses of grey matter derived from the alar and basal plates and crura cerebri formed by marginal layer ventrally.

ventral midline portions (Fig. 15.16A). The alar plates and the roof plates form together the *tectum,* and the basal plates and floor-plates constitute the *tegmentum* of midbrain.

Basal plates or ventral laminae give rise to motor neurons which are arranged in two columns—general somatic efferent and general visceral efferent (Fig. 15.16B):

- ***General somatic efferent* (GSE)** is represented by oculomotor nucleus rostrally, and caudally by the trochlear nucleus (Table 15.1). The trochlear nucleus is developed from the isthmus rhombencephali which is incorporated into the mesencephalon.

- ***General visceral efferent (GVE)*** is represented by *Edinger-Westphal nucleus* of oculomotor nerve, which conveys preganglionic parasympathetic fibres to the sphincter pupillae and ciliary muscle.

Alar plates or dorsal laminae give rise to sensory neurons. The neuroblasts of alar plate form following nuclei:

- *General somatic afferent (GSA)* component is represented by the mesencephalic nucleus of trigeminal nerve. It receives proprioception from the muscle of mastication, facial and ocular muscles.

- *Special somatic afferent (SSA)* is represented by the superior and inferior colliculi, the elevated structures formed or either side of the midline by neuroblasts of alar laminae. Initially these form one mass which later becomes subdivided by a transverse fissure. The superior colliculi function as correlation and reflex center for the visual impulses; and the inferior colliculi serve as synaptic relay stations for auditory reflexes.

- *Red nucleus and substantia nigra* is formed by the neuroblasts of alar plates which migrate ventrally (Fig. 15.16B).

Marginal layer

The marginal layer overlying the basal plates in the ventral part of the mesencephalon enlarges and forms the *crus cereberi* (Fig. 15.16B). These crura cereberi serve as pathways for nerve fibres descending from cerebral cortex to lower center in the pons (cortico pontine), medulla (corticobulbar) and spinal cord (cortico spinal).

DEVELOPMENT OF FOREBRAIN

Forebrain develops from prosencephalon which consists of:

- Diencephalon and
- Telencephalon.

Diencephalon

The diencephalon consists of a central neural cavity bounded by a thin roof-plate, two thick lateral walls and floor plates (Fig. 15.17A). The central cavity develops into *third ventricle.* The diencephalon gives rise to optic cup and stalk, posterior pituitary, thalamus, hypothalamus and pineal body.

Derivatives of lateral wall

The lateral wall of the diencephalon is very thick and is formed by the *alar plate* (basal plate is not formed in the diencephalon). The *hypothalamic* sulcus divides the lateral wall into a dorsal and a ventral region (Fig. 15.17A).

Thalamus is formed by the dorsal region. The various nuclei of thalamus are formed by multiplication of neuroblasts of mantle layer forming the alar plates.

Hypothalamus develops from the ventral region of the lateral wall of diencephalon. The neuroblasts in this region differentiate into a number of nuclear areas that regulate the visceral functions including sleep, digestion, body temperature and emotional behaviour.

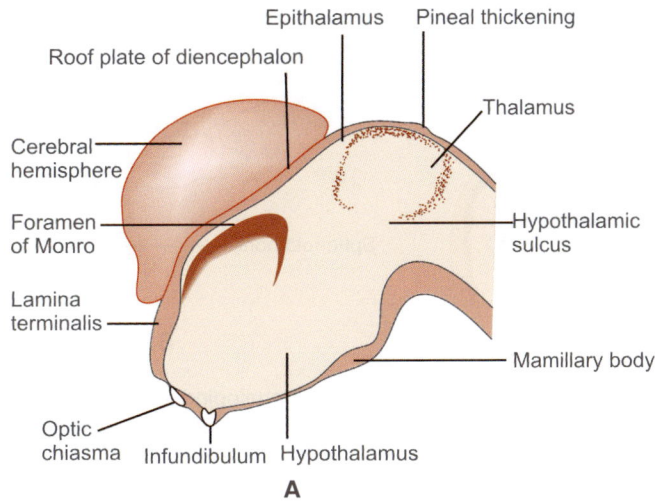

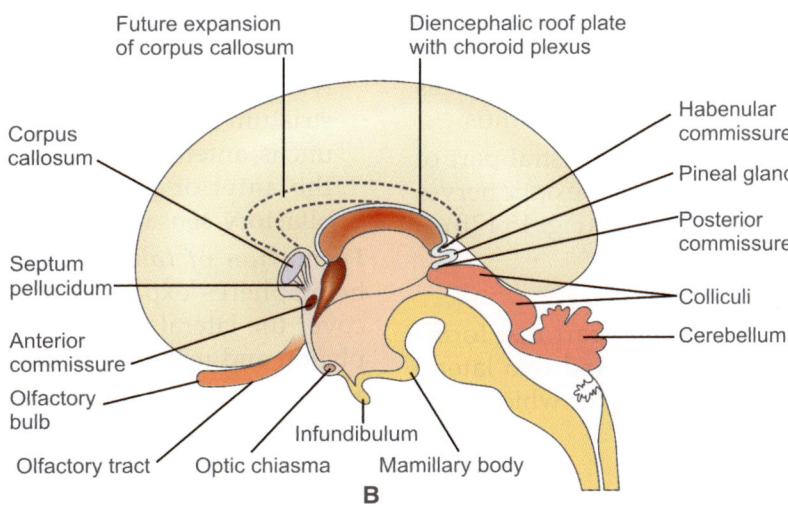

Fig. 15.17: Derivatives of diencephalon: A, inner view of right lateral wall of diencephalon; note hypothalamic and epithalamic sulci dividing it into epithalamus, thalamus and hypothalamus; B, medial surface of the right half of brain depicting structures derived from the roof plate (tela choroidea and choroid plexus, and pineal body), floor plate (mamillary body, infundibulum, and optic chiasma). Also note the commissures.

Derivatives from roof plate

The roof plate of the diencephalon is continuous rostrally with the *lamina terminalis* and from anterior to posterior form the following structures (Fig. 15.17B):

Tela choroidea is formed by the thin ependymal layer forming roof plate along with the vascular mesenchyme covering it externally. From the tela choroidea the vascular capillaries project into the third ventricle and constitute the choroid plexuses.

Pineal body or epiphysis, a median elevation, develops from the most caudal part of the roof of diencephalon. Just anterior to the pineal body in the upper part of lateral wall are formed trigonum habenular and

posterior commissure and the three collectively are named as *epithalamus*. The epithalamic sulcus separates the epithalamus from the thalamus (Fig. 15.17B).

Derivatives of floor plates

The floor plate of diencephalon exhibits the following features from behind forward (Fig. 15.17B):

Mammillary bodies, one on each side of the midline, project on the ventral surface of the hypothalamus.

Infundibulum, a downward extension from diencephalon grows caudally dorsal to the *Rathke's pouch.* The Rathke's pouch is an ectodermal upgrowth from the stomodaeum. The two together forms the hypophysis or pituitary gland. Thus, the hypophysis develops as below (Fig. 15.18):

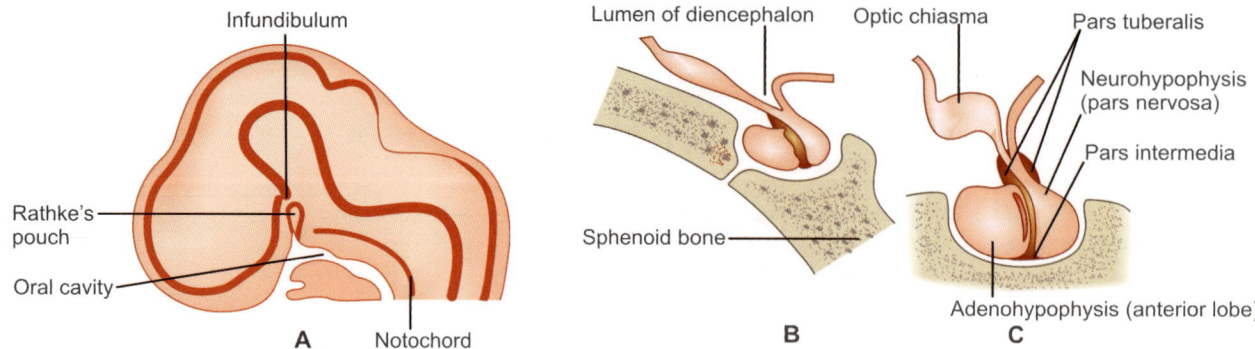

Fig. 15.18: Sagittal section through the sucessive stages of developing embryo depicting development of pituitary gland (hypophysis): A, at 6th week; B, at 11th week; and C, at 16th week of development.

- *Adenohypophysis,* the intermediate lobe, and pars tuberalis develop from Rathke's pouch, and
- *Neurohypophysis* or posterior lobe of the hypophysis (stalk and pars nervosa) develops from the infundibulum. It is composed of neuroglial cells and receives nerve fibres from hypothalamus.

Optic stalks are attached to the most rostral part of the floor plate. Here the nasal fibres of the optic nerves decussate and form the optic chiasma (Fig. 15.17B).

Telencephalon

Telencephalon consists of a median part that forms the anterior part of third ventricle, and two lateral diverticulae known as cerebral vesicles which form the cerebral hemispheres.

Histogenesis and development of cerebral hemispheres

The wall of the developing cerebral vesicles like any other parts of neural tube consists of from interior to exterior of ependymal layer a mantle and a marginal layer and encloses, a cavity which later forms the lateral ventricles. Initially in the development the wall of each cerebral vesicle is thin in the superior part and thick in the basal part (Fig.15.19A). Further histogenesis and development of the cerebral hemispheres can be summarized as below:

Formation of cerebral cortex

Some neuroblasts migrate from the mantle layer of thick basal part to the overlying marginal layer and proliferate to form the cerebral cortex. Developmentally the cerebral cortex can be divided into three parts (Fig. 15.19B):

- *Hippocampal cortex* forms the hippocampus and indusium griseum.
- *Neocortex* develops from the *neopallium* (part of the wall of cerebral vesicle between hippocampus and paleopallium) and forms the major part of cerebral cortex.
- *Pyriform cortex* develops from the *paleopallium* or archipallium (part of the wall of cerebral vesicle lying immediately lateral to the developing corpus striatum (Fig. 15.19B). Pyriform cortex includes the uncus, anterior part of parahippocampal gyrus and the anterior perforated substance. It receives olfactory sensations.

Formation of lobes, sulci and gyri: The cerebral hemispheres expand extensively on all sides and cover the lateral aspects of diencephalon, mesencephalon and metencephalon.

- *Lobes* of the cerebral hemispheres, frontal, temporal, parietal and occipital are formed as a result of continuous growth.
- *Gyri and sulci:* Due to greater expansion of the cerebral cortex than that of the underlying structures of hemisphere the cortex becomes folded on itself. As a result of this folding the sulci and gyri are formed.

Formation of corpus striatum

The neuroblasts remaining in the mantle layer of thick basal parts of the wall of developing cerebral vesicles proliferate and form a thick nuclear mass the *corpus striatum* (Fig. 15.19B). Soon this nuclear mass is divided into following two parts by the bundle of nerve fibres *(internal capsule)* passing to and from the cerebral cortex to the lower centres (pons, medulla, cerebellum and spinal cord) (Fig. 15.19C):

Caudate nucleus refers to the part of the corpus striatum that comes to lie deep or medial to the internal capsule. With the fusion of medial wall of the hemisphere and lateral wall of the diencephalon the caudate nucleus and thalamus come into close contact (Fig. 15.19C).

Lentiform nucleus refers to the part of corpus striatum lying superficial or lateral to the internal

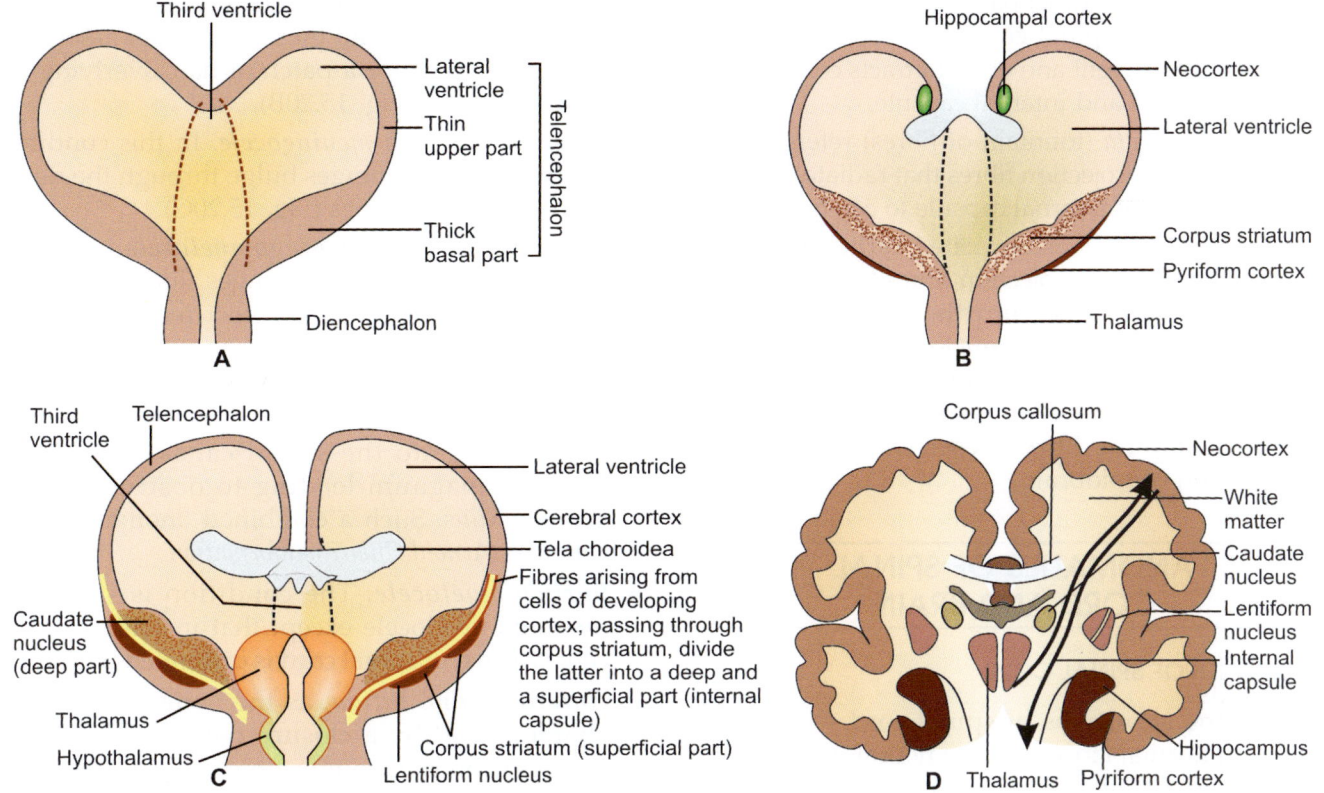

Fig. 15.19: Coronal section through telencephalon depicting histogenesis and development of cerebral hemispheres: A, note the thin upper and thick basal (parts of the wall of cerebral vesicles; B, formation of corpus striatum and early differentiation of cerebral cortex. Note hippocampal, cortex, neocortex and pyriform cortex; C, formation of caudate and lentiform nuclei, internal capsule and further; D, subdivision of lentiform nucleus and further differentiation of cerebral cortex.

capsule. It is later subdivided into two parts (Fig. 15.19D):

- Putamen, and
- Globus pallidus

Formation of white matter of cerebrum

Axons passing through, between and around the subcortical masses of grey matter of cerebrum form the tracts of white matter. The white matter of cerebrum consists of three types of fibres—association fibres, commissural fibres, and projection fibres.

1. **Association fibres** are those axons which connect the different gyri of the same hemisphere.
2. **Commissural fibres** are those which connect the corresponding parts of two cerebral hemispheres. *Lamina terminalis* (the part of the wall of neural tube that closes the cranial end of prosencephalon and later lies in the anterior wall of third ventricle) becomes thickened to form the *commissural plate* and facilitates the passage of fibres from one hemisphere to the other. The bundle of commissural fibres formed are (Fig. 15.17B):
   - *Anterior commisure* is the first to develop. It consists of the fibres which are connecting the

olfactory bulb and related brain areas of the two hemispheres.

- *Hippocampal commissure* or *fornix commissure* is the second to develop. Its fibres arise in the hippocampus and converse to lamina terminalis and terminate in the mammillary body and the hypothalamus.
- *Corpus callosum* is the most important commissure. It appears by last week of development and initially forms a small bundle in the lamina terminalis lying anterior to the diencephalon. However, soon it progresses forward and backward, and presents rostrum, genu, body and splenium.
- *Habenular commissure* is formed just below and rostral to the stalk of the pineal gland.
- *Posterior commissure* is also formed below and rostral to the pineal body.
- *Optic chiasma* appears in the rostral wall of diencephalon. It contains fibres from the medial halves of retinae.

3. **Projection fibres** which make white matter of the cerebrum are those which connect the cerebral

hemispheres with other parts of CNS, e.g. thalamus, brainstem and spinal cord. The projection fibres include the afferent and efferent tracts contained in corona radiata and internal capsule.

- *Corona radiata* (fountain of fibres) refers to that part of the projection fibres that radiate from the upper end of internal capsule to cerebral cortex.
- *Internal capsule,* as described earlier, is a thick curved band of projection fibres (ascending and descending) that occupy the space between the thalamus and caudate nucleus medially and the lentiform nucleus laterally (Fig. 15.19C). Superiorly it fans out as corona radiata, and inferiorly the fibres descend into the crura cereberi of midbrain.

ANOMALIES OF SPINAL CORD AND BRAIN

ANOMALIES OF SPINAL CORD

Most of the anomalies of spinal cord result from defects in normal closure of the neural tube and are thus termed as *neural tube defects (NTDs)*.

Common causes of NTDs reported are:

- Hyperthermia
- Teratogenic drugs including hypervitaminosis A
- Genetic predisposition (positive family history).

Prevention. Administration of folic acid (folate) in the dose of 400 mg/day beginning 2 months prior to conception and continuing throughout gestation is reported to reduce the incidence of NTDs by 70%.

Common varieties of NTDs can be grouped as below:

- Rachischisis,
- Spina bifida, and
- Spina bifida anterior.

Rachischisis

Rachischisis refers to a condition in which the neural groove fails to close and is exposed to surface (Fig. 15.20A). The condition involving spinal cord is also called *spina bifida with myeloschisis.*

Spina Bifida

Spina bifida is a type of NTD in which the vertebral arches are splitted and unable to cover the spinal cord dorsally. Depending upon the associated involvement of underlying structure the spina bifida may be of following types:

1. *Spina bifida occulta.* The defect usually involves vertebral arches of 2 to 3 vertebrae in the lumbo-sacral region. The defect in vertebral arches is covered with skin and there is no other associated anomaly except for a patch of hair overlying the affected region (Fig. 15.20B).

2. *Spina bifida with meningocele.* In this condition the fluid filled meninges bulge through the defect in the vertebral arches (Fig. 15.20C).

3. *Spina bifida with meningomyelocele* is characterized by protusion of meninges along with spinal cord tissue through the defect in the vertebral arches (Fig. 15.20D).

   Meningomyelocele is often associated with downward shift of medulla and some part of cerebellum into the spinal canal through the foramen magnum leading to obstruction and *hydrocephalus.* Such a combined anomaly is also called as *Arnold Chiari malformation.*

4. *Syringomyelocele.* The condition is similar to meningo-myelocele except that in this condition central canal of spinal cord is distended with fluid.

5. *Anterior spina bifida*, as the name indicates, is characterized by a closure defect affecting the vertebral body through which spinal meninges protrude ventrally (Fig. 15.20E).

ANOMALIES OF BRAIN

A few of the anomalies involving brain are described below:

1. *Anencephaly* also known as *exencephaly* results due to failure of the anterior neuropore to close. It is characterized by absence of cranial vault, exposed malformed brain (which later degenerates). Such fetuses lack swallowing reflex, therefore, the last 2 months of pregnancy are characterized by hydramnios.

   Antenatal diagnosis of the condition can be made by ultrasonography in later part of pregnancy and estimation of α-fetoprotein levels of the aminioic fluid. It is advisable to terminate the pregnancy, when anencephaly is diagnosed.

   Prevention: Like spina bifida, administration of 400 mg of folic acid /day before and during pregnancy can prevent about 70% cases of anencephaly.

2. *Microcephaly* is characterised by a small sized brain and a smaller cranial vault, usually associated with mental retardation.

   Causes may be genetic (autosomal recessive or acquired) such as prenatal infections, exposure to teratogenic drugs or other substances.

3. *Hydrocephalus* refers to a condition in which excessive CSF is accumulated in the skull.

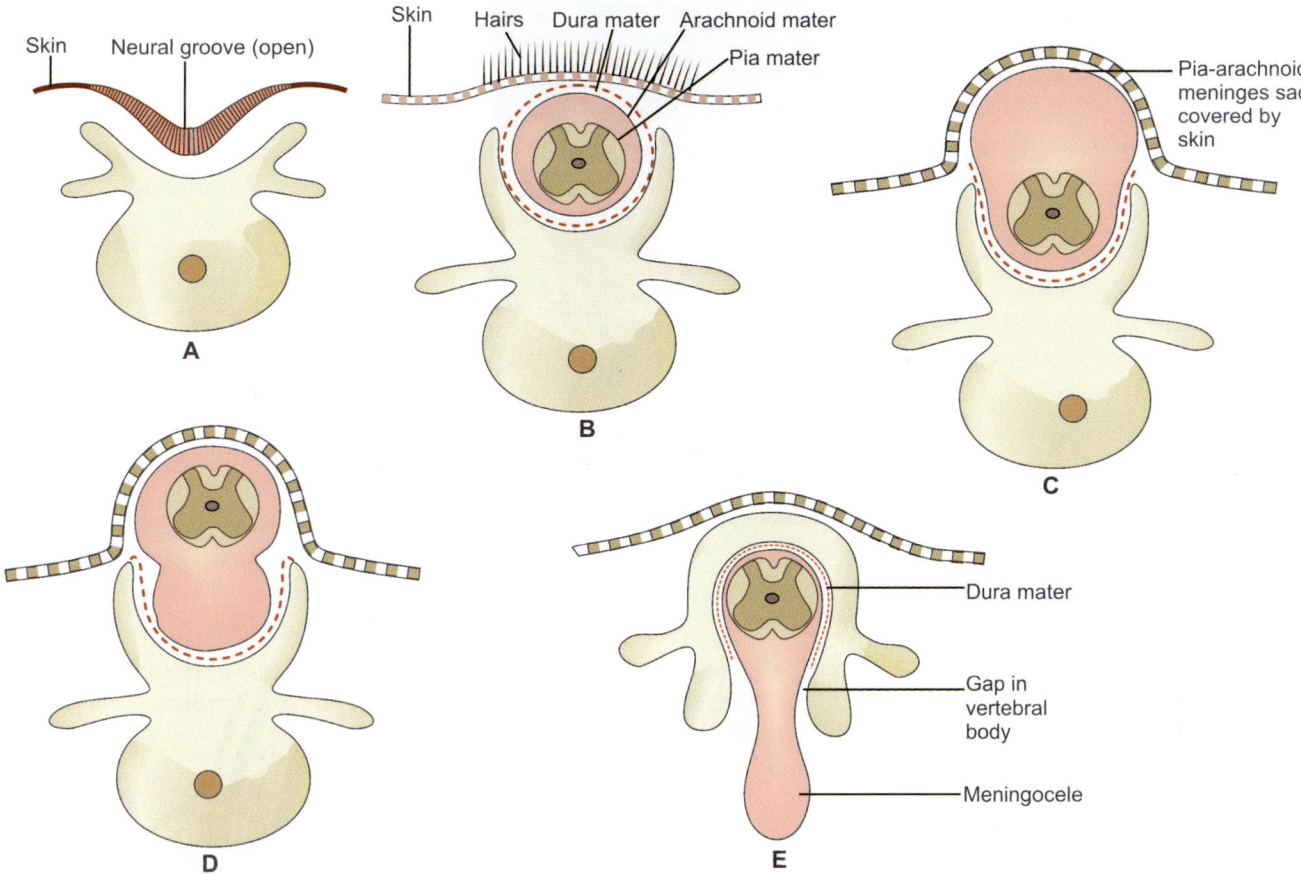

Fig. 15.20: Anomalies of spinal cord: A, rachischisis; B, spina bifida occulta; C, spina bifida with meningocele; D, spina bifida with meningomyelocele; E, anterior spina bifida.

Causes: Hydrocephalus can be of two types:

i. *Communicating type:* In this condition the CSF appears in the cisterna magna but fails to reach the supratentorial space for absorption into the dural sinuses.

ii. *Non-communicating type* hydrocephalus is characterized by obstruction to the passage of CSF at any of the following places:

- Foramen of Monro,
- Aqueduct of Sylvius,
- Foramen in the ependymal roof of fourth ventricle, or
- Foramen magnum (e.g. Arnold-Chiari malformation). *Features* include dilatation of ventricular system of brain, expansion of cranial vault, and separation of cranial bones at suture (Fig. 15.21A).

4. *Meningocele, meningoencephalocele* and *meningohydroencephalocele* are all caused by a ossification defect in the skull bones, frequently the squamous part of occipital bone.

- *Meningocele* is characterized by herniation of meninges of brain through the defect in skull bones (Fig. 15.21B).
- *Meningoencephalocele* occurs when the defect is large. In this condition along with meninges, part of brain is also prolapsed (Fig. 15.21C).
- *Meningohydroencephalocele* occurs in advanced cases, when a part of ventricle of the brain is incorporated in the herniated mass (Fig. 15.21D).

5. *Absence of corpus callosum,* partial or complete may occur without any functional defect.

6. *Absence of cerebellum,* partial or complete, may occur with only slight disturbance of co-ordination.

7. *Functional defects* in the form of severe mental retardation may occur in the absence of gross morphological defects. Some of the causes are:
- Down's syndrome (trisomy 21),
- Klinefelter syndrome (47 XXY),
- Maternal alcohol abuse,
- Phenylketonuria,
- Exposure to teratogens and
- Infections (e.g. rubella, cytomegalovirus, and toxoplasmosis).

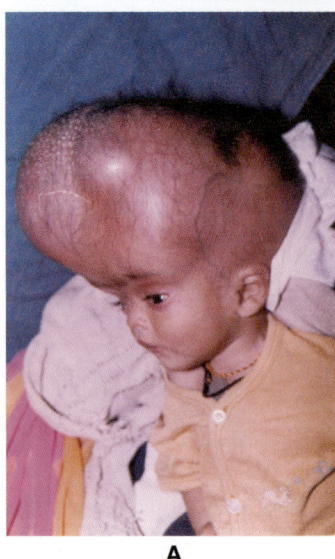

A

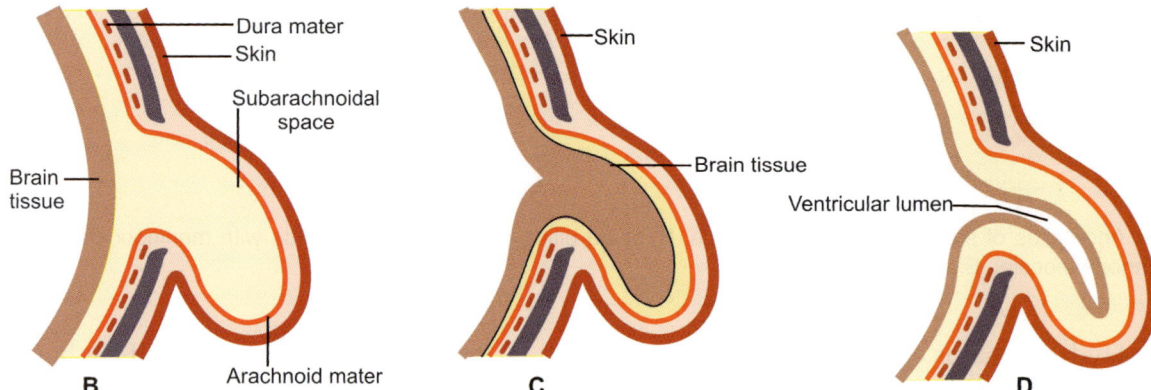

Fig. 15.21: Some anomalies of brain: A, a case of hydrocephalus; B, meningocele; C, meningoencephalocele; D, meningo-hydro-encephalocele.

DEVELOPMENT OF AUTONOMIC NERVOUS SYSTEM

The autonomic nervous system include:
- Sympathetic nervous system (thoracolumbar outflow), and
- Parasympathetic nervous system (cranio-sacral outflow).

SYMPATHETIC NERVOUS SYSTEM

Sympathetic nervous system consists of:
- Sympathetic preganglionic neurons,
- Sympathetic ganglia, and
- Sympathetic postganglionic neurons.

Sympathetic preganglionic neurons

The sympathetic preganglionic neurons develop from the neuroblasts located near the sulcus limitans in the mantle layer of thoracic and upper three lumbar segments of spinal cord (Fig. 15.22).

Cell bodies of these neurons form the *intermediolateral horns of spinal cord* from T_1 to L_3 segments and thus constitute the thoracolumbar outflow.

Axons of these visceral motor neurons are myelinated, and as shown in Fig. 15.22 after leaving the spinal cord via ventral root pass via the white rami communicantes to paravertebral ganglia of sympathetic trunk (which are simultaneously developed from neural crest cell as described below).

After reaching the sympathetic trunk preganglionic fibres may pass to one of the following three destinations:

- They may terminate in the ganglion at the level of entrance by synapsing with an excitor cell in the ganglion (Fig. 15.22).

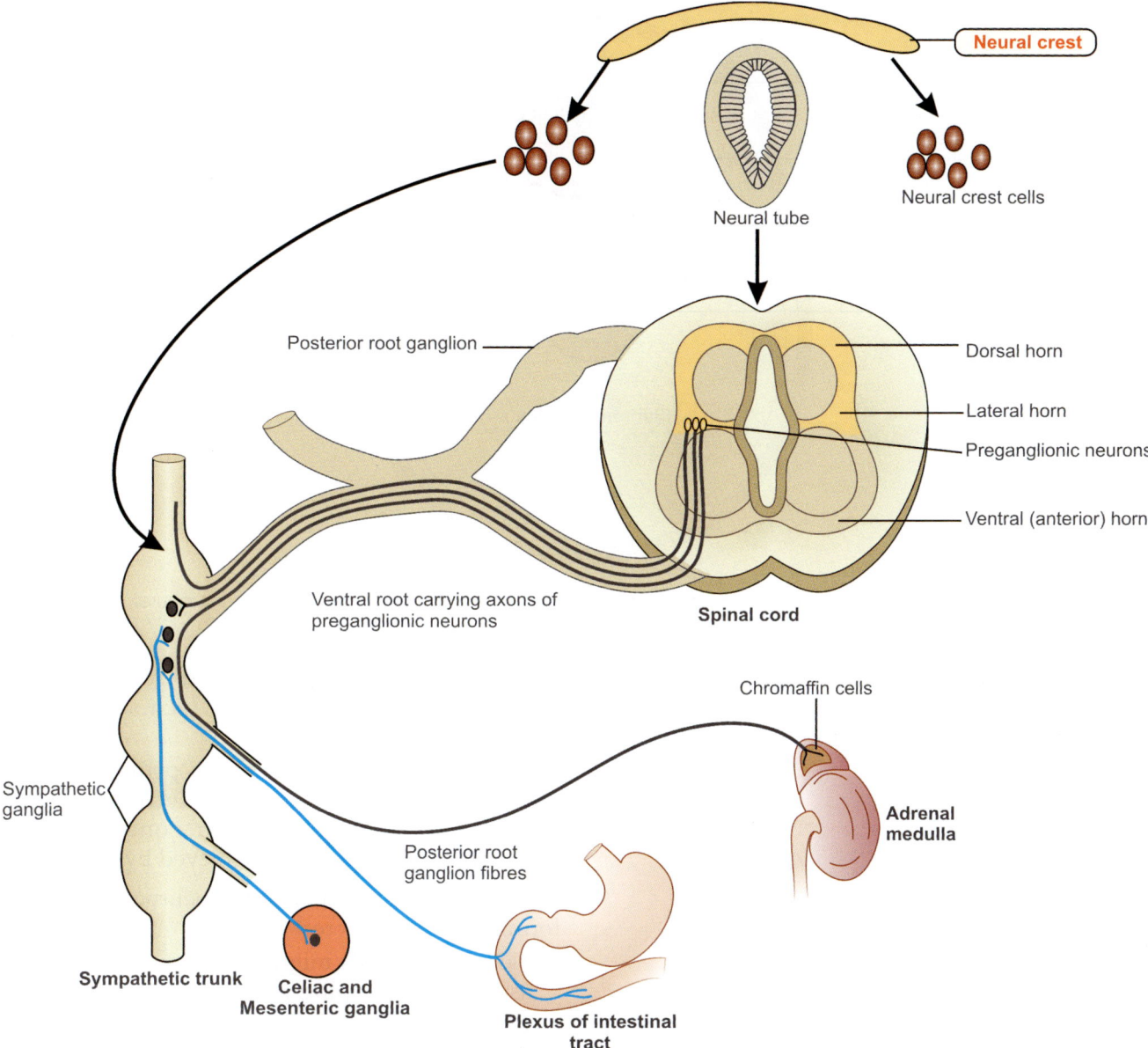

Fig. 15.22: Development of preganglionic and postganglionic sympathetic neurons.

- They may travel up or down in the sympathetic trunk to terminate in the ganglia located at a higher or lower level (Fig. 15.22).
- They may travel through sympathetic trunk and exit without synapsing via splanchnic nerve and terminate in a prevertebral or peripheral ganglia (Fig. 15.22).

Sympathetic ganglia

Three types of sympathetic ganglia which develop from *neural crest cells* are as below:

1. *Paravertebral ganglia.* During the 5th week neural crest cells in the thoracic region migrate along each side of spinal cord and proliferate to form paravertebral sympathetic ganglia (Fig. 15.23).

Then ganglia get connected by longitudinal nerve fibres to form two *sympathetic trunks* (right and left) placed on either side of the vertebral column. These paravertebral ganglia include:

- *Cervical ganglia* three in number — superior, middle and inferior.
- *Thoracic ganglia,* 12 in number, and
- *Lumbar ganglia,* 4 in number.

2. *Prevertebral (preaortic) ganglia.* Some neural crest cells migrate ventral to the aorta and form preaortic ganglia (Fig. 15.23). These include:

- Celiac ganglion,
- Inferior mesenteric ganglion, and
- Superior mesenteric ganglion.

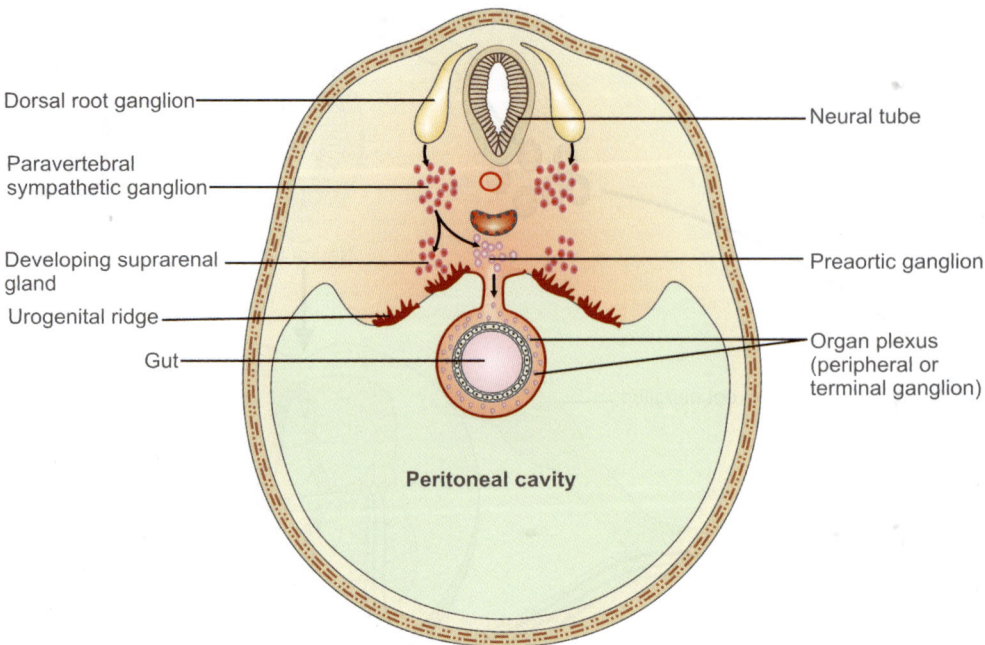

Fig. 15.23: Formation of paravertebral, preaortic and peripheral (terminal) sympathetic ganglia from the neural crest cells and development of suprarenal gland.

3. ***Peripheral or terminal ganglia.*** Other neural crest cells migrate to the peripheral area and form terminal ganglia near the following structures supplied by them:

- Heart,
- Bronchi,
- Pancreas,
- Gastrointestinal tract, and
- Urinary bladder.

Postganglionic neurons and axons

Cell bodies of postganglionic neurons, as described above are located in the sympathetic ganglia. Their axons supply the viscera, blood vessels, smooth muscles, sweat gland, etc.

Development of suprarenal gland

Each suprarenal gland consists of two parts:
- Cortex, and
- Medulla

Cortex of suprarenal gland is developed from the mesodermal cells located near the developing gonad.

- *Primitive cortex* or fetal cortex is first formed during 5th week, when mesothelial cells between the roof of mesentery and developing gonad begin to proliferate and penetrate the underlying mesenchyme (Fig. 15.23). These cells differentiate into large acidophilic cells which form primitive cortex.

- *Definitive cortex* is then formed by second wave from the mesothelial cells which surround the primitive cortex.

- *Adult cortex:* After birth, the primitive cortex regresses rapidly and the definitive cortex differentiates into reticular zone. The adult structure of the cortex is achieved by puberty.

Medulla is developed from the neuroectoderm cells forming the neural crest cells:

- Neural crest cells migrate and invade the medial aspect of developing primitive cortex (Figs 15.23 and 15.24A).

- These cells are then arranged in cords and cluster and form the medulla of suprarenal gland (Fig. 15.24B). The cells forming medulla are called *chromaffin cells,* as they stain yellow brown with chrome salts.

DEVELOPMENT OF PARASYMPATHETIC SYSTEM

Parasympathetic nervous system consists of:
- Parasympathetic preganglionic neurons,
- Parasympathetic ganglia, and
- Parasympathetic postganglionic fibres.

Parasympathetic preganglionic neurons

These include:
- Cranial parasympathetic preganglionic neurons, and
- Sacral parasympathetic preganglionic neurons.

Chromaffin cells migrating from neural crest
Acidophilic fetal cortex (primitive cortex)
A
Adult cortex
Zona glomerulosa
Zona fasciculata
Zona reticularis
Medulla
Primitive cortex
Definitive cortex
B

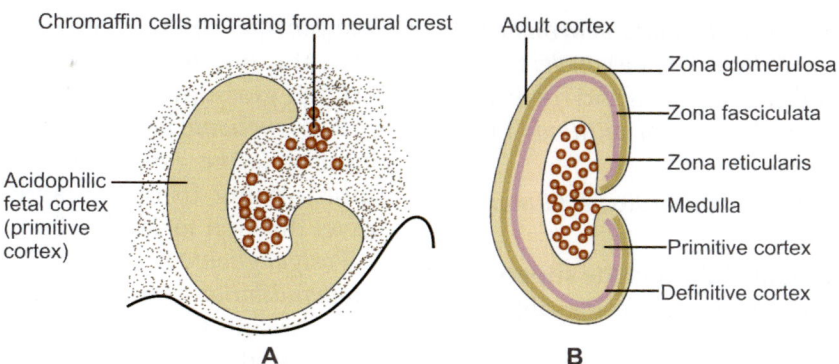

Fig. 15.24: Development of suprarenal gland: A, invasion of primitive cortex by neural crest cells; B, definitive cortex surrounding the medulla formed by chromaffin cells.

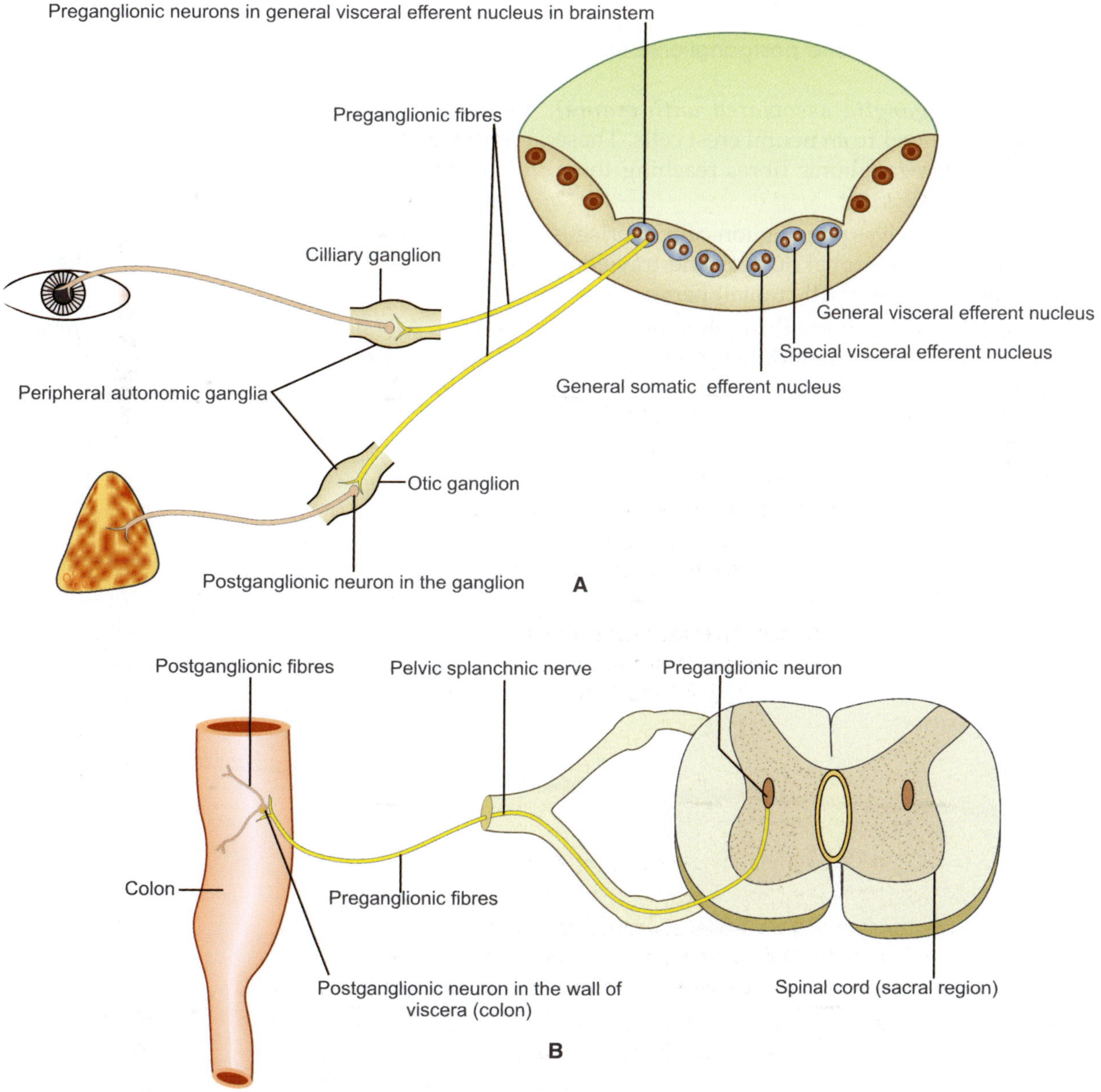

Preganglionic neurons in general visceral efferent nucleus in brainstem
Preganglionic fibres
Cilliary ganglion
Peripheral autonomic ganglia
General visceral efferent nucleus
Special visceral efferent nucleus
General somatic efferent nucleus
Otic ganglion
Postganglionic neuron in the ganglion
A
Postganglionic fibres
Pelvic splanchnic nerve
Preganglionic neuron
Colon
Preganglionic fibres
Postganglionic neuron in the wall of viscera (colon)
Spinal cord (sacral region)
B

Fig. 15.25: Development of preganglionic and postganglionic parasympathetic neurons: A, cranial outflow; B, sacral outflow.

Cranial parasympathetic preganglionic neurons are developed as *general visceral efferent* (GVE) *nuclei* from the mantle layer in mid brain (page 256) and medulla (page 251) and constitute the *cranial outflow* (Fig. 15.25A):

- GVE nucleus developed in midbrain is *Edinger-Westphal nucleus*, and
- GVE nuclei developed in medulla include superior, salivary nucleus, lacrimal nucleus, inferior salivary nucleus, and dorsal vagal nucleus.

Sacral parasympathetic preganglionic neurons are developed from the neuroblasts of mantle layer and form the *intermediolateral grey horn* of 2nd, 3rd and 4th sacral segments (S_2 to S_4) of spinal cord. These constitute the sacral outflow (Fig. 15.25B).

Parasympathetic ganglia and postganglionic fibres

Parasympathetic ganglia associated with cranial outflow are developed from neural crest cells. These ganglia and the preganglionic fibres reaching them are as below (Fig. 15.25A):

- *Ciliary ganglion* receives preganglionic fibres arising from the Edinger-Westphal nucleus and travelling through the oculomotor (III cranial) nerve.
  - *Postganglionic fibres* pass through short ciliary nerves (branches of oculomotor nerves) and supply ciliary muscle.

- *Otic ganglion* receives preganglionic fibres arising from the *inferior salivary nucleus* which travel through glossopharyngeal (IX cranial) nerve.
  - *Postganglionic fibres* supply the parotid gland.
- *Sphenopalatine ganglion* receives preganglionic fibres arising from the lacrimal nucleus which travel through facial (VII cranial) nerve.
  - *Postganglionic fibres* supply the lacrimal gland.
- *Submandibular ganglion* receives preganglionic fibres arising from the superior salivary nucleus travelling through facial (VII cranial) nerve.
  - *Postganglionic fibres* pass to submandibular and sublingual salivary glands.
- *Ganglia (or nerve plexus) closely related to the visceral organs* (head, lungs GIT) receive preganglionic fibres arising from the dorsal nucleus of vagus nerve travelling through vagus (X cranial) nerve.
  - *Post ganglionic fibres* supply smooth muscle and glands of the viscera (e.g. heart, lungs and GIT).

Parasympathetic ganglia associated with sacral outflow are in the form of *pelvic autonomic plexus*. These neurons are located in the wall of pelvic viscera and receive preganglionic fibres arising from S_2 to S_4 intermediolateral grey horns which travel through the spinal nerves and their branches the pelvic splanchnic nerves.

- *Postganglionic fibres* arising from these neurons supply the pelvic viscera and the distal part of colon (Fig. 15.25B).

Development of Eye and Ear

DEVELOPMENT OF THE EYE

The eyeball and its related structures are derived from the following primordia:

1. An outgrowth from prosencephalon called optic vesicle (neuroectodermal structure).
2. A specialized area of surface ectoderm called lens placode and the surrounding surface ectoderm.
3. Mesoderm surrounding the optic vesicle.
4. Visceral mesoderm of maxillary process.

Before going into the development of individual structures, it will be helpful to understand the formation of optic vesicle, lens placode, optic cup and changes in the surrounding mesoderm, which play a major role in the development of the eye and its related structures.

FORMATION OF OPTIC VESICLE AND OPTIC STALK (FIG. 16.1)

The area of neural plate (Fig.16.1A) which forms the prosencephalon develops a linear thickened area on either side (Fig.16.1B), which soon becomes depressed to form the optic sulcus (Fig.16.1C). Meanwhile the neural plate gets converted into prosencephalic vesicle. As the optic sulcus deepens, the walls of the prosencephalon overlying the sulcus bulge out to form the *optic vesicle* (Figs 16.1D to F). The proximal part of the optic vesicle becomes constricted and elongated to form the *optic stalk* (Figs 16.1G and H).

FORMATION OF LENS VESICLE

The optic vesicle grows laterally and comes in contact with the surface ectoderm. The surface ectoderm,

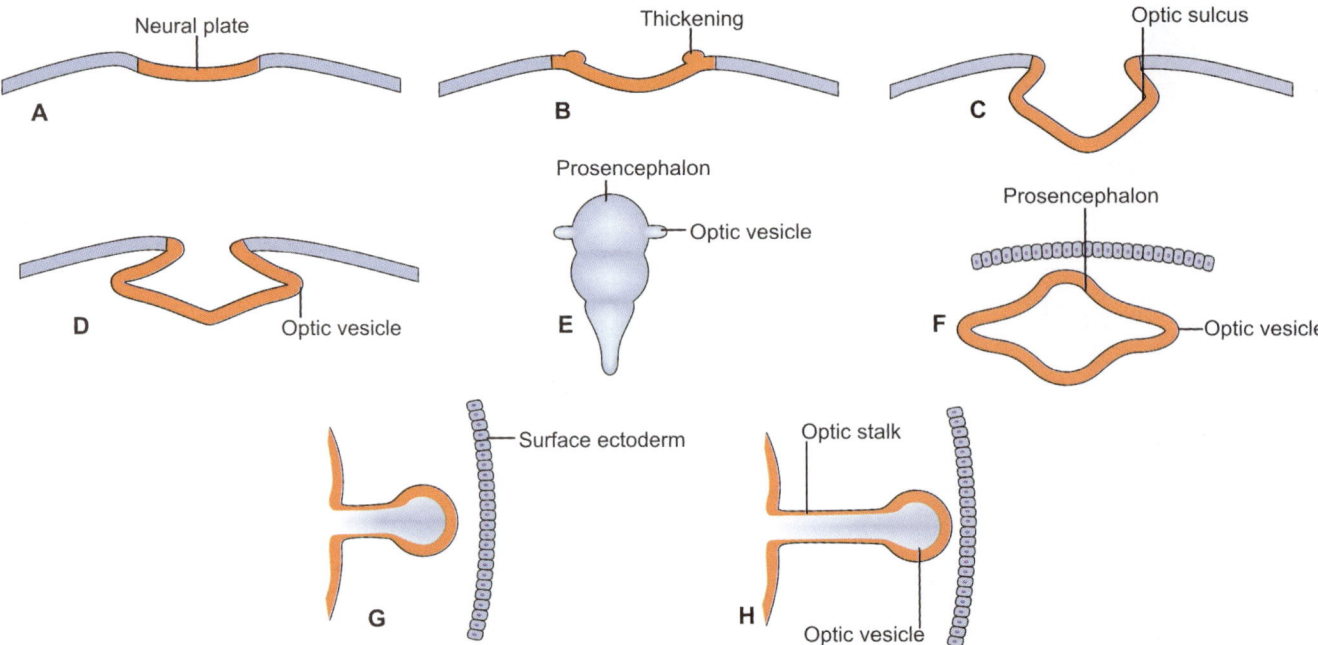

Fig. 16.1: Formation of the optic vesicle and optic stalk.

overlying the optic vesicle becomes thickened to form the lens placode (Fig. 16.2A) which sinks below the surface and is converted into the lens vesicle (Fig. 16.2B and C). It is soon separated from the surface ectoderm (Fig. 16.2D).

FORMATION OF OPTIC CUP

The optic vesicle is converted into a double-layered *optic cup*. It appears from Fig. 16.2 that this has happened because the developing lens has invaginated itself into the optic vesicle. In fact conversion of the optic vesicle to the optic cup is due to differential growth of the walls of the vesicle. The margins of optic cup grow over the upper and lateral sides of the lens to enclose it. However, such a growth does not take place over the inferior part of the lens, and therefore the walls of the cup show deficiency in this part. This deficiency extends to some distance

along the inferior surface of the optic stalk and is called the *choroidal or fetal fissure* (Fig. 16.3).

CHANGES IN THE ASSOCIATED MESODERM

The developing neural tube (from which central nervous system develops) is surrounded by mesoderm, which subsequently condenses to form meninges. An extension of this mesoderm also covers the optic vesicle. Later, this mesoderm differentiates to form a superficial fibrous layer (corresponding to dura) and a deeper vascular layer (corresponding to pia-arachnoid) (Fig. 16.4).

With the formation of optic cup, part of the inner vascular layer of mesoderm is carried into the cup through the choroidal fissure. With the closure of this fissure, the portion of mesoderm which has made its way into the eye is cut off from the surrounding mesoderm and gives rise to the hyaloid system of the vessels (Fig. 16.5).

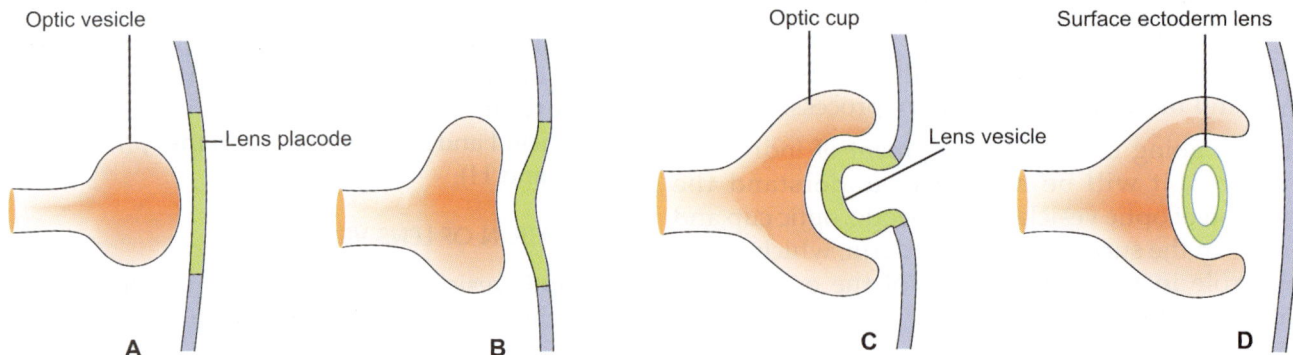

Fig. 16.2: Formation of lens vesicle and optic cup.

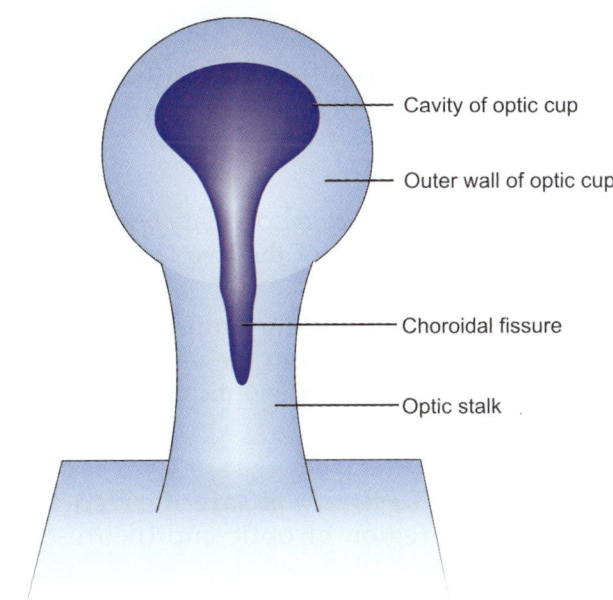

Fig. 16.3: Optic cup and stalk seen from below to show the choroidal fissure.

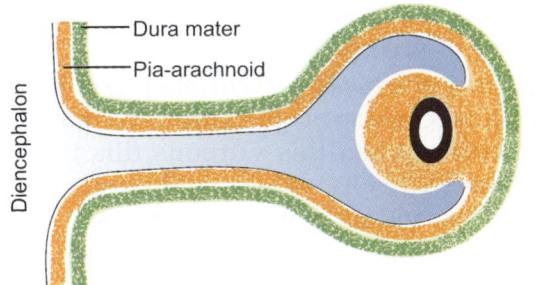

Fig. 16.4: Developing optic cup surrounded by mesoderm.

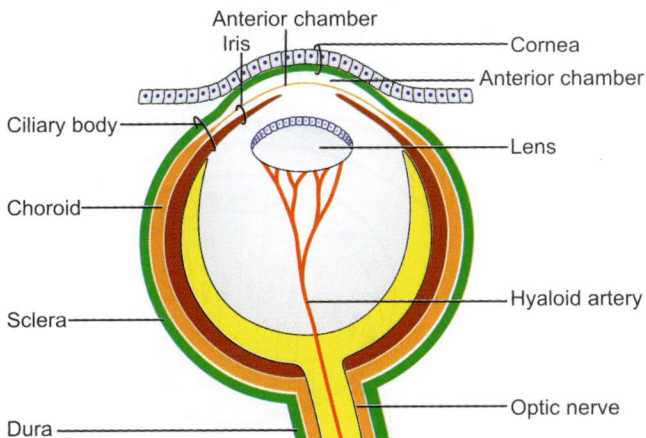

Fig. 16.5: Derivation of various structures of the eyeball.

The fibrous layer of mesoderm surrounding the anterior part of optic cup forms the cornea. The corresponding vascular layer of mesoderm becomes the iridopupillary membrane, which in the peripheral region attaches to the anterior part of the optic cup to form the iris. The central part of this lamina is pupillary membrane which also forms the tunica vasculosa lentis (Fig. 16.5).

In the posterior part of optic cup the surrounding fibrous mesoderm forms sclera and extraocular muscles, while the vascular layer forms the choroid and ciliary body.

DEVELOPMENT OF VARIOUS OCULAR STRUCTURES

Retina

Retina is developed from the two walls of the optic cup, namely: (a) nervous retina from the inner wall, and (b) pigment epithelium from the outer wall (Fig. 16.6).

a. *Nervous retina.* The inner wall of the optic cup is a single-layered epithelium. It divides into several layers of cells which differentiate into the following three layers (as also occurs in neural tube):

　1. *Matrix cell layer:* Cells of this layer form the rods and cones.

　2. *Mantle layer:* Cells of this layer form the bipolar cells, ganglion cells, other neurons of retina and the supporting tissue.

　3. *Marginal layer:* This layer forms the ganglion cells, axons of which form the nerve fibre layer.

b. *Outer pigment epithelial layer.* Cells of the outer wall of the optic cup become pigmented. Its posterior part forms the pigmented epithelium of retina and the anterior part continues forward in ciliary body and iris as their anterior pigmented epithelium.

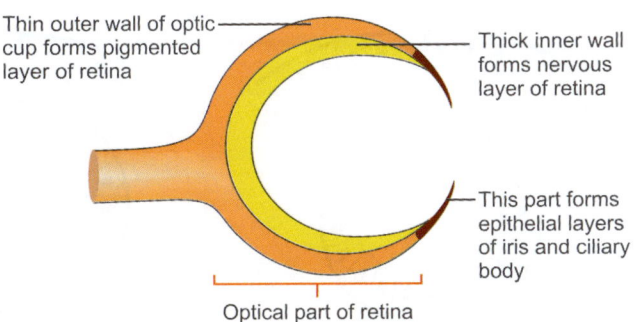

Fig. 16.6: Development of the retina.

Optic nerve

It develops in the framework of optic stalk as below:

1. Fibres from the nerve fibre layer of retina grow into optic stalk by passing through the choroidal fissure and form the *optic nerve fibres.*
2. The epithelial cells forming the walls of optic stalk develop into *glial system* of the nerve.
3. The fibrous *septa* of the optic nerve are developed from the vascular layer of mesoderm which invades the nerve at 3rd fetal month.
4. *Sheaths of optic nerve* are formed from the layers of mesoderm like meninges of other parts of central nervous system.
5. *Myelination of nerve* fibres takes place from brain distally and reaches the lamina cribrosa just before birth and stops there. In some cases this extends up to around the optic disc and presents as congenital opaque nerve fibres. These develop after birth.

Crystalline lens

It is formed from the lens vesicle. The cells of the posterior wall elongate to form the lens fibres. Rest of the fibres are formed from equatorial cells of anterior epithelium which remain active throughout life (Fig. 16.7).

Cornea (Fig. 16.5)

1. *Epithelium* is formed from the surface ectoderm.
2. *Other layers viz.* endothelium, Descemet's membrane, stroma and Bowman's layer are derived from the fibrous layer of mesoderm lying anterior to the optic cup.

Sclera

Sclera is developed from the fibrous layer of mesoderm surrounding the optic cup (corresponding to dura of CNS).

Choroid

It is derived from the inner vascular layer of mesoderm that surrounds the optic cup.

Ciliary body

1. The two layers of *epithelium* of ciliary body develop from the anterior part of the two layers of optic cup (neuroectodermal).
2. *Stroma of ciliary body,* ciliary muscle and blood vessels are developed from the vascular layer of mesoderm surrounding the optic cup.

Iris

1. Both layers of *epithelium* are derived from the marginal region of optic cup (neuro-ectodermal).
2. *Sphincter and dilator pupillae* muscles are derived from the anterior epithelium (neuro-ectodermal).
3. *Stroma and blood vessels* of the iris develop from the vascular mesoderm present anterior to the optic cup.

Vitreous

1. *Primary or primitive vitreous* is mesodermal in origin and is a vascular structure having the hyaloid system of vessels.
2. *Definitive or secondary or vitreous proper* is secreted by neuroectoderm of optic cup. This is an avascular structure. When this vitreous fills the cavity, primitive vitreous with hyaloid vessels is pushed anteriorly and ultimately disappears.
3. *Tertiary vitreous* is developed from neuroectoderm in the ciliary region and is represented by the ciliary zonules.

Eyelids

Eyelids are formed by reduplication of surface ectoderm above and below the cornea (Fig. 16.8). The folds enlarge and their margins meet and fuse with

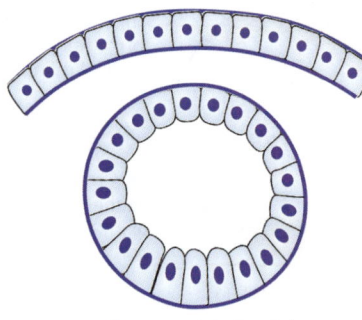
Lens vesicle (early)

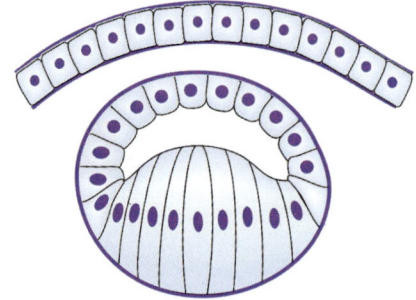
Lens vesicle (late)

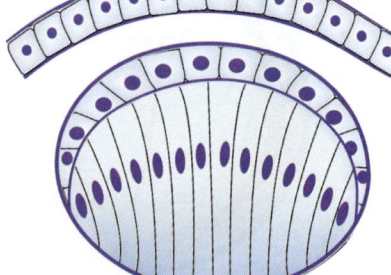
Lens vesicle (nucleus)

Fig. 16.7: Development of the crystalline lens.

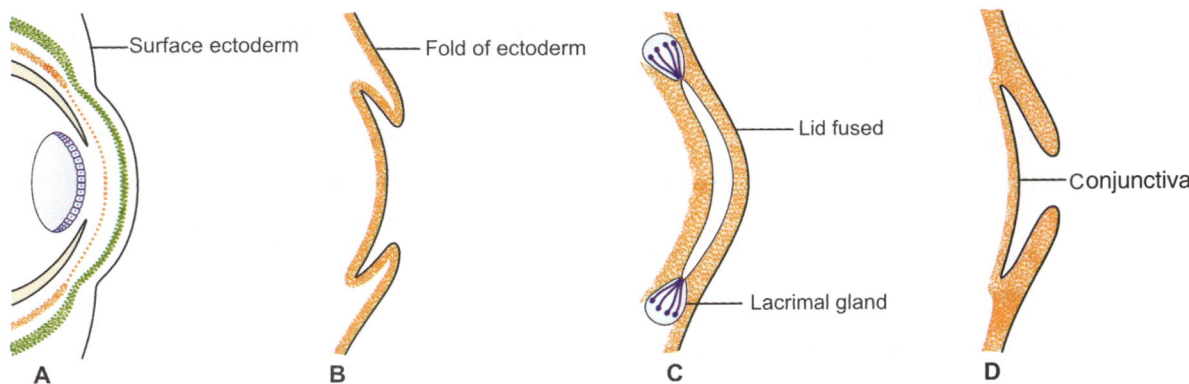

Fig. 16.8: Development of the eyelids, conjunctiva and lacrimal gland.

each other. The lids cut off a space called the conjunctival sac. The folds thus formed contain some mesoderm which would form the muscles of the lid and the tarsal plate. The lids separate after the seventh month of intrauterine life.

Tarsal glands are formed by ingrowth of a regular row of solid columns of ectodermal cells from the lid margins.

Cilia develop as epithelial buds from lid margins.

Conjunctiva

It develops from the ectoderm lining the lids and covering the globe (Fig. 16.8).

Conjunctival glands develop as growth of the basal cells of upper conjunctival fornix. Fewer glands develop from the lower fornix.

The lacrimal apparatus

Lacrimal gland is formed from about 8 cuneiform epithelial buds which grow by the end of 2nd month of fetal life from the superolateral side of the conjunctival sac (Fig. 16.8).

Lacrimal sac, nasolacrimal duct and canaliculi: These structures develop from the ectoderm of nasolacrimal furrow. It extends from the medial angle of eye to the region of developing mouth. The ectoderm gets buried to form a solid cord. The cord is later canalised. The upper part forms the lacrimal sac. The nasolacrimal duct is derived from the lower part as it forms a secondary connection with the nasal cavity. Some ectodermal buds arise from the medial margins of eyelids. These buds later canalise to form the canaliculi.

Extraocular muscles

All the extraocular muscles develop in a closely associated manner by mesenchymal condensation. This probably corresponds to preotic myotomes,

hence the triple nerve supply (III, IV and VI cranial nerves).

STRUCTURES DERIVED FROM THE EMBRYONIC LAYERS

Based on the above description, the various structures derived from the embryonic layers are given below:

1. *Surface ectoderm*
   - The crystalline lens,
   - Epithelium of the cornea,
   - Epithelium of the conjunctiva,
   - Lacrimal gland,
   - Epithelium of eyelids and its derivatives viz., cilia, tarsal glands and conjunctival glands.
   - Epithelium lining the lacrimal apparatus.

2. *Neural ectoderm*
   - Retina with its pigment epithelium,
   - Epithelial layers of ciliary body,
   - Epithelial layers of iris,
   - Sphincter and dilator pupillae muscles,
   - Optic nerve (neuroglia and nervous elements only),
   - Melanocytes,
   - Secondary vitreous, and
   - Ciliary zonules.

3. *Associated paraxial mesoderm*
   - Blood vessels of choroid, iris, ciliary vessels, central retinal artery, other vessels.
   - Primary vitreous,
   - Substantia propria, descemet's membrane and endothelium of cornea,
   - The sclera,
   - Stroma of iris,
   - Ciliary muscle,
   - Sheaths of optic nerve,
   - Extraocular muscles,

- Fat, ligaments and other connective tissue structures of the orbit,
- Upper and medial walls of the orbit,
- Connective tissue of the upper eyelid.

4. *Visceral mesoderm of maxillary process below the eye*
   - Lower and lateral walls of orbit, and
   - Connective tissue of the lower eyelid.

IMPORTANT MILESTONES IN THE DEVELOPMENT OF THE FETAL EYE

Stage of growth	Development
2.6 mm (3 weeks)	Optic pits appear on either side of cephalic end of forebrain.
3.5 mm (4 weeks)	Primary optic vesicle invaginates.
10 mm (6 weeks)	Retinal layers differentiate, lens vesicle formed.
20 mm (9 weeks)	Sclera, cornea and extraocular muscles differentiate.
25 mm (10 weeks)	Lumen of optic nerve obliterated.
50 mm (3 months)	Optic tracts completed, pars ciliaris retina grows forwards, pars iridica retina grows forward.
60 mm (4 months)	Hyaloid vessels atrophy, iris sphincter is formed.

Eye at birth

- Anteroposterior diameter of the eyeball is about 16.5 mm (70% of adult size which is attained by 7–8 years).
- Corneal diameter is about 10 mm. Adult size (11.7 mm) is attained by 2 years of age.
- Anterior chamber is shallow and angle is narrow.
- Lens is spherical at birth. It grows throughout life.
- Apart from macular area the retina is fully differentiated. Macula differentiates 4–6 months after birth.
- Myelination of optic nerve fibres has reached the lamina cribrosa.
- Newborn is usually hypermetropic by +2 to +3 D.
- Orbit is more divergent (50°) as compared to adult (45°).

MOLECULAR REGULATION OF EYE DEVELOPMENT

Gene playing key role in the development of eye is PAX6 a member of paired pox (PAX) family. It is expressed in the single eye field at the neural plate stage. Other genes involved are PAX$_2$. SOX2, SIX3, PROXD AND FOX3.

Signaling molecules which plays role are:
- *Sonic hedghog (SHH)* protein separates the single eye field area on the neural plate into two optic primordia. It upregulates PAX2 expression in the optic stalk, while down regulating PAX6, restricting the gene's expression to the optic cup and lens.
- *Fibroblast growth factors (FGFs)* from the surface ectoderm promote differentiation of the neural (inner layer) of retina.
- *Transforming growth factor β (TGF β)*, secreted by surrounding mesenchyme, controls formation of pigmented layer of retina.
- *Bone morphogenetic protein 4 (BMP 4)* is another signaling molecule involved in the development of eye.

Epithelial mesenchymal interactions between the prospective lens ectoderm, optic vesicle, and surrounding mesenchyme play most essential role in the lens and optic cup differentiation.

ANOMALIES OF THE OCULAR STRUCTURES

Anomalies of the eyeball

1. *Anophthalmos*, refers to absence of eyeball, i.e. entire eyeball fails to develop rarely.
2. *Microphthalmos* refers to small sized eyeball.
3. *Cyclopia*, this is a rare anomaly in which only a single eyeball lodged in the single orbit is present in the median position. The rudimentary nose known as proboscis lies above the median eye.
4. *Congenital coloboma of uveal tract*, congenital coloboma (absence of tissue) of iris, ciliary body and choroid may be seen in association or independently. Coloboma may be typical or atypical.
   - *Typical coloboma* is seen in the inferonasal quadrant and occurs due to defective closure of the embryonic fissure.
   - *Atypical coloboma* is occasionally found in other positions.

   Complete coloboma extends from pupil to the optic nerve, with a sector-shaped gap occupying about one-eighth of the circumference of the retina, choroid, ciliary body, iris, and causing a corresponding indentation of the lens where the zonular fibres are missing (Fig. 16.9A).
5. *Congenital anomalies of iris and pupil* include:
   - Congenital aniridia (iridremic), i.e. absence of iris.

- Persistent pupillary membrane (PPM),
- Corectopia, i.e. eccentric placed pupil,
- Polycoria, i.e. presence of more than one pupil.

6. ***Congenital anomalies of crystalline lens include:***
   - Coloboma of the lens
   - Congenital ectopia lentis, i.e. congenital subluxation of the lens (Fig. 16.9B).
   - Lenticonus, i.e. cone shaped elevation of anterior (Fig. 16.9C) or posterior pole of the lens.
   - *Microspherophagic*, i.e. small and spherical lens instead of normal biconvex lens.
   - *Congenital cataract* (Fig. 16.9D), i.e. congenital opacification of the lens may occur due to many causes. Common causes are hereditary, rubella infection of mother during pregnancy.

7. ***Congenital anomaly of vitreous,*** seen commonly is *persistent hyperplastic primary vitreous* (PHPV). It results from failure of the primary vitreous structure to regress combined with the hypoplasia of the posterior portion of vascular meshwork.

Anomalies of accessory structures of eye

I. ***Anomalies of lids*** include:
   - *Congenital ptosis,* i.e. drooping down of upper eyelid (Fig. 16.10A).
   - *Congenital coloboma of eyelid,* i.e. a full thickness gap in the tissues of lid (Fig. 16.10B).
   - *Epicanthus,* i.e. presence of a semicircular fold of skin over the medial canthus.
   - *Cryptophthalmos,* i.e. failure of lids to separate (Fig. 16.10C).

II. ***Anomalies of lacrimal apparatus***
   - *Lacrimal gland* may be absent, hypoplasic or ectopic in position.
   - *Punctal atresia,* i.e. congenital absence of lacrimal puncta.

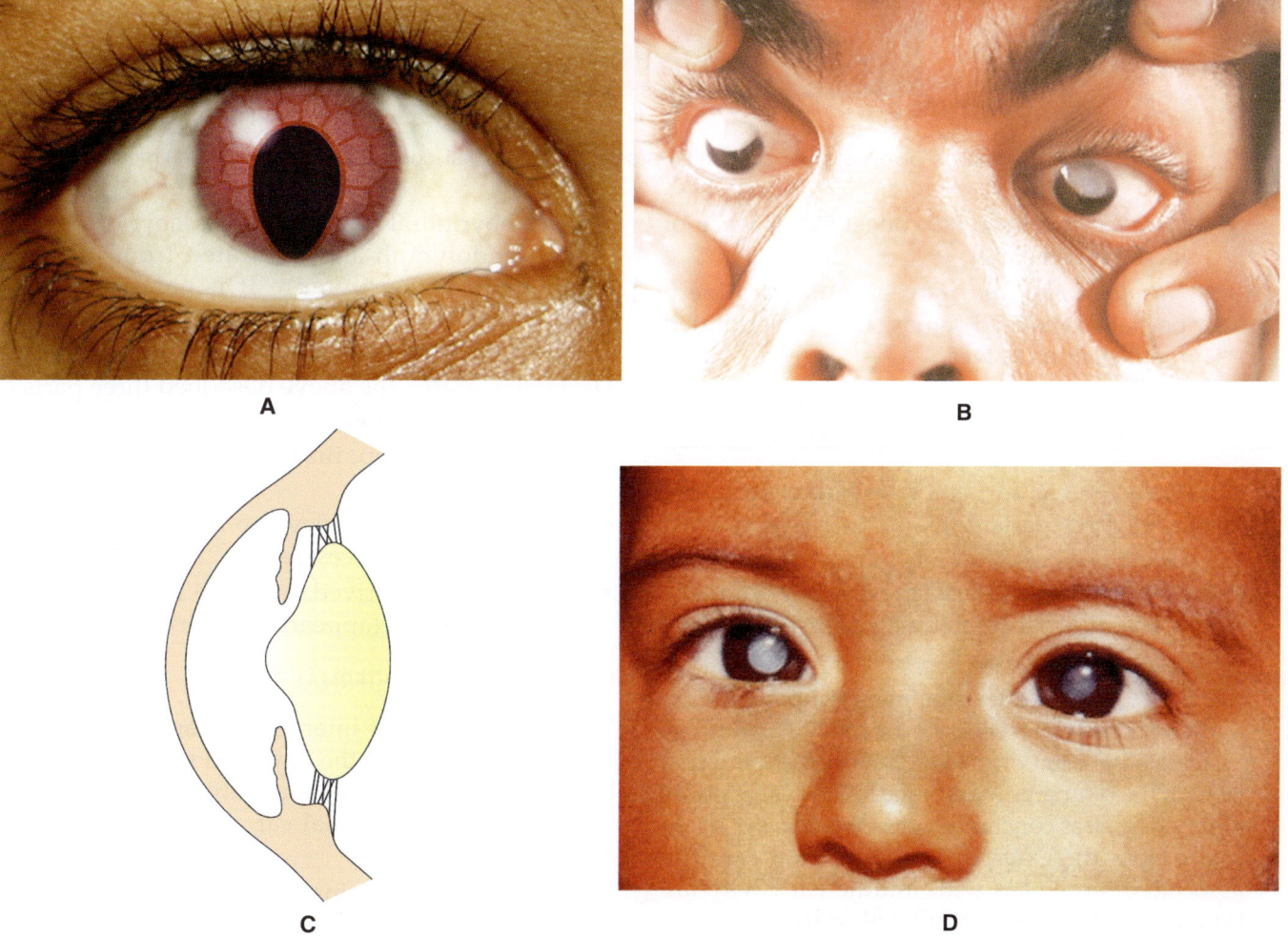

A   B

C   D

Fig. 16.9: Some congenital anomalies of eyeball: A, coloboma of iris; B, congenital ectopia lentis in a child with Marfan's syndrome; C, lenticonus anterior; D, total congenital cataract.

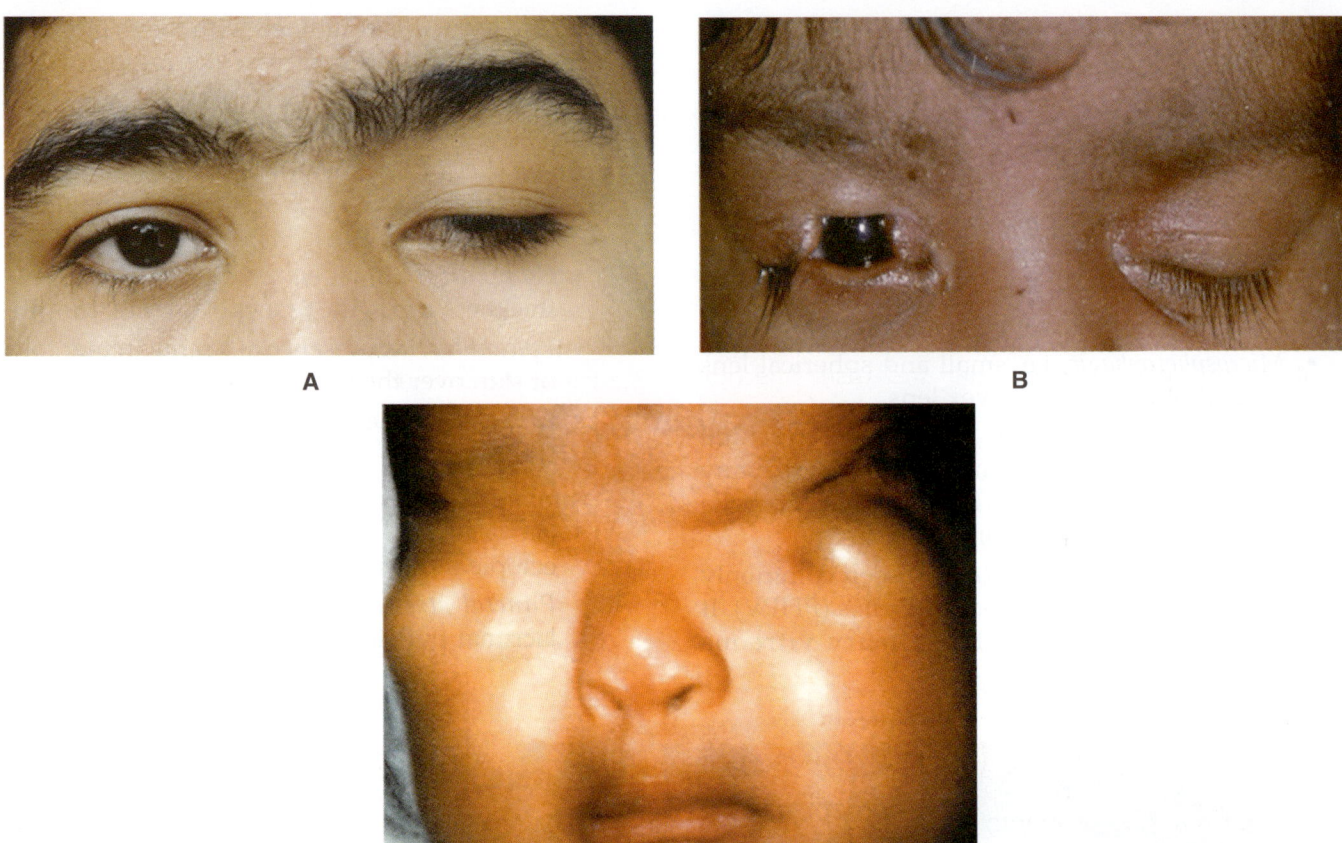

Fig. 16.10: Anomalies of eyelids: A, congenital ptosis; B, congenital coloboma; C, cryptophthalmos.

- *Canalicular atresia,* i.e. congenital absence of lacrimal canaliculi.
- *Nasolacrimal duct* may be non-canalized, partially canalized or may show imperforated membranous valves.

DEVELOPMENT OF THE EAR

Structurally the ear forms a continuous structure consisting of three parts:

- *External ear* comprises auricle (pinna), the external auditory meatus, and external layer of tympanic membrane. It is concerned with *collection of sound waves.*

- *Middle ear* consists of air-containing tympanic cavity, auditory tube and a set of three movable auditory ossicles (small ear bones) which connect the internal layer of the tympanic membrane to the oval window of inner ear. It is concerned with *conduction of sound waves* from the external to the internal ear. The associated structures with middle ear cavity are tympanic antrum and mastoid air cells.

- *Internal ear* includes vestibulocochlear organ consisting of membranous labyrinth lodged in the bony labyrinth. The membranous labyrinth is filled with endolymph and separated from the bony labyrinth by perilymph. It is concerned with *conversion of sound waves into nerve impulses* and maintenance of equilibrium.

Developmentally, the above described three parts of the ear are independent:

- *Internal ear* develops first of all from the ectodermal vesicle the otocyst,
- *Middle ear,* is next to develop from the endoderm of tubotympanic recess, and
- *External ear* is derived from the first ectodermal pharyngeal cleft (appears last).

DEVELOPMENT OF INTERNAL EAR

The development of internal ear can be considered to commence around the day 22nd when the embryo has eight pairs of somites and is about 2 mm in length. The structures of internal ear are derived from the following primordia:

- *Otic vesicle,* an invagination from surface ectoderm, gives rise to membranous labyrinth, and
- *Mesenchyme* surrounding the otic vesicle forms the bony labyrinth.

Membranous labyrinth

Formation of otic vesicle

- *Otic placode,* an ectodermal thickening, appears on each side in the region of developing rhombencephalon, early in the 4th week (Fig. 16.11A and B).
- *Otic pit* is soon formed by invagination of the otic placode into underlying mesenchyme (Fig. 16.11C).
- *Otic vesicle* (otocyst) is then formed when the edges of the otic pit come together and fuse. The otic vesicle detaches from the surface ectoderm and soon develops diverticulum, (Fig. 16.11D). The otocyst migrates inwards and comes to lie near the ventrolateral aspect of the alar plate of the developing rhombencephalon.

Formation of endolymphatic duct and utricular and saccular parts of otic vesicle

- *Endolymphatic duct* grows as a diverticulum from the otic vesicle. Its distal end dilates to form sac (saccule) (Fig. 16.12A and B).
- *Division of otic vesicle* (primordial membranous labyrinth) occurs soon into two parts (Fig. 16.12C)
    - *Dorsal utricular part* gives rise to the utricle, semicircular ducts, and endolymphatic duct.
    - *Ventral saccular part,* form the saccule and cochlear duct.

The partition extends towards the endolymphatic duct. The communication persists as Y-shaped utriculosaccular duct.

Formation of utricle, and semicircular ducts

- *Three disc-like evaginations* arise during 6th week from the utricular part of the primordial membra-nous labyrinth at right angles to each other. These discs fuse with each other (Fig. 16.12D and E)
    - *Semicircular ducts* are then formed when the central parts of three discs disappear (Fig. 16.12E). Superior semicircular duct appear first followed by lateral and posterior.
- *Ampullae,* localized dilatations, at one end of each semicircular canal (Fig. 16.12F).
- *Cristae ampullaris,* specialized receptor areas then differentiate in the three ampullae and also in the utricle and saccule (maculae utriculi and sacculi) (Fig. 16.13).
- *Crus commune* is then formed by union of the non-ampullated ends of the superior and posterior semicircular ducts. Thus, the three semicircular ducts open into the utricle by five openings (Fig. 16.12F).

Formation of saccule, cochlear duct and organ of corti

- *Cochlear duct,* a tubular diverticulum, arises from the saccular part of the otic vesicle (Fig. 16.12E) and elongates spirally for 2.75 turns in the surrounding mesenchyme during the 8th week (Fig. 16.12F).
- *Ductus reuniens* is soon formed as narrow connection between the cochlea and the saccule (Fig. 16.12F).
- *Organ of corti,* consisting of a tectorial membrane and hair cells (sensory cells of auditory system), differentiate from the cells in the wall of cochlear duct (Fig. 16.13).

Development of innervation of internal ear

Vestibulocochlear ganglion is formed from some cells which break away from the otocyst wall along with the neural crest cells. The cells forming the ganglion are bipolar neurons (Fig. 16.13).

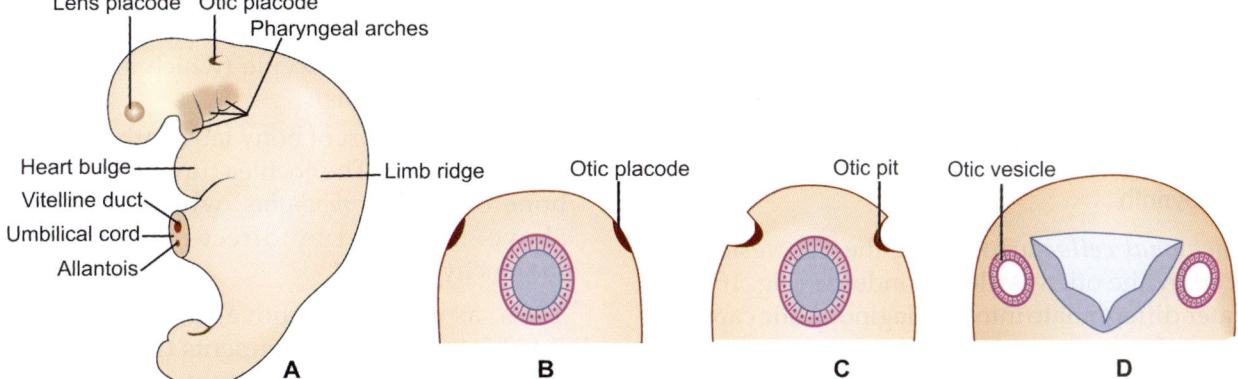

Fig. 16.11: Formation of otic vesicle: A, location of otic placode in an embryo (4 weeks) B, C, D, transverse sections depicting otic placode, otic pit, and otic vesicle, respectively.

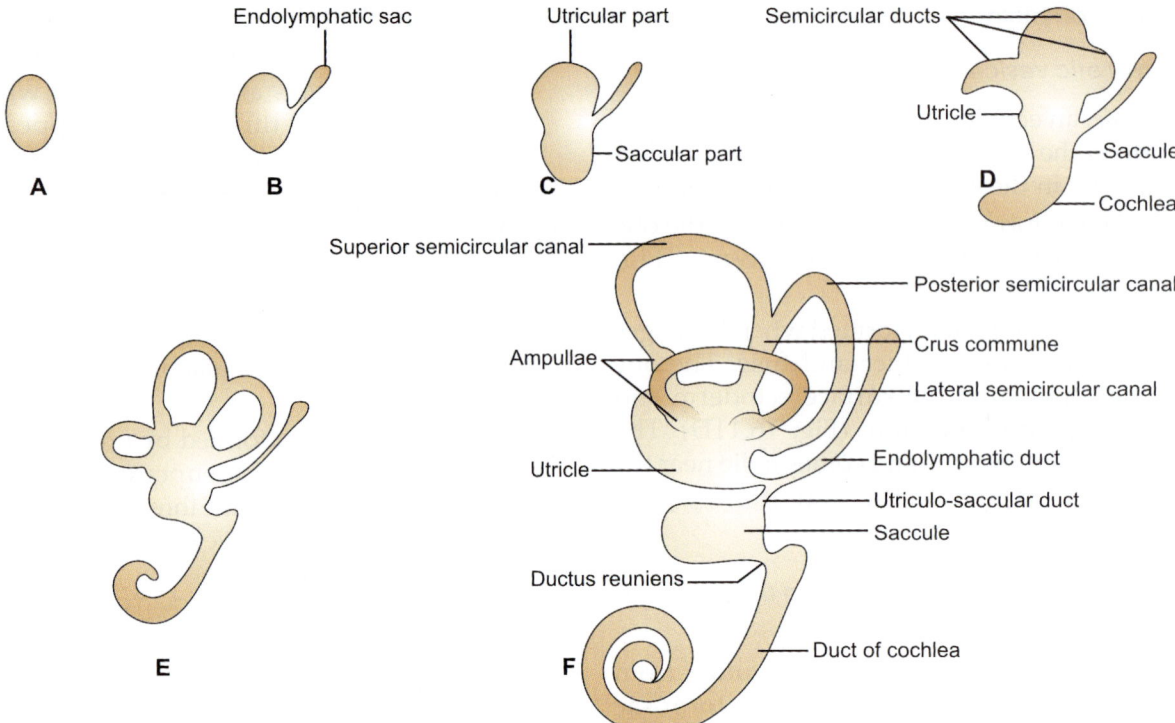

Fig. 16.12: Formation of membranous labyrinth: A, rounded otic vesicle; B, origin of endolymphatic duct and sac; C, division of otic vesicle into vestibular (utricular) part and cochlear (saccular) part; D, formation of three semicircular discs; E, formation of semicircular canals and cochlear duct; F, completion of membranous labyrinth.

- *Peripheral processes* of these bipolar neurons reach the wall of otocyst in the region of saccule, utricle and semicircular ducts, conveying sense of equilibrium.
- *Central processes* terminate in the vestibular nucleus as vestibular nerve.

Spiral ganglion (cochlear ganglion) is formed by the ganglion cells of VIII cranial nerve which migrate along the coils of the membranous cochlea (Fig. 16.13).

- *Peripheral processes* of bipolar cells forming spiral ganglion terminate in the hair cells of organ of corti and convey sense of hearing.
- *Central processes* form the cochlear nerve which terminates in the cochlear nucleus.

Note: The vestibular and cochlear nerve fibres run together as vestibulocochlear nerve.

Bony labyrinth

Mesenchymal cells surrounding the otic vesicle are induced by the otic vesicle to condense (Fig. 16.14A) and later differentiate into cartilaginous otic capsule (Fig. 16.14B).

Perilymphatic spaces filled with perilymph are formed between the membranous labyrinth and the cartilaginous otic capsule by de-differentiation of the adjoining cartilage cells (Fig. 16.14C). The perilymphatic spaces which communicate with each other at the apex of cochlea through an opening called helicotrema are:

- *Scala tympani* which is separated from the cochlear duct by basilar membrane, and
- *Scala vestibuli* which is separated from the cochlear duct by vestibular or Reissner's membrane.

Cartilaginous otic capsule then ossifies to form the bony labyrinth. The modiolus of the cochlea directly ossifies from the mesenchyme (Fig. 16.14D).

Bony labyrinth, so formed, consists of three parts:

- *Semicircular canals* enclose the semi circular ducts.
- *Vestibule* is the part of the bony labyrinth which lodge, utricle and saccule (which are collectively called *otolith organs*).
- *Cochlea* is that part of bony labyrinth which lodges duct of cochlea. The cochlea turns around a central bone called the *modiolus,* which, as mentioned above, is formed by direct ossification of the mesenchyme.

Thus, as described above, the bony cochlea is divided into three compartments (Fig. 16.14D):

- *Scala vestibuli* (filled with perilymph),
- *Scala media* (membranous cochlear duct filled with endolymph), and

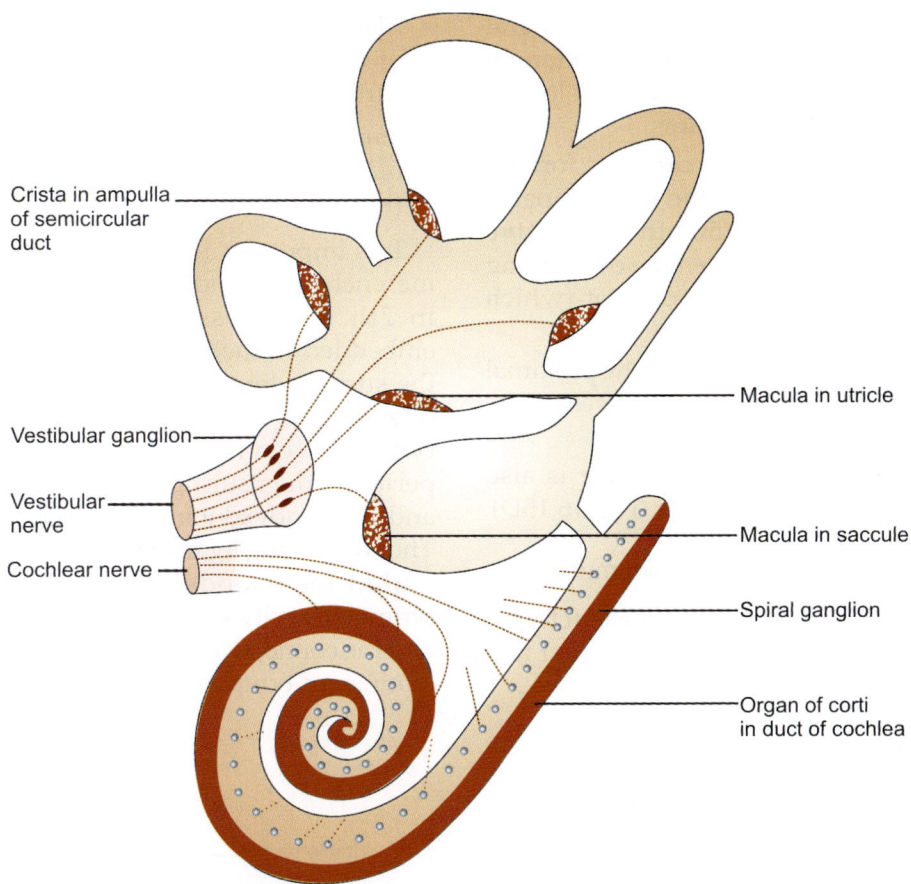

Fig. 16.13: The development of crista ampullaris, maculae in utricle and saccule, and organ of corti, and the innervation of the inner ear.

- *Scala tympani* (filled with perilymph and continuous with scala vestibuli through helicotrema).

DEVELOPMENT OF MIDDLE EAR

As mentioned earlier, the middle ear and associated structures include:
- Tympanic cavity,
- Auditory tube,
- Ear ossicles and associated muscles,
- Tympanic antrum, and
- Mastoid air cell.

Formation of tympanic cavity and auditory tube

Tympanic cavity and auditory tube develop from the endoderm of first pharyngeal pouch (Fig. 16.15A) as below:

Tubotympanic recess is first formed by elongation and expansion of the first pharyngeal pouch during

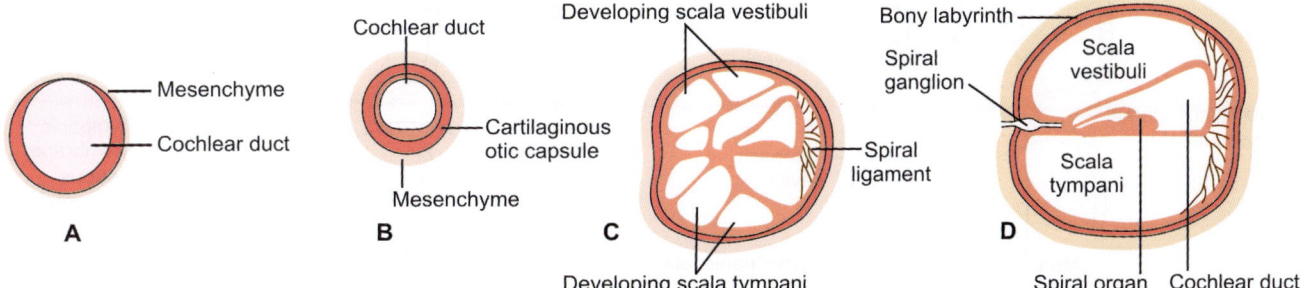

Fig. 16.14: Schematic transverse section of one coil of cochlear duct to depict formation of bony labyrinth and three compartments of bony cochlea: A, mesenchymal condensation around the cochlear duct; B, formation of cartilaginous otic capsule; C, formation of perilymphatic space by de-differentiation of some part of cartilagenous capsule, D, ossification of cartilagenous capsule, formation of modiolus, and three compartments of cochlea (scala vestibuli, scala media, and scala tympani).

5th week (Fig. 16.15B). The recess expands in lateral direction and comes in contact with the ectodermal floor of the first pharyngeal cleft which is developing into primary external auditory meatus.

Primitive tympanic or middle ear cavity is formed by the distal widened portion of the tubotympanic recess. As shown in Fig. 16.15C, the primitive tympanic cavity is placed in between the developing external auditory meatus and the otocyst (which forms internal ear).

Auditory (eustachian) tube is formed by the proximal narrow portion of the tubotympanic recess (Fig. 16.15D).

Endodermal lining of tympanic membrane is also derived from the tubotympanic recess (Fig. 16.15D).

Formation of ear ossicles and associated muscles

Ear ossicles are derived from the mesenchyme destined to form the skeletal derivatives of first and second pharyngeal arches (Fig. 16.15B):

- *Malleus and incus* are derived from the dorsal end of cartilage of first pharyngeal pouch (Meckle's cartilage), (Figs 16.15D and 16.16), and

- *Stapes* develops from the dorsal end of the cartilage of second pharyngeal arch (Reichert's cartilage) (Fig. 16.15D and 16.16).

It is important to note that the ossicles appear as mesenchymal condensations in 4th week, chondrify in 7th week, ossify in 4th month but remain embedded in the mesenchyme till 8th month, when the surrounding tissue dissolves. When the ossicles become free, the endodermal lining of the primitive tympanic cavity coats the ossicular chain like peritoneum ensuring a blood supply to the ossicles and the synovial joints between them (Fig. 16.15D). The supporting ligaments of the ossicles later develop within the endodermal lining. Expansion of the tympanic cavity sandwiches the handle of the malleus and the connective tissue between the inner and outer laminae of tympanic membrane.

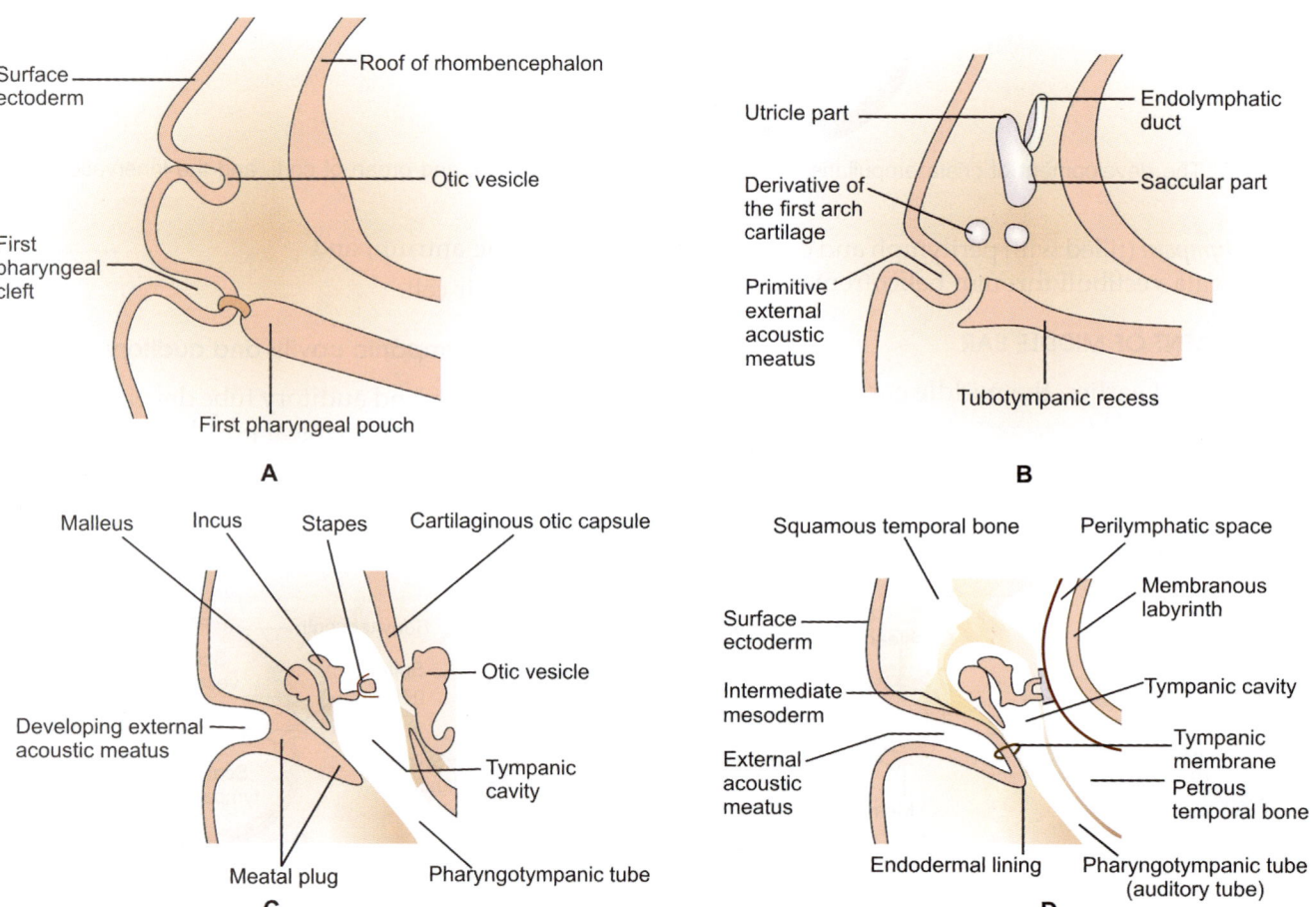

Fig. 16.15: Schematic drawing depicting formation of middle ear, tympanic membrane and external auditory meatus: A, note relation of otic vesicle with first pharyngeal arch, pouch and cleft; B, formation of tubotympanic recess and primitive external auditory meatus; C, formation of primitive tympanic cavity, auditory tube and meatal plug; D, formation of definitive tympanic cavity, auditory tube, tympanic membrane and external auditory meatus.

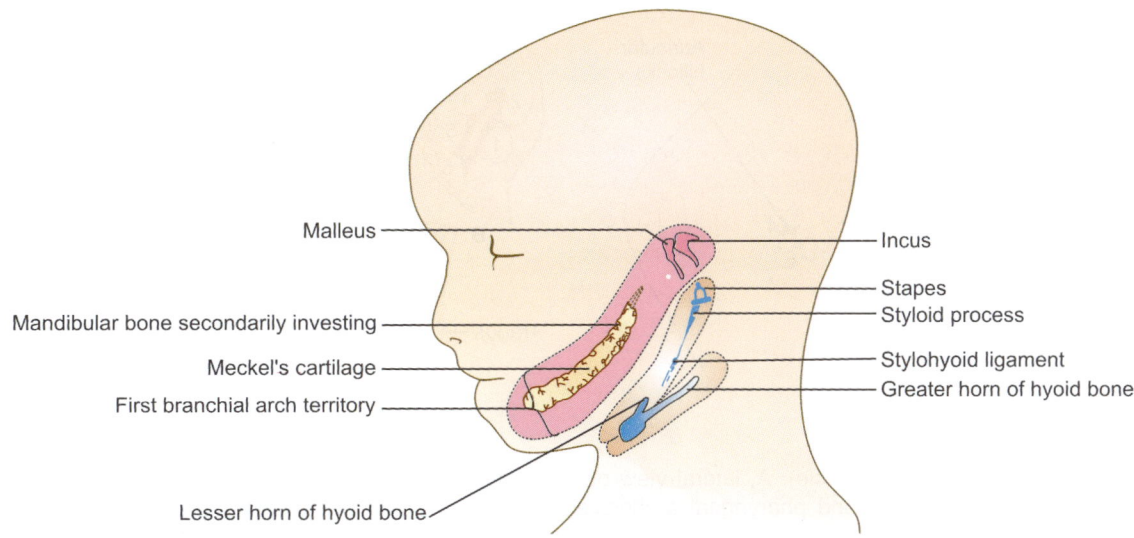

Fig. 16.16: Derivation of malleus and incus from dorsal end of Meckle's (first arch) cartilage and stapes from dorsal end of second arch cartilage.

Muscles associated with ear ossicles are developed from the mesenchyme as below:

- *Tensor tympani,* the muscle associated with malleus, is derived from the mesenchyme of first pharyngeal arch and is thus supplied by mandibular branch of trigeminal nerve.
- *Stapedius,* the muscle attached to stapes, is derived from the mesenchyme of 2nd pharyngeal arch and is supplied by the facial nerve.

Formation of tympanic (mastoid) antrum and mastoid air cells

Tympanic (mastoid) antrum, is formed during fetal life, when the tympanic cavity expands dorsally by vacuolization of the surrounding tissue.

Mastoid air cells are well developed after birth at about 2 year of age forming conical mastoid processes. Later, most of the mastoid air cells come in contact with antrum and tympanic cavity. It is important to note that because of this close proximity, the infections of middle ear cavity may involve the antrum and mastoid air cells.

DEVELOPMENT OF EXTERNAL EAR

The external ear consists of:
- External auditory meatus
- Tympanic membrane, and
- Pinna or auricle.

Formation of external auditory meatus

The external auditory (acuostic) meatus develops from the dorsal part of the Ist pharyngeal cleft (Fig. 16.15A) as below:

Primitive meatus is first formed by a funnel-shaped ectodermal invagination from the dorsal part of Ist pharyngeal cleft (Fig. 16.15B).

Meatal plug, a solid epithelial plate, is then formed by proliferation of the epithelial cells from the floor of primitive meatus at the beginning of third month (Fig. 16.15C).

Definitive (secondary) meatus is formed in the seventh month by dissolution of the epithelial meatal plug. The cells at the bottom of meatus participate in the formation of definitive tympanic membrane (Fig. 16.15D).

Formation of tympanic membrane (ear drum)

The definitive tympanic membrane consists of three layers which develop from three different sources (Fig. 16.15A to D):

Outer cuticular layer develops from the ectoderm of the first pharyngeal pouch. Epithelial cells left after dissolution of meatal plug proliferate to form this layer.

Inner mucous layer is derived from the endoderm of the tubotympanic recess, a derivative of the first pharyngeal pouch.

Intermediate fibrous layer develops from the adjoining mesoderm of first and second pharyngeal arches. The handle of the malleus and chorda tympani nerve extend into the tympanic membrane between the fibrous and mucous layers.

DEVELOPMENT OF PINNA (AURICLE)

Mesodermal auricular hillocks (six in number), which appear three each on the dorsal ends of the

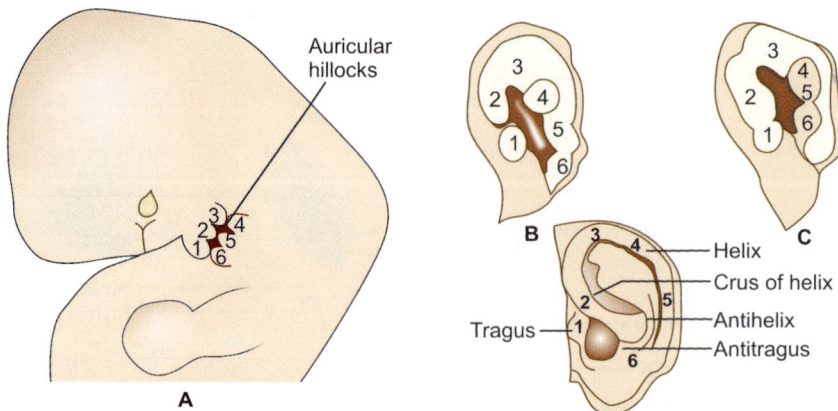

Fig. 16.17: Development of pinna (auricle): A, lateral view of the head of embryo showing six auricular hillocks (three each on the dorsal ends of first and second pharyngeal arches, surrounding the first pharyngeal cleft; B, C and D, fusion and progressive development of auricular hillocks into the adult pinna. Note, hillock 1 forms tragus, 2 crus of helix, 3 helix, 4 and 5 bifurcate anti-helix and 6 antitragus.

first and second pharyngeal arches surrounding the first pharyngeal cleft (which forms external auditory meatus from the primordia of the pinna (Fig. 16.17A). *Fusion of auricular hillocks,* which are numbered cyclically 1 to 6, leads to formation of the pinna (Figs 16.17B to D). The probable contribution of each hillock is a below (Fig. 16.17D):

- *Hillock 1 :* Tragus,
- *Hillock 2 :* Crus of helix.
- *Hillock 3 :* Helix
- *Hillock 4 and 5 :* The bifurcate antihelix, and
- *Hillock 6 :* Antitragus

Lobule of the ear develops late in fetal life.

Muscles of the pinna develop from the myoblasts of second pharyngeal arch and are supplied by the posterior auricular branch of the facial, the nerve of hyoid arch.

Location of the external ears, initially is in the lower neck region (Fig. 16.17A), but with development of the mandible, they ascend to the side of head at the level of eyes.

ANOMALIES OF THE EAR

Congenital deafness

Congenital deafness is usually associated with mutism. It may be:

1. *Congenital conductive deafness* occurs due to following anomalies which interfere with the conduction of sound from external ear to cochlea:
   - Failure of canalization of metal plate.
   - Congenital stenosis or atresia of the external auditory meatus.

- Congenital malformation of auditory ossicles and eardrum.
- Absence of external meatus and tympanic cavity (rare).

2. *Congenital sensorineural deafness* may occur due to:
   - Abnormal development of membranous labyrinth as a whole or cochlea only.
   - Failure of auditory nerve to make contact with developing otocyst.
   - Damage to hearing apparatus by prenatal and perinatal factors.

Anomalies of the auricle

Anomalies of auricle are not rare. These include:

1. *Absence of pinna.* Pinna (auricle) may be completely or partly absent.

2. *Preauricular appendages and pits* refers to skin tags and shallow depressions, respectively, anterior to the pinna. Preauricular appendages result from accessory hillocks, while pits occur due to abnormal development of hillocks. These may be associated with other malformation, e.g. in Goldenhar syndrome.

3. *Aural fistula* refers to a narrow tract seen between the tragus and crus of helix due to incomplete fusion of the tubercle.

4. *Otocephaly.* In this condition the two auricles fuse in the mid-ventral line of neck. It is associated with failure of mandible to grow as in mandibulofacial dysostosis.

Applied Embryology

Section 3

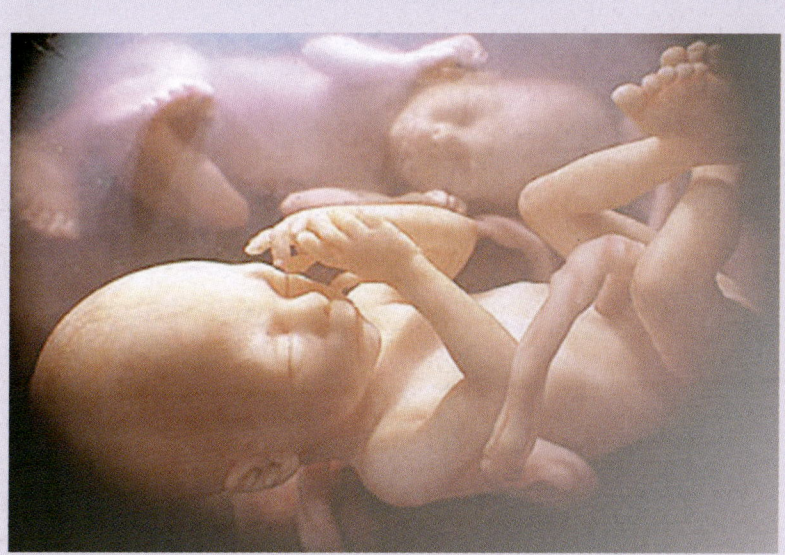

17

Teratology, Prenatal Diagnosis and Fetal Therapy

TERATOLOGY
General Considerations
- Teratology : Definition
- Factors responsible for teratogenesis
- Principles of teratogenesis

Congenital anomalies
- Terminologies used for congenital anomalies

- Incidence
- Common congenital anomalies produced by genetic and environmental factors

PRENATAL DIAGNOSIS AND FETAL THERAPY
- Indications of prenatal diagnosis
- Methods of prenatal diagnosis
- Fetal therapy

TERATOLOGY

GENERAL CONSIDERATIONS

Teratology: Definition

Teratology or dysmorphology refers to that branch of science which deals with the study of causes, mechanisms, and patterns of abnormal development leading to congenital anomalies.

Factor responsible for teratogenesis

Teratogenesis refers to abnormal embryonic and fetal development. Factors responsible for teratogenesis include:

1. *Genetic factors* such as:

Chromosomal abnormalities inherited through the genes in the ovum or sperm affecting:
- Autosomes, or
- Sex chromosomes

Mutation of genes, may lead to:
- Autosomal dominant traits,
- Autosomal recessive traits, or
- X-linked recessive traits.

Homeobox genes are groups of regulatory genes that control the expression of other genes involved in the normal development, growth and differentiation. Teratogens like retinoic acid can activate these genes to cause abnormal gene expression.

2. *Environmental factors* having teratogenic effect on the developing embryo and fetus are called *teratogens.* These can be grouped as below:
- *Physical factors* such as X-rays, radiations and hyperthermia.
- *Chemical factors* include the teratogenic drugs used by the pregnant mothers. Food and Drug Administration (FDA) authority in United States have grouped the drugs into A, B, C, D and X-categories depending upon the associated risk of teratogens (Table 17.1)

Table 17.1: Risk categories of drugs and medications for teratogenicity during pregnancy

Category	Definition
A	Controlled studies in humans have failed to demonstrate a fetal risk.
B	Animal studies indicate no fetal risk but controlled studies in human do not exist or adverse effects in animals have been demonstrated but not in well controlled human studies.
C	Animal studies have shown adverse effects but controlled studies in human do not exist or adequate studies in animals and human do not exist.
D	There is evidence of fetal risk but benefits are thought to outweigh the risks.
X	Proven fetal risks clearly outweigh any benefits. The drug should be considered contraindicated in woman who are or who may become pregnant. Drugs in the group are: Alcohol, ACE inhibitors, lithium, methotrexate, valproic acid, mifepristone, danazol, isotretinoin, radioactive iodine and others.

From: Food and Drug Administration (FDA), Drug Bulletin (1980).

- *Nutritional factors* such as maternal malnutrition, hyper-or hypovitaminosis, mineral excess or deficiency.
- *Hormonal factors:* Metabolic and endocrinal disorders such as maternal diabetes, use of synthetic progesterones, oestrogens, cortisone, etc.
- *Maternal infections* such as rubella, cytomegalo-virus, toxoplasmosis, HIV, syphlis, etc.
3. *Multifactorial:* Most of the malformations probably result from delicate and complex interactions between genetic predisposition and altered environmental factors, the nature of which remains obscure in majority of cases.

PRINCIPLES OF TERATOGENESIS

Factors influencing effects of teratogens

1. *Genetic factors*

Genotype of the conceptus affects the susceptibility to teratogens:
- An agent teratogenic for one species may not be so for another species.
- The manner in which genetic composition of the conceptus interacts with the environment is an essential factor.
- Teratogenic substances may exaggerate the frequency of the incidence when an abnormal hereditary trait appear sporadically.

Maternal genome is also important with respect to drug metabolism, resistance to infection and other biochemical and molecular processes that affect the conceptus.

2. *Developmental stage at the time of exposure to teratogen: Periods of susceptibility*

Period of vulnerability to teratogens vis-a-vis stage of development is as follows (Fig. 17.1):
- *First two weeks of development,* i.e. fertilization to formation of bilaminar disc is usually not sensitive period for teratogens. In fact, during this period the teratogens have all-or-none effect, i.e. the conceptus either does not survive or survives without anomalies. Thus, during this phase lethality rate may be high.

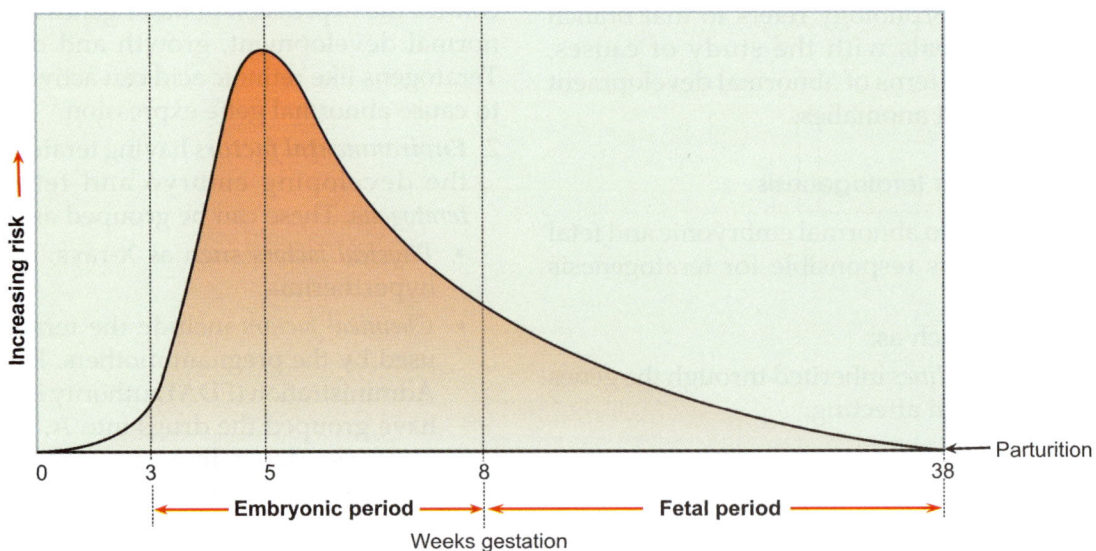

Fig. 17.1: Relationship of risk of developing congenital anomalies with stage of development at the time of exposure to teratogens.

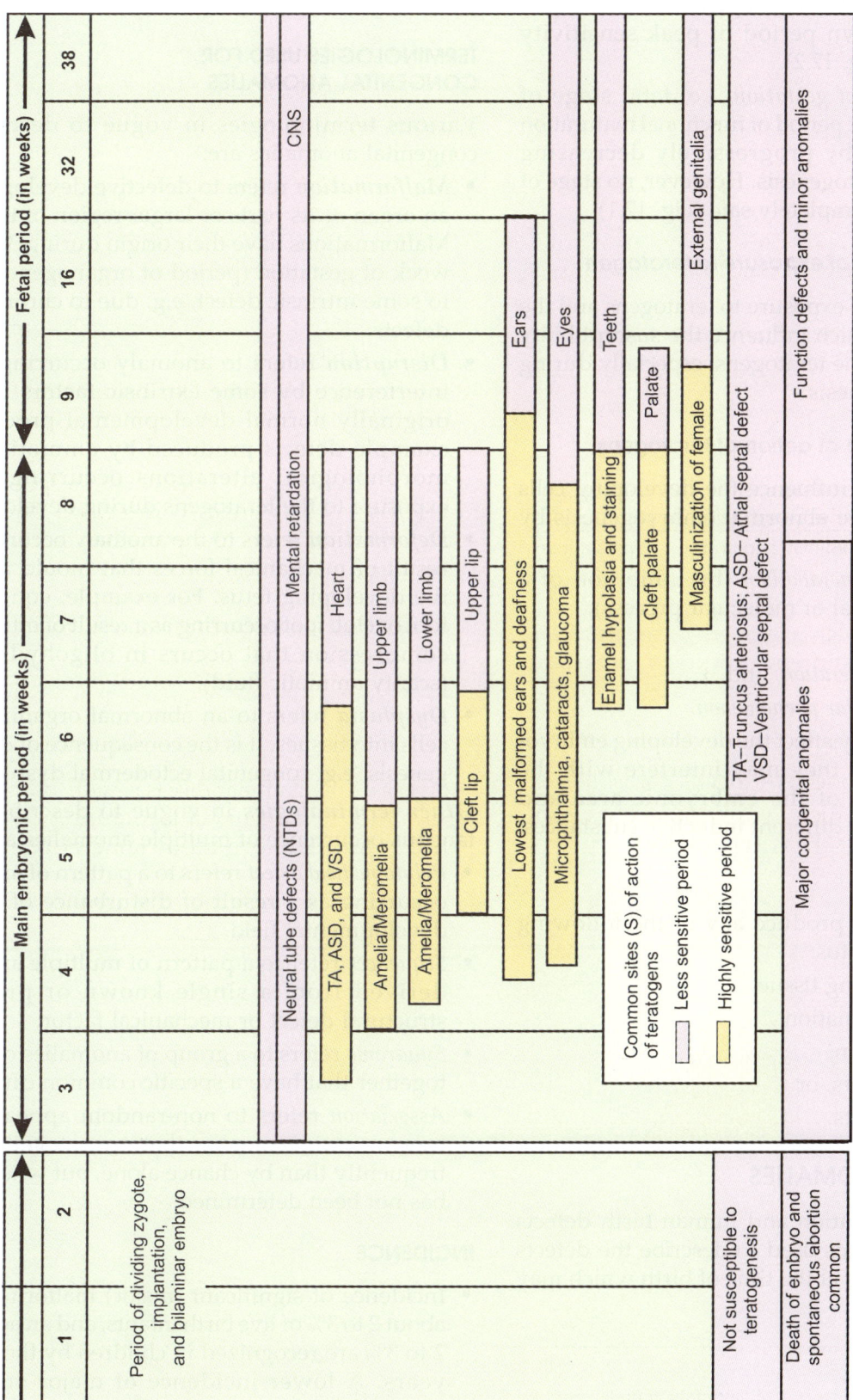

Fig. 17.2: Critical periods in human prenatal development.

- *3rd to 8th week of development,* i.e. period of embryogenesis (organogenesis) is the period of *greatest sensitivity* for teratogenesis. Each organ system has its own period of peak sensitivity (*critical period*) (Fig. 17.2).

- *9th to 38th week of gestation,* i.e. fetal stage of development or the period of functional maturation is characterised by progressively decreasing sensitivity for teratogenesis. However, no stage of development is completely safe (Fig. 17.1).

3. *Dose and duration of exposure to teratogen*

Dose and duration of exposure to teratogens and the important factors which influence the susceptibility of the conceptus to the teratogens, especially during period of embryogenesis.

Modes (mechanisms) of action of teratogens

The teratogens may influence the developing cells and tissues to initiate abnormal embryogenesis by following mechanisms:

- *Altering cellular metabolism* (by inhibition of a specific biochemical or molecular process),
- *Cell death,*
- *Decreased cell proliferation,* and
- *Altering other cellular phenomenon.*

The teratogens may affect the developing embryonic area directly or they may interfere with the organising centres of the embryonic area and elaborate all together different inductive substances.

Effects of teratogens

The teratogens may produce any of the following effects on the conceptus:
- Death of developing tissue,
- Structural malformation,
- Growth retardation,
- Metabolic disorders, or
- Behavioural defects.

CONGENITAL ANOMALIES

Congenital malformation and human birth defects are synonymous terms used to describe the defects present in a newborn at the time of birth which may be:
- Structural defects,
- Functional defects,
- Metabolic disorders, or
- Behavioral defects.

Developmental defects—This term, in addition to the defects present at birth, also includes those defects which express later in life.

TERMINOLOGIES USED FOR CONGENITAL ANOMALIES

Various terminologies in vogue to describe the congenital anomalies are:

- *Malformation* refers to defective development of an organ or its parts or larger region of the body. Malformations have their origin during 3rd to 8th week of gestation (period of organogenesis), due to some intrinsic defect, e.g. due to chromosomal defects.

- *Disruption* refers to anomaly occurring due to interference by some extrinsic factors with the originally normal developmental process. For example defects produced by amniotic bands, morphological alterations occurring due to exposure to the teratogens during development.

- *Deformation* refers to the anomaly occurring as a result of mechanical forces that mould a part of the developing fetus. For example, equinovarus foot or club foot occurring as a result of intrauterine compression that occurs in oligohydramnios (scanty amniotic fluid).

- *Dysplasia* refers to an abnormal organization of cells into tissues. It is the consequence of dyshistogenesis, e.g. congenital ectodermal dysplasia.

Other terminologies in vogue to describe simultaneous occurrence of multiple anomalies are:

- *Polytopic field defect* refers to a pattern of anomalies occurring as a result of disturbance of a single developmental field.

- *Sequences* refer to a pattern of multiple anomalies derived from a single known or presumed structural defect or mechanical factor.

- *Syndrome* refers to a group of anomalies occurring together that have a specific common cause.

- *Association* refers to non-random appearance of two or more anomalies that occur together more frequently than by chance alone, but where cause has not been determined.

INCIDENCE

- Incidence of significant (major) malformations is about 2 to 3% of live birth infants, and an additional 2 to 3% are recognized in children by the age of 5 years. A lower incidence of major structural anomalies (1 in 500 live births) is, however, reported from the hospital statistics of India.

- Minor anomalies occur in about 15% of newborns. Infants with one minor anomaly have 3% chance of having associated major malformation, those with two minor anomalies have a 10% chance and those with three or more minor anomalies have a 20% chance.
- In Western countries, major fetal anomalies account for about 20% of prenatal deaths and many survivors are physically and or mentally handicapped.
- About 50% cases of malformations involve central nervous system.

Etiological incidence of congenital anomalies is as below (Fig. 17.3):

- Idiopathic, i.e. unknown cause: 40 to 60%
- Genetic factors: 15%
- Environmental factors: 10%
- Multifactorial inheritance: 20 to 25%
- Twinning: 0.5 to 1%.

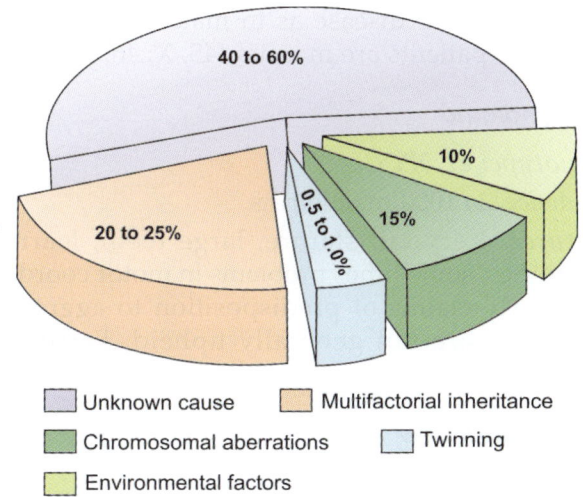

Fig.17.3: Graphical representation of the causes of human birth defects.

COMMON CONGENITAL ANOMALIES

Common congenital anomalies produced by genetic and environmental factors are described briefly.

ANOMALIES CAUSED BY GENETIC FACTORS

These include:

- Anomalies caused by chromosomal abnormalities, and
- Anomalies caused by mutant genes.

ANOMALIES CAUSED BY CHROMOSOMAL ABNORMALITIES

Chromosomal abnormalities include:

- Abnormal number of chromosomes, and
- Structural abnormalities of chromosomes.

Abnormal number of chromosomes

Euploidy means that the chromosome number per body cell is an integral multiple of the haploid number, N = 23.

Aneuploidy means that it is other than an integral multiple. Aneuploidy is usually ascribed to *failure of conjugation* of chromosomes in meiosis I: or *non-disjunction, premature disjunction* or *anaphase lag* (delayed separation) in meiosis II. The frequency of chromosomal errors in oocytes increases dramatically with *maternal* age.

Diploidy describes the normal situation, a typical body cell in humans having 2N = 46 chromosomes. Women have 23 similar pairs, including a pair of X chromosomes, their *karyotype* formula being **46, XX**. In normal men there is a X and a Y-chromosome, their karyotype being **46,XY**.

Polyploidy refers to multiples of the haploid number (e.g. *triploidy* 3N = 69).

- *Trisomy* (2N+1) refers to the presence of three copies of one chromosome. Possession of only a single copy of an autosome (2N–1) is called monosomy.
- *Mosaic* individuals contain two different cell lines derived from one zygote. A chimaera also contains two different cell lines, but is derived by fusion of two zygotes (e.g. a 46, XX/46, XY hermaphrodite). Mosaics can be caused by chromosomal non-disjunction during *mitosis*.

Possibly as many as 25% of conceptions involve a chromosomal disorder, but this is reduced to 0.6% at birth by natural loss, mainly during the first trimester.

The non-sex chromosomes are called autosomes. Trisomies 21, 18 and 13 are the only autosomal trisomies compatible with survival to birth and only Trisomy 21 with life beyond infancy.

Down syndrome, Trisomy 21

Karyotype. Trisomy 21 (**47, XX, +21** or **47, XY, +21)** accounts for about 96% of cases of Down syndrome. The remaining 4% have translocations between 21 and another chromosome. Some patients are mosaics.

Incidence. About 1/700 live births.

Features. Typically there are *epicanthal folds* and a flat, broad face. Other features include a large gap between first and second toes, webbing of toes 2 and 3, general *hypotonia* (poor muscle tone), flat *occiput* (back of skull), short stature, *Brushfield spots* in irides, *single transverse crease* in the palm, single fold on and *clinodactyly* of fifth digit, open mouth with protruding tongue that lacks a central fissure, hearing deficit (60–80%), increased risk of infection, *leukaemia* (80%), congenital heart defects (40–50%), and *epilepsy* (5–10%). IQ is 25–75, with typically a happy temperament, but Alzheimer-like dementia may occur in upto 50% in mid-life and there is often early-onset *atheromatous* (i.e. with fatty deposits) degenera-tion of the cardiovascular system, Hirschprung disease and hypothyroidism (15–20%).

Life expectancy. Due to heart defects, for some it is less than 50 years.

Edward syndrome, Trisomy 18

Karyotype. 47, XX, +18 or 47, XY, + 18.

Incidence. About 1/3000 live births.

Features. Clenched fists with index and fifth fingers overlapping the rest; 'rocker bottom' feet with prominent heels; low-set, malformed ears; micro-gnathia (small lower jaw); single palmar crease; growth deficiency; cardiac and renal abnormalities; prominent occiput and general hypotonia.

Mean survival time. About 2 months; 30% die within a month; only 10% survive beyond a year.

Patau syndrome, Trisomy 13

Karyotype. 47,XX,+13 or 47,XY,+13.

Incidence. About 1/5000 live births.

Features. Microcephaly (small head) with sloping forehead; holo-prosencephaly (failure of formation of paired cerebral hemispheres); 'rocker-bottom' feet, microphthalmia, anophthalmia, cyclopia or hypo-telorism (i.e. small or absent eyes, a single central eye or closely spaced eyes); cryptorchidism (undescended testicles); simian crease; heart defects' cleft lip and palate; micrognathia and postaxial polydactyly (sixth finger present).

Survival rate. Similar to Edward syndrome, with rather more (50%) dying within the first month.

Klinefelter syndrome

Karyotype. **47,XXY** (or **48, XXXY: 49, XXXXY,** etc).

Incidence. About 1/500 male births.

Features. Phenotype is basically male, but with gynaecomastia (breasts) and feminine body hair distribution (but masculine facial hair); small genitalia and infertility. They are tall, with elongated lower legs and forearms. There may be learning difficulties, scoliosis (spinal curvature), emphysema (gaseous distension of lung tissues), osteoporosis (skeletal breakdown) and varicose veins; 8% have diabetes mellitus.

Turner syndrome

Karyotype. 45, X

Incidence. 1/5000 female births. (The fetus aborts in over 95% of cases).

Features. Phenotype is basically female, but patients fail to mature sexually. There is often also *lympho-edema* (excess fluid) in the hands and feet of newborns; excess skin forming a web between neck and shoulders and low posterior hairline; heart-shaped face with micrognathia, epicanthal folds and *strabismus* (squint); short stature; short fourth metacarpals; many *naevi* (moles), shield-shaped chest with widely spaced nipples; increased 'carrying angle' at elbow (*cubitus valgus).* Intelligence is normal. There is congenital heart disease in 20%, unexplained *hypertension* (high blood pressure) in 30%, kidney malformations and *thyroiditis.* They may develop X-linked recessive disease as in males. Some Turner syndrome patients are mosaics (45, X; 46,XY).

XYY syndrome

Karyotype: **47, XYY.**

Incidence. 1/1000 male births.

Features. Very tall stature, large teeth, learning disabilities, some times problems in motor coordination. Early claims of predisposition to aggressive behaviour are not generally upheld. Fertility is normal.

Triple X syndrome

Karyotype: **47, XXX.**

Incidence. 1/1000 female births.

Features. Generally tall with some learning problems and difficulty in interpersonal relationships. Claims of reduced fertility are now sometimes ascribed to 45, X oocytes in 45. X/47, XXX mosaics.

Structural abnormalities of chromosomes

Structural aberrations include *translocations, deletions, ring chromosomes, duplications, inversions, isochromo-somes* and *centric fragments.* Most of these result from unequal exchange between homologous repeated sequences on the same or different chromosomes, or when two chromosome breaks occur close together and enzymic repair mechanisms link the wrong ends.

Translocations

A translocation involves exchange of chromosomal material between chromosomes. Three types are recognized : *centric fusion* or *'Robertsonian'*, *reciprocal* and *insertional*.

Centric fusion or 'Robertsonian' translocations

Centric fusion arises from breaks at or near the centromeres of two chromosomes, followed by their fusion. The long arms of chromosomes 13, 14, 15, 21 and 22 are most commonly involved, especially 13 with 14 and 14 with 21. These are all *acrocentric* chromosomes with very small short arms the latter carrying multiple copies of the ribosomal RNA genes.

Although centric fusion involves loss of rRNA genes, sufficient intact copies remain for no serious consequence to result. The carrier of a pair of centrically fused chromosomes may therefore have only 45 chromosomes, but be quite healthy as the overall loss is insignificant. This is a *balanced translocation*.

When centrically fused chromosomes pair during meiosis a *trivalent* structure is formed allowing contact between homologous chromosome segments. At anaphase six possible gametic combinations can then be formed : one normal, one abnormal but balanced and four unbalanced. However, selection of gametes and pregnancy loss result in a lower than expected frequency of unbalanced offspring.

Down syndrome: About 4% of cases of Down syndrome are due to Robertsonian translocation between the long arms of chromosome 21 and any other acrocentric, usually 14. In some cases one parent has a balanced version of the same translocation.

Reciprocal Translocations

Reciprocal translocation involves interchromosomal exchange. Either arm of any chromosome can be involved and the carriers are usually healthy. The medical significance is therefore usually for *future* generations, as carriers can produce chromosomally unbalanced fetuses.

Insertional Translocations

Insertional translocation involves insertion of a deleted segment interstitially at another location. It is extremely rare and balanced carriers are usually healthy, but may produce chromosomally unbalanced off-spring with either a duplication or a deletion.

Deletions

Deletion of part of a chromosome can be *interstitial or terminal*. Deletions can arise from two breaks, followed by faulty repair, from unequal crossing over in a previous meiosis, or as a consequence of a translocation in a parent.

The smallest deletions detectable by *high-resolution banding* are of about 3000 Kb (i.e. 3 million base pairs) and are generally characterized by mental handicap and multiple congenital malformations.

Several syndromes are ascribed to microscopically invisible *microdeletions*. When several genes are deleted together the term *contiguous gene syndrome* is applied.

Examples of Deletions

Prader-Willi and Angelman syndromes. The combined incidence of *Prader-Willi and Angelman syndromes* is 1/25000 live births. Around 70% of patients have a deletion in the long arm of chromosome 15: in Prader-Willi this is the paternal copy, in Angelman the maternal.

Cri-du-chat syndrome is so called because the malformed larynxes of these babies cause them to cry with a sound like a cat. They have profound learning disability, *hypertelorism* (widely spaced eyes), epicanthal folds, *strabismus*, low-set ears, low birth weight and failure to thrive. The cause is terminal deletion of the short arm of chromosome 5 and it occurs in about 1/50000 births.

Wolf-Hirschhorn syndrome also occurs in about 1/50000 births, also with profound cognitive impairment, hypertelorism, epicanthal folds and low-set ears. Patients typically have a broad and prominent nose, cleft lip and palate, microcephaly, heart defects, convulsions and *hypospadias* (non-closure of the penile urethra). It is caused by terminal deletion of the short arm of chromosome 4.

Ring chromosomes

If two breaks occur in the same chromosome the broken ends can fuse as a ring. Acentric rings are lost, but if the ring contains a centromere it can survive subsequent cell division. Clinically a ring represents two deletions. They can double by sister chromatid exchange, leading to effective trisomy, or be lost, resulting in monosomy.

Duplications

Duplication is the presence of two adjacent copies of a chromosomal segment and can be either *direct* or *inverted*. Duplications may originate by unequal crossing-over in a previous meiosis, or as a consequence of translocation, inversion or presence of an iso-chromosome in a parent. Duplications are more common, but generally less harmful than deletions.

Inversions

Inversions arise from two chromosomal breaks with end-to-end switching of the intervening segment. If this includes the centromere it is *pericentric;* if not, the inversion is *paracentric.* The medical significance of inversions lies in their capacity to lead to chromosomally unbalanced gametes following crossing-over.

Isochromosomes

An isochromosome has a deletion of one chromosome arm, with duplication of the other. In live births the commonest involves the long arm of the X, resulting in Turner syndrome due to short arm monosomy (despite long arm trisomy). Most isochromosomes cause spontaneous abortion.

ANOMALIES CAUSED BY MUTANT GENES

Anomalies caused by mutation of genes can be divided into three groups:
- Autosomal dominant trait anomalies.
- Autosomal recessive trait anomalies, and
- X-linked recessive trait anomalies.

Autosomal dominant trait anomalies

Characteristics of autosomal dominant inheritance
- *Both males and females* express the allele and can transmit it equally to sons and daughters.
- *Vertical transmission,* i.e. trait is transmitted from one generation to other. In other words every affected person has an affected parent.
- *Risk of transmission* is 50% when one of the parent is affected.
- *Unaffected members* do not transmit the trait further.
- *Degree of expression* of abnormal trait may vary in different family members.
- *Mode of expression* is alteration of structural proteins.
- When both parents are not affected, all the children are unaffected.

Pedigree chart. Symbols used in a pedigree chart are shown in Fig. 17.4 and the pedigree chart of autosomal dominant trait is shown in Fig. 17.5.

Examples of autosomal dominant traits include:
- Achondroplasia
- Angioneurotic oedema
- Acute intermittent porphyria
- Brachydactyly

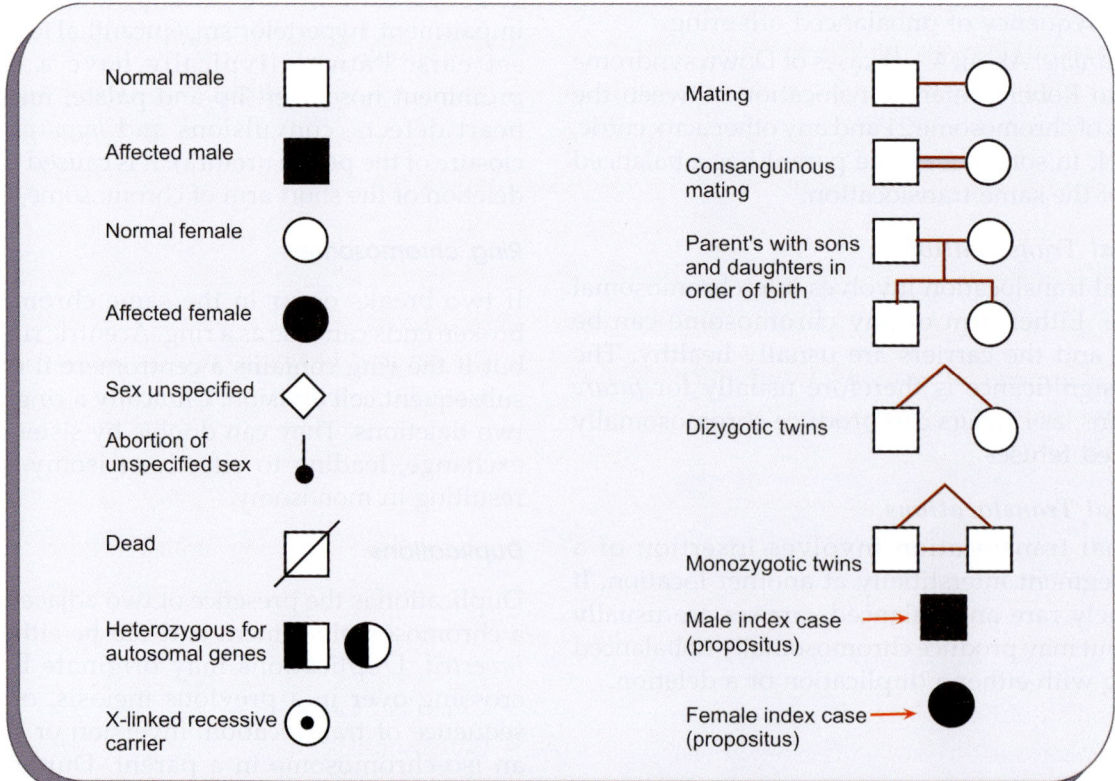

Fig.17.4: Symbols used in pedigree chart.

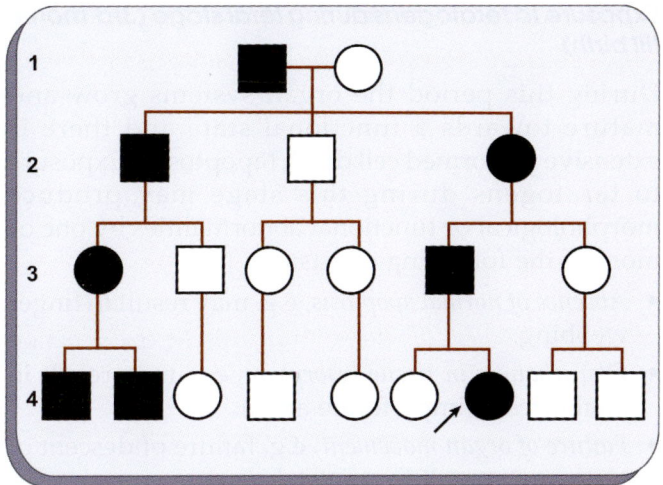

Fig. 17.5: Pedigree chart of autosomal dominant trait.

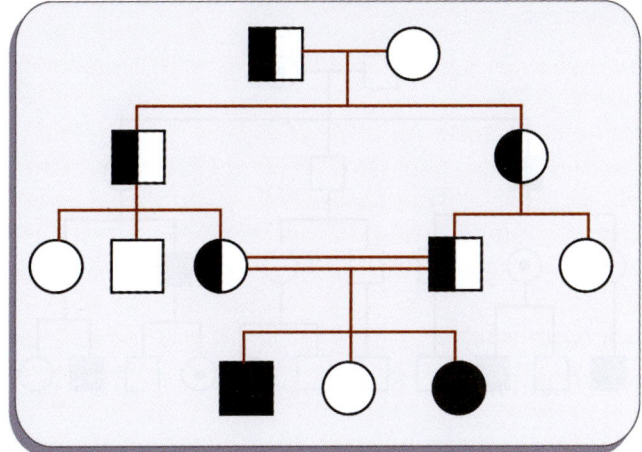

Fig. 17.6: Pedigree chart of autosomal recessive trait.

- Huntington's chorea
- Marfan's syndrome
- Multiple neurofibromatosis
- Osteogenesis imperfecta.

Autosomal recessive trait anomalies

Characteristics of Autosomal Recessive Inheritance

- *Both sexes* (males and females) are equally affected.
- *Transmitted* by a couple, of whom one is carrier of one abnormal gene, but are themselves healthy, because the other allele is normal.
- *Pattern of expression* is horizontal, i.e. siblings are affected while the parents are normal.
- *Risk of having affected child* by a carrier couple is 25%.
- *When both parents are affected,* all the children are affected.
- *Affected individual with normal partner,* will have all the children normal.

Pedigree chart of autosomal recessive inheritance is shown in Fig. 17.6

Example of autosomal recessive inheritance include:

i. *Inborn errors of metabolism*
   - Albinism
   - Alkaptonuria,
   - Galactosaemia,
   - Phenylketonuria
   - Tay-Sachs disease.
ii. *Haemoglobinopathies*
   - Sickle cell anaemia
   - Thalassemia major in homozygotes
   - Thalassemia minor in hetrozygotes.
iii. *Other examples*
   - Cystic fibrosis

- Spinal muscular atrophy
- Congenital deafness.

X-linked recessive trait anomalies

Characteristics of X-linked recessive traits are:

- Females are carriers and males are sufferers. Therefore, incidence of disease is very much higher in males than females.
- Mutant allele is passed from an affected man to all of his daughters, but they do not express it.
- Heterozygous carrier women passes the allele to half her sons, who express it and half of her daughter's who do not.
- The mutant allele is never passed from father to son.

Pedigree chart of X-linked recessive inheritance is shown in Fig. 17.7.

Examples of X-linked recessive inheritance are :

- Haemophilia
- Red-Green blindness
- Becker and Duchencen muscular dystrophies
- G-6-PD deficiency.

ANOMALIES CAUSED BY ENVIRONMENTAL FACTORS

Specific effects of common teratogens

The environmental factors acting as teratogens can be grouped as below:

- Physical factors,
- Chemical factor,
- Nutritional factors,
- Hormonal factors, and
- Maternal infections.

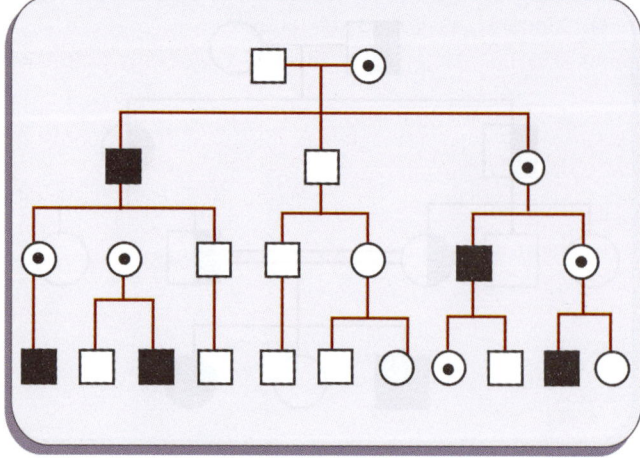

Fig. 17.7: Pedigree chart of X-linked recessive trait, when affected mother reproduce.

Specific effects of common teratogens are summarised in Table 17.2.

Teratogenic effects depending upon the stage of development

Exposure to teratogens during pre-embryo stage of development (First 2 weeks)

During this period teratogens have all-or-none effect, i.e. the conceptus either dies resulting in *spontaneous abortion* or survives without anomalies. The exceptional teratogenic effects produced at his stage are:

- Monozygotic twinning, and
- Germ layer defects, e.g. ectodermal dysplasias affecting skin, nails, hair, teeth and stature.

Exposure to teratogens during embryo stage of development (3rd to 8th week)

This is the most *critical period,* for teratogenic effects (Fig. 17.2). Exposure to teratogens during this period may produce major congenital anomalies by one or more of the following effects:

- *Failure of cell migration,* e.g. of neural crest cells resulting Waarden Burg syndrome.
- *Failure of embryonic induction,* e.g. anophthalmia (absence of eyes)
- *Failure of tube closure,* e.g. failure of neural tube closure in anterior part may result is anencephaly and in lumbar region may result in spina bifida.
- *Developmental arrests,* e.g. cleft palate
- *Failure of tissue fusion,* e.g. occurrence of cleft palate.
- *Defective morphogenetic fields,* e.g. sirenomelia (mermaid life fusion of legs).

Exposure to teratogens during fetal stage (3rd month till birth)

During this period the organ systems grow and mature towards a functional state and there is extensive preformed cell death (apoptosis). Exposure to teratogens during this stage may produce morphological or functional abnormalities by one or more of the following effects:

- *Absence of normal apoptosis,* e.g. may result in finger webbing.
- *Disturbances in tissue resorption,* e.g. may result in anal atresia (imperforate anus).
- *Failure of organ movement,* e.g. failure of descent of testis may result in *cryptorchidism.*
- *Destruction of formed structures,* e.g. due to interference in blood supply of limb buds may result in *phocomelia* (seal-like arms).
- *Hypoplasia* may occur due to reduced proliferation of cells, e.g. *achondroplasia.*
- *Hyperplasia* may occur due to enhanced proliferation, e.g. *macrosomia* (large body size) due to maternal diabetes.
- *Constriction by amniotic bands,* e.g. may result in limb amputation.
- *Restriction of movement,* e.g. talipes (club foot).
- *Disturbance of ossification centres* may result in skeletal anomalies.
- *Abnormalities in the ordering of neural connection* due to exposure to high level of radiations and infectious agents may cause *mental retardation.*

PRENATAL DIAGNOSIS AND FETAL THERAPY

INDICATIONS OF PRENATAL DIAGNOSIS

In addition to routine assessment of normal growth of conceptus and to screen for the various congenital malformations, prenatal diagnosis with special tests is indicated in *high risk pregnancies* which include:

Maternal risk factors

- Advanced maternal age (>35 years)
- Family history or previous child with neural tube defects.
- Previous gestation with chromosomal abnormalities.
- One or both parents carrier of X-linked or autosomal traits.
- A child born with an unbalanced translocation.
- History of recurrent miscarriages.

Table 17.2: Congenital anomalies produced by teratogens (environmental factors)

Teratogenic factors	Common congenital anomaly produced
1. *Physical agents*	
• Radiations from X-rays	Microcephaly, anencephaly, mental retardation, cleft palate, skeletal anomalies, growth retardation, cataracts and limb defects.
• Hyperthermia	Anencephaly, microcephaly, mental retardation, spina bifida, limb defects, facial defects, cardial abnormalities.
2. *Drugs*	
• *Abortifacients,* e.g. Aminopterin (folic acid antagonist)	IUGR, skeletal defects, CNS malformations, especially meroanencephaly.
• *Antiabortifaciens,* e.g. diethylstilbestrol	Malformations of reproductive organs, e.g. of the uterus, vagina, cervical erosions.
• *Anticonvulsants* Diphenyl-hydantoin, Phenytoin	Fetal hydantoin syndrome (FHS), microcephaly, IUGR, Mental retardation.
• *Sedatives and tranquilizers*	Facial defects
- Thalidomide	Limb defects (meromelia, i.e. partial absence or amelia, i.e. complete absence). Heart malformation.
- Lithium	Cardiovascular malformations.
• *Anticancer drugs,* e.g.	
- Methotrexate	IUGR, skeletal defects.
- Aminopterin	CNS malformation.
• *Antibiotics,* e.g.	
- Streptomycin	Inner ear deafness.
- Tetracyclins	Inhibit skeletal calcification stained teeth, hypoplasia of enamel.
• *Anticoagulants,* e.g.	
- Warfarin	Nasal hypoplasia, hypoplastic phalanges, mental retardation, ocular anomalies chondrodysplasia, microcephaly.
• *Antihypertensive agents,* e.g. ACE inhibitors	Growth retardation, fetal death.
• *Antithyroid drugs*	Congenital goiter.
• *Vitamin A analogues,* e.g.	
- Retinoids	Craniofacial dysmorphism, cleft palate, cardiovascular anomalies and neural tube defects
• *Alcohol*	Fetal alcohol syndrome, mental retardation, heart defects. IUGR, short palpebral, fissures, ocular anomalies, joint anomalies.
• *Cocaine*	IUGR, prematurity, microcephaly, behavioral abnormalities
• *Valproic acid*	Craniofacial anomalies, neural tube defects, heart anomalies, limb anomalies.
3. *Chemicals*	
• Organic mercury	Cerebral atrophy, seizures, mental retardation.
• Lead	IUGR, neurological disorders.
• Industrial solvents	Low birth weight, craniofacial and neural tube defects.
4. *Hormones*	
• Androgens	Masculanization of female genitalia, fused labia, clitoral hypertrophy.
• Diethylstilbestrol (DES)	Malformation of reproductive organs.
• Maternal diabetes	Heart and neural tube defects.
• Maternal obesity	Heart defects, omphalocele.
5. *Infectious agents*	
Viral infections	
• Rubella virus	IUGR, cardiovascular defects, deafness, cataract, glaucoma.
• Cytomegalo virus (CMV)	Microcephaly, mental retardation, blindness, chorioretinitis.
• Herpes simplex virus	Microphthalmia, microcephaly, retinal dysplasia.
• HIV	IUGR, microcephaly, facial anomalies.
• Varicella virus	Mental retardation, muscle atrophy, limb hypoplasia.
Protozoal infections	
• Toxoplasmosis	Hydrocephalus, cerebral calcification, microphthalmia, mental retardation, hearing loss.
Bacterial infections	
• Syphilis	Hydrocephalus, congenital deafness, mental retardation, anomalies of teeth and bone.

Prenatal risk factors

- Oligohydramnios,
- Polyhydramnios,
- Decreased fetal activity,
- Severe intrauterine growth retardation,
- Presence of soft tissue markers of chromosomal anomaly on routine ultrasonography.

METHODS OF DIAGNOSIS

I. Pre-implantation genetic diagnosis (PGD)

Following techniques are used whenever indicated:

- Polar body biopsy,
- Blastomere biopsy (from 6 to 8 cell stage) and
- Trophectoderm biopsy.

II. Prenatal diagnostic techniques

1. ***Ultrasonography:*** It is a non-invasive technique used for routine antenatal check up to assess fetal growth as well as to detect structural abnormalities whenever indicated.

   Assessment of fetal growth is done by serial ultrasonography for following parameters:

   - Fetal age and growth is assessed by crown rump length (CRL) during 5th to 10th week of gestation.
   - Other parameters which help in assessment of fetal growth are biparietal diameter (BPD) of the skull, femur length and abdominal circumference.

   Congenital malformations that can be determined by ultrasonography include the:

   - Neural tube defects (anencephaly and spina bifida)
   - Abdominal wall defects such as omphalocele and gastroschisis.
   - Heart defects, and
   - Facial defects including cleft lip and cleft palate.

   Soft tissue markers for chromosomal anomalies: When observed on ultrasonography, fetal Karyotyping is indicated for confirmation.

Blood flow velocity

Blood flow velocity is measured in the Doppler ultrasonography to detect the vascular resistance secondary to fetal hypoplasia and IUGR.

2. ***Maternal serum screening tests*** recommended to search for *biochemical markers* of fetal status are:

   i. *Serum α-fetoprotein levels*
      - *Elevated* in twinning, neural tube defects, intestinal atresia, and fetal demise.
      - *Lowered* in trisomies and aneuploidy
   ii. *Human chorionic gonadotropins (HCG)* levels are also lowered in trisomies and aneuploidy.
   iii. *Circulating fetal cells in maternal blood* for molecular DNA genetic analysis.

3. ***Amniocentesis.*** In this technique about 20–30 ml of amniotic fluid is withdrawn with the help of a needle inserted into the amniotic cavity transabdominally under ultrasound guidance. It is indicated to perform following tests:

   - *Biochemical analysis* for α-fetoprotein and acetyl choline esterase.
   - *Karyotyping* (cytogenetics) from the fetal cells present in the fluid.
   - *Molecular genetic* DNA diagnosis genome detection etc by using various tests including polymerase chain reaction (PCR).
   - *Fetal maturity assessment* from the levels of creatinine and lecithin.

4. ***Cordocentesis,*** i.e. percutaneous umbilical cord blood sampling is used for:

   - *Fetal blood disorders* such as anaemia, hemoglobinopathies, thrombocytopenia, polycyathemia.
   - *Response to infection* by IgM antibody levels in fetal blood.
   - *Rapid karyotyping* and *molecular* DNA genetic diagnosis.

5. ***Fetal tissue biopsies*** indicated in certain specific conditions are as below:

   - *Chorionic villus sampling* (CVS) involves transabdominally needle aspiration of about 5 to 30 mg of villus tissue from the placenta. The material obtained is used for karyotyping, molecular DNA genetic analysis and enzyme analysis.
   - *Fetal skin biopsy* is indicated with history of hereditary skin disorders.
   - *Fetal liver biopsy* may sometimes be required for enzyme essay.

6. ***Fetal urine analysis*** is needed to comment on prognosis in obstructive uropathy.

7. ***Antepartum biophysical monitoring (ABM)*** required for fetal distress and hypoxia include:

   - Nonstress test,
   - Contraction stress test, and
   - Biophysical profile (BPP).

III. Postnatal tests to detect congenital malformations

1. *Clinical evaluation at birth.* Gross anomaly can be seen on routine clinical examination of newborn. Look specifically for:
   - Imperforate anus, and
   - Tracheoesophageal fistulae.
2. *Imaging techniques* like ultrasonography, MRI, radiography, etc can be employed in a newborn if indicated to detect:
   - Anomalies of gastrointestinal tract like oesophageal or duodenal atresia, extent of imperforate anus,
   - Cardiac abnormalities,
   - Intracranial abnormalities and
   - Gross skeletal abnormalities.

FETAL THERAPY

Modern prenatal diagnostic techniques have made it possible to diagnose and treat some fatal diseases. Following modes of therapy are in vogue for fetal diseases:

1. *Medical therapy to mother* for prevention as well as treatment of certain fetal disorders being used are:
   - *Administration of folic acid* before and during pregnancy has markedly reduced the incidence of neural tube defects.
   - *Administration of steroids to mother* to accelerate fetal lung maturation and decrease the incidence of respiratory distress syndrome during the risk of premature delivery.
   - *Medical treatment* of fetal infections, cardiac arrhythmias, compromised thyroid functions, anaemias, can be done successfully.
2. *Fetal transfusion* through umbilical cord vein (ultrasound guided cordocentesis) is recommended in cases of fetal anaemia produced by maternal antibodies or other causes.
3. *Fetal surgery* in most advanced ultramodern centers is possible for following conditions with guarded risk to mother and fetus:
   - Obstructive urinary diseases to prevent renal damage,
   - Congenital diaphragmatic hernia,
   - Cystic lesions in the lungs,
   - Neural tube defects (spina bifida).
4. *Stem cell transplantation and gene therapy* still under research includes:
   - *Transplantation of hematopoietic stem cells* for treatment of immunodeficiency and hematologic disorders.
   - *Gene therapy* for inherited metabolic disorders such as Tay Sachs disease and cystic fibrosis.

Note. Tissue or cell transplantation is possible before 18 weeks of gestation, as before this time fetus does not develop any immunocompetence.

Multiple Choice Questions

CHAPTER 1

1. Gene is defined as:
   a. All the DNA on one chromosome
   b. All the DNA and RNA of the nucleus
   c. A segment of DNA which is responsible for production of a polypeptide or a protein
   d. All the DNA in the nucleus

2. Number of human chromosome as 46 was shown in the year:
   a. 1956
   b. 1970
   c. 1900
   d. 1888

3. All the statements about RNA are true *except*:
   a. It is double stranded
   b. The sugar molecule is ribose
   c. The base is uracil
   d. It is composed of nucleotides, comprising of base, sugar and phosphate

4. Human genome project started in 1990, got completed in:
   a. 2000 AD
   b. 2003 AD
   c. 2006 AD
   d. 2010 AD

5. Which is the correct nitrogenous base pairing in the DNA molecule?
   a. $C = A$
   b. $G = A$
   c. $A \equiv T$
   d. $G a \equiv C$

6. The codon or genetic code consists of:
   a. Duplet of bases
   b. Triplet of bases
   c. One base pair
   d. Tetraplet of bases

7. Different amino acid in human are:
   a. 6
   b. 10
   c. 20
   d. 80

8. How many autosomes are present in a single haploid set of chromosomes?
   a. 22
   b. 23
   c. 44
   d. 46

9. Which of the following statement regarding second meiotic division is correct?
   a. DNA synthesis occurs prior to division
   b. Bivalents are formed by pairing
   c. Chiasma formation and exchange of chromatid segments occurs
   d. The end of second meiotic division results in 2 daughter cells each with 23 single stranded chromosome

10. In meiotic division I, which is the correct statement:
    a. DNA duplication occurs before this division
    b. Pairing of homologous chromosomes does not occur
    c. Crossing and exchange of chromatid segment does not occur
    d. The end result is two daughter cells each with 23 single stranded chromosomes

CHAPTER 2

1. Chromosomal constitution of spermatid is:
   a. 23 X or 23 Y
   b. 23 XY
   c. 46 XY
   d. 44 XY

2. Acrosomal cap of the sperm is formed by:
   a. Endoplasmic reticulum
   b. Nucleus
   c. Golgi apparatus
   d. Mitochondria

3. Sheath of middle piece of sperm is formed by:
   a. Mitochondria
   b. Golgi apparatus
   c. Centriole
   d. Nucleus

4. Parts of mature spermatozoon are:
   a. Head
   b. Neck
   c. Tail
   d. All of the above

5. **Primary oocyte lie in a prolonged phase of 1st meiotic division for 12–35 years:**
   a. Metaphase
   b. Prophase
   c. Telophase
   d. Anaphase

6. **During 20–28 weeks of development, the approximate total number of germ cells including oogonia, primary oocytes and primordial follicles are:**
   a. 5 million
   b. 10 million
   c. 7 million
   d. 2 million

7. **Which statement about mature ovum is correct?**
   a. Mature ovum are not formed after birth
   b. Prophase of 1st meiotic division gets completed after ovulation
   c. Ovum is not the largest cell of the body
   d. 2nd polar body is extruded at ovulation

8. **Which is the fundamental reproductive unit of ovary?**
   a. Primordial follicle
   b. Primary follicle
   c. Secondary follicle
   d. Graafian follicle

9. **Main hormone responsible for ovulation is:**
   a. FSH
   b. LH
   c. Estradiol
   d. Progesterone

10. **Which is the first corpus to develop after ovulation?**
    a. Corpus haemorrhagicum
    b. Corpus luteum
    c. Corpus albicans
    d. Corpus luteum of pregnancy

CHAPTER 3

1. **The development of new individual involves following phases:**
   a. Pre-embryo phase
   b. Embryo phase
   c. Fetal phase
   d. All of the above

2. **Fertilization occurs in:**
   a. Isthmus of uterine tube
   b. Uterine cavity
   c. Ampulla of uterine tube
   d. Pelvic cavity

3. **Mature ovum usually dies after ovulation within:**
   a. 8–12 hours
   b. 12–24 hours
   c. 24–36 hours
   d. 36–72 hours

4. **Motility of sperms is aided by the following *except*:**
   a. Acidic medium of vaginal fluid
   b. Oestrogens which make secretions thin and watery
   c. Normal body temperature
   d. Release of oxytocin hormone

5. **Sperm capacitation in female genital tract takes:**
   a. 10 minutes
   b. 1–10 hours
   c. 7 days
   d. 40 seconds

6. **Fusion of gametes involves following steps:**
   a. Chemoattraction
   b. Penetration of sperm through ovum coverings
   c. Fusion of two gametes
   d. All of the above

7. **First week of development involves all steps *except*:**
   a. Cleavage of zygote
   b. Formation of morula and blastocyst
   c. Implantation of blastocyst
   d. Formation of three germ layers

8. **Implantation occurs in:**
   a. Posterior wall of junction of body with fundus of uterus
   b. In lower part of body of uterus
   c. At level of internal os
   d. In the fallopian tube

9. **Implantation or embedding of the blastocyst occurs at about the .... days after fertilization:**
   a. 1–3 day
   b. 6–7 day
   c. 10–12 day
   d. 12–15 day

10. **In vitro fertilization involves all steps *except*:**
    a. Maturation of ovarian follicles by administration of gonadotropins
    b. Collection of oocytes
    c. Fertilization of oocytes by sperms
    d. Transfer of blastocyst in the uterine cavity

11. **Main changes occurring during 2nd week are following *except*:**
    a. Formation of epiblast and hypoblast
    b. Formation of amniotic cavity and yolk sac
    c. Formation of somatic and splanchnopleuric layers of extraembryonic mesoderm
    d. Non-differentiation of trophoblast into cytotrophoblast and syncytiotrophoblast

12. **Changes during 3rd week of development are following *except*:**
    a. Formation of primitive streak
    b. Formation of intraembryonic mesoderm
    c. Formation of notochord
    d. Formation of buccopharyngeal and cloacal membranes

13. **Neurulation involves following steps *except*:**
    a. Formation of neural plate, neural groove
    b. Formation of neural tube
    c. Formation of neural crest
    d. Neurulation is regulated by activation of bone morphogenetic protein 4 (BMP 4)

14. **Somite differentiation occurs by all genes *except*:**
    a. Sonic hedgehog from notochord for sclerotome formation
    b. PAX 1 expressed by sclerotome cells for regulation of vertebral development
    c. PAX 3 regulated by WNT proteins for dermomyotome differentiation
    d. Fibroblast growth factor (FGF) causes myogenic differentiation

CHAPTER 4

1. **All of the following structures are formed from mesoderm *except*:**
   a. Prostatic utricle
   b. Suprarenal cortex
   c. Trigone of urinary bladder
   d. Gametes in both sexes

2. **All of the following epithelia are endodermal in origin *except*:**
   a. Respiratory epithelium
   b. Gastric epithelium
   c. Pancreatic epithelium
   d. Parotid gland epithelium

3. **Which of the following epithelia are mesodermal in origin:**
   a. Epithelium of tongue
   b. Epithelium of stomach
   c. Respiratory epithelium
   d. Urothelium

4. **Neural tube gives rise to following *except*:**
   a. Central nervous system
   b. Retina
   c. Pineal gland
   d. Anterior part of hypophysis cerebri

5. Neural crest gives rise following *except*:

   a. Suprarenal cortex
   b. Pigment cells
   c. Cranial and sensory nerves and their ganglia
   d. Pharyngeal arch cartilages

6. Intraembryonic mesoderm gets divided into:

   a. Paraxial   b. Intermediate
   c. Lateral plate   d. All of the above

7. Fetal causes of intrauterine growth retardation are all *except*:

   a. Chromosomal anomalies   b. Multiple pregnancies
   c. Anaemic mother   d. Infections

8. Aim of prenatal diagnosis is:

   a. Medical termination of pregnancy if necessary
   b. Assurance to the parents
   c. Medical/surgical treatment if necessary
   d. All of the above

CHAPTER 5

1. Weight of fetus by the end of 5th month is:

   a. Less than 500 gm   b. 600 gm
   c. 800 gm   d. About 1000 gm

2. Weight of fetus is as follows during third month:

   a. 20–60 gm   b. 10–45 gm
   c. 25–80 gm   d. 20–100 gm

3. Head and body length ratio reduced to one of the following levels during 4th month:

   a. 1:3   b. 1:2   c. 1:4   d. 1:5

4. When do active fetal movements begin:

   a. End of 3rd month   b. End of 4th month
   c. End of 5th month   d. End of 6th month

CHAPTER 6

1. Following are the fetal membranes *except*:

   a. Placenta   b. Umbilical cord
   c. Amnion   d. Amniotic fluid

2. Following are the parts of decidua:

   a. Decidua basalis   b. Decidua parietalis
   c. Decidua capsularis   d. All of the above

3. Amount of liquor amni in the amniotic cavity at term is usually about:

   a. 0.2 litre   b. 0.5 litre
   c. 1.0 litre   d. 2 litres

4. The average length of the umbilical cord at term is about:

   a. 10 cm   b. 50 cm
   c. 100 cm   d. 200 cm

5. Placenta develops from which of the decidua:

   a. Decidua basalis   b. Decidua parietalis
   c. Decidua capsularis   d. All of the above

6. Following layers form the placental barrier *except*:

   a. Endothelium and basement membrane
   b. Connective tissue
   c. Cytotrophoblast
   d. Syncytiotrophoblast and its basement membrane

7. Following are the contents of umbilical cord at term *except*:

   a. Two umbilical arteries   b. One umbilical vein
   c. Wharton's jelly   d. Yolk sac

8. Foetal membranes include following *except*:

   a. Placenta and umbilical cord
   b. Amnion and chorion
   c. Yolk sac
   d. Decidua

9. Following statements about dizygotic twins are true *except*:

   a. These result from fertilization of two oocytes
   b. They bear greater resemblance to one another than other siblings
   c. Each embryo develops in its own chorionic sac
   d. Each twin is different in its constitution

10. Placenta overlying the internal os of the cervix is called as:

    a. Placenta praevia   b. Battledore placenta
    c. Placenta increta   d. Placenta percreta

CHAPTER 7

1. Haemopoiesis occurs in the following organs *except*:

   a. Liver   b. Spleen
   c. Kidney   d. Bone marrow

2. Formula of hydroxyapatite crystal is:

   a. $[Ca_8(PO_4)_6(OH)_3]$
   b. $[Ca_{10}(PO_4)_6(OH)_2]$
   c. $[Ca_{10}(PO_4)_4(OH)_4]$
   d. $[Ca_{10}(PO_4)_2(OH)_4]$

3. Following are the types of bone cells:

   a. Osteoblast   b. Osteoclast
   c. Osteocyte   d. All of the above

4. Following hormones affect growth of bone *except*:

   a. Growth hormone
   b. Oestrogen and androgen
   c. Thyroid hormone
   d. Antidiuretic hormone

5. Following muscles develop from mesoderm *except*:

   a. Skeletal muscle   b. Cardiac muscle
   c. Muscles of iris   d. Smooth muscle

6. Intraembryonic coelom forms the following cavity:

   a. Pericardial
   b. Pleural
   c. Peritoneal including cavity of tunica vaginalis
   d. All of the above

7. All of the following are derived from ectoderm *except*:

   a. Muscles of middle ear
   b. Myoepithelial cells of mammary gland
   c. Myoepithelial cells of sweat gland
   d. Muscles of iris

8. Dorsal mesogastrium forms the following ligaments *except*:

   a. Greater omentum
   b. Lineorenal ligament
   c. Gastrosplenic ligament
   d. Falciform ligament

9. Diaphragm develops from following structures *except*:

   a. Septum transversum
   b. Pleuroperitoneal membranes
   c. Dorsal and ventral mesenteries of foregut
   d. Muscular growth from lateral body wall

10. Length of phrenic nerve in adults is about:

    a. 10 cm   b. 20 cm
    c. 30 cm   d. 40 cm

CHAPTER 8

1. **Which part of skin is developed from dermatome:**
   a. Dermis
   b. Epidermis
   c. Sebaceous gland
   d. Hair follicle

2. **If breast enlarges in males, the condition is known as:**
   a. Polymastia
   b. Gynaecomastia
   c. Amastia
   d. Polythelia

3. **Melanocytes of skin are derivatives of:**
   a. Dermamyotome
   b. Ectoderm
   c. Mesoderm
   d. Neural crest

4. **Keratohyaline granules are present in one of the following layers of epidermis:**
   a. Stratum basale
   b. Stratum spinosum
   c. Stratum granulosum
   d. Stratum corneum

5. **Appendages of skin are:**
   a. Hair follicle
   b. Sweat and sebaceous glands
   c. Nails
   d. All of the above

CHAPTER 9

1. **Following muscles are developed from mesoderm of upper limb bud** *except*:
   a. Trapezius
   b. Deltoid
   c. Pectoralis major
   d. Brachioradialis

2. **Which of the following muscle shows active migration during its development:**
   a. Deltoid
   b. Pectoralis minor
   c. Latissimus dorsi
   d. Brachialis

3. **Early closure of sagittal suture of skull causes:**
   a. Acrocephaly
   b. Scaphocephaly
   c. Microcephaly
   d. Plagiocephaly

4. **Preotic somites give rise to:**
   a. Muscles of tongue
   b. Muscles of iris
   c. Prevertebral muscles
   d. Extraocular muscles

5. **Statements about upper limb bud development are correct** *except*:
   a. The bud rotates laterally
   b. Takes foetal position by 8th week
   c. Preaxial border becomes medial
   d. Dorsal surface becomes posterior

6. **Oxycephaly results due to premature closure of:**
   a. Sagittal suture
   b. Coronal suture
   c. Coronal suture of one half of skull
   d. All of the above sutures

7. **Remnant of notochord are:**
   a. Nucleus pulposus of intervertebral disc
   b. Annulus fibrosis of intervertebral disc
   c. Whole of intervertebral disc
   d. Vertebral bodies

8. **Nucleus pulposes begins to degenerate and may protrude at:**
   a. Six years of life
   b. After 20th year
   c. 60 years
   d. 10 years

9. **Bones formed by membranous ossification of skull include all of the following** *except:*
   a. Frontal and parietal
   b. Squamous part of temporal
   c. Interparietal part of occipital bone
   d. Ethmoid

10. **Bones formed by endochondral ossification of skull include all** *except:*
    a. Ethmoid and sphenoid
    b. Petrous temporal
    c. Base of occipital bone
    d. Maxilla

11. **Which one of the following bones is not a dermal bone**
    a. Frontal
    b. Squamous part of temporal
    c. Parietal
    d. Sphenoid

CHAPTER 10

1. **Which arch is called hyoid arch?**
   a. First
   b. Second
   c. Third
   d. Fourth

2. **Which nerve supplies musculature of third pharyngeal arch?**
   a. Mandibular
   b. Facial
   c. Glossopharyngeal
   d. Vagus

3. **All of the following structures are derived from first pharyngeal arch** *except*:
   a. Malleus
   b. Incus
   c. Stapes
   d. Sphenomandibular ligament

4. **Which of the following cartilage develops from sixth pharyngeal arch?**
   a. Arytenoid
   b. Thyroid
   c. Cricoid
   d. Lower part of body of hyoid bone

5. **Which muscle is not derived from first pharyngeal arch?**
   a. Tensor veli palatini
   b. Tensor tympani
   c. Muscles of mastication
   d. Levator veli palatini

6. **Pretrematic nerve of first pharyngeal arch is a branch of:**
   a. Glossopharyngeal
   b. Facial
   c. Trigeminal
   d. Vagus

7. **Palatine tonsil is derived from:**
   a. First pharyngeal cleft
   b. First pharyngeal pouch
   c. Second pharyngeal pouch
   d. Second pharyngeal cleft

8. **Components of pharyngeal arches are:**
   a. Skeletal
   b. Muscular
   c. Artery and nerve
   d. All of the above

9. **Tympanic membrane is formed by all** *except:*
   a. Ectoderm of first pharyngeal cleft
   b. Endoderm of first pouch
   c. Intervening mesoderm
   d. Neural crest cells

10. **Just after head fold formation, stomodeum is bounded caudally by:**
    a. Cardiac prominence
    b. Septum transversum
    c. Forebrain
    d. Mandible

11. **Which of the following arch does not contribute to formation of the tongue?**

    a. First arch
    b. Second arch
    c. Third arch
    d. Fourth arch

12. **All of the following nerves carry taste from tongue except:**

    a. Chorda tympani
    b. Maxillary
    c. Glossopharyngeal
    d. Superior laryngeal

13. **Which germinal layer gives rise to submandibular and sublingual salivary glands?**

    a. Ecotderm
    b. Endoderm
    c. Mesoderm
    d. All of the above

14. **Deciduous teeth pass through the following stages during their development:**

    a. Dental lamina
    b. Dental bud and dental cap stage
    c. Dental bell stage
    d. All of the above

15. **Pharynx comprises:**

    a. Nasopharynx
    b. Oropharynx
    c. Laryngopharynx
    d. All of the above

16. **Third pharyngeal pouch from ventral wing gives rise to:**

    a. Thymus
    b. Inferior parathyroid
    c. Superior parathyroid
    d. Thyroid

17. **The downgrowth of thyroglossal duct is visualised between:**

    a. Lingual swellings and tuberculum impar
    b. Tuberculum impar and cupola
    c. Lingual swellings and tuberculum impar
    d. Cupola from 2nd of 3rd arches and cranial dorsal and part of hypobranchial eminence (from 4th arch)

18. **Posterior one-third of tongue is derived from:**

    a. Cupola (cranial part of hypobranchial eminence)
    b. Tuberculum impar
    c. Caudal part of hypobranchial eminence
    d. Lingual swellings

19. **Face is formed by processes:**

    a. One frontonasal process
    b. A pair of maxillary processes
    c. A pair of mandibular processes
    d. All of the above

20. **Following molecules play role in facial development except:**

    a. Bone morphogenetic protein 7 (BMP)
    b. Fibroblast growth factor 8 (FGF8)
    c. Sonic hedgehog (SHH) proteins
    d. Hox genes

21. **Following bones contain paranasal sinuses except:**

    a. Frontal   b. Parietal   c. Ethmoid   d. Maxilla

CHAPTER 11

1. **All of the following parts are derived from cranial part of foregut except:**

    a. Pharynx
    b. Tongue
    c. Lower respiratory passages
    d. Spleen

2. **All of the following parts develop from caudal part of foregut except:**

    a. Oesophagus
    b. Stomach
    c. Pancreas
    d. Whole of duodenum

3. **Precaecal segment of midgut gives rise to the following structures except:**

    a. Jejunum
    b. Ileum
    c. 3rd and 4th parts of duodenum
    d. Whole of 2nd part of duodenum

4. **Post-caecal segment gives rise to the following structures except:**

    a. Caecum
    b. Vermiform appendix
    c. Ascending colon
    d. Whole of transverse colon

5. **Preallantoic part of hind gut gives rise to all of the following structures except:**

    a. Distal one-third of transverse colon
    b. Splenic flexure
    c. Descending and sigmoid colon
    d. Rectum

6. **Post allantoic part of hindgut gives rise to all structures except:**

    a. Rectum
    b. Whole of anal canal
    c. Most of urinary bladder
    d. Proximal part of urethra

7. **Molecular regulation of gut tube development is done by following molecules except:**

    a. Sonic hedgehog
    b. Hox genes
    c. Parahox
    d. Fibroblast growth factor

8. **Development of stomach shows following milestones except:**

    a. Fusiform dilatation
    b. Differential growth
    c. Rotation along anteroposterior axis
    d. Rotation along transverse axis

9. **Ventral mesogastrium gives rise to all except:**

    a. Lesser omentum
    b. Gastrosplenic ligament
    c. Coronary ligament
    d. Falciform ligament

10. **Zygosis occurs during development of all following organs except:**

    a. Duodenum
    b. Pancreas
    c. Stomach
    d. Kidney

11. **Molecular regulator of liver is done by following factor except:**

    a. Fibroblast growth factor
    b. BMP
    c. Hepatocyte nuclear transcription factors
    d. Sonic hedgehog

12. **Dorsal pancreatic bud forms:**

    a. Most of the head of pancreas
    b. Uncinate process
    c. Neck
    d. Body and tail of pancreas

13. **Cells expressing both homeobox genes PAX4 and PAX6 control development of the following endocrine cells except:**

    a. β cells (insulin secreting)
    b. Somatostatin secreting
    c. Pancreatic polypeptide secreting
    d. Glucagon secreting

14. **Viewed from ventral side, the midgut loops shows rotation of:**

    a. 90 degree clockwise
    b. 90 degree anticlockwise
    c. 270 degree clockwise
    d. 270 degree anticlockwise

15. **Physiological umbilical hernia occurs between:**

    a. 6th–10th week
    b. 7th –11th week
    c. 6th –12th week
    d. 7th–12th week

16. Congenital megacolon occurs due to:
    a. Increased thickness of muscles of colon
    b. Imperforate anus
    c. Non-development of nerve plexuses in wall of colon
    d. Dilation of colon

17. Non return of physiological umbilical hernia is called:
    a. Volvulus   b. Exomphalos
    c. Umbilical sinus   d. Diverticulum ilei

18. Hepatic bud grows from endoderm at the junction of:
    a. Upper and lower halves of foregut
    b. Midgut and hindgut
    c. Foregut and midgut
    d. Upper and lower halves of hindgut

19. Anal canal is lined by:
    a. Lower part by endoderm, upper part by ectoderm
    b. Lower part by ectoderm, upper part by endoderm
    c. Upper part by endoderm, lower part by mesoderm
    d. Upper part by ectoderm, lower part by mesoderm

CHAPTER 12

1. The developing kidney in human is called as:
   a. Pronephros   b. Mesonephros
   c. Metanephros   d. All of the above

2. Metanephros develops in which of the following region:
   a. Lumbar   b. Sacral
   c. Cervical   d. Thoracic

3. Metanephros forms one of the following structures:
   a. Excretory tubules   b. Collecting tubules
   c. Glomerulus   d. Ureter

4. Before rotation, the hilum of kidney faces:
   a. Posteriorly   b. Anteriorly
   c. Laterally   d. Medially

5. Horehoe kidney is the anomaly of development of kidney where:
   a. Two kidneys are on one side and the adjacent poles are fused.
   b. Two kidney form one mass lying in midline
   c. The lower poles of kidneys are fused by connective tissue
   d. Kidneys are lobulated

6. Failure of joining the excretory tubules of metanephros with the collecting tubules causes:
   a. Hydronephrosis   b. Polycystic kidney
   c. Horseshoe shaped kidney d. Pancake kidney

7. Which structures of urinary bladder develops from endoderm:
   a. Adventitia   b. Musculature
   c. Whole epithelium   d. Epithelium of trigone

8. Which one of the following parts of intraembryonic mesoderm is responsible for the development of urogenital system:
   a. Paraxial
   b. Intermediate cell mass
   c. Somatic layer of lateral plate mass
   d. Splanchnic layer of lateral plate mass

9. Ectopia vesicle is defined when:
   a. Urinary bladder communicates with rectum
   b. Urinary bladder is duplicated
   c. Its mucous membrane is exposed due to absence of its anterior wall and absence of anterior abdominal wall as well
   d. It is divided into 2 compartments

10. Which of the following is an autosomal recessive disorder:
    a. Multicystic dysplastic kidney
    b. Polycystic kidney
    c. Horseshoe shaped kidney
    d. Floating kidney

11. Mesonephric duct in make does not form one of the following structures:
    a. Ureteric bud
    b. Epididymis and vas deferens
    c. Seminal vesical and ejaculatory duct
    d. Duct of Gartner

12. Following factors are responsible for descent of testis except:
    a. Mullerian inhibiting substance causing atrophy of paramesonephric duct
    b. Enlargement of process vaginalis
    c. Gubernaculum
    d. Oestrogens

13. Paramesonephric duct in female forms all the following structures except:
    a. Fallopian tube
    b. Uterus
    c. Ureter
    d. Upper two-thirds of vagina

14. Following are stages in formation of vagina except:
    a. Formation of sinovaginal bulb
    b. Formation of vaginal plate
    c. Formation of Gartner's duct
    d. Formation of vaginal canal

15. Indifferent external genitalia include all except:
    a. Urogenital membrane   b. Cloacal folds
    c. Urethral swellings   d. Genital tubercle

CHAPTER 13

1. Molecular control of respiratory development occurs due to following factors except:
   a. Transcription factor TBX 4
   b. Fibroblast growth factor FGF 10
   c. Sonic hedgehog SHH
   d. Hox genes

2. Larynx develops from all the following structures except:
   a. 4th and 6th pharyngeal arches
   b. Uppermost part of laryngotracheal tube
   c. Caudal part of hypobranchial eminence
   d. Hyoid bone

3. Number of generations of subdivision of bronchial tree to form respiratory bronchioles:
   a. 10–12   b. 17–18
   c. 18–20   d. 24–26

4. Following stages occur during maturation of lung except:
   a. Pseudoglandular
   b. Canalicular
   c. Subalveolar
   d. Terminal saccular and alveolar stage

5. Number of alveoli at the age of 8–10 yr child in both the lungs is about:
   a. 300 million   b. 500 million
   c. 20 million   d. 100 million

CHAPTER 14

1. **Development of cardiovascular system occurs during:**
   a. 3rd–7th week of pregnancy
   b. 4th–8th week
   c. 5th–10th week
   d. 2nd–6th week

2. **Veins associated with primordial heart are:**
   a. Vitelline veins
   b. Umbilical vein
   c. Common cardinal vein
   d. All of the above

3. **Left horn of sinus venosus contributes to the development of:**
   a. Left atrium
   b. Coronary sinus
   c. Right atrium
   d. Superior vena cava

4. **Myoepicardial mantle forms following systems *except*:**
   a. Epicardium
   b. Myocardium
   c. Endocardium
   d. Parietal pericardium

5. **Limbus fossa ovalis represents free lower margin of:**
   a. Septum primum
   b. Septum intermedium
   c. Septum secondum
   d. Septum spurium

6. **The right venous valve of sinuatrial opening forms following structures *except*:**
   a. Valve of inferior vena cava
   b. Interatrial septum
   c. Crista terminalis
   d. Valve of coronary sinus

7. **All of the following structures contribute to the development of left artrium *except*:**
   a. Part of common atrial chamber
   b. Sinus venosus
   c. Atrioventricular canal
   d. Absorbed proximal parts of 4 pulmonary veins

8. **Aortic and pulmonary valves are derived from:**
   a. Atrioventricular cushions
   b. Bulbar ridges
   c. Spiral septum
   d. Endocardial cushions

9. **Fallot's tetrology comprises all of the following defects *except*:**
   a. Pulmonary stenosis
   b. Hypertrophy of left ventricle
   c. Overriding of aorta
   d. Interventricular septal defect

10. **Right ventricle develops from:**
    a. Primitive ventricle
    b. Proximal and mid portions of bulbus cordis
    c. Sinus venosus
    d. Distal part of truncus arteriosus

11. **Aortic valve has following 3 cusps:**
    a. One posterior and two anterior
    b. One anterior and two posterior
    c. One anterior, one posterior and one septal
    d. One posterior, one anterior, and one superior

12. **Genes and molecules involves in cardiac development are all of the following *except*:**
    a. NKX 2
    b. HAND 1
    c. HAND 2
    d. Sonic hedgehog

13. **Which of the following arch arteries disappear during development *except*:**
    a. Third
    b. First
    c. Second
    d. Fifth

14. **Ductus arteriosus is formed by one of the following arch artery:**
    a. Right sixth
    b. Right fourth
    c. Left sixth
    d. Left fifth

15. **Ligamentum teres is remnant of:**
    a. Left umbilical vein
    b. Left umbilical artery
    c. Right umbilical vein
    d. Right umbilical artery

16. **Foetus receives oxygenated blood from placenta via:**
    a. Umbilical arteries
    b. Umbilical vein
    c. Vitelline vein
    d. Vitelline artery

17. **Umbilical arteries after birth form internal iliac and which of the following artery:**
    a. Inferior vesical
    b. Superior vesical
    c. Superior rectal
    d. Middle rectal

18. **Second part of vertebral artery develops from:**
    a. Dorsal ramus of 7th intersegmental artery
    b. Postcostal anastomosis
    c. Spinal branch of first intersegmental artery
    d. Preneural division

19. **Arch of aorta is formed by all following parts *except*:**
    a. Left aortic sac
    b. Left IV aortic arch
    c. Fused dorsal aortae
    d. Left dorsal aorta

20. **Which of the following structures help to form inferior vena cava:**
    a. Sinus venosus
    b. Right vitelline vein
    c. Right umbilical vein
    d. Right common cardinal vein

21. **Ligamentum teres of the liver is a remnant of:**
    a. Left umbilical artery
    b. Left umbilical vein
    c. Sinus venosus
    d. Ductus arteriosus

22. **Fetus receives oxygenated blood from the placenta through:**
    a. Vitelline vein
    b. Right umbilical artery
    c. Left umbilical vein
    d. Vitelline artery

23. **Following lymph sacs with their numbers are recognized:**
    a. Two jugular lymph sacs
    b. Two retroperitoneal lymph sacs
    c. Two iliac lymph sacs
    d. Single cisterna chyli

24. **Thoracic duct receives lymph from following areas *except*:**
    a. Left upper limb
    b. Both lower limbs
    c. Right upper limb
    d. Left side of head and neck

CHAPTER 15

1. **Which one is the signalling molecule for development of nervous system?**
   a. Transforming growth factor b (TGF b) family
   b. BMP 2
   c. BMP 4
   d. Cresent produced by endodermal cells

2. **Neural crest forms following cells *except*:**
   a. Sympathetic trunk cells
   b. Parasympathetic ganglia
   c. Chromaffin cells
   d. Stratum spinosum of the epidermis

3. **Spinal cord at puberty ends at the level of:**
   a. Lower border of lumbar one vertebra
   b. Lower border of lumbar two vertebra
   c. Upper border of lumbar three vertebra
   d. Junction of lower border of lumbar two and upper border of lumbar three vertebra

4. **Which of the following flexures appear much later during development:**

   a. Cervical flexure
   b. Mesencephalic flexure
   c. Pontine flexure
   d. Telencephalic flexure

5. **Following structures develop from neural crest** *except*:

   a. Cortex of suprarenal
   b. Melanoblast
   c. Schwann cells
   d. Chromaffin cells

6. **Cavity of mesencephalic vesicle gives rise to:**

   a. Third ventricle
   b. Lateral ventricle
   c. Aqueduct of Sylvius
   d. Fourth ventricle

7. **Mesoderm gives rise to which one of the following cells:**

   a. Astrocyte
   b. Microglia
   c. Oligodendrocyte
   d. Schwann cells

8. **Optic vesicles are derived from:**

   a. Rhombencephalon
   b. Diencephalon
   c. Telencephalon
   d. Mesencephalon

9. **Basal plates of medulla oblongata gives rise to following columns** *except*:

   a. General somatic efferent (GSE)
   b. Special visceral efferent (SVE)
   c. General visceral efferent (GVE)
   d. All of the above

10. **Alar plates give rise to sensory neurons arranged in four columns. These are all following** *except*:

    a. General somatic afferent (GSA)
    b. Special visceral afferent (SVA)
    c. General somatic efferent (GSE)
    d. Special somatic afferent (SSA)

11. **Neocerebellum regulates and performs one of the following:**

    a. Regulate tone and posture
    b. Regulate equilibrium and posture
    c. Perform motor activities
    d. Perform skillful motor acts with precision

12. **Cerebellum is connected to the components of brainstem by:**

    a. Midbrain to cerebellum by superior cerebellar peduncle
    b. Pons to cerebellum by middle cerebellar peduncle
    c. Medulla oblongata to cerebellum by inferior cerebellar peduncle
    d. All of the above

13. **Migration of neurons (neurobiotaxis) occurs in:**

    a. From mantle layer of thick basal part to overlying marginal layer of cerebral vesicle
    b. Neuroblast from mantle layer migrate through the marginal zone to form external granular layer which forms Golgi, granular, Purkinje cells, etc.
    c. Neurons of facial nerve nucleus migrate close to nucleus of spinal tract of trigeminal nerve in the pons
    d. All of the above

14. **Derivatives of diencephalon are:**

    a. Thalamus
    b. Hypothalamus
    c. Epithalamus
    d. Otic vesicle

15. **Development of cerebral cortex is divided into following parts:**

    a. Hippocampal cortex
    b. Neocortex
    c. Pyriform cortex
    d. All of the above

16. **Sympathetic nervous system has following features** *except*:

    a. Preganglionic fibres are short
    b. Postganglionic fibres are long
    c. It is called thoracolumbar outflow
    d. Postganglionic neurons are situated in the wall of the viscera

CHAPTER 16

1. **Surface ectoderm form following parts of eyeball** *except*:

   a. Lens
   b. Conjunctiva
   c. Surface epithelium of cornea
   d. Vitreous body

2. **Mesoderm forms following parts of the eyeball** *except*:

   a. Sclera
   b. Choroid
   c. Part of ciliary body
   d. Epithelium of cornea

3. **During accommodation of eye for reading, following changes occur** *except*:

   a. Contraction of ciliary muscles
   b. Relaxation of suspensory ligament of lens
   c. Increased curvature of anterior surface of lens
   d. Increased curvature of posterior surface of lens

4. **Neuroectoderm gives rise to the following structures** *except*:

   a. Retina
   b. Sphincter and dilator pupillae muscles
   c. Optic nerve
   d. Cornea

5. **Following genes are involves in development of eye:**

   a. PAX 6
   b. PAX 2
   c. SOX 2
   d. BMP 4

6. **Tubotympanic recess forms all the following structures** *except*:

   a. Middle ear cavity
   b. Pharyngotympanic tube
   c. Endodermal lining of tympanic membrane
   d. Mesodermal layer between first and second pharyngeal arches

7. **Bony labyrinth consists of:**

   a. Semicircular canals
   b. Vestibule
   c. Cochlea
   d. All of the above

8. **Bony cochlea is divided into following compartments:**

   a. Scala vestibuli
   b. Scala tympani
   c. Scala media
   d. All of the above

9. **Branches of VII nerve within internal ear are all** *except*:

   a. Greater petrosal nerve
   b. Nerve to stapedius
   c. Chorda tympani
   d. Posterior auricular

CHAPTER 17

1. **After which week of development, the gonads acquire female/male structural features:**

   a. Sixth
   b. Seventh
   c. Ninth
   d. Eleventh

2. **Klinefelter's syndrome shows the following pattern:**

   a. 47 XYY
   b. 47 XXX
   c. 45 XO
   d. 47 XXY

3. **Karyotype in testicular feminization is one of the following:**

   a. 46 XY
   b. 47 XXY
   c. 46 XX/46 XY
   d. 46 XY

4. **When phenotypic appearance masks the genotypic sex, the condition is called:**

   a. Pseudohermaphroditism
   b. Gonadal dysgenesis
   c. Klinefelter's syndrome
   d. True hermaphroditism

5. If primordial germ cells fail to migrate to the developing gonad, the condition is called:

 a. Turner's syndrome
 b. Pure gonadal dysgenesis
 c. Klinefelter's syndrome
 d. Pseudohermaphrodite

6. Characteristics of autosomal dominant inheritance are following *except*:

 a. Both male and female express the allele and can transmit it equally to daughter/son
 b. Tract is transmitted from one generation to the other, i.e. vertical transmission

 c. Pattern of expression is horizontal, i.e. siblings are affected while parents are normal
 d. Mode of expression is alteration of structural proteins

7. Characteristics of autosomal recessive trait are following *except*:

 a. Both sexes are equally affected
 b. Risk of having affected child by a carrier couple is 25%
 c. Affected individual with normal partner will have all normal children
 d. Mode of expression is vertical

8. Following are examples of X-linked recessive trait *except*:

 a. Haemophilia
 b. Red-green blindness
 c. G6PD deficiency
 d. Albinism

ANSWERS

Chapter 1

| 1. c | 2. a | 3. a | 4. b | 5. c | 6. b | 7. c |
| 8. a | 9. d | 10. a | | | | |

Chapter 2

| 1. a | 2. c | 3. a | 4. d | 5. b | 6. c | 7. a |
| 8. a | 9. b | 10. a | | | | |

Chapter 3

| 1. d | 2. c | 3. b | 4. a | 5. b | 6. d | 7. d |
| 8. a | 9. b | 10. d | 11. d | 12. a | 13. d | 14. d |

Chapter 4

| 1. d | 2. d | 3. d | 4. d | 5. a | 6. d | 7. c |
| 8. d | | | | | | |

Chapter 5

| 1. a | 2. b | 3. a | 4. b |

Chapter 6

| 1. d | 2. d | 3. c | 4. b | 5. a | 6. d | 7. d |
| 8. d | 9. b | 10. a | | | | |

Chapter 7

| 1. c | 2. b | 3. d | 4. d | 5. c | 6. d | 7. a |
| 8. d | 9. c | 10. c | | | | |

Chapter 8

| 1. a | 2. b | 3. d | 4. c | 5. d |

Chapter 9

| 1. a | 2. c | 3. b | 4. d | 5. c | 6. b | 7. a |
| 8. b | 9. d | 10. d | 11. d | | | |

Chapter 10

1. b	2. c	3. c	4. a	5. d	6. b	7. c
8. d	9. d	10. a	11. b	12. b	13. b	14. d
15. d	16. a	17. b	18. a	19. a	20. d	21. b

Chapter 11

1. d	2. d	3. d	4. d	5. d	6. b	7. d
8. d	9. b	10. c	11. d	12. b	13. d	14. d
15. a	16. c	17. b	18. c	19. b		

Chapter 12

1. c	2. a	3. b	4. c	5. c	6. b	7. c
8. b	9. c	10. b	11. d	12. d	13. c	14. c
15. c						

Chapter 13

| 1. d | 2. d | 3. b | 4. c | 5. a |

Chapter 14

1. a	2. d	3. b	4. d	5. c	6. b	7. b
8. d	9. b	10. b	11. b	12. d	13. a	14. c
15. a	16. b	17. b	18. b	19. c	20. b	21. b
22. c	23. b	24. c				

Chapter 15

1. a	2. d	3. a	4. d	5. a	6. c	7. b
8. b	9. d	10. c	11. d	12. d	13. d	14. d
15. d	16. d					

Chapter 16

| 1. d | 2. d | 3. d | 4. d | 5. d | 6. d | 7. d |
| 8. d | 9. d | | | | | |

Chapter 17

| 1. b | 2. d | 3. a | 4. a | 5. b | 6. c | 7. d |
| 8. d | | | | | | |

Index